Essential Dental MICROBIOLOGY

Essential Dental MICROBIOLOGY

Norman P. Willett, PhD
Professor and Dental Education Coordinator
Department of Microbiology and Immunology
Temple University Schools of Medicine and Dentistry
Philadelphia, Pennsylvania

Robert R. White, PhD
Professor
Department of Microbiology
University of Texas Health Science Center at Houston
Dental Branch
Houston, Texas

Samuel Rosen, PhD
Professor of Oral Biology and Microbiology
Section of Oral Biology, College of Dentistry
Department of Microbiology, College of Biological Sciences
Ohio State University
Columbus, Ohio

APPLETON & LANGE
Norwalk, Connecticut/San Mateo, California

0-8385-2453-2

Notice: Our knowledge in clinical sciences is constantly changing. As new information becomes available, changes in treatment and in the use of drugs become necessary. The authors and the publisher of this volume have taken care to make certain that the doses of drugs and schedules of treatment are correct and compatible with the standards generally accepted at the time of publication. The reader is advised to consult carefully the instruction and information material included in the package insert of each drug or therapeutic agent before administration. This advice is especially important when using new or infrequently used drugs.

92 93 94 95 / 10 9 8 7 6 5 4 3 2

Prentice Hall International (UK) Limited, *London*
Prentice Hall of Australia Pty. Limited, *Sydney*
Prentice Hall Canada, Inc., *Toronto*
Prentice Hall Hispanoamericana, S.A., *Mexico*
Prentice Hall of India Private Limited, *New Delhi*
Prentice Hall of Japan, Inc., *Tokyo*
Simon & Schuster Asia Pte. Ltd., *Singapore*
Editora Prentice Hall do Brasil Ltda., *Rio de Janeiro*
Prentice Hall, *Englewood Cliffs, New Jersey*

Library of Congress Cataloging-in-Publication Data
Essential dental microbiology / [edited by] Norman P. Willett, Robert White, Samuel Rosen.
p. cm.
ISBN 0-8385-2453-2
1. Mouth—Microbiology. 2. Medical microbiology. [1. Mouth--microbiology.] I. Willett, Norman P. II. White, Robert, 1936– III. Rosen, Samuel, 1923–
[DNLM: QW 65 E78]
QR47.E86 1990
617.5′22—dc20
DNLM/DLC
for Library of Congress

90-890
CIP

ISBN 0-8385-2453-2

90000

9 780838 524534

Acquisitions Editor: William R. Schmitt
Production Editor: Susan Meiman
Designer: Janice Barsevich

PRINTED IN THE UNITED STATES OF AMERICA

Contributors

Carl M. Allen, DDS, MSD
Associate Professor
Section of Diagnostic Services
Oral Diagnosis and Oral Medicine
Ohio State University College of Dentistry
Columbus, Ohio

George H.W. Bowden, PhD
Professor
Faculty of Dentistry
Department of Oral Biology
University of Manitoba
Winnipeg, Manitoba
Canada

P.H. Chandrasekar, MD
Assistant Professor
Division of Infectious Diseases
Detroit Receiving Hospital
Detroit, Michigan

James Crawford, PhD
Professor
Department of Endontics
University of North Carolina
School of Dentistry
Chapel Hill, North Carolina

Memory Elvin-Lewis, PhD
Professor
Department of Microbiology
Washington University
School of Dental Medicine
St. Louis, Missouri

Paul A. Farber, DDS, PhD
Professor
Department of Pathology
Temple University Schools of Medicine and Dentistry
Philadelphia, Pennsylvania

Mary Ann Gerenscer, PhD
Research Associate
Department of Microbiology and Immunology
Health Sciences Center North
West Virginia University
Morgantown, West Virginia

Vincent F. Gerenscer, PhD
Associate Professor
Department of Microbiology
Health Sciences Center North
West Virginia University
Morgantown, West Virginia

James D. Kettering, PhD
Professor and Assistant Chairman
Department of Microbiology
University of California, Loma Linda School of Medicine
Loma Linda, California

Robert Kolstad, PhD
Department of Microbiology
Baylor University Dental School
Dallas, Texas

Thomas T. Lillich, PhD
Professor and Chairman
Department of Oral Health Science
University of Kentucky School of Dentistry
Lexington, Kentucky

Walter K. Long, PhD
Associate Professor
Department of Microbiology and Immunology
Temple University School of Medicine
Philadelphia, Pennsylvania

John A. Mayo, PhD
Associate Professor
Department of Microbiology, Immunology, and Parasitology
Louisiana State University School of Dentistry
New Orleans, Louisiana

Virginia A. Merchant, MS, DMD
Associate Professor
Department of Microbiology and Biochemistry
University of Detroit School of Dentistry
Detroit, Michigan

Chris H. Miller, PhD
Professor and Chairman
Department of Oral Microbiology
Indiana University School of Dentistry
Indianapolis, Indiana

John A. Molinari, PhD
Professor and Chairman
Department of Biomedical Sciences
University of Detroit School of Dentistry
Detroit, Michigan

Peggy A. O'Neill, DDS, PhD
Professor
Department of Peridontics
Department of Microbiology
University of Texas Health Science Center at Houston
Dental Branch
Houston, Texas

Samuel Rosen, PhD
Professor of Oral Biology and Microbiology
Section of Oral Biology, College of Dentistry
Department of Microbiology, College of Biological Sciences
Ohio State University
Columbus, Ohio

Robert R. White, PhD
Professor
Department of Microbiology
University of Texas Health Science Center at Houston
Dental Branch
Houston, Texas

Norman P. Willett, PhD
Professor and Dental Education Coordinator
Department of Microbiology and Immunology
Temple University Schools of Medicine and Dentistry
Philadelphia, Pennsylvania

Contents

Preface ix

1. Bacterial Structure 1
   Thomas T. Lillich

2. Bacterial Physiology 17
   Thomas T. Lillich

3. Bacterial Genetics 39
   John A. Mayo

4. Disinfection and Sterilization 55
   Robert Kolstad and Robert R. White

5. Antibiotics and Chemotherapy 67
   Norman P. Willett and James Crawford

6. Antigens, Antibodies, and Complement 85
   Robert R. White and Peggy A. O'Neill

7. The Immune Response 103
   Robert R. White and Peggy A. O'Neill

8. Immune Protection and Injury 119
   Robert R. White and Peggy A. O'Neill

9. Host-Parasite Interactions 135
   Norman P. Willett

10. Staphylococci 153
    Robert R. White

11. Streptococci 157
    Robert R. White

12. *Neisseria* 165
    John A. Molinari and P.H. Chandrasekar

13. Corynebacteria 169
    Robert R. White

14. *Clostridium* 173
    Mary Ann Gerenscer and Vincent F. Gerenscer

15. Mycobacteria 181
    John A. Molinari and P.H. Chandrasekar

16. Enterobacteriaceae and Related Gram-Negative Bacteria 189
    Chris H. Miller

17. *Bacteroides* 197
    Vincent F. Gerenscer and Mary Ann Gerenscer

18. Spirochetes 201
    John A. Molinari and Virginia A. Merchant

19. Actinomycetes 209
    George H.W. Bowden

20. Rickettsiae, Chlamydiae, and Mycoplasmas 215
    Chris H. Miller

21. Anaerobic Infections 223
    Robert R. White

22. Miscellaneous Organisms of Public Health Significance 229
    Samuel Rosen, John A. Molinari, and Norman P. Willett

23. Medical Mycology 237
    Carl M. Allen

24. Basic Virology 251
    James D. Kettering

25. The Herpesviruses 265
    Paul A. Farber

26. Adenoviruses, Papovaviruses, Parvoviruses, and Poxviruses 275
    Paul A. Farber

27. Orthomyxoviruses and Paramyxoviruses 283
    Walter K. Long

28. Picornaviruses, Coronoviruses, and Reoviruses 291
    Walter K. Long

29. Togaviruses and Rhabdoviruses 297
Walter K. Long

30. Hepatitis Viruses 303
Walter K. Long

31. Tumor Viruses, Human Immunodeficiency Virus, and Slow Viruses 311
Walter K. Long

32. Oral Microflora 319
Samuel Rosen and Memory Elvin-Lewis

33. Dental Caries 341
Samuel Rosen

34. Periodontal Microbiology 357
Chris H. Miller

35. Microbiology of Pulp and Periapical Infections 385
Robert R. White

Index 391

Preface

The complex interactions of the microbial flora that frequent the body and the impact of these organisms on oral medicine make it imperative that dental practitioners understand the significance of microbiology to themselves and to their patients. It has been the editors' purpose to produce a book that presents this science in a way that will facilitate dental students' mastery of this knowledge and enhance their ability to apply it to dental practice.

Although many factors contributed to the genesis of this text, perhaps the most fundamental was the exponential increase in new information not only in microbiology, but also in other fields such as molecular biology and immunology. Diseases such as AIDS, Lyme disease, and Hepatitis C, previously unknown or undetected, have emerged rapidly. The etiologic agents of some such as human immunodeficiency viruses have had a profound effect on the practice of dentistry. In addition, the application of new technology such as genetic engineering and monoclonal antibodies have contributed to the information explosion in medical and dental microbiology.

It has become apparent that it is no longer practical to present a broad nonselective course, but rather, in order to best use the limited time available to dental students, all instructors must be more discriminating in their coverage of their respective fields; they must concentrate on the essential facts and concepts needed to produce a well-rounded, competent, dental professional. To this end, many of the authors initially collaborated in developing a document describing the essential material for dental school microbiology courses. This was circulated for review by the dental school microbiology community throughout the United States and Canada, and based on the responses, was modified to produce a core curriculum for a dental school microbiology course. Subsequently this document was used by the Microbiology Section of the American Association of Dental Schools as the basis for writing the Curricular Guidelines for Microbiology (*J Dent Ed*. 1984;84:109.). The knowledge and experience gained from these efforts led to this textbook, which parallels these documents in scope, but has been expanded and updated as additional information and concepts critical to the education of future dental practitioners became apparent.

A factor of equal significance to the development of this text was the need to hold the dental students' interest. Therefore, we have included and emphasized oral and/or dental aspects throughout the text, beginning with the basic microbiology chapters and including the immunology and applied medical microbiology chapters. Oral applications are cited throughout each chapter, and most chapters include a special section on oral significance to emphasize or summarize the material of dental interest. The essential material in each chapter is supplemented by suggested contemporary readings for more advanced students or those who wish to pursue a topic in more detail.

The editors wish to express their thanks to the contributing authors, to the various editors at Appleton & Lange who encouraged us in what seemed a never-ending task, and to all of the reviewers who provided constructive and helpful suggestions.

Norman P. Willett, PhD

Robert R. White, PhD

Samuel Rosen, PhD

CHAPTER 1

Bacterial Structure

Thomas T. Lillich

INTRODUCTION

BACTERIAL SIZE AND SHAPE

BACTERIOLOGIC METHODS
- Staining Techniques
- Brightfield Microscopy
- Darkfield Microscopy
- Phase Contrast Microscopy
- Electron Microscopy

BACTERIAL ULTRASTRUCTURE
- Bacterial Cell Surfaces
- Bacterial Cell Envelope
- Bacterial Cytoplasm

ORAL ASPECTS

SUGGESTED READINGS

INTRODUCTION

Bacteria are a ubiquitous, nutritionally and environmentally diverse group of microscopic, unicellular prokaryotic organisms. They are members of the kingdom Protista, which also includes algae, fungi, protozoa, and viruses. There are two major subdivisions of the Protista, prokaryotes and eukaryotes, based primarily on the presence or absence of a nuclear membrane. Bacteria are prokaryotes and do not have a nuclear membrane. The eukaryotes, which include algae, fungi, and protozoa, do have a membrane surrounding their genetic material. Viruses are not included in this classification because they are chemically and structurally different from the other four groups of Protista. Bacteria are also different from some eukaryotes in that they are unicellular. They may be found in groups or clusters, but there is no differentiation within the population—no cellular specialization that is characteristic of plant and animal cells. Each bacterial cell retains its autonomy, that is, its ability to metabolize, grow, and reproduce apart from the other cells. Animal and plant cells, on the other hand, survive only as part of the larger, multicellular organism.

Classification of bacteria makes it possible to identify the etiologic agents of infectious diseases. Taxonomy is the means of classifying microbes. The species is the basic unit of classification. A bacterial species is a group of organisms that share a set of characteristics. Some of the characteristics used to determine relatedness among bacteria are shown in Table 1–1. Phenotypic analysis includes microscopic examination of individual bacteria or their colonies and the study of their metabolic traits. A thorough genetic analysis is essential for accurate classification because the sequence and arrangement of nucleotide basepairs on the bacterial chromosome determine all other cellular characteristics. Additional information can be obtained from analysis of bacterial metabolic requirements and capabilities and from serologic studies that reveal similarities in the surface structures of bacteria that bind the same immunoglobulin molecules.

The most important aids to bacterial classification are the genetic and biochemical characteristics of the microorganisms. As new techniques and tests become available, the classification of some bacteria changes. For example, when they were first isolated in 1921, all black-pigmented *Bacteroides* were included in the same genus, *Bacteroides melaninogenicus*. Since

TABLE 1–1. BACTERIAL CHARACTERISTICS USED IN TAXONOMY

- Phenotype
- DNA analysis
  - Guanine + cytosine content (%)
  - DNA–DNA hybridization
- Chemical analysis
  - Lipids
  - Cell wall polymers
  - Isoprenoid quinones
  - Cytochromes
  - Enzymes
- Serology

Adapted from Zambon JJ. Bacterial Classification. In: Newman MG, Nisengard R, eds. Oral Microbiology and Immunology. *Philadelphia: WB Saunders; 1988.*

then, more detailed studies using biochemical and molecular biologic techniques have resulted in the division of this genus into six species, several of which are found in the mouth. Numerical taxonomy is an approach to classification that uses information about bacterial phenotype, genotype, metabolism, and serology in a different way. As much information as possible is collected about each organism. Each characteristic is assigned a value, often the same one, and a similarity profile is constructed. Organisms are grouped according to their similarity profiles. Those with 90% or greater similarity in characteristics usually are considered to be the same species.

Bacteria are named according to the binomial system of nomenclature that uses two names with Latin endings to describe a species. The first word indicates the genus, the second the species. Both describe characteristics based on metabolism, shape, color of colony, site from which isolated, or the individual who first described the microbe.

This chapter provides a description of bacteria and those structures that are important in their growth and reproduction. It begins with a general discussion of morphology and cellular arrangement. Brief mention is then made of some of the analytic techniques used to study them. The rest of the chapter is devoted to a description of bacterial structure. Groundwork is laid here for a more detailed treatment of structure–function relationships in subsequent chapters.

BACTERIAL SIZE AND SHAPE

Bacteria are the smallest organisms that have the capability to metabolize, grow, and reproduce independently of other cells. Table 1–2 is a listing of weights and measures used to describe bacteria and their environments.

Bacteria can be divided morphologically into spheres, rods, and spirals (Fig 1–1). Each shape may occur in several variations, as illustrated in Fig 1–2. Spherical bacteria, also called cocci, average about 1.0 μm in diameter, although they can range from 0.4 μm to 2.0 μm. They may exist as single cells or as pairs (diplococci), chains (streptococci), clusters (staphylococci), or tetrads (sarcinae), which result from incomplete separation of daughter cells that arise by division of the mother cell in one or more planes. Bacterial rods, or bacilli, usually have the same diameter as cocci but range in length from 2 μm to 20 μm. Bacilli not much longer than they are wide are called coccobacilli. Those that grow very long are filamentous forms. The ends of bacilli may be either tapered or blunt. Rod-shaped bacteria also may be curved, either gently into a comma or more severely into a helix that appears to have several

TABLE 1–2. WEIGHTS AND MEASURES

Unit	Symbol	Conversion				
		nm	μm	mm	cm	m
Nanometer (millimicron)[a]	nm ($m\mu$)	1	10^{-3}	10^{-6}	10^{-7}	10^{-9}
Micrometer (micron)	μm (μ)	10^{2}	1	10^{-3}	10^{-4}	10^{-6}
Millimeter	mm	10^{6}	10^{3}	1	10^{-1}	10^{-3}
Centimeter	cm	10^{7}	10^{4}	10	1	10^{-2}
Meter	m	10^{9}	10^{6}	10^{3}	10^{2}	1
		ng	**μg**	**mg**	**g**	**kg**
Nanogram	ng	1	10^{-3}	10^{-6}	10^{-9}	10^{-12}
Microgram (gamma)	μg (γ)	10^{3}	1	10^{-3}	10^{-6}	10^{-9}
Milligram	mg	10^{6}	10^{3}	1	10^{-3}	10^{-6}
Gram	g	10^{9}	10^{6}	10^{3}	1	10^{-3}
Kilogram	kg	10^{12}	10^{9}	10^{6}	10^{3}	1

[a]Parentheses indicate former designation.

sinusoidal waves when viewed through a microscope. The shape and arrangement of bacteria in clinical specimens are important aids in the diagnosis and treatment of infectious diseases.

BACTERIOLOGIC METHODS

There is a variety of methods used to study bacteria. Although many sophisticated techniques are finding their way into diagnostic laboratories, one of the most useful aids in the diagnosis and treatment of bacterial diseases remains visual observation of living or heat-fixed, stained specimens with a light microscope.

Staining Techniques

One of the most useful techniques was developed by the nineteenth century Danish bacteriologist, Christian Gram. The value of the Gram stain is its ability to differentiate most bacteria into two major groups, gram positive or gram negative, based on their color after staining. This distinction is important diagnostically because gram-positive and gram-negative bacteria differ in their susceptibility to antibiotics. The staining procedure consists of the following steps carried out on a specimen that has been air dried and heat fixed to a clean microscope slide: (1) the specimen is stained with a crystal violet solution, (2) the slide is flooded with Gram's iodine solution, which

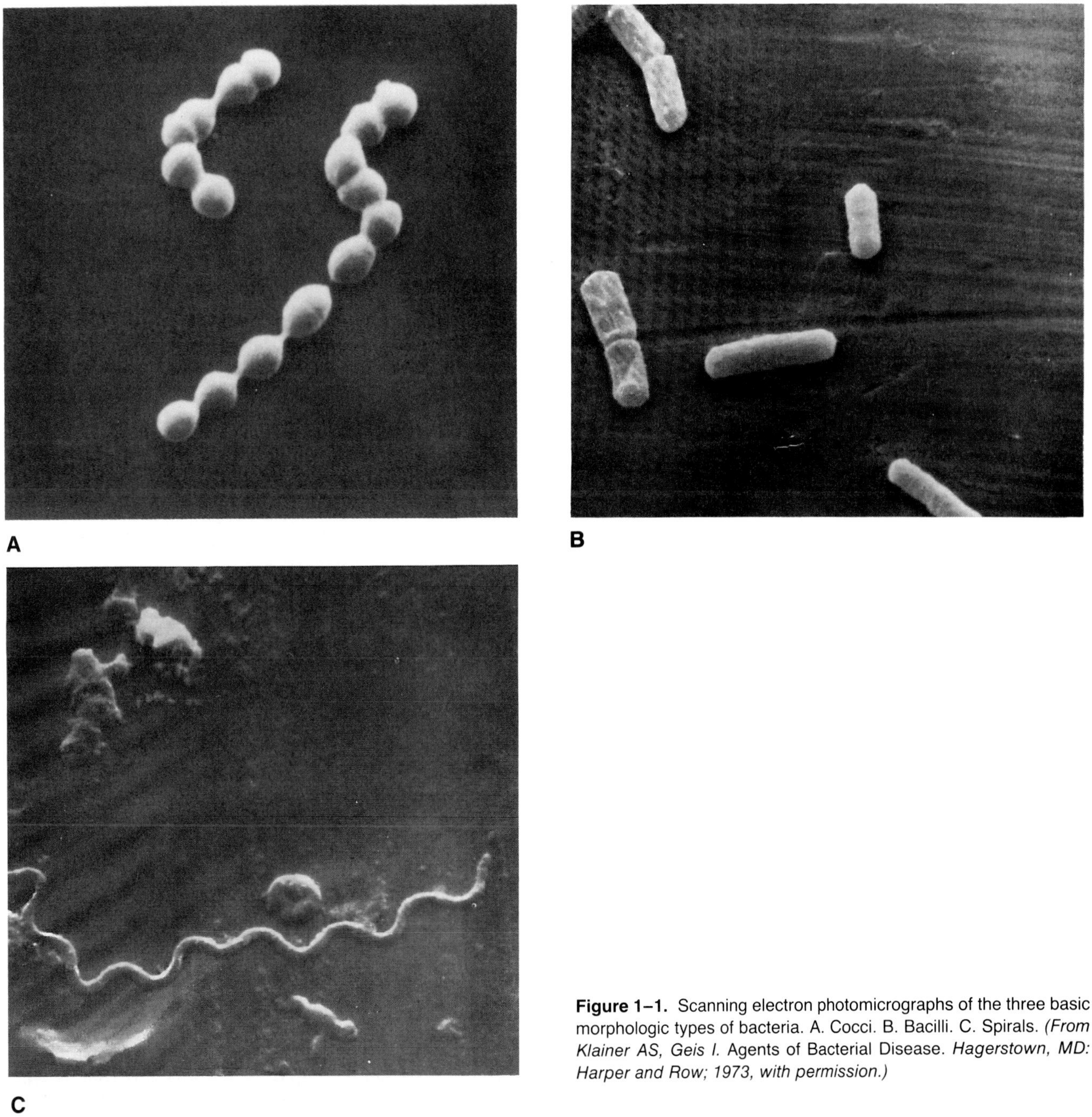

Figure 1–1. Scanning electron photomicrographs of the three basic morphologic types of bacteria. A. Cocci. B. Bacilli. C. Spirals. *(From Klainer AS, Geis I.* Agents of Bacterial Disease. *Hagerstown, MD: Harper and Row; 1973, with permission.)*

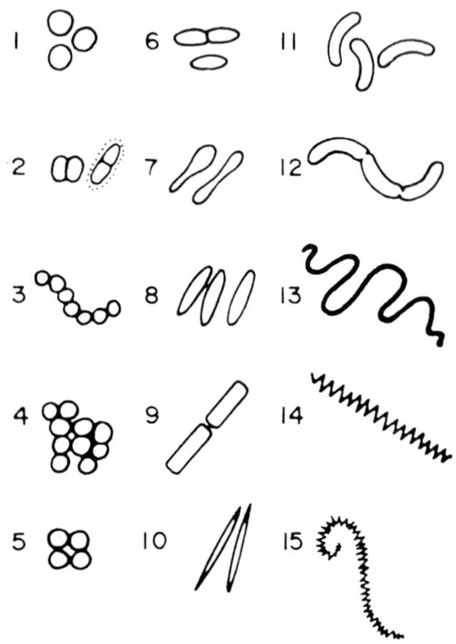

Figure 1–2. Variations in basic bacterial morphology. 1. Single cocci. 2. Pairs of cocci. 3. Chains of cocci. 4. Clusters of cocci. 5. Cocci in tetrads. 6. Coccobacilli. 7. Club-shaped bacilli. 8. Bacilli with rounded ends. 9. Bacilli with square ends. 10. Bacilli with tapered ends (fusiforms). 11. Vibrios. 12. *Spirillum*. 13. *Borrelia*. 14. *Treponema*. 15. *Leptospira*. *(From Joklik WK, Willett HP, Amos DB, eds.* Zinsser Microbiology, *19th ed. E. Norwalk, CT: Appleton Lange 1984:25.)*

acts as a mordant, (3) the specimen is decolorized with alcohol, and (4) a counterstrain, usually safranin, is applied. In the light microscope, gram-positive cells appear violet, and gram-negative cells are red. The difference in reaction is due to the different permeability of the cell walls to the crystal violet–potassium iodide complex formed during the staining procedure. Gram-positive cell walls are impermeable to the complex and retain the primary crystal violet stain. The complex is readily removed, however, from gram-negative cells by an alcohol wash, rendering them colorless and making possible expression of the counterstain color, in this case the red of safranin.

Acid-fast staining is another common differential staining method. This technique is used to differentiate members of the genera *Mycobacterium* and *Nocardia* from other bacteria. Clinical specimens, often sputum or lung aspirates, are placed on a microscope slide, stained with phenolic carbolfuchsin, decolorized with dilute mineral acid, and counterstained with methylene blue. Bacteria that retain the red primary carbolfuchsin stain after the acid rinse are classified as acid fast. Nonacid-fast organisms are decolorized by acid alcohol and appear blue after counterstaining. Mycobacterial acid fastness is due to the unique cell wall lipid content of members of the genus. The presence of acid-fast organisms in the sputum of an individual is a very important clue in the diagnosis of tuberculosis and other mycobacterial diseases.

There are several other staining techniques used to determine bacterial structure and morphology. Special techniques have been developed to demonstrate bacterial structures, such as flagella, endospores, capsules, and nuclear material.

Brightfield Microscopy

The compound brightfield microscope is a basic tool of microbiology. It is compound because it has three lens systems and brightfield because it uses visible light passing directly through the specimen to the observer's eye. Image magnification up to 1000× is possible using an oil immersion lens to reduce light scatter as it passes from the specimen into the objective lens. Maximum magnification is limited by the ability to distinguish between two objects that are a certain distance apart. This ability is called the resolving power and is a function of the wavelength of light used and the angle at which the light enters the objective lens. Under optimum conditions, using blue light and oil immersion, objects can be resolved if they are no closer than 0.2 μm. Since they are transparent, it is very difficult to observe unstained bacteria with a brightfield microscope because there is so little contrast between the microorganisms and the background. Most specimens are stained before observation using one of the techniques described earlier in this chapter.

Darkfield Microscopy

Because staining a bacterial culture or clinical specimen precludes studying living cells, techniques involving darkfield and phase contrast microscopy have been developed to observe unstained preparations in an aqueous environment. Both techniques are being used by dental practitioners for patient education and to monitor the effectiveness of treatment.

Darkfield microscopes use a method of illumination that makes possible the observation of bacteria and bacterial structures that are too thin to be seen with a brightfield microscope but long enough to have a characteristic shape. This technique is particularly useful for observing spirochetes that have a diameter of 0.1 to 0.15 μm and flagella that are invisible by more conventional brightfield techniques. Darkfield illumination uses a substage condenser that produces an inverted, hollow cone of light that does not pass directly into the objective lens. Only light that is dif-

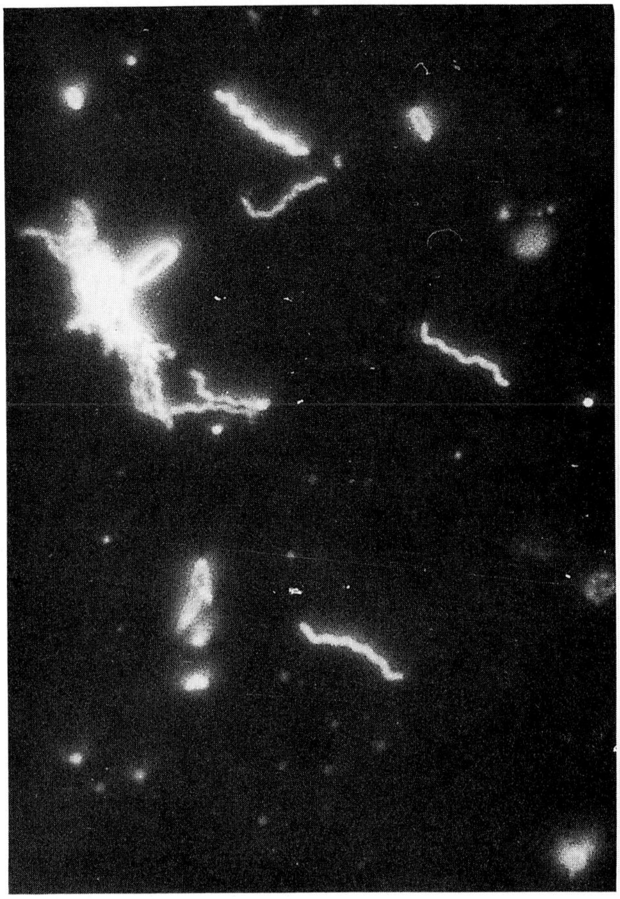

Figure 1–3. Darkfield photomicrograph of gingival debris showing several curved bacteria. ×1000. *(Courtesy of Dr. Max A. Listgarten, University of Pennsylvania School of Dental Medicine.)*

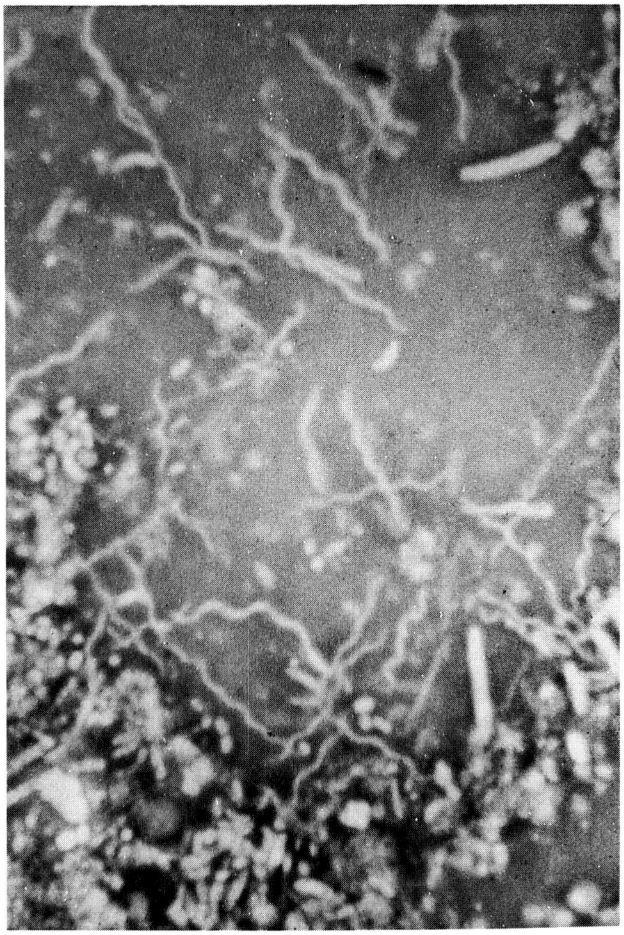

Figure 1–4. Phase contrast photomicrograph showing mixed gingival crevice microflora. ×1000. *(Courtesy of Dr. William Briner, The Procter and Gamble Company.)*

fracted while passing through the specimen reaches the objective. Consequently, bacteria or other particles that deflect the light rays appear as bright white or silver objects against a black background (Fig 1–3). Darkfield microscopy is a rapid, noninvasive method of evaluating the bacteriologic status of oral tissues, particularly the periodontium, where this technique allows visualization of the spirochetes and other delicate gram-negative bacteria that comprise a significant proportion of the flora, especially in diseased sites.

Phase Contrast Microscopy

Another technique by which microorganisms can be observed in unstained preparations is phase contrast microscopy. This method also can be used to observe intracytoplasmic organelles. The technique uses special microscope condensers and objectives to increase the contrast between cells and their environment or between cytoplasmic organelles by accentuating the differences in densities (Fig 1–4). Microorganisms can appear either darker or lighter than the background depending on the equipment used.

Nomarski microscopy is based on the same principles as phase contrast microscopy but uses polarized light. Contrast is greatest in parts of the specimen where there are large changes in light absorption over a large area. Consequently, Normarski optics are useful to visualize the outlines of cells or intracytoplasmic organelles, such as the nucleus.

Electron Microscopy

The development of the electron microscope has made possible a much more detailed look at the subcellular structure of fixed, stained bacteria. With these instruments, it is possible to increase resolution from 2×10^{-1} to 5×10^{-4} m because electrons are used instead of light waves to create an image of the specimen on a fluorescent screen. Direct magnifications of up to 1×10^{6} are possible. There are two kinds of electron microscopes, transmission electron microscopes (TEM) and scanning electron microscopes (SEM). TEMs are used to study whole cells that have been either stained, fixed, and cut into very thin sections or frozen, freeze-fractured, and stained. These instruments make possible the detailed study of in-

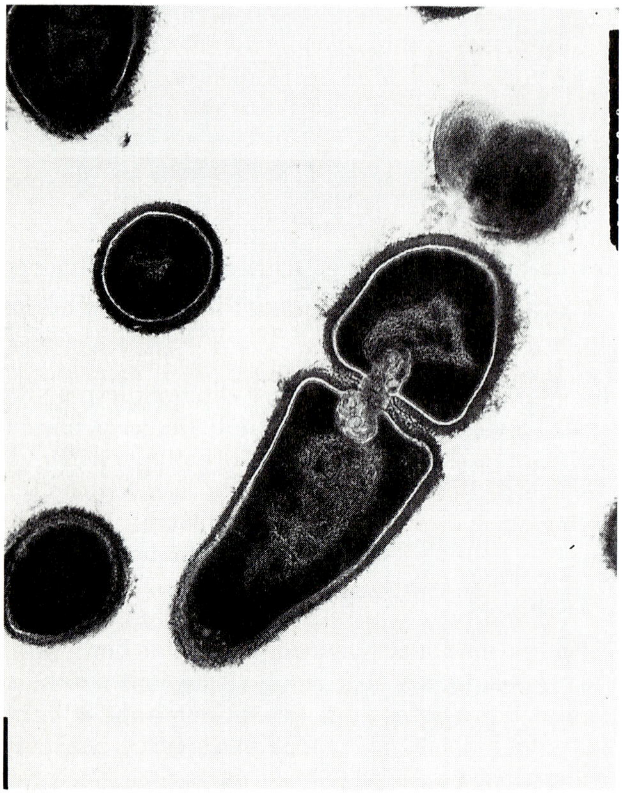

Figure 1–5. Electron photomicrograph of *Leptotrichia dentium*, showing septal mesosomes. *(Courtesy of Dr. M.A. Listgarten, University of Pennsylvania School of Dental Medicine.)*

tracellular and cell surface organelles and have become valuable tools in examining the relationships between bacterial structure and function. Figure 1–5 is a TEM of an oral spirochete *Leptotrichia dentium*, showing some internal structures.

SEMs provide a three-dimensional image of the specimen as opposed to the two-dimensional view from a transmission microscope. Specimens are coated with heavy metal and then scanned with an electron beam. SEM is particularly useful to study bacterial surface structures and the interrelationships between organisms in complex, heterogeneous microenvironments, such as dental plaque. Figure 1–6 illustrates the image created by SEM of dental plaque grown in vitro on hydroxyapatite.

BACTERIAL ULTRASTRUCTURE

Because of their size and light refractive properties, information gained from routine light microscopic examination of bacteria is limited to gross morphology and differential staining characteristics. Although such knowledge is helpful in the diagnosis of infectious diseases, little information is gained about cellular structure and organization. Such information is necessary to understand fully how bacteria colonize host tissue and how the resulting association between host and parasite ultimately may cause disease. Detailed studies of bacterial ultrastructure have been undertaken during the past 35 years aided by increasingly sophisticated electron microscopic and immunochemical techniques. Figure 1–7 is a composite drawing of an idealized bacterium, showing the more common, although not universal, structures. Note that the left side depicts a gram-positive bacterium, and the right side shows a gram-negative cell. The following sections discuss bacterial ultrastructure and the role of these structures in disease.

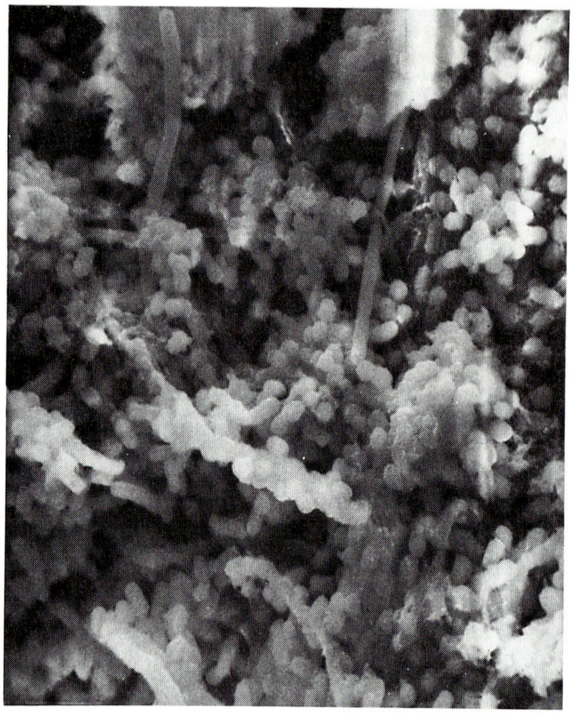

Figure 1–6. Scanning electron photomicrograph of 48-hour plaque from the gingival area. Note the three-dimensional appearance of the specimen and the presence of rods, filaments, cocci, and several corncobs. ×4000. *(From Lie T.* J Periodont Res. *1977;12:85, with permission.)*

Bacterial Cell Surfaces

Capsule and Slime Layer or Glycocalyx. The outermost layers of bacteria are important for survival and as virulence factors because it is through these that the microbe interacts with its environment. Most bacteria synthesize polymers that are associated with the cell envelope. If this material has a well-defined outer limit and adheres firmly to the cell wall, it is called a capsule. If its outer limit is less well defined, or if it is easily separated from the cell wall, it is called a slime layer or glycocalyx. These structures usually are carbohydrate heteropolymers or homopolymers. They are immunogenic, and antigenic differences exist in cap-

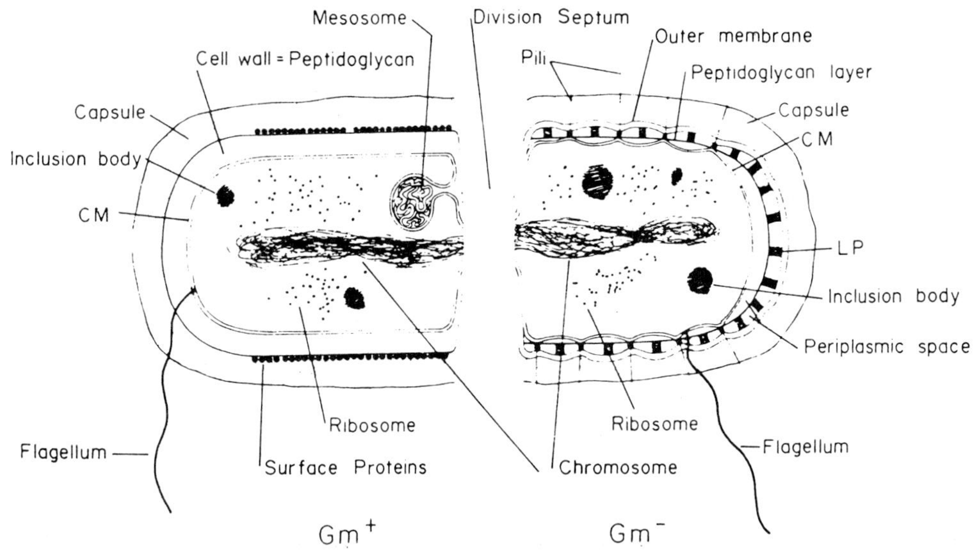

Figure 1–7. Drawing of idealized gram-positive (Gm+) and gram-negative (Gm−) bacteria showing structural similarities and differences. *(From Joklik WK, Willett HP, Amos DB, eds.* Zinsser Microbiology, *18th ed. E. Norwalk, CT: Appleton Lange 1984:24.)*

sules within a species. There are more than 80 serotypes of *Streptococcus pneumoniae,* for example, based on differences in capsular sugars. These differences are useful in identifying the strain causing a particular infection. *Streptococcus mutans,* one of the normal oral microflora, is another bacterium that produces extracellular polysaccharide capsules. It produces polymers of glucose (glucan) and fructose (fructan) from sucrose. These polymers are important in the accumulation of dental plaque and are discussed in detail in Chapter 33. Extracellular polymers may also be composed of protein. Strains of *Bacillus anthracis,* the etiologic agent of anthrax, have polypeptide capsules of D-glutamic acid polymers.

Extracellular polymers are not obligatory for bacterial survival but are important virulence factors because they enable organisms to stick to surfaces and because they reduce the efficiency of phagocytosis, one of the most important internal host defense mechanisms. Encapsulated bacteria are usually extracellular parasites. They owe their pathogenicity to the ability to grow in tissue spaces outside host cells. Capsules, by reducing the efficiency of phagocytosis, enable the bacteria to remain in tissue spaces, increase in numbers, and cause disease.

Flagella. Flagella are long, threadlike structures that are the organs of motility in bacilli, most vibrios, and spirilla. They are composites of several strands of a globular, contractile protein called flagellin, which can extend out from the cell from 3 μm to 12 μm. Flagellin is immunogenic; it is called the H antigen. The diameter of a typical flagellum is 0.01 μm. They can be seen with an electron microscope or with a darkfield microscope but not in a heat-fixed, stained preparation. The proximal end of each flagellum is anchored in the bacterial cell wall and membrane by specialized structures called a hook and a basal body (Fig 1–8). Motion is due to rotation of the flagella around the fixed anchorpoint in the cell wall. Because of their tertiary protein structure, flagella have regular sinusoidal curves with a wavelength that is a species characteristic.

Because bacterial flagella are arranged in several genetically stable patterns, their location can help distinguish between the two bacterial orders, Eubacteriales and Pseudomonadales. Eubacteriales have peritrichous flagella that can occur anywhere on the cell. Pseudomonadales have flagella at the cell poles. If a pseudomonad has a single polar flagellum, it is monotrichous. If there is one at each pole, it is amphitrichous. Some pseudomonads have tufts of lophotrichous flagella at one or both cell poles. Recently, periodontal microbiologists proposed another

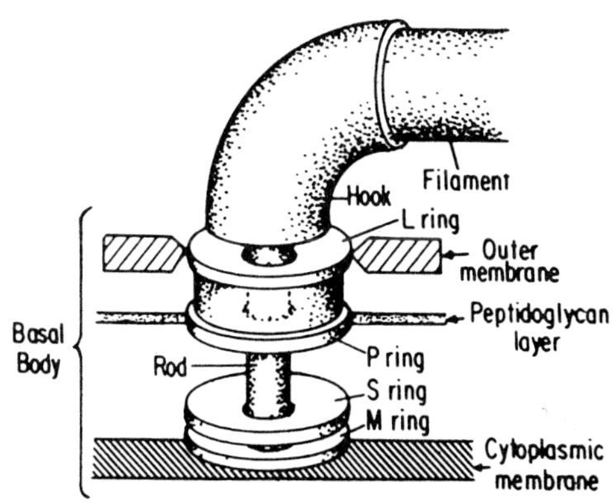

Figure 1–8. Drawing of the structures that anchor the flagellum to the bacterial cell wall and membrane. *(Modified from DePamphlis ML, Adler,* J Bacteriol. *1971;105:396.)*

category of flagellar arrangement, called helicotrichous. This classification is based on the isolation of gram-negative, anaerobic rods from patients with periodontitis. These bacteria, named *Centipeda periodontii,* are long, serpentine cells with a linear zone of flagella that form a helical spiral around the cell body, giving them a centipedelike appearance.

As an alternative to flagellar motility, some gram-negative bacteria, most notably spirochetes, have from 2 to more than 10 fibers, called axial filaments, attached at each pole and wound tightly around the entire length of the cell between the outer and cytoplasmic membranes (Fig 1–9). Movement is due to the alternate contraction and relaxation of these filaments, causing the cell to bend and then straighten.

Other gram-negative bacteria (eg, *Capnocytophaga ochraceus*) exhibit motility by gliding on a solid surface, such as agar. This type of motility seems to be associated with the presence of proteinaceous rotary assemblies in the cell envelope, although the actual mechanism of locomotion remains unknown.

The in vivo role of motility in the pathogenesis of infectious disease is unclear. Intuitively, it is reasonable to assume that the mechanisms described, in conjunction with chemotaxis, would enable bacteria to gain access to anatomic sites conducive to their growth and reproduction and may therefore serve as virulence factors. Whether or not the environmental conditions necessary for motility exist in many body sites is moot. The oral cavity is one anatomic site that is aqueous enough for some form of motility to play a role in the spread of bacteria. It has been suggested that many of the organisms found in the unattached dental plaque of periodontal pockets gain entrance to this site either by their own motility or by being transported passively while attached to species that are motile.

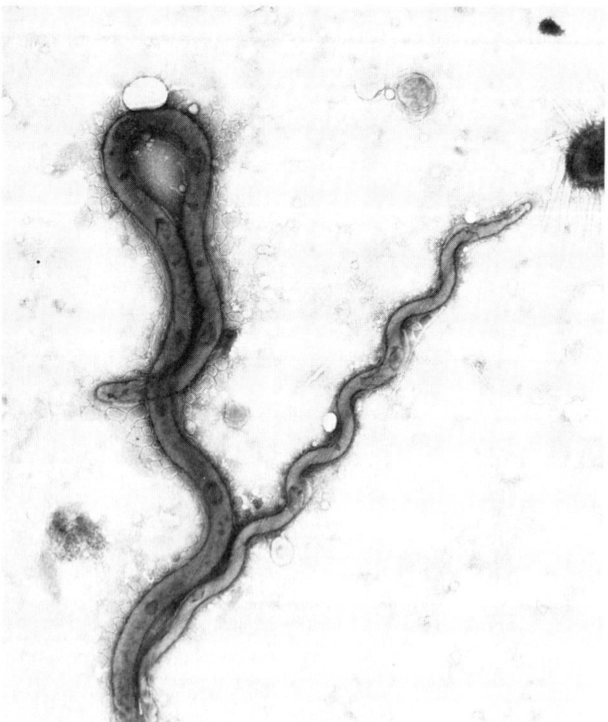

Figure 1–9. Axial filaments of oral spirochetes. *(From Listgarten MA, Socransky SS.* J Bacteriol. *1964;88:1087, with permission.)*

Pili. These fine, hairlike, proteinaceous appendages, also called fimbriae, are most often found on gram-negative bacteria. They are shorter, thinner, and straighter than flagella and have no role in motility. There are two types, each with its own function. Conjugal, or sex, pili are found on the male cell of conjugating bacterial pairs. These structures mediate the transfer of genetic material between cells by conjugation and episome transfer. The other type, somatic pili, mediate bacterial adsorption to host tissues.

Pili increase the pathogenic potential of bacteria. Conjugal pili facilitate the transfer of genetic material between members of the same or closely related species. A consequence of this promiscuity is the spread of antibiotic resistance among closely related bacteria, with the associated treatment complications. Somatic pili also give bacteria an ecologic advantage by enabling them to adsorb to host tissues. Adsorbed organisms subsequently may colonize the tissue if environmental conditions are suitable for their growth and reproduction. Furthermore, somatic pili have been associated with virulence in many bacteria, most notably *Neisseria gonorrhoeae* and *Actinomyces viscosus,* a periodontal pathogen. Gnotobiotic rats monoinfected with an *A. viscosus* strain with numerous pili suffered severe alveolar bone loss, whereas animals infected with a strain with far fewer pili did not (Fig 1–10).

Bacterial Cell Envelope

The bacterial cell envelope is composed of the cell wall and the cytoplasmic membrane. The structure and chemical composition of the cell envelope vary from one genus to another. Several general comments can be made about these variations that explain some of the differences observed among bacteria. First, variation in the chemical composition and consequent permeability of the cell envelope, particularly the cell wall, allow separation of bacteria into gram-positive and gram-negative cells. Closer examination of the cell envelopes of these two major bacterial subgroups reveals some important chemical and structural differences (Fig. 1–11). Gram-negative envelopes are generally more chemically and structurally complex than are those of gram-positive cells. They are multilayer structures consisting of a cytoplasmic membrane surrounded by a relatively thin peptidoglycan layer en-

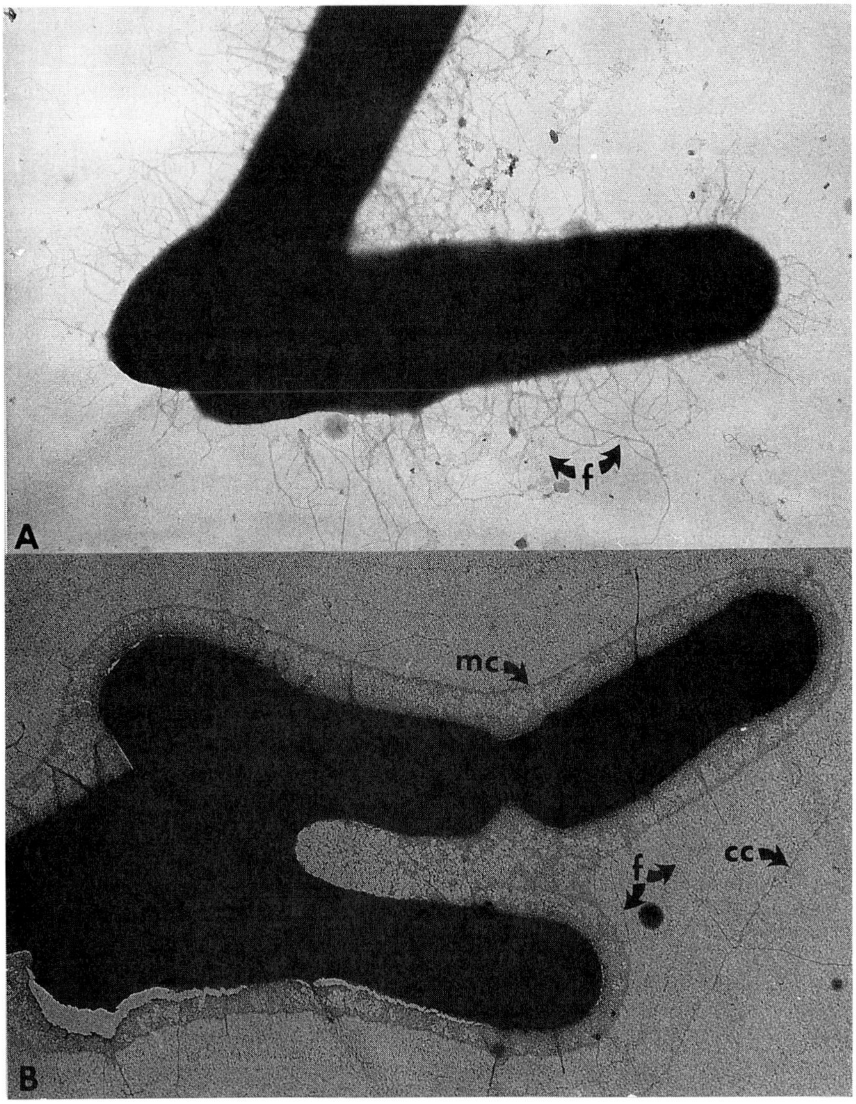

Figure 1–10. Electron photomicrographs of oral *Actinomyces viscosus*. A. Virulent *A. viscosus* strain T14-Vi with numerous pili (f) that facilitate attachment to oral surfaces. B. Avirulent *A. viscosus* strain T14-Av, which has fewer pili and is enclosed in a cell-associated capsule (mc). Both factors decrease the ability of this strain to colonize the mouth. *(From Lillich TT. Oral microbiology. In Roth GI, Calmes R.* Oral Biology. *St. Louis, MO: CV Mosby Co; 1981, with permission.)*

closed by a phospholipid outer membrane containing an endotoxin. Gram-positive envelopes usually consist of just two layers, the plasma membrane and a peptidoglycan wall that might be quite thick relative to gram-negative cells.

These differences in cell envelope structure and composition have important consequences for the host response to the bacterium and for chemotherapy. Endotoxin in gram-negative bacterial envelopes can cause widespread inflammation and shock, depending on the amount present and the intensity of the host response. Differences in cell envelope also have chemotherapeutic implications. Gram-positive cells, for example, are sensitive to penicillin and lysozyme, both of which are active against peptidoglycan. Gram-negative cells are not as sensitive to these compounds perhaps because their access to the peptidoglycan layer is limited by the outer membrane. Gram-negative bacteria also are generally less sensitive to antibiotics because their outer membrane acts as a barrier restricting antibiotic access to the cell wall, membrane, and cytoplasm.

Bacterial Cell Walls. Cell walls are present on all bacteria except mycoplasmas. They are located immediately outside the plasma membrane and protect the cell from lysis resulting from osmotic pressure differences or mechanical damage. They also give the cell its characteristic shape, determine its gram stain reaction, and impart antigenic characteristics.

Gram-positive Cell Walls. Electron microscopic examination of gram-positive cell walls reveals a single, 15 to 80 nm thick, uniform, electron-dense layer closely associated with the outer surface of the plasma membrane (Fig 1–12A). The electron-dense material is peptidoglycan, a polysaccharide that constitutes the rigid backbone of the cell wall (Fig 1–13). Peptidoglycan is composed of repeating units of the sugars N-acetylglucosamine (NAG) and N-acetylmuramic acid

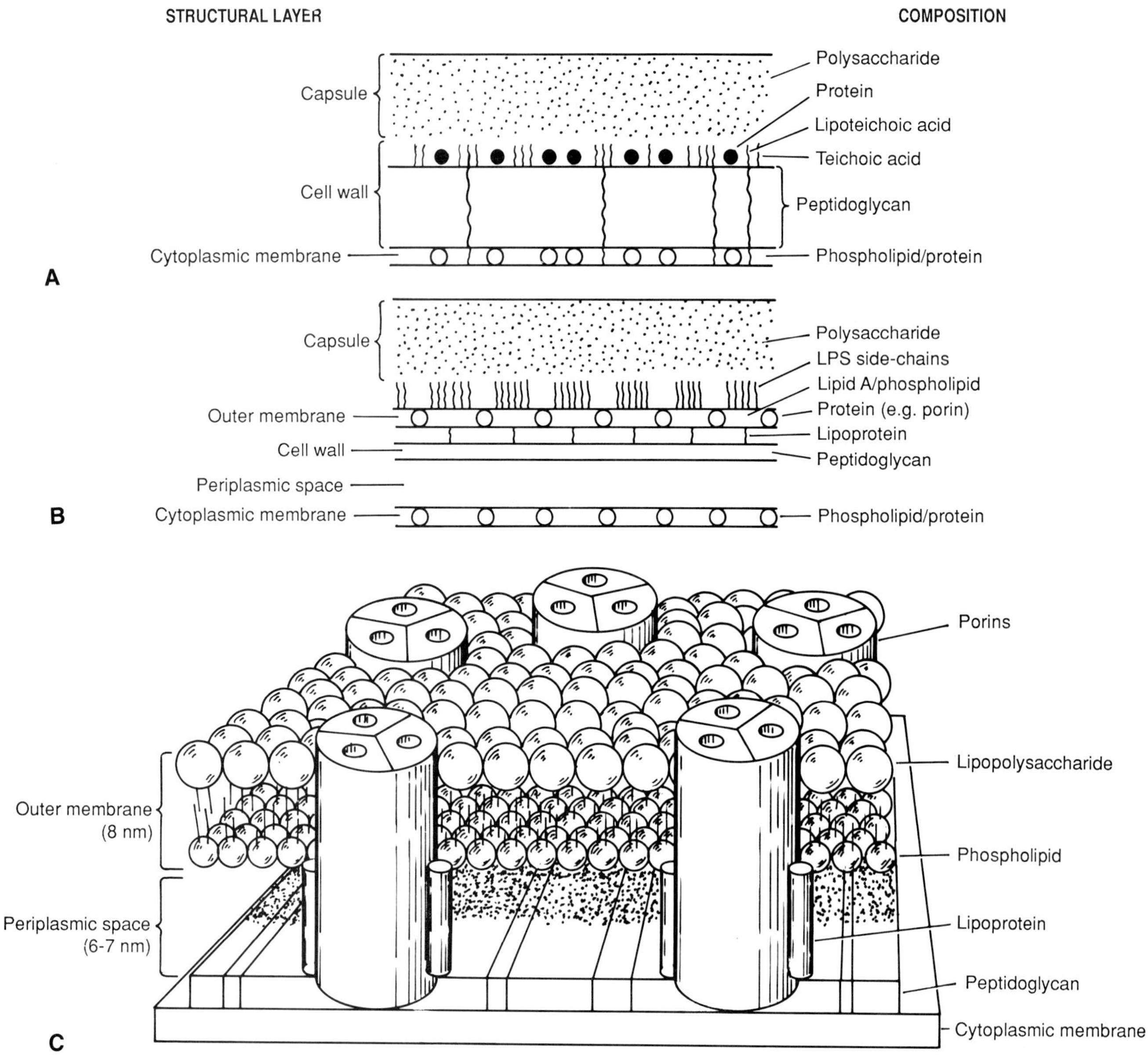

Figure 1–11. Diagram of gram-positive and gram-negative bacterial cell envelopes. **A.** Gram-positive. **B.** Gram-negative. **C.** Detail of the gram-negative envelope. *(A and B modified from Taussig MJ.* Processes in Pathology and Microbiology, *2nd ed. Oxford: Blackwell Scientific Publications; 1984:393. C from Boyd RF,* General Microbiology. *St. Louis, MO: Times Mirror/Mosby College Publishing, 1984:157.)*

(NAM) linked by $\beta(1\rightarrow4)$ bonds. This polymer is crosslinked to a three-dimensional mesh by peptide bridges, the amino acid content of which varies from one bacterial genus to another. The percentage of crosslinking between the NAM–NAG polymers also varies with the organism being studied—from as little as 25% in some gram-negative bacteria to as much as 75% in gram-positive bacteria such as *Staphylococcus aureus.* In some gram-positive bacteria, there can be as many as 40 peptidoglycan layers all crosslinked into a single three-dimensional cell wall.

Gram-positive bacterial cell walls contain uronic acids in addition to peptidoglycan. Teichoic, teichuronic, and uronic acids are the most common. These molecules are linear polymers of glycerol or ribitol linked by phosphodiester bonds (Fig 1–11A). They may have sugars or amino acids attached to them. Uronic acids are negatively charged and mediate the attachment of gram-positive bacteria, such as streptococci, to tooth surfaces, red blood cells, epithelium, and other positively charged surfaces through adhesin-like activity. They are also major surface antigens of some bacterial species (eg, the group D streptococci).

Closely associated with the external side of gram-positive cell walls are a variety of periplasmic proteins and exoenzymes that are synthesized in the cell and secreted into the environment. These proteins perform a variety of functions. First, they convert imper-

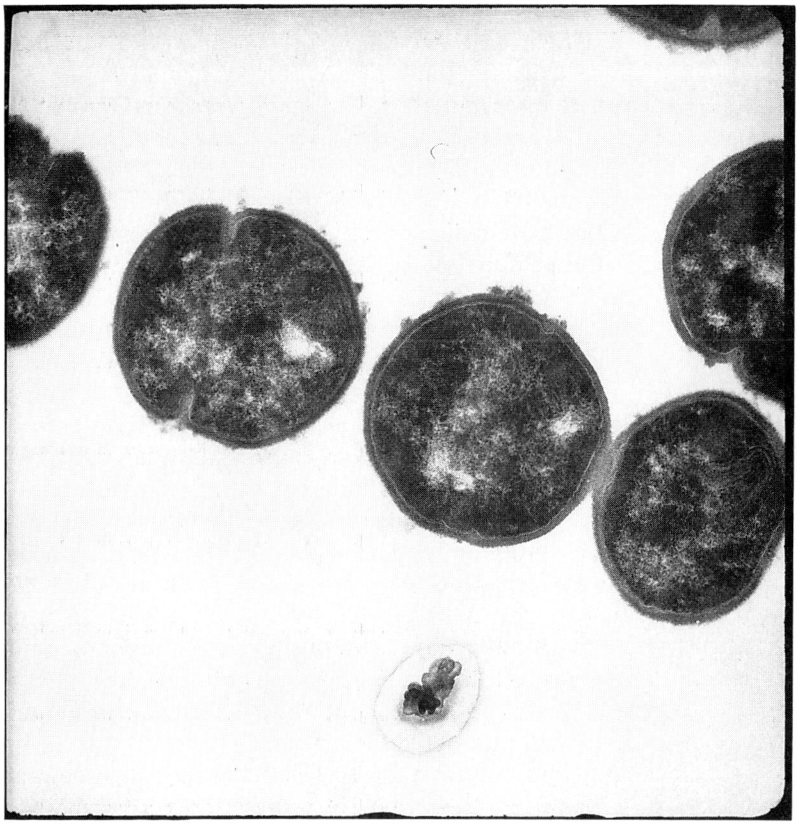

A

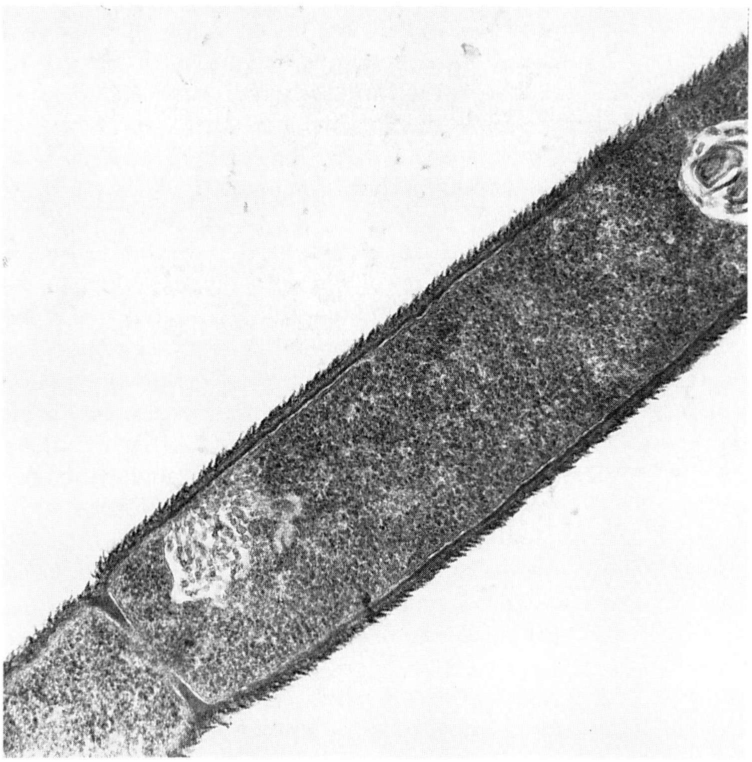

B

Figure 1–12. Electron photomicrographs of gram-positive and gram-negative bacteria. **A.** Oral streptococci illustrating the uniform, dense gram-positive bacterial cell wall (cw). ×60,000. *(Courtesy of Dr. J. Theilade, Royal Dental College, Aarhus, Denmark.)* **B.** *Leptotrichia buccalis,* illustrating the complex gram-negative cell envelope (C.E.). ×70,000. *(Courtesy of Dr. M.A. Listgarten, University of Pennsylvania School of Dental Medicine.)*

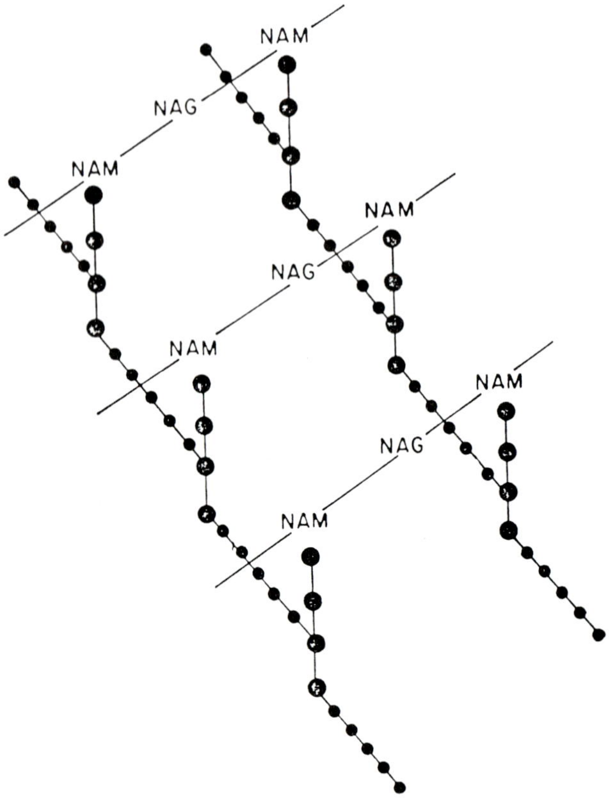

Figure 1–13. Diagram of the peptidoglycan layer in gram-positive cell walls. Tetrapeptides (large circles) attached to muramic acid (NAM) are covalently linked to NAM in adjacent chains by pentapeptides (small circles). NAM, N-acetylmuramic acid: NAG, N-glucosamine. *(From Boyd RF,* General Microbiology. *St. Louis, MO: Times Mirror/Mosby College Publishing; 1984, with permission.)*

meable substances into smaller molecules that can be transported into the cell and used as food or building blocks. Second, they detoxify or destroy potentially harmful substances. Some bacteria, for example, synthesize enzymes that degrade antibiotics, thus rendering the organism resistant to those antimicrobial agents. Finally, periplasmic proteins (eg, exotoxins) may serve as virulence factors, increasing the pathogenic potential of the bacterium.

Gram-negative Cell Envelope. Electron micrographs of gram-negative cell walls reveal a much more complex structure than those of gram-positive bacteria (Fig 1–12B). There are two layers outside the cytoplasmic membrane. The first, very closely associated with the membrane itself, is a relatively thin peptidoglycan layer, which has a similar chemical composition and physical structure and performs the same functions as that in gram-positive organisms. Immediately external to and closely associated with the peptidoglycan layer is a lipopolysaccharide (LPS) outer membrane (Fig 1–11B,C). This structure exhibits the typical lipid bilayer arrangement of all biologic membranes and is tightly bound to the peptidoglycan backbone by lipoprotein and protein bridges. LPS imparts several important characteristics to gram-negative cells. First, its outermost portion is the site of cellular somatic or O antigens, variable regions of sugars attached to the LPS core that stimulate an antibody response when injected into animals. O antigens are characteristic of particular species and are useful in the serologic identification of such bacteria as *Salmonella*. They are also bacterial virulence factors that inhibit the phagocytic ability of host leukocytes. Second, the gram-negative cell envelope contains lipid A, a toxic component capable of inducing inflammation in the host. Finally, LPS functions as a molecular sieve, allowing diffusion of molecules through protein pores.

Porins are trimeric proteins arranged in pores that extend across the outer membrane. They permit nonspecific diffusion of molecules less than 800 MW. Another type of outer membrane protein forms pores that allow penetration of specific carbohydrates, nucleosides, and amino acids. The permeability of the outer membrane of gram-negative bacteria is in contrast to the cytoplasmic membrane, which excludes all hydrophilic molecules but water itself unless there is a transport mechanism specific for the substance in question. The outer membrane is much less permeable to hydrophobic or amphipathic molecules, thereby accounting for the fact that gram-negative bacteria are, on the whole, less susceptible to antibiotics than are gram-positive cells.

Gram-negative bacteria secrete proteins into the periplasmic space between the cell wall and the outer membrane. These enzymes degrade and detoxify as do those secreted into the environment by gram-positive cells. In this respect, the gram-negative periplasmic space can be considered the bacterial equivalent of eukaryotic lysosomes.

Protoplasts and Spheroplasts. In a hypotonic environment, blockage of peptidoglycan synthesis or enzymatic digestion of peptidoglycan will result in cell lysis. This demonstrates that an intact cell wall is required for osmotic stability. If, however, similar cells are treated in an isotonic solution, they will survive as osmotically sensitive spheres that maintain full respiratory activity as well as the ability to synthesize protein and nucleic acid. Gram-positive cells treated in this manner do not retain any cell wall material and are called protoplasts. Gram-negative cells treated similarly are called spheroplasts and retain part of the outer membrane.

Bacterial Cell Membranes. The cell or cytoplasmic membrane constitutes the innermost structure of the cell envelope. It is composed of 60 to 70% protein and 20 to 30% lipid, with a trace of carbohydrate. The lipids are primarily phosphatides that are arranged in

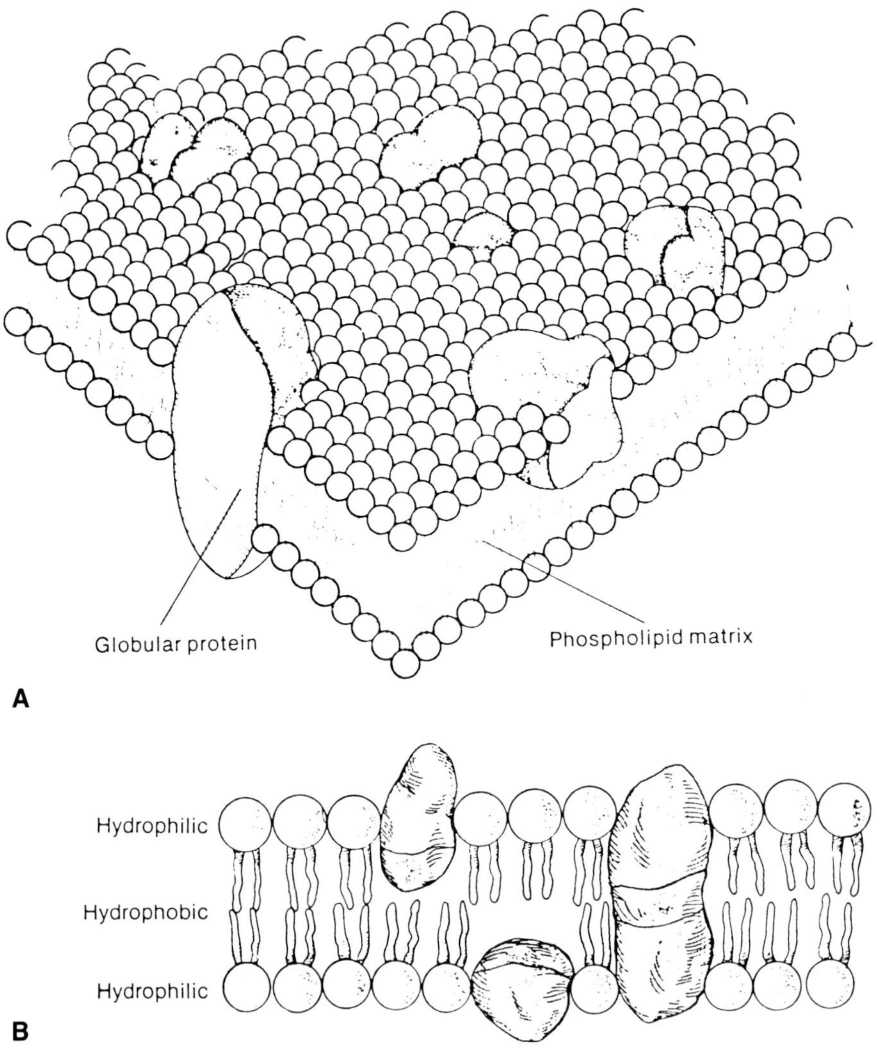

Figure 1–14. Drawing of the bacterial cytoplasmic membrane. **A.** The fluid mosaic model of membrane structure showing globular proteins imbedded in the phospholipid bilayer. *(From Singer, Nicholson.* Science. *1972;175:720.)* **B.** The arrangement of hydrophobic and hydrophilic moieties based on the fluid mosaic model. *(From Boyd RF.* General Microbiology. *St. Louis, MO: Times Mirror/Mosby College Publishing; 1984, with permission.)*

a typical bilayer (Figs 1–12, 1–14). There are no sterols in bacterial membranes except those of *Mycoplasma.* The proteins, which can constitute up to 20% of the entire cell protein, have lipophilic regions that allow them to be incorporated into the lipid. They either are enzymes or participate in transport of molecules across the membrane. Such transport systems are necessary because this lipoprotein membrane is the boundary between the cell and its environment. It is an osmotic barrier that enables the bacterium to achieve required physiologic concentrations of substrates, ions, and cofactors within the cytoplasm while excluding unneccessary or harmful substances. Unlike the outer membrane of gram-negative bacteria, which is permeable to molecules up to about 800 MW, the cytoplasmic membrane is impervious to most molecules except those for which specific transport systems exist. The membrane has little or no mechanical strength. Its integrity is maintained by a balance between the high cytoplasmic osmotic pressure and the opposing force of the rigid peptidoglycan backbone of the cell wall that tightly surrounds it.

The cytoplasmic membrane can be pictured as a phospholipid osmotic barrier breached at intervals by proteins that participate in a variety of functions essential to the survival of the cell. Protein involvement in substrate transport systems has been mentioned. Other activities ascribed to membrane proteins include electron transport and oxidative phosphorylation, synthesis of lipids and cell wall constituents, DNA replication, ribosome binding, and protein secretion. Membrane proteins also can serve as receptor sites for chemotactic agents.

In some gram-positive and gram-negative genera there are large, irregular invaginations of the cytoplasmic membrane, called mesosomes (Fig 1–5). Careful electron photomicrographic studies show that mesosomes are contiguous with the cytoplasmic membrane and are connected to the periplasmic space. Their function is unclear, but circumstantial evidence suggests that they may be involved in cell division and in secretion. Evidence for the role of mesosomes in cell division comes from observations of their intimate association with septum formation. Mesosomes also may be involved in segregation of daughter strands of DNA as a prelude to cell division. The association of mesosomes with secretion is the reesult of studies of penicillinase production by *Bacillus licheniformis*. Organisms induced to synthesize this enzyme have an increased number of mesosomes not associated with the septal region of the cell but continuous with the periplasmic space. These mesosomes contain most of the cellular penicillinase, which can be released into the environment to protect the bacteria from penicillin.

Bacterial Cytoplasm

Nucleus. The bacterial nucleus, also called the nuclear body, chromatin body, or nucleoid, appears as a compact, electron-transparent, centrally located region in the bacterial cytoplasm (Fig 1–5). It is composed of 60% DNA, 30% RNA, and 10% protein and can occupy as much as 10% of the entire cell volume. Cells often contain two or more such areas because cell division usually lags behind nuclear division. Although it clearly performs many of the same functions, the bacterial nucleus varies from nuclei of eukaryotic cells in several important respects. (1) It is not separated from the rest of the cytoplasm by a nuclear membrane. (2) Discrete chromosomes cannot be observed. The hereditary material of bacteria is a single, closed, circular duplex of DNA around which the genes are arranged in a linear fashion. The length of the DNA is many times that of the nucleus, so it is folded back on itself, an arrangement called supercoiling that results in the parallel strands often seen in bacterial nuclei. (3) There are no basic proteins (histones) associated with the DNA. (4) There is no mitotic apparatus.

Some bacteria also contain extrachromosomal DNA. This DNA may be in the form of either episomes or plasmids—circular, double-stranded DNA that can replicate autonomously or in synchrony with DNA. Plasmids are transferred between susceptible bacteria by transducing phage. They are not incorporated into the bacterial genome but are found in the cytoplasm. Episomes are plasmids that become part of the recipient cell chromosome. They are transferred between bacterial mating pairs via conjugal pili. Extrachromosomal genetic elements have important chemotherapeutic implications because it is through them that antibiotic resistance can be transferred between bacteria, particularly members of the Enterobacteriaceae.

Ribosomes. The ground substance of the bacterial cytoplasm appears in electron micrographs as a homogeneous, uniformly textured, stippled area (Fig 1–12) because of the presence of numerous ribosomes, the sites of protein synthesis. Bacterial ribosomes are dense, spherical particles composed of 70% RNA and 30% protein. Each particle consists of a 30S (S=Svedberg unit, a unit related to molecular size that defines the sedimentation rate of a macromolecule in a centrifugal field) and a 50S subunit. The complete ribosome sediments at 70S. Although some ribosomes are free in the cytoplasm, 80% of them are grouped into polysomes along an mRNA strand. Polysomes can be floating in the cytosol, or they may be attached to the cytoplasmic membrane. They are the sites where amino acid-charged tRNA is paired with the code contained in mRNA to ensure accurate synthesis of multiple copies of protein.

Inclusion Granules. Many bacteria contain intracytoplasmic polymer granules that are reserves of energy and raw materials stored in a form that will not upset the osmotic balance of the cell. Their synthesis is a response to growth conditions, often to an environmental imbalance, such as the decrease in an essential nutrient, for example, nitrogen. Such an imbalance can trigger a decrease in DNA and protein synthesis and an increase in synthesis of storage polymers. Granules containing many kinds of storage materials have been reported, but the most common are metachromatic granules, polysaccharide granules, and poly-β-hydroxybutyrate granules.

Metachromatic granules, also called volutin or Babes-Ernst granules, are linear polymers of orthophosphate. They are not membrane bound. Their purpose is to conserve phosphate for biosynthesis.

Polysaccharide granules, also called glycogen or starch granules, contain high molecular weight polymers of glucose. They usually are not membrane bound, although in some genera they are enclosed in a single-layer protein membrane. Polysaccharide granules are depots of carbon and energy.

Poly-β-hydroxybutyrate (PBHB) granules are widely distributed in bacteria. They consist of polymers of esterified β-hydroxybutyric acid enclosed in a single-layer protein membrane. PBHB is unique to prokaryotes and is analogous to neutral fats in eukaryotic cells. These granules are depositories of energy and carbon.

Cytoplasmic Solutes. The typical bacterium is about 75% water. The water content of the cytoplasm is even higher—up to 80% in some genera. Dissolved in the cytoplasmic water or cytosol are many enzymes, small molecules, and inorganic ions that make up a pool from which the bacterium can draw raw materials necessary for generation of energy and for biosynthesis of cellular constituents and products.

Endospores. Bacterial endospores are refractile, dehydrated, oblate spheroids produced by the genera

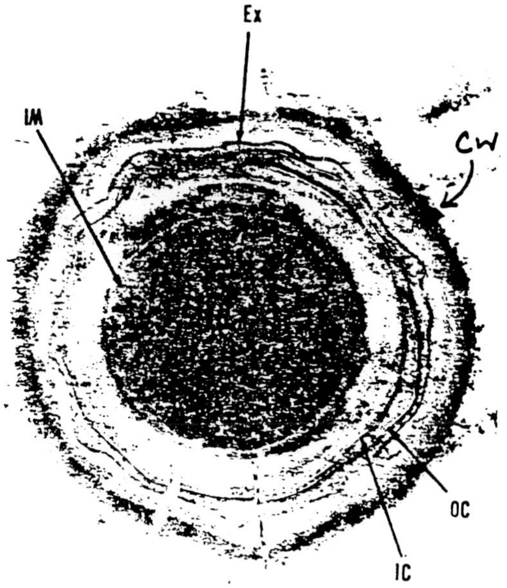

Figure 1–15. Electron photomicrograph of a mature *Bacillus cereus* endospore prior to release from the parent cell. Ex, exosporium; IM, inner membrane; R, ribosomal aggregates; OC, outer coat; IC, inner coat; CM, parent cell membrane. *(From Ellar, Lundgrin.* J Bacteriol. *1966;92:1748.)*

Bacillus, Clostridium, Desulfotomaculum, Sporolactobacillus, and *Thermoactinomyces* (Fig 1–15). Those produced by *Bacillus* and *Clostridium* are the most important in disease. Endospores are not part of the normal vegetative growth cycle of these organisms. Their production is triggered by change in the nutritional environment of the mother cell or sporangium. Sporulation is not a reproductive cycle, since only one spore is produced from each vegetative cell. Spores have no detectable metabolic activity and appear to be adapted to survive for long periods under adverse environmental conditions. They are relatively resistant, compared to their vegetative counterparts, to killing by heat, freezing, chemicals, radiation, and, most importantly, desiccation. They are, therefore, an important consideration in designing protocols for sterilization of materials and supplies and for disinfection of environmental surfaces.

Endospore formation is a multistage sequence of events that results in the production of one mature spore per cell (Fig 1–16). Sporulation usually begins at the end of the exponential growth phase. The initial events resemble cell division. At this point, each vegetative cell contains two nuclear bodies, which condense and coalesce into an axial filament. A transverse septum begins to form near one pole as the chromosomes separate and move toward the cell termini. The septum divides the cell into two unequal parts, the smaller of which ultimately will become the endospore. Unlike normal cell division, there is no transverse cell wall laid down along the septum. Instead, the membrane of the larger cell grows around the smaller cell, engulfing it and creating a forespore that is surrounded by two sets of unit membranes, its own and that of the larger protoplast. The spore cortex is next laid down between the two membranes, followed rapidly by the layers of protein coat. This is a time of great metabolic activity, with rapid synthesis and deposition of the unique spore structures and chemical constituents. It is also during this time that the spore matures, although it is not yet resistant to

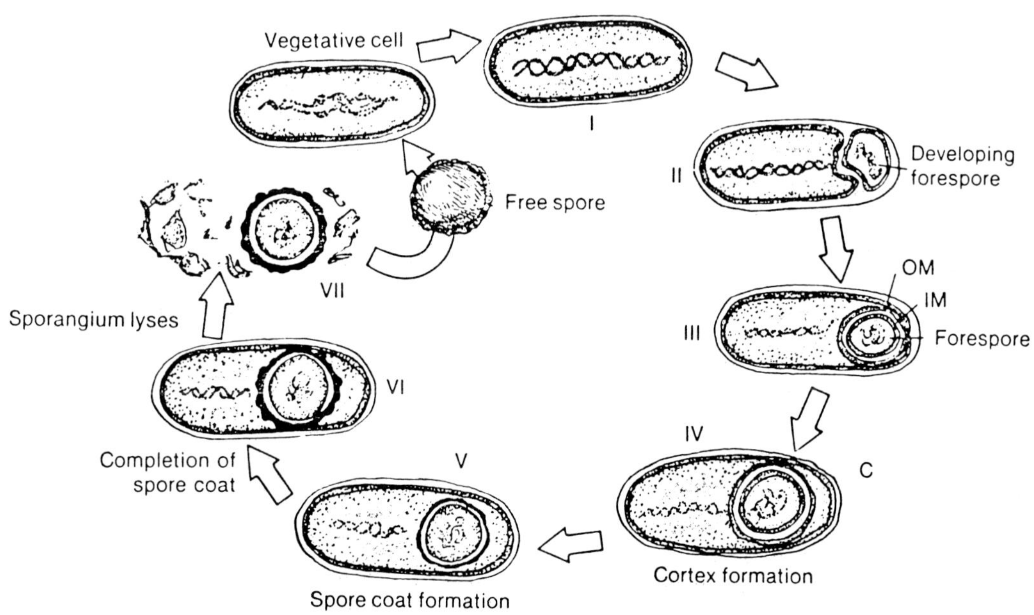

Figure 1–16. Stages in the formation of bacterial endospores. *(From Boyd RF,* General Microbiology. *St. Louis, MO: Times Mirror/ Mosby College Publishing; 1984, with permission.)*

environmental extremes. During maturation, there is the accumulation of high concentrations of calcium and the synthesis of dipicolinic acid, events that are closely related to resistance, especially to heat. The culmination of these events is the release 6 to 8 hours after initiation of a mature endospore from the sporangium.

ORAL ASPECTS

Oral infections such as dental caries and periodontal disease are called endogenous infections because they are caused by members of our own oral microflora. The normal flora is composed of a heterogeneous group of microorganisms that we acquire gradually, beginning at birth, and that stay with us for life with little variation unless there are major changes in the oral environment. These organisms are able to colonize our oral surfaces because the environment in this anatomic site satisfies their chemical and physical requirements. To survive in an econiche like the mouth, an organism must be able to adapt to the existing physical conditions and then use the nutrients available to grow and reproduce. We have studied in this chapter the physical structures of bacteria. Although they are neither as numerous nor as elegant as those of eukaryotic cells, it is clear that they are sufficient to enable bacteria to establish themselves on or in host tissues. In Chapter 2, we will study the mechanisms by which bacteria carry out the metabolic processes necessary to remain a part of the oral microflora. A thorough understanding of the organization and physiology of bacteria is essential to appreciate how this heterogeneous group of microbes can colonize the oral cavity and how, through poor oral hygiene or damage to host defenses, they can cause dental diseases.

SUGGESTED READINGS

Benz R. Structure and function of porins from gram-negative bacteria. *Annu Rev Microbiol.* 1988;42:359–393.

Brock TD. The bacterial nucleus: A history. *Microbiol Rev.* 1988;52:397–411.

Burchard RP. Gliding motility of procaryotes: Ultrastructure, physiology and genetics. *Annu Rev Microbiol.* 1981;35:497–529.

Costerton JW. The role of electron microscopy in the elucidation of bacterial structure and function. *Annu Rev Microbiol.* 1979;33:459–479.

Costerton JW, Irvin RT, Cheng KJ. The bacterial glycocalyx in nature and disease. *Annu Rev Microbiol.* 1981;35:299–324.

Coykendall AL. Classification and identification of the viridans streptococci. *Clin Microbiol.* 1989;2:315–328.

DeGraaf FK, Mooi FR. The fimbrial adhesins of *Escherichia coli. Adv Microbiol Physiol.* 1986;28:65–145.

Doetsch RN, Sjoblad RD. Flagellar structure and function in eubacteria. *Annu Rev Microbiol.* 1980;34:69–108.

Fischer W. Physiology of lipoteichoic acids in bacteria. *Adv Microbiol Physiol.* 1988;29:233–302.

Gest H. *The World of Microbes.* Menlo Park, CA: Benjamin/Cummings; 1987.

Hanson RS. The physiology and diversity of bacterial endospores. In: Parish JH, ed. *Developmental Biology of Procaryotes.* Berkeley, CA: University of California Press; 1979.

Holt JG, ed. *Bergey's Manual of Systematic Bacteriology.* Baltimore: Williams & Wilkins; 1984.

Joklik WK, ed. *Zinsser Microbiology,* 19th ed. E. Norwalk, CT: Appleton & Lange, 1988.

Paranchych W, Frost LS. The physiology and biochemistry of pili. *Adv Microbiol Physiol.* 1988;29:53–114.

Seifert HS, So M. Genetic mechanisms of bacterial antigenic variation. *Microbiol Rev.* 1988;52:327–336.

Shockman GD, Barrett JF. Structure, function, and assembly of cell walls of gram-positive bacteria. *Annu Rev Microbiol.* 1983;37:501–527.

Stanier RY, Rogers HH, Ward JB, eds. *Relations Between Structure and Function in the Prokaryotic Cell.* Cambridge: Cambridge University Press, 1978.

Sutherland IW. Biosynthesis and composition of gram-negative bacterial extracellular and wall polysaccharides. *Annu Rev Microbiol.* 1985;39:243–270.

van Iterson W, ed. *Inner Structures of Bacteria.* New York: Van Nostrand/Reinhold; 1984.

van Iterson W, ed. *Outer Structures of Bacteria.* New York: Van Nostrand/Reinhold; 1984.

Ward JB. Teichoic and teichuronic acids: Biosynthesis, assembly, and location. *Microbiol Rev.* 1981;45:211–243.

Woese CJ. Bacterial evolution. *Microbiol Rev.* 1987;51:221–271.

CHAPTER 2

Bacterial Physiology

Thomas T. Lillich

INTRODUCTION

GROWTH
- Classification
- Chemical Requirements of Chemoheterotrophs
- Physical Requirements of Chemoheterotrophs
- Nutrient Uptake of Chemoheterotrophs
- Growth in Cultures of Chemoheterotrophs

ENERGY PRODUCTION
- Role of ATP
- Other High Energy Compounds
- Metabolic Role of Pyridine Nucleotides
- Energy From Carbohydrates
- Energy from Proteins and Amino Acids
- Energy from Other Sources
- Terminal Oxidation

MACROMOLECULAR BIOSYNTHESIS
- Cell Wall Peptidoglycan Biosynthesis
- Lipopolysaccharide Biosynthesis
- Polysaccharide Biosynthesis
- DNA and Protein Synthesis

METABOLIC REGULATION
- Regulation of Enzyme Activity
- Regulation of Enzyme Synthesis
- Regulation of DNA and RNA Synthesis

ORAL ASPECTS

SUGGESTED READINGS

INTRODUCTION

Bacterial physiology is the study of life processes, those chemical and physical conditions and events that make possible the growth and reproduction of bacteria. It includes studies of cell morphology, structure, growth, and the dynamics of cell populations as functions of the cell's physical and chemical environment. Central to a study of physiology are several metabolic pathways by which bacteria systematically extract the intrinsic chemical energy contained in substrates, conserve this energy in a biologically useful form, and use it to drive the synthesis of macromolecules.

There are several kinds of metabolic pathways. Catabolic pathways systematically break down substrates and cellular constituents, resulting in the production of energy and small molecules that can be used as biosynthetic precursors. Anabolic pathways are the routes by which bacteria synthesize cellular constituents and products. They use the energy produced by catabolism to synthesize macromolecules. A third type of metabolic pathway functions in either a catabolic or a biosynthetic mode depending upon cellular needs. These are called amphibolic pathways. The tricarboxylic acid (TCA), or Krebs, cycle is an example of an amphibolic pathway in that it catabolizes 2- and 3-carbon compounds to generate energy and also produces intermediates used in the biosynthesis of amino acids, porphyrins, and other compounds essential for cell growth and reproduction. Finally, anapleurotic pathways function in certain situations to replenish intermediates of the other pathways that are used in biosynthesis. If, for example, there were no anapleurotic pathways associated with the TCA cycle, use of pathway intermediates for biosynthesis would soon shut down the pathway and prevent the cell from efficiently metabolizing sources of carbon and energy. All of these pathways are regulated to ensure maximum efficiency and coordination in substrate use and in production of energy and biosynthetic precursors necessary for survival and growth.

Understanding the pathways by which bacteria extract energy and precursors from their environment for use in synthesis of protoplasm is the key to understanding disease. Disease is predicted on two events: (1) a microbe has colonized the host, and (2) the microbe has avoided host defenses long enough to reach a population size sufficient to cause disease. Both of these events depend on bacterial metabolic capabilities. Colonization depends on the adsorption of bacteria to a surface, followed by growth and reproduction. The microbe must be able to use host components for energy and as building blocks for its own cellular constituents. Only then can it persist in that econiche. Resistance to host defenses often involves production of extracellular products that are toxic to host cells and tissues or that reduce the efficiency of nonspecific host defenses such as phagocytosis. These allow bacteria to spread from their original site and increase in numbers, with consequent damage to the host. The result is the onset of the clinical signs and symptoms of diseases, such as dental caries, periodontal disease, endodontal infections, and mixed infections of the head and neck, all a direct result of bacterial metabolism and growth in tissues.

This chapter emphasizes four aspects of bacterial physiology: (1) nutrition and growth, (2) mechanisms of energy production, (3) selected pathways of macromolecular biosynthesis, and (4) mechanisms of metabolic regulation.

GROWTH

Growth is the coordinated increase of all cellular constituents leading to replication of individual cells and, consequently, to an increase in the cell population. Like all living things, bacteria require a suitable chemical and physical environment to grow and reproduce. Physical requirements include proper temperature, pH, redox potential, and oxygen concentration. Chemically, there must be a reliable source of energy, and basic nutritional requirements must be provided. Energy can be produced by fermentation, metabolism with organic compounds serving both as electron donors and acceptors, or by respiration, in which oxygen or another inorganic molecule serves as the electron receptor. In addition, all living things require sources of carbon, nitrogen, sulfur, phosphorus, several metals, vitamins, and water. Bacteria are a nutritionally heterogeneous group of organisms. Some genera grow on a few inorganic salts and a source of carbon and energy. Others are much less biosynthetically sophisticated and require many precursors supplied preformed before they can grow.

Classification

There are four categories of bacteria based on their carbon and energy sources: (1) photoautotrophs, (2) photoheterotrophs, (3) chemoautotrophs, and (4) chemoheterotrophs. Photoautotrophs obtain energy from photosynthesis and most of their carbon from CO_2. Photoheterotrophs also produce energy from light, but they obtain carbon from organic molecules. Chemoautotrophs derive energy from chemical oxidation-reduction reactions and carbon primarily from CO_2. Chemoheterotrophs also use chemical oxidation-reduction reactions for energy but obtain carbon primarily from organic sources. They may also require trace amounts of CO_2 for optimum growth. Most medically and dentally important bacteria are chemoheterotrophs.

Chemical Requirements of Chemoheterotrophs

Chemoheterotrophs require organic compounds both as biosynthetic precursors and for energy-producing oxidation-reduction reactions. Carbon is supplied most often by carbohydrates, although some genera can use amino acids. Nitrogen usually is obtained from a complex source, such as amino acids, proteins, or peptides. Other organic compounds, such as vitamins, specific amino acids, purines and pyrimidines and porphyrin, a constituent of bacterial cytochromes, often must be supplied by adding digests, infusions, or extracts of animal or plant tissues.

Inorganic molecules, also required for growth, occur naturally as salts and are taken into the cell as ions. Sulfur, for example, usually is acquired as sulfate. Once inside, it is reduced to sulfide for use in biosynthesis. Nitrogen, carbon, oxygen, and hydrogen also can be assimilated in inorganic form, although chemoheterotrophs prefer organic sources. There are many other inorganic compounds that act as activators, cofactors, or structural stabilizers of specific enzymes.

Physical Requirements of Chemoheterotrophs

A physical environment with the appropriate temperature, pH, gases, and oxidation-reduction potential is required for growth. Bacteria are divided into three classes, psychrophiles, mesophiles, and thermophiles, based on their optimum growth temperature (Table 2–1). Differences in growth at temperature extremes have been attributed to variation in protein stability, the proteins of thermophiles, for example, being much more resistant to thermal denaturation than are similar proteins from mesophiles.

Most bacteria grow at a neutral or slightly alkaline pH, although many will tolerate a pH between 5 and 9. Intracellular pH is maintained close to neutrality despite external conditions. Internal neutrality is necessary to protect constituents such as nucleic acids and high energy compounds that are susceptible to either acid or alkali. Environmental pH is one condition that is altered readily by bacterial metabolic activity, with consequences that can be beneficial or detrimental to either the bacteria or the host. The pH of a site colonized by bacteria can be lowered by acid products of fermentation or raised by ammonia released through deamination of nitrogen-containing compounds such as amino acids. The resulting pH changes can have a direct effect on the host, as in the demineralization of tooth enamel at pH 5.5 and below, or it can have a more subtle effect by altering environmental conditions so that there is a change in the microflora at a particular site. The change may allow a potential pathogen to become established or, conversely, may preclude such establishment. The pH of oral mucosal and mineralized tissues is controlled by saliva flow and buffering capacity. Alterations in either or in access of saliva (eg, to tooth surfaces coated with plaque) compromises this defense mechanism and predisposes the host to oral disease.

The presence of carbon dioxide (CO_2) and oxygen (O_2) also can affect bacterial growth. Because CO_2 is directly incorporated into several metabolic pathways, atmospheric levels of this gas (about 0.03%) are sometimes not enough to allow even heterotrophic organisms to start growing. This requirement can be satisfied by the organism's own metabolism once growth begins, but many bacteria grow better in an atmosphere enriched with CO_2. The role of CO_2 in metabolism is discussed later in this chapter.

TABLE 2–1. CLASSES OF BACTERIA BASED ON GROWTH TEMPERATURE

Class	Optimum Temperature (°C)	Range (°C)
Psychrophiles	20	0–30
Mesophiles[a]	37	10–45
Thermophiles	50–55	25–90

[a]Contains most human pathogens.

Bacteria vary widely in their response to oxygen, a gas that has important implications for the survival and growth of bacteria and, hence, for pathogenesis. Bacteria are grouped into four categories based on the effect of oxygen on their growth and metabolism. (1) Obligate aerobes, such as *Pseudomonas,* have an absolute requirement for oxygen because they produce energy by respiration. Also in this classification are the microaerophiles, organisms that grow best at oxygen concentrations below that of air. (2) Obligate anaerobes, are organisms either inhibited or killed by molecular oxygen. (3) Facultative anaerobes, such as *Escherichia coli,* grow fermentatively under anaerobic conditions but respire in the presence of oxygen. (4) Aerotolerant anaerobes either grow fermentatively when oxygen is available or not or have a limited capacity to detoxify partial reduction products of oxygen. This category contains many important dental pathogens, such as streptococci, lactobacilli, *Bacteroides* spp., *Fusobacterium nucleatum* and *Campylobacter sputorum.* Oxygen tolerance is essential for survival of these bacteria in the normally aerobic oral environment and is a characteristic that predisposes oral soft tissues to disease if the partial pressure of oxygen falls to where the bacteria can grow and reproduce. Some medically important bacteria and their growth in different oxygen concentrations are shown in Table 2–2.

Oxygen and its reduction products can be very toxic to bacteria. Many enzymes in anaerobes are inhibited by oxygen-containing products, which cause rapid death of the microbe. Oxygen metabolites also can affect bacterial structure. Even obligate aerobes can be harmed by oxygen concentrations above that normally found in air. All bacteria have enzymes that react with oxygen, often with the production of toxic intermediates. For example, incomplete oxygen reduction produces powerful oxidizing agents such as hydrogen peroxide (H_2O_2) and superoxide radical (O_2^-) that are toxic because they damage the cytoplasmic membrane. Metabolic pathways must exist to completely reduce oxygen to two water molecules. The aerotolerance of a bacterium depends on its ability to carry out these reactions.

Superoxide dismutase, catalase, and peroxidase are enzymes that play an important role in reducing oxygen to nontoxic end products. The most crucial role is that of superoxide dismutase (SOD), which catalyzes the reduction of superoxide free radicals to hydrogen peroxide.

TABLE 2–2. OXYGEN SENSITIVITY OF SOME ANAEROBIC BACTERIA

	Percent Oxygen in Atmosphere												
Species	**0**	**0.01**	**0.03**	**0.05**	**0.07**	**1.0**	**2.0**	**3.0**	**4.0**	**6.0**	**8.0**	**10**	**12**
Treponema macrodentium	+2[a]	+2	0	0									
Treponema denticola	+2	+2	0	0									
Selenomonas ruminatium	+2	+2	+1	+1	0	0							
Butyrivibrio fibrisolvens	+2	+2	+2	+1	0	0							
Succinivibrio dextrinosolvens	+2	+2	+2	+1	0	0							
Megasphaera eldensii	+2	+2	+2	+2	+2	+2	+1	0	0				
Bacteroides oralis	+2	+2	+2	+2	+2	+2	+2	+2	+1[b]	+1[b]	0	0	
Bacteroides melaninogenicus	+2	+2	+2	+2	+2	+2	+2	+2[b]	+2[b]	+1[b]	+1[b]	0	0
Fusobacterium nucleatum	+2	+2	+2	+2	+2	+2	+2	+2	+2	+2[b]	+1[b]	0	0
Bacteroides fragilis	+2	+2	+2	+2	+2	+2	+2	+2	+2	+1[a]	+1[b]	0	0
Campylobacter sputorum	+1	+1	+1	+2	+2	+2	+2	+2	+2	+2	+2	+2	+1[b]
Campylobacter fetus	+1	+1	+1	+2	+2	+2	+2	+2	+2	+2	+2	+2	+2

[a] +2 = growth; +1 = slight growth; 0 = no growth.
[b]Growth varied with strain or incubation time.
Modified from Loesche WJ. Appl Microbiol. *1969;18:723.*

$$2O_2^- + 2H^{2+} \xrightarrow{SOD} O_2 + H_2O_2$$

Most bacteria also contain catalase, which cleaves two molecules of hydrogen peroxide to water and oxygen.

$$2H_2O_2 \rightarrow 2H_2O + O_2$$

Bacteria such as lactobacilli, which lack catalase, detoxify hydrogen peroxide with peroxidases. This family of enzymes catalyzes the oxidation of organic compounds by hydrogen peroxide, with its concomitant reduction to water and oxygen.

$$\text{Oxidized organic compound} + H_2O_2 \rightarrow \text{reduced organic compound} + H_2O + O_2$$

The SOD concentration in a bacterium determines its degree of oxygen tolerance. Obligate anaerobes lack both this enzyme and catalase. Other bacteria, including aerotolerant anaerobes, have varying concentrations of this enzyme. Thus, bacteria fall on a continuum based on their ability to detoxify partial reduction products of oxygen. At one extreme are obligate anaerobes unable to metabolically neutralize any toxic oxygen containing metabolic product. At the other extreme are the obligate aerobes that readily reduce those compounds to nontoxic end products. Anaerobiosis is, therefore, a relative concept.

The final physical aspect of the environment that affects growth is the oxidation-reduction (redox) potential, a measure of the tendency of a solution to lose, donate, or give up electrons. The redox potential (Eh) of an environment is measured in millivolts and often is expressed relative to that of a hydrogen electrode under standard conditions. The more negative the value, the greater the tendency to donate electrons, thus creating a protective, reduced environment for anaerobes. Conversely, the more positive the value, the greater the tendency to accept electrons, thus oxidizing the environment and making it less favorable for anaerobes. Compounds that donate electrons are reducing agents and will decrease Eh. Compounds such as oxygen, that accept electrons are oxidizers and will increase the Eh.

The redox potential, then, is a function of the kinds and concentrations of solutes in the environment. In vivo, Eh also depends on the anatomy of a site and on the cohabiting microflora. Eh is an important criterion for growth of different bacterial genera. Dental plaque has, for example, an initial Eh of +270 mV. The microflora of such plaque is predominantly gram-positive cocci that are aerotolerant anaerobes. As plaque grows, there is a decrease in Eh so that at 7 days it is about −126 mV. Concomitant with this decrease and other environmental and nutritional changes is a change in the plaque microflora. Seven day plaque is much more microbiologically heterogeneous and contains many more obligate anaerobes than younger plaque. Figure 2–1 illustrates the increase in two genera of oral anaerobic bacteria as a function of decreasing plaque Eh. Left undisturbed, plaque Eh will continue to fall. The potential measured in gingival crevices of volunteers with experimental gingivitis approaches −250 mV, a value observed in anaerobic cultures. The implication is that the plaque microflora is altering the environment (Eh is only one aspect), thus creating conditions conducive to establishment or ascendency of an anaerobic microflora with pathogenic potential that is manifest clinically as gingivitis.

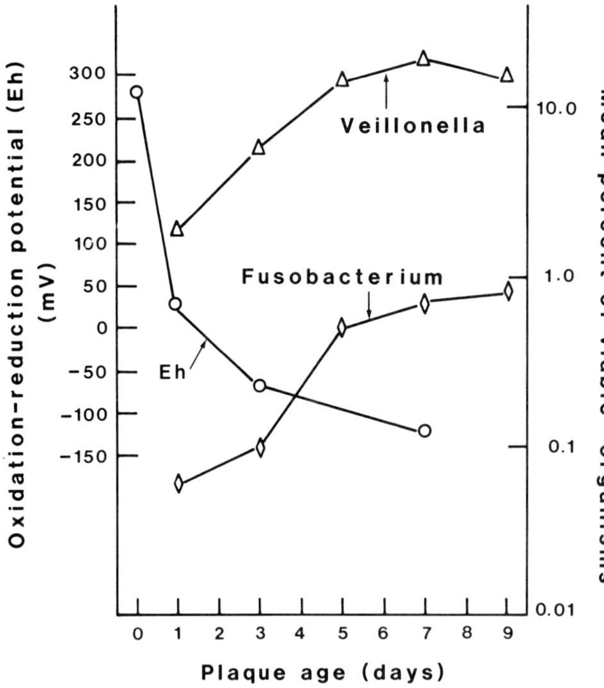

Figure 2–1. The relationship between redox potential (Eh) and the percentage of two anaerobic genera in accumulating dental plaque. *(Modified from Kenney EB, Ash MM. J* Periodontol. *1969;40:630–633; and Ritz HL.* Arch Oral Biol. *1967;12:1561–1568.)*

Nutrient Uptake of Chemoheterotrophs

The cytoplasmic membrane is the boundary between a bacterial cell and its environment. It is a lipid bilayer containing pores and other passages through which low molecular weight substances pass in a selective, highly regulated manner. In order for most substances to traverse the cytoplasmic membrane, they must be carried across by specific transport mechanisms. The cytoplasmic membrane is the osmotic barrier that allows intracellular solutes to reach concentrations many times those in the environment—concentrations essential to efficient cell growth and reproduction. It is through this regulatory structure that nutrients and end products must pass if the cell is to survive.

Many bacterial nutrients exist as complex macromolecules that must be degraded before they can enter the cell. Carbohydrates, for example, which are preferred sources of both carbon and energy by many chemoheterotrophs, often exist as polysaccharides that are impermeable to the cell membrane. Likewise, amino acids that serve as metabolic precursors themselves often are found as peptides or proteins that must be degraded. Both gram-positive and gram-negative bacteria secrete enzymes that degrade these and other macromolecules into compounds that can traverse the cell membrane. Those secreted by gram-positive cells are true exoenzymes that are released from the cell into the environment. The extracellular enzymes of gram-negative bacteria also may be released but more often remain associated with the inner or outer membrane in the periplasmic space. Exoenzymes have been implicated as bacterial virulence factors. Their secretion causes disruption of tissue integrity around the infection site, which can compromise host defenses and allow the infection to spread. Tissue destruction accompanying an infection can be viewed in these instances as a side effect of the bacterial search for nutrients rather than a preplanned strategy by the parasite.

Bacteria have four mechanisms by which nutrients can cross the cytoplasmic membrane: passive diffusion, facilitated diffusion, active transport, and group translocation.

Passive Diffusion. Passive diffusion occurs only if there is a concentration gradient across the membrane, that is, if the solute concentration is higher on one side of the membrane than on the other. The rate of movement is directly proportional to the magnitude of the gradient. As the solute diffuses, there is a decrease in the gradient between the cell cytoplasm and the environment until there is no longer sufficient difference for diffusion to continue. Passive diffusion is nonspecific and does not require energy. Water is the most important substance transported this way.

Facilitated Diffusion. Facilitated diffusion is a mechanism by which substances are transported from an area of high concentration to one of relatively low concentration without energy expenditure. Facilitated diffusion is specific because it is mediated by membrane-bound proteins, called permeases, that bind molecules on the outer surface, carry them through the membrane, and release them unchanged into the cytoplasm (Fig 2–2). It is also faster than passive diffusion. This mechanism is relatively common in eukaryotes but is rare in prokaryotes.

Active Transport. Active transport is a common mechanism of substrate uptake that allows solutes to enter the cell against a concentration gradient via specific membrane-bound permeases. With this mechanism, nutrients can be accumulated in the bacterial cytoplasm up to 1000 times their environmental concentration. The ability to concentrate nutrients intracellularly is important in the dilute, aqueous environment in which most bacteria live so that substrates are present in concentrations that make enzymatic reactions thermodynamically favorable. Active transport requires the expenditure of energy that is used to decrease the substrate affinity of the permease on the inside of the cell relative to that on the external surface.

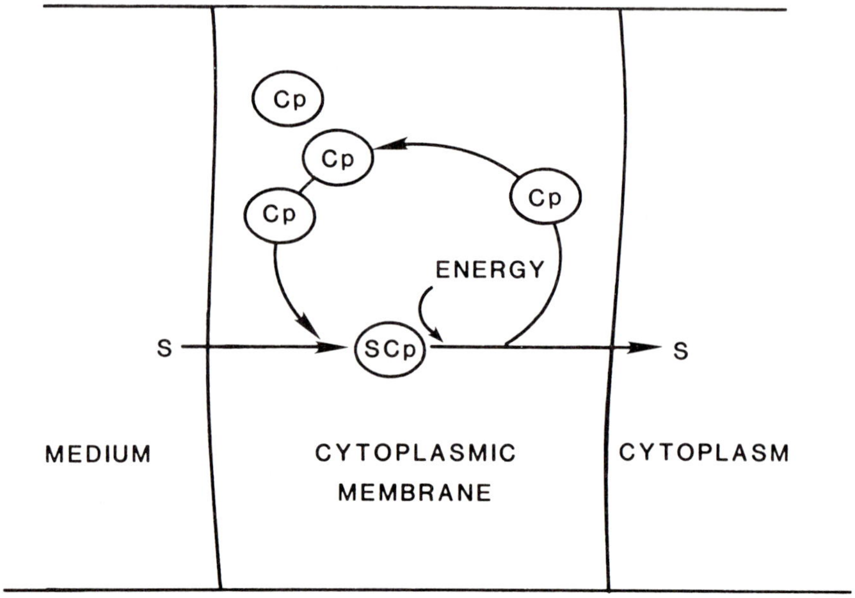

Figure 2–2. Facilitated diffusion. Solutes are transported from a region of high concentration to an area of low concentration by specific protein permeases in the cell membrane. The solute is not chemically altered during transport. *(Modified from Boyd RF.* General Microbiology. *St. Louis: Times-Mirror/Mosby College Publishing; 1984.)*

Therefore, more substrate is transported into the cell than out, and the intracytoplasmic substrate concentration increases. The substrate is released unmodified into the cytoplasm and can then be activated to enter catabolic or biosynthetic pathways. The energy to drive active transport, called the proton motive force, is produced by the membrane-bound electron transport system in aerobic bacteria or via hydrolysis of adenosine triphosphate (ATP) by a membrane-bound ATPase in anaerobes (Fig 2–3). In both cases, cellular metabolism establishes both an ion gradient and an electrical potential difference across the membrane. This transmembrane potential is the energy that drives substrate transport into the cytoplasm. Active transport is one important mechanism in which metabolic energy is converted into osmotic work.

Group Translocation. Group translocation is a transport mechanism in which the substrate is modified chemically on its way into the cell to a form that cannot pass back out of the cytoplasm (Fig 2–4). It requires energy expenditure, but unlike active transport, there is very little increase in the cytoplasmic concentration of unmodified substrate. What accumulates is the modified form, often a phosphorylated derivative. The process begins by the relatively nonspecific phosphorylation of substrates. These modified compounds are transported across the membrane by specific permeases and are released into the cytoplasm. Many bacteria transport sugars in this manner using a sugar-phosphoenolpyruvate (PEP) phosphotransferase system. During transport, sugars are phosphorylated using energy from PEP. The phosphorylated derivatives of the sugars are released into the cytoplasm. What accumulates in the cell is not the free sugar but sugar phosphate. Group translocation is more efficient than active transport because the phosphorylated derivatives released into the cytoplasm are ready to participate in many metabolic reactions without further chemical activation. Substrates

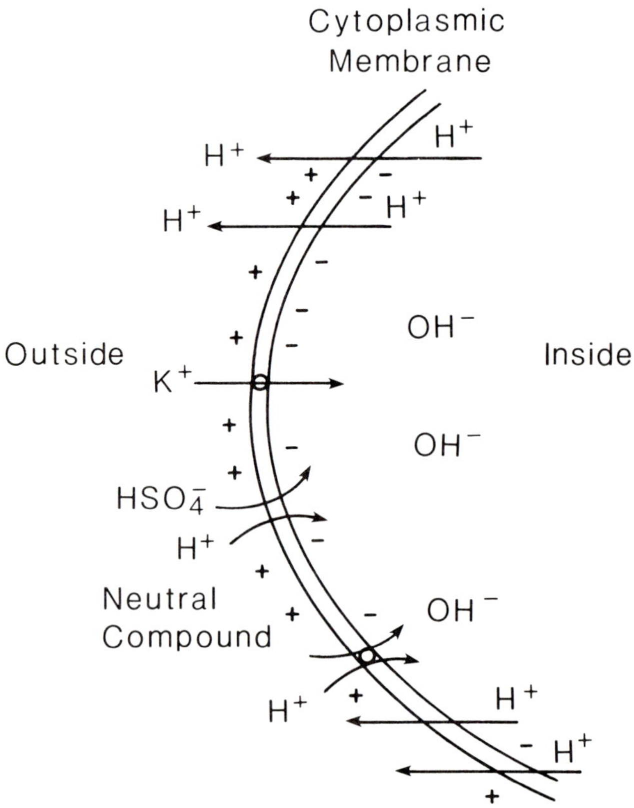

Figure 2–3. Active transport. An ion and electrical potential gradient called the proton motive force, created by electron transport or by membrane-bound ATPases, is used to power the selective uptake of solutes. *(Modified from Brock TD.* Biology of Microorganisms. *Englewood Cliffs, NJ: Prentice-Hall; 1974.)*

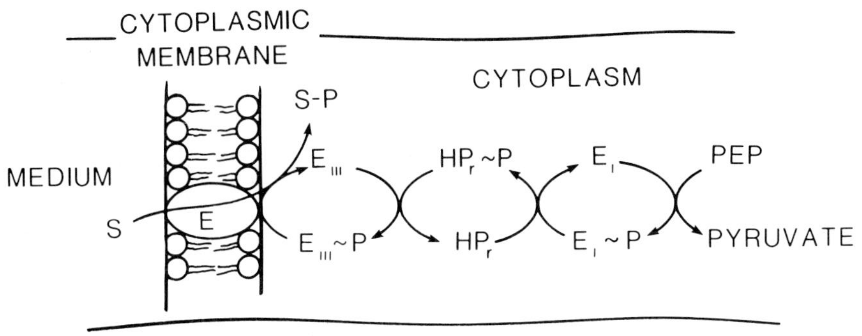

Figure 2–4. Group translocation. Substrate is transported across the cytoplasmic membrane by specific permeases and is modified chemically during the process before being released into the cytoplasm. This mechanism commonly is used by bacteria to transport sugars by phosphorylating them through an enzymatic couple to phosphoenolpyruvate (PEP). This is the sugar-phosphoenolpyruvate phosphotransferase system. *(Modified from Boyd RF.* General Microbiology. *St. Louis: Times-Mirror/Mosby College Publishing; 1984.)*

transported via active transport, on the other hand, require activation by further expenditure of energy before they can be metabolized. The efficiency of group translocation is especially important in fermentations where ATP is at a premium. It is the primary mechanism of transport in fermentative bacteria.

Growth in Cultures of Chemoheterotrophs

The inoculation of bacteria into a suitable physical and chemical environment eventually will result in the growth of those organisms—the orderly increase in all chemical components of the individual cells. Growth results in an increase in size and weight of individual cells, usually as a prelude to cell division. Because individual bacteria are so small, studies of bacterial growth usually are made with populations, or cultures, of cells. Population growth is a consequence of individual cell growth and division. This section describes methods commonly used to measure growth of pure cultures of bacteria.

Growth Measurement. There are two common ways of measuring in vitro bacterial growth: cell mass and cell number. Both assume that the culture is in balanced growth, that is, that all cellular constituents are being synthesized at equal rates, and therefore, any one can be used to measure growth.

Cell mass can be measured directly by determining the dry weight of cell material in a known volume of culture medium. This method is tedious and often inaccurate, so cell mass is usually measured indirectly with a spectrophotometer or nephalometer. These instruments use optical methods to measure the amount of light scattered by a cell suspension. The amount scattered is directly proportional to the concentration of bacteria in the suspension. Under controlled conditions, the cell concentration measured optically can be related to the dry weight of a similar suspension by use of a standard curve. Another measure of bacterial cell mass is cell yield, defined as the cell mass produced per unit of a limiting nutrient, such as glucose. When expressed relative to the amount of substrate used, it is an indication of the efficiency of substrate conversion into bacterial mass.

Numbers of bacteria in a culture also can be determined directly or indirectly. Direct measurement involves either manual counting of bacteria in a small, known volume of culture fluid or electronic counting using a device such as a Coulter counter that will give both the numbers and size distribution of bacteria in a sample. These methods measure both living and dead cells. Values tend to be higher, therefore, than those obtained with a direct plate count, another method of measuring cell numbers. The direct plate count or viable count is accomplished by diluting a culture and plating aliquots on a solid medium. The theory behind the technique is that, at appropriate dilutions, bacteria will be deposited individually at isolated spots on the agar surface. Each colony that grows on the agar is theoretically a clone arising from a single cell in the dilution that was plated. The number of viable bacteria in the original culture can be calculated from the dilution used and the amount plated. The culture medium and environmental conditions must be chosen carefully to ensure optimum growth of the bacteria under study. Plate counts actually may underestimate the bacterial population because (1) microorganisms that grow in chains form a single colony from more than one cell, and (2) culture media often do not support growth of all organisms.

Growth in Liquid Medium. Bacterial growth studies are based on the reproduction of individual cells by binary fission. Beginning with a single cell, the population increases geometrically as long as sufficient nutrients are available in the environment to support growth.

$$1 \rightarrow 2 \rightarrow 2^2 \rightarrow 2^3 \rightarrow 2^4 \rightarrow 2^5 \rightarrow 2^n$$

The time required for cells to divide, for the population to double, is called the generation time. Generation time is a function of both the bacterium and the environment in which it is growing. Bacteria such as *E. coli* and some species of *Streptococcus* and *Staphylococcus*, divide every 20 minutes under optimum laboratory conditions. Other species, such as *Mycobacterium tuberculosis,* which has an in vitro generation time of 24 hours, grow much more slowly even under the best laboratory conditions. In experiments designed to more closely approximate the in vivo environment, however, *E. coli* innoculated into a section of guinea pig intestine along with a normal mixed intestinal flora doubled every 6 hours, presumably because of competition for nutrients and production of inhibitory substances by other members of the microflora. Similar results were obtained using a *Salmonella typhimurium* strain with an optimal in vitro generation time of 30 minutes. When grown in mouse spleen cells, these bacteria doubled every 5 to 12 hours. Results of in vitro growth experiments, therefore, are not necessarily accurate predictors of bacterial behavior in vivo, where host defenses and the physical and chemical environment may cause variations from anticipated values.

In vitro bacterial growth can be studied using batch cultures, continuous cultures, or synchronous growth techniques in which all cells in a culture are maintained in the same phase of the cell cycle. Batch cultures involve inoculation of bacteria into a fixed volume of culture fluid to which nothing is subsequently added or removed except by bacterial metabolism. Conditions are relatively constant initially, but as the culture grows and the population (cell numbers) increases, there are alterations in the environment that eventually cause a decline, first in the rate of growth and finally in the viability of the culture. Growth measurement in batch culture results in a four phase curve, shown in Fig 2–5. The first phase (A) is called the lag phase, a period of adjustment in which there is intense physiologic activity as bacteria inoculated into the medium adapt to their new environment. The population size remains constant during this time. The lag phase may be short or long depending on the physiologic condition of the cells and the suitability of the medium. At the end of this phase, the cells divide, but they are not in synchrony, so there is a gradual increase in the population as the culture enters the exponential phase (B). Cells in an exponential phase culture are dividing steadily, and the population increases at a constant rate, called the generation time. During the exponential phase, the growth rate is maximal, and the population is most nearly uniform in chemical composition and metabolic activity. The culture is in a balanced state. Since batch cultures are closed systems, an exponential culture soon will change its own environment by depleting essential nutrients and by producing end products that adversely affect the cells. The effect of this change is a slower growth rate, reflected in the third phase of the curve, the stationary phase (C). During this time, the population remains constant due to a balance between the number of cells dividing and those dying. The final phase of the growth curve, the death phase (D), reflects an increasing number of cells dying relative to living, multiplying cells.

Continuous cultures keep bacteria in balanced, exponential, or steady state growth for long periods of time. Cells are grown in a turbidostat or chemostat, which automatically monitors growth, adds fresh medium, and removes spent medium, thus replenishing nutrients and removing toxic end products. Continuous cultures are used industrially to achieve maximum yields of desired end products from bacterial cultures. In some respects, the oral cavity operates like a biologic chemostat. Bacteria adhering to oral epithelium or occupying the outermost layer of dental plaque are bathed by saliva, which supplies nutrients and removes metabolic end products much like the in vitro conditions in a chemostat.

Growth on Solid Medium. Solid media are prepared by the addition of a solidifying agent, such as agar, a galactose polymer that is not metabolized by most

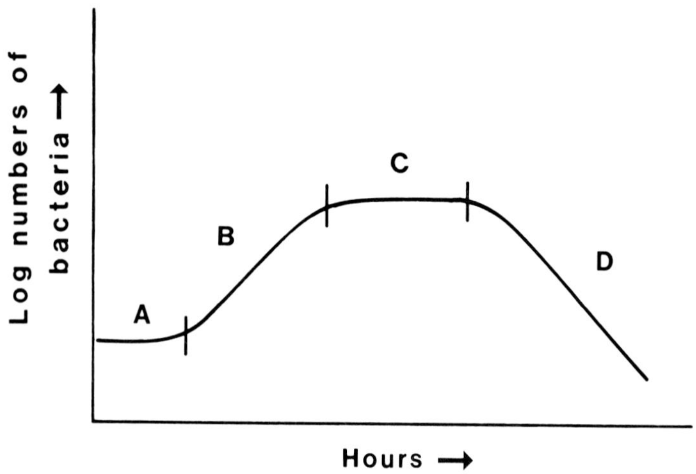

Figure 2–5. Growth curve of a bacterial batch culture. A, log phase; B, exponential phase; C, stationary phase; D, death phase.

bacteria, to liquid media. Such media have a number of advantages over fluid media, particularly in diagnostic microbiology. Solid media allow the isolation of individual cells from mixtures, the determination of viable bacteria in cultures, and the presumptive identification of bacteria based on size, shape, color, opacity, and texture of their colonies. Additives such as blood, dyes, and other ingredients in agar enhance the ability of clinical microbiologists to identify pathogens in a specimen. Rapid, accurate identification is essential to effective treatment of infectious diseases. There are four types of special purpose media that are used in solid or liquid form in a diagnostic laboratory: defined, enriched, differential, and selective.

A defined medium is one in which all the chemical constituents are known. These media are prepared using highly purified, chemically defined ingredients. Usually, such media are suitable only for bacteria with relatively simple nutritional requirements. They do not fulfill all the nutritional requirements for more fastidious bacteria, so they are often enriched by the addition of blood, serum, or extracts of various plant and animal tissues. The essential nutrients present in these additives often are unknown but may include heme, vitamins, or other cofactors. Differential media contain chemicals that allow desired species of bacteria to be distinguished from others in the specimen. Blood agar, for example, which is both differential and enriched, makes possible the identification of streptococcal species based on their effect on the blood cells in the medium. Selective media contain substances that inhibit certain bacteria while allowing others to grow. Dyes such as crystal violet and brilliant green, are examples of selective agents used in this kind of medium. Other inhibitors, such as antibiotics, also may be used. Some media are both selective and differential. Mitis-salivarius agar, used routinely in studies of oral streptococci, is an example. It contains the selective agent crystal violet that inhibits gram-negative bacteria. The inclusion of sucrose makes possible the differentiation of *Streptococcus mutans*, *Streptococcus sanguis*, and *Streptococcus salivarius* colonies based on colonial morphology, extracellular polysaccharide synthesis, and attachment to the agar surface.

Special Considerations for Growth of Anaerobes. Because of the nutritional and environmental fastidiousness of anaerobic bacteria, their laboratory growth always has created a challenge for research and clinical microbiologists. Only in the past several years, using rigorous techniques for processing samples, has in vitro recovery of anaerobes approached the numbers predicted by direct microscopic counts of samples. The study of anaerobes always has been hampered by technical difficulties in maintaining the proper redox potential during sampling, laboratory manipulations, and growth. This has been a particular problem when studying oral bacteria. Many of these problems have been overcome by the addition of reducing agents, such as thioglycollate, dithiothreitol, cysteine, or ascorbic acid to media, by using fresh medium that has not yet absorbed oxygen from the environment, by incubating cultures under anaerobic conditions in Brewer jars, glove boxes, or in the GasPak system, or by growing bacteria in roll tubes. The necessary redox potential is maintained in nature by a combination of reduced access by oxygen because of anatomic barriers and the scavenging of oxygen by cohabiting microflora and host tissues.

ENERGY PRODUCTION

Much of the metabolic effort of bacteria is devoted to the stepwise degradation of substrates so that their intrinsic bond energy is conserved in a biologically useful form. This catabolic arm of metabolism provides the energy needed to synthesize nucleic acids, proteins, lipids, polysaccharides, and heteropolymers that make up cellular form and substance. The total energy contained in an organic substrate can be released only by its complete oxidation to CO_2. The amount of energy available in an organic substrate is a function of how close its oxidation level is to that of CO_2. The closer it is, the less energy is available.

The bacterial classifications described in the section on oxygen requirements are used here to separate organisms according to the catabolic, energy-generating pathways available to them. Obligate aerobes, such as *Pseudomonas aeruginosa*, require molecular oxygen because they depend on aerobic respiration for their energy needs. They use molecular oxygen as the terminal oxidizer in the energy-producing pathways. Anaerobes, such as *F. nucleatum*, on the other hand, use fermentative pathways of energy production that are less efficient than respiration but that do not involve oxygen. They must avoid oxygen because they are not able to detoxify the harmful partial reduction products of oxygen produced during respiration. Aerotolerant anaerobes, such as *S. mutans*, continue to ferment substrates even in the presence of oxygen. By not reducing oxygen during metabolism, these bacteria avoid producing toxic oxygen-containing intermediates. Facultative bacteria, such as *E. coli*, switch between respiration and fermentation depending on the availability of oxygen. These bacteria contain the enzymes necessary to detoxify partial reduction products of oxygen.

Respiration is a much more efficient means of generating energy than is fermentation. Respiration releases more energy from a substrate than fermentation because the compound is oxidized more completely. An aerobe theoretically can produce 38 mol of ATP for each 1 mol of substrate (glucose) consumed. Fermentative organisms, in contrast, produce only 4 mol of ATP for each 1 mol of glucose. This gives aerobes a competitive advantage over fermentative bacteria in an aerobic environment.

Role of ATP

Adenosine triphosphate is the universal energy currency of biologic systems. It is the primary carrier of biologically useful energy (Fig 2–6). All energy requiring biologic reactions is coupled directly or indirectly to the hydrolysis of ATP to ADP and inorganic phosphate. In this reaction, the phosphate from ATP is donated to a large number of metabolic intermediates. The energy transferred from ATP during phosphorylation increases the energy state of these intermediates and enables them to participate in biochemical reactions that otherwise would be thermodynamically unfavorable.

ATP is the link between catabolic pathways that produce energy and anabolic pathways that use energy to drive macromolecular synthesis, nutrient uptake, cell division, and other essential cell functions. Energy for ATP synthesis is derived from coupled oxidation-reduction reactions by which bacteria catabolize substrates. The bond energy of the substrates is conserved as electrons are transferred from a donor, which becomes oxidized to an acceptor that is reduced. Electrons flow from donors of low redox potential to acceptors with relatively high potentials until a terminal acceptor is reached. The terminal acceptor may be oxygen, as in obligate aerobes, other inorganic molecules such as nitrogen or sulfur, or an organic molecule as in fermentative bacteria. At certain key places during the electron flow, there is enough energy conserved and there exist the enzymes for ATP to be produced from ADP and inorganic phosphate. There are two basic mechanisms of ATP synthesis: electron transport phosphorylation and substrate level phosphorylation.

Electron transport phosphorylation occurs via a series of closely associated, membrane-bound, iron-containing proteins. Electrons are accepted from organic donors and transported through the protein chain by the alternate reduction and oxidation of the iron molecule in the core of each protein. Flow occurs in the direction of increasing redox potential until electrons are transferred to a terminal acceptor, either oxygen or another inorganic molecule. Flow is coupled to ATP synthesis at several points. A detailed discussion of ATP synthesis via the electron transport chain will be found later in this chapter (see also Fig 2–13).

Substrate level phosphorylation occurs during the catabolism of organic compounds in which a small number of intermediates are formed that have high energy phosphoryl bonds. These intermediates are 1,3-diphosphoglyceric acid, phosphoenolpyruvic acid, and acetylphosphate. Further metabolism of these compounds is coupled with the transfer of a high energy phosphate bond to ADP (Fig 2–7).

Other High Energy Compounds

Although ATP is the primary form of biologic energy storage and transfer, there are several other metabolites with high energy bonds that provide energy for specialized cellular biosynthetic reactions. Some of these compounds and the biosynthetic events in which they participate are shown in Table 2–3.

Metabolic Role of Pyridine Nucleotides

Oxidation, removal of electrons from the donor in an oxidation-reduction pair, is accompanied by the simultaneous removal of two protons. The electron donor is, therefore, both oxidized and dehydrogenated. Conversely, reduction of the electron acceptor is often

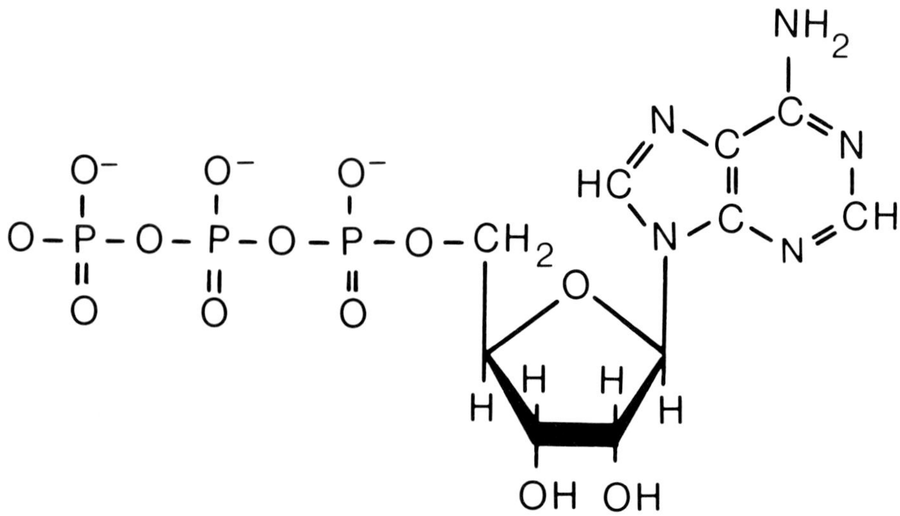

Figure 2–6. Structural formula for adenosine-5′-triphosphate (ATP).

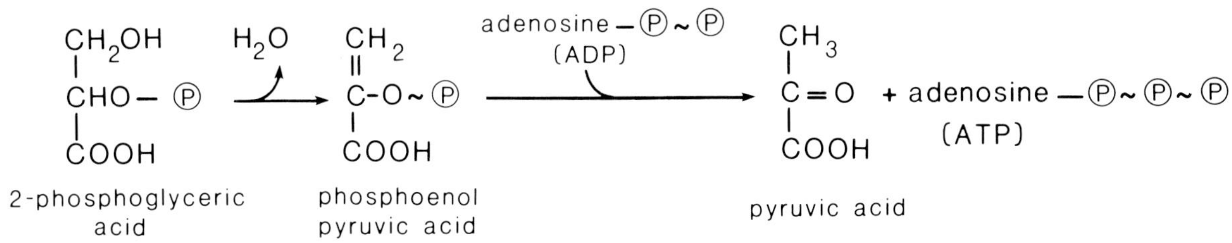

Figure 2–7. An example of substrate level phosphorylation. The low energy bond of phosphate in 2-phosphoglyceric acid is converted by dehydration to a high energy bond in phosphoenolpyruvic acid. This phosphate bond energy is conserved by transfer to ADP, with the production of one ATP molecule.

accompanied by acceptance of the protons, or hydrogenation. The pyridine nucleotides nicotinamide adenine dinucleotide (NAD) and nicotinamide adenine dinucleotide phosphate (NADP) are mediators of biologic redox reactions in that they accept protons from dehydrogenated electron donors and transfer them to the electron acceptor in the redox pair. They thus function in the transfer of reducing power (hydrogen and electrons) by coupling dehydrogenation with electron transport through the electron transport system or between redox pairs.

Energy from Carbohydrates

Carbohydrates are the most common bacterial energy sources. Pathways of carbohydrate metabolism also provide the cell with essential biosynthetic intermediates. As described previously, macromolecules must be hydrolyzed before they can be transported and metabolized. Many bacteria secrete extracellular enzymes, such as amylases or cellulases, that perform this hydrolysis. Internal storage polysaccharides are hydrolyzed by phosphorylases that conserve ATP by producing phosphorylated monosaccharides ready for catabolism without further activation.

Hexoses play a key role in the metabolism of many bacteria by serving both as sources of energy and as biosynthetic precursors for bacterial cell walls, capsules, slime layers, and intracellular storage polymers. The use of most hexoses as energy sources involves their conversion to glucose-6-phosphate, which is metabolized to pyruvate with the production of ATP. Likewise, the common dietary disaccharides sucrose and lactose are metabolized as hexoses after hydrolysis.

$$\text{Sucrose} \xrightarrow[\text{invertase}]{} \text{glucose} + \text{fructose}$$

$$\text{Lactose} \xrightarrow[\beta\text{-galactosidase}]{} \text{glucose} + \text{galactose}$$

Pentoses are also important biosynthetic precursors and energy sources in many bacteria. They are constituents of nucleic acids and such molecules as ATP and NAD. Extracellular pentose polymers, like their polyhexose counterparts, are hydrolyzed by exoenzymes to monomers than can transverse the cytoplasmic membrane. Once inside the cell, they are phosphorylated and converted to xylulose-5-phosphate, a molecule that occupies a position in pentose metabolism analogous to that of glucose-6-phosphate in hexose catabolic pathways. Some bacteria can synthesize pentoses from other precursors, thus eliminating the need for preformed 5-carbon sugars in their environment.

Bacteria use three pathways to catabolize sugar: (1) the Embden-Meyerhof-Parnas pathway, also called the glycolytic pathway, (2) the pentose phosphate pathway, or hexose monophosphate shunt, and (3) the Entner-Doudoroff pathway. Depending on the bacterium and the environmental conditions, various combinations of these pathways are used to provide the organism with energy and biosynthetic intermediates. All of these pathways eventually yield pyruvic acid, a key metabolic intermediate.

Embden-Meyerhof-Parnas Pathway. This pathway is shown schematically in Fig 2–8. This pathway is present in virtually all bacteria that use carbohydrates as carbon and energy sources. Bacteria must initially expend 2 mol of ATP converting glucose to fructose 1,6-diphosphate, an intermediate that is at a high enough energy state to enable subsequent reactions to occur. Fructose 1,6-diphosphate is cleaved by

TABLE 2–3. HIGH ENERGY COMPOUNDS OTHER THAN ATP AND THEIR BIOSYNTHETIC ROLES

Compound	Role
Guanosine triphosphate (GTP)	Ribosome function and protein synthesis
Uridine triphosphate (UTP)	Synthesis of bacterial cell wall peptidoglycan
Cytidine triphosphate (CTP)	Phospholipid synthesis
Deoxythymidine triphosphate (dTTP)	Synthesis of bacterial cell wall lipopolysaccharide
Acetylcoenzyme A	Fatty acid synthesis

Adapted from Stanier RY, Adelberg EA, Ingraham J. The Microbial World, *4th ed. Englewood Cliffs, NJ: Prentice-Hall; 1976.*

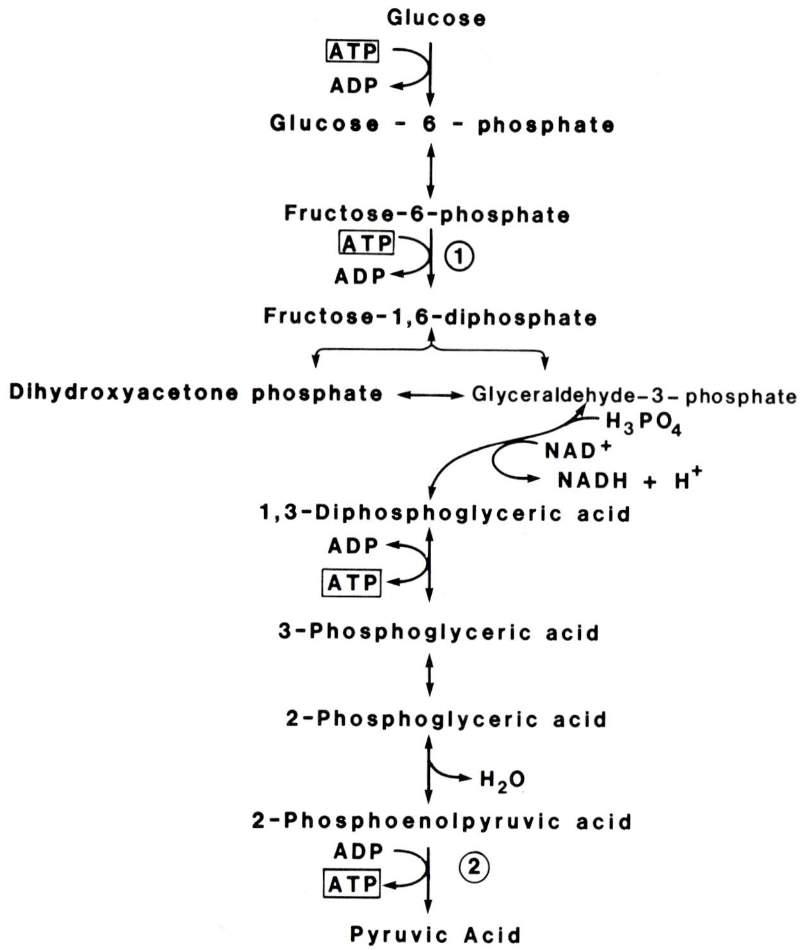

Figure 2–8. The Embden-Meyerhof-Parnas, or glycolytic, pathway. The numbered reactions are catalyzed by allosteric enzymes that are important regulatory points in hexose metabolism. 1, phosphofructokinase; 2, pyruvate kinase.

aldolase to two freely interconvertible molecules, glyceraldehyde 3-phosphate and dihydroxyacetone phosphate. No electrons have been transferred yet, although the cell has used 2 ATP molecules. The first oxidation-reduction reaction occurs with oxidation of the triosephosphate and the concomitant reduction of NAD. During the oxidation, inorganic phosphate is incorporated into a high energy ester in the product, 1,3-diphosphoglyceric acid. This reaction is a substrate level phosphorylation (Fig 2–7). The subsequent conversion of 1,3-diphosphoglyceric acid to pyruvate allows transfer of both phosphates to ADP, thus producing 2 moles of ATP per mole of triose. On balance, this pathway produces a net gain of 2 moles of ATP per mole of glucose catabolized.

Pentose Phosphate Pathway. The pentose phosphate pathway, or hexose monophosphate shunt, shown in Fig 2–9, is a cyclic pathway that produces (1) reduced NADP needed for biosynthesis and (2) ribose 5-phosphate for nucleic acid and coenzyme synthesis. Bacteria that do not have a nutritional requirement for pentoses use all or part of this pathway to synthesize the 5-carbon sugars they need for biosynthesis. Enteric streptococci, *Streptococcus faecalis* and *Streptococcus faecium,* that are found in small numbers in the oral cavity have been shown to use this pathway.

Entner-Doudoroff Pathway. The Entner-Doudoroff pathway, shown in Fig 2–10, is used primarily by aerobic bacteria such as the pseudomonads that are able to metabolize a wide variety of substrates. It yields 2 mol of acetyl-CoA for each hexose used. The acetyl-CoA can then enter the TCA cycle for terminal oxidation. The pathway is characteristic of gram-negative bacteria that use respiration to generate energy and is seldom used in hexose fermentation. However, some of the heterofermentative lactobacilli that colonize the oral cavity have been reported to use this pathway.

The Central Role of Pyruvate. Pyruvic acid is a junction point in bacterial metabolism. It can serve either as a substrate for additional redox reactions, yielding more energy and a variety of end products, or it can serve as a precursor for the biosynthesis of many cellular components. Some of the reactions in which pyruvate can participate are shown in Fig 2–11. In

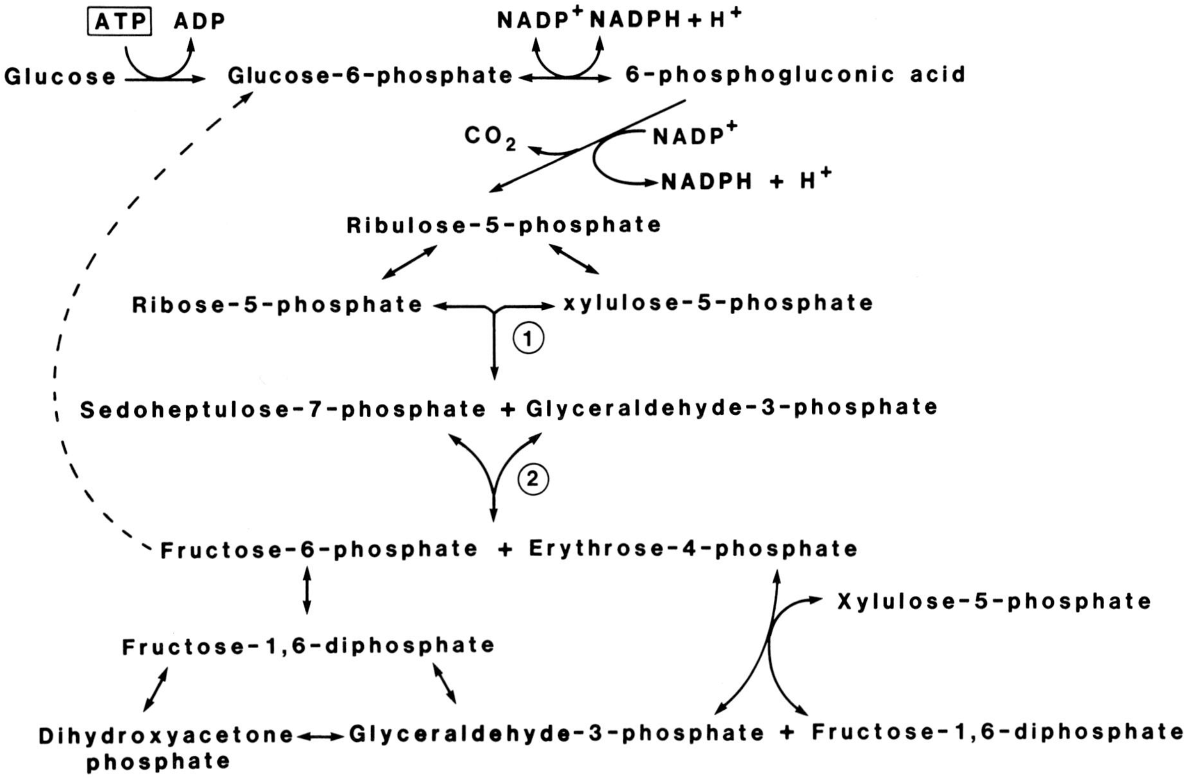

Figure 2–9. The pentose phosphate pathway or hexose monophosphate shunt. Steps 1 and 2 are catalyzed by the enzymes transketolase and transaldolase, respectively, and ultimately result in synthesis of hexose.

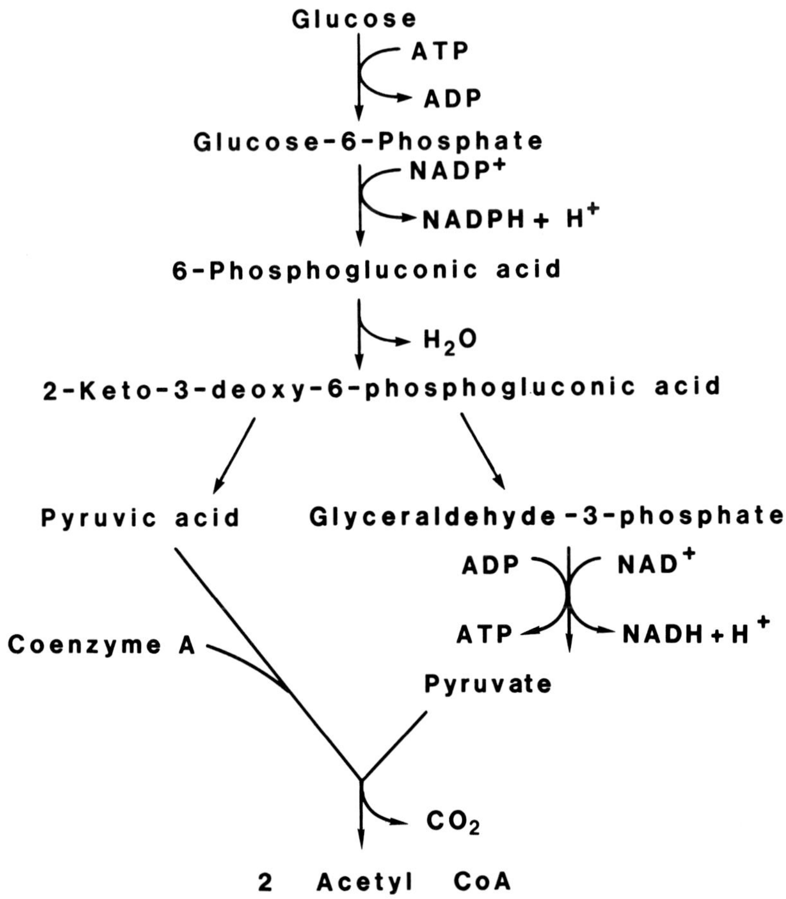

Figure 2–10. The Entner-Doudoroff pathway.

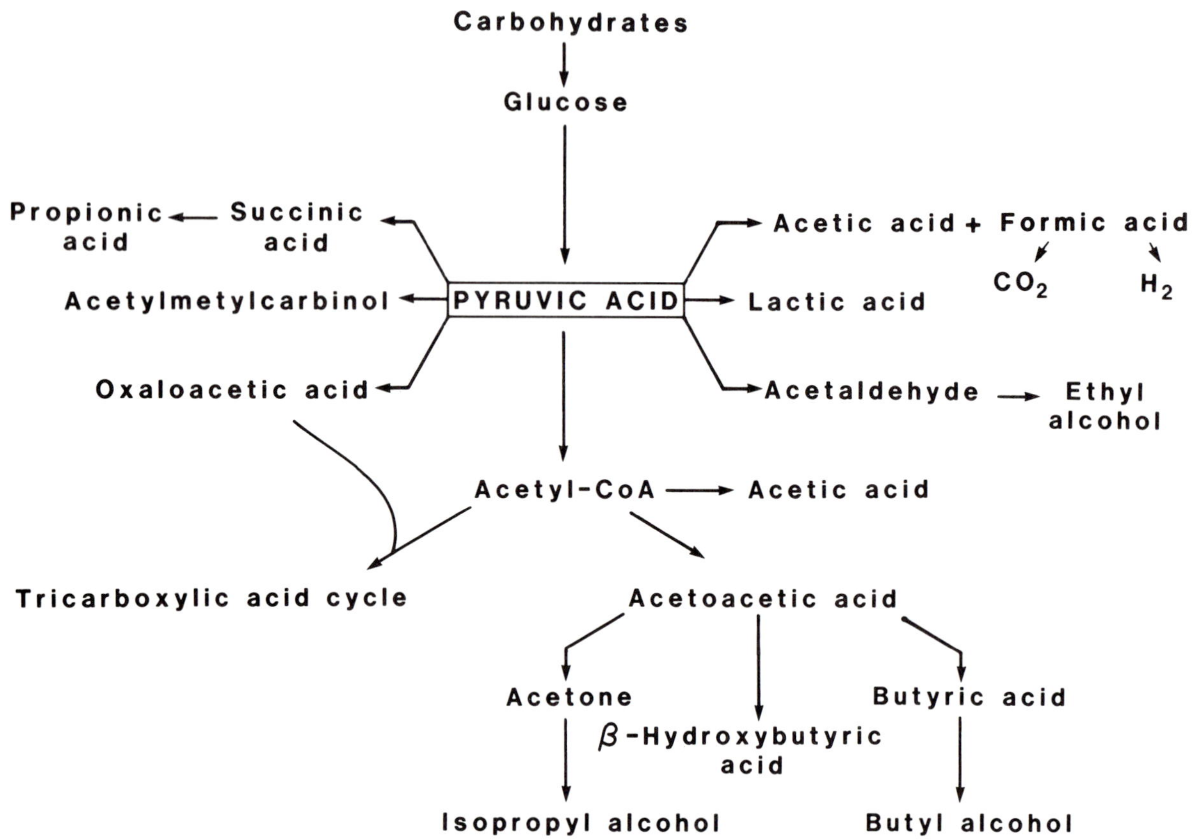

Figure 2–11. The metabolic fate of pyruvic acid.

aerobic bacteria, pyruvate is completely oxidized to CO_2 and water via the TCA cycle. Pyruvate is oxidized in the presence of a high energy cofactor, coenzyme A (CoA). Carbon dioxide is released, and the high energy intermediate acetyl-CoA is formed. Acetyl-CoA enters the TCA cycle and is completely oxidized to CO_2 and H_2O. In the process, energy is conserved by oxidative phosphorylation as electrons pass through a membrane-bound electron transport chain to oxygen. Both the TCA cycle and oxidative phosphorylation are described in greater detail later in this chapter.

Fermentative bacteria produce a variety of products from pyruvate by using it in oxidation-reduction reactions. Some bacteria, such as lactobacilli and streptococci, use pyruvate as a terminal electron acceptor, reducing it to lactic acid and other organic acids. Others produce ethyl alcohol and CO_2 via alcoholic fermentations. Still others produce butylene glycol, butyl alcohol, isopropyl alcohol, β-hydroxybutyrate, propionic acid, or acetic acid. These organisms all produce pyruvate by glycolysis. They differ in the pathways by which they use pyruvate as an electron acceptor to balance the overall oxidation-reduction equation for carbohydrate metabolism. Some anaerobes synthesize ATP by the anaerobic degradation of pyruvate, a reaction known as the phosphoroclastic cleavage.

$$\text{Pyruvate} + \text{coenzyme A} \rightarrow \text{acetyl-CoA} + CO_2 + H_2$$
$$\text{Acetyl-CoA} + P_i \rightarrow \text{acetyl-P} + \text{coenzyme A}$$
$$\text{Acetyl-P} + \text{ADP} \rightarrow \text{acetate} + \text{ATP}$$

Acetyl-P synthesis is a substrate level phosphorylation analogous to those in the glycolytic pathway. The hydrogen produced in the first step of this cleavage is dependent on the presence of an iron-containing protein called ferredoxin and a dehydrogenase, which combine electrons from pyruvate with protons to produce hydrogen gas.

$$\text{Pyruvate} \xrightarrow{\text{oxidation}} 2e^- \rightarrow \text{ferredoxin} \xrightarrow{\text{dehydrogenase}} 2H^+ \rightarrow H_2$$

Pyruvate also serves as a biosynthetic precursor of many essential cellular components. It can be carboxylated to form the carbon skeleton of TCA cycle intermediates and amino acids. It can be aminated to form the amino acid alanine. Its decarboxylation product acetyl-CoA is essential in fatty acid biosynthesis. It also can serve as a precursor for synthesis of capsules, intracellular storage materials, and cell walls.

Synthesis of some of these polymers is described later in this chapter.

Energy from Proteins and Amino Acids

Some bacteria can use proteins and polypeptides as energy sources. A general rule is that the substrate must be readily convertible to an intermediate that can either be metabolized via the TCA cycle or participate in substrate level phosphorylation. Like polysaccharides, these polymers must be degraded to subunits that can be transported into the cell before they can be used.

Aerobes that use amino acids as energy sources usually do so by deaminating them to organic acids that are metabolized via the TCA cycle. Deamination is accomplished in three ways. One is transamination, in which the amino group on the amino acid to be metabolized is transferred to a keto group on another molecule, thus producing a new amino acid and a keto acid that can enter the TCA cycle. A second alternative is dehydrogenation, an oxidation-reduction reaction usually involving NAD in which the amino acid is converted into a keto acid, with release of the amino group as ammonia. The final possibility is decarboxylation of the amino acid to an amine, with subsequent loss of the amine group and metabolism of the carbon skeleton.

Obligate anaerobes, particularly members of the genus *Clostridium*, ferment pairs of amino acids by the Stickland reaction. One amino acid serves as the electron donor, the other as the acceptor. The classic reaction involves alanine and glycine. Alanine is oxidatively deaminated to pyruvate, which is decarboxylated to acetyl-CoA and CO_2. The energy contained in acetyl-CoA is used to synthesize ATP from ADP and inorganic phosphate. NAD, the electron acceptor for the oxidative steps, is reoxidized by the reductive deamination of glycine to acetic acid. The net reaction is 1 mole of ATP synthesized for every 3 moles of amino acid consumed.

$$\text{Alanine} + 2\ \text{Glycine} + \text{ADP} + P_i \rightarrow 3\ \text{acetate} + 3\ NH_3 + CO_2 + \text{ATP}$$

The Stickland reaction is advantageous for anaerobes growing in high protein environments because energy can be obtained from most amino acids in this way.

A few anaerobes can ferment single amino acids, although this ability is not so widespread nor versatile as the Stickland reaction. A common substrate is glutamic acid that is ultimately metabolized to acetate and butyrate with pyruvate as an intermediate. ATP is produced during the conversion of pyruvate to butyrate.

Energy from Other Sources

Theoretically, all natural compounds can serve as energy sources for some genera or species of bacteria. Some of the more common substrates, other than carbohydrates and proteins, are fatty acids, fats, phospholipids, hydrocarbons, heterocyclic compounds, and single-carbon compounds.

Fatty acids are metabolized aerobically by a process called β-oxidation in which carbons are removed from the parent compound 2 at a time to form acetyl-CoA, which is further oxidized via the TCA cycle or the glyoxylate shunt. Electrons reduced during degradation are transferred first to flavin adenine dinucleotide (FAD) or NAD and then to the electron transport chain, where ATP is produced via oxidative phosphorylation.

Fats are composed of fatty acids esterified to a glycerol backbone. Phospholipids have a similar structure except that they also contain one polar nonfatty acid molecule, such as serine, choline, or inositol, esterified to one of the glycerol carbons. These complex molecules are metabolized by hydrolyzing the ester bonds and releasing the 3-carbon glycerol moiety from the side chains. Glycerol enters the glycolytic pathway, and the fatty acids are metabolized by β-oxidation.

Hydrocarbons are organic compounds that contain only carbon and hydrogen. They can occur as straight chains, branched chains, or aromatic rings. Their degradation is limited to relatively few bacteria and is a strictly aerobic process. The pathway is not understood completely, but the products are acetate subunits that are oxidized by the TCA cycle.

Some bacteria are able to oxidize heterocyclic compounds such as purines and pyrimidines. These organisms secrete nucleases that degrade nucleic acids into continuent bases that are transported into the cell and degraded. Purines are metabolized to ammonia and CO_2 via a pathway with urea as an intermediate. The pyrimidine pathway also yields ammonia and CO_2 but with alanine as an intermediate. The heterocyclic amino acids phenylalanine and tyrosine are metabolized via the homogentisic acid pathway to TCA cycle intermediates.

Terminal Oxidation

The final steps of substrate oxidation in aerobic bacteria are carried out by two pathways, the TCA, or Krebs, cycle and the electron transport system (ETS). These pathways ensure the complete oxidation of substrates to CO_2 and H_2O with maximum conservation of energy.

Tricarboxylic Acid Cycle. The TCA cycle is the primary pathway of pyruvate oxidation in aerobes. Much of the energy in substrates such as glucose is still locked in pyruvate. Further oxidation by the TCA cycle extracts much of this remaining energy. The energy can then be converted into ATP by the ETS. Pyruvate carbon enters the TCA cycle via acetyl-CoA, as shown in Fig 2–12. The TCA cycle releases protons and electrons that are captured by carriers such as NAD, NADP, and FAD and produces intermediates such as oxaloacetate, α-glutarate, and succinyl-CoA that are important in the synthesis of cellular constituents. Most anaerobic bacteria have a partial TCA cycle, so they can synthesize these biosynthetic precursors. The anaerobic pathway cannot oxidize pyruvate, however, because there is an enzyme missing, often that catalyzes the step between α-ketoglutarate and succinate.

Associated with the TCA cycle is an anaplerotic pathway called the glyoxalate shunt, or bypass (Fig 2–12). This pathway operates in bacteria growing on two carbon substrates such as acetate or on fatty acids that are converted to acetyl-CoA, and enter the TCA cycle without going through pyruvate. Bacteria using these substrates cannot synthesize oxaloacetate by carboxylating pyruvate or phosphenolpyruvate as do many organisms. Consequently, they would quickly run out of oxaloacetate if it were not for this pathway that results in the net conversion of 2 molecules of acetyl-CoA in this important intermediate.

Electron Transport System. The electron transport system carries out the final stage of respiration, in which the substrate is fully oxidized and the electrons released are transferred to a terminal acceptor, most commonly oxygen.

Bacterial ETS are complex structures of iron-containing enzymes and cofactors organized in rigid, lipid-containing matrices called electron transport particles associated with the cytoplasmic membrane. The ETS has three functions: (1) to accept electrons from a donor and transfer them to an acceptor, (2) to conserve energy released by this electron transfer as ATP, and (3) to create an electrochemical potential gradient between the inside and the outside of the cell that can be used to perform work.

Recall that electrons released during substrate oxidation are captured by acceptors such as NAD, NADP, and FAD. These molecules are cofactors that work in association with dehydrogenases. Electrons are transferred from them to the ETS, a series of membrane bound flavoprotein, cytochrome, and quinone carriers (Fig 2–13). The first carrier in most prokaryotic systems is a flavoprotein with either flavin adenine mononucleotide (FMN) or FAD as a prosthetic group. Flavoproteins accept both protons (hydrogen atoms) and electrons from NAD reduced during substrate oxidation and transfer them to quinones. Pro-

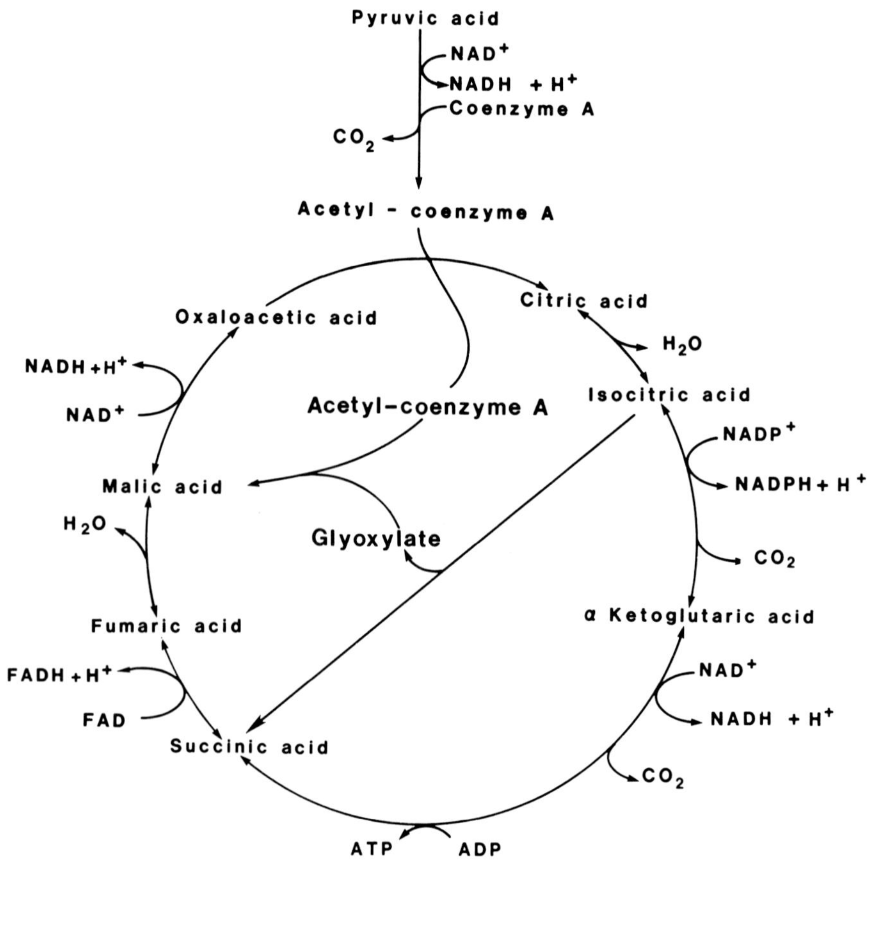

Figure 2–12. The tricarboxylic acid (TCA) cycle, including reactions of the glyoxylate shunt within the circle.

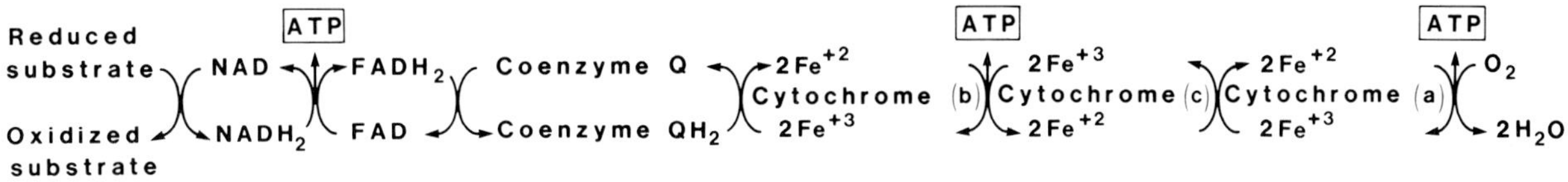

Figure 2–13. The electron transport system linking the dehydrogenation of an oxidizable substrate with the production of water from molecular oxygen. Concomitant transfer of electrons through the cytochrome pigments creates sufficient oxidation-reduction potential to generate ATP at three points.

tons are released into the environment from the quinones; electrons are transferred to membrane bound enzymes called cytochromes. These proteins, designated by letters, can undergo reversible oxidation and reduction through an atom of iron bound to a porphyrin prosthetic group in each molecule. Each cytochrome has its own standard oxidation-reduction potential expressed in volts. Electrons flow through this system from cytochromes with more negative potentials to those with more positive until they reach a terminal acceptor. In aerobic respiration, this acceptor is oxygen. Some bacteria can respire under anaerobic conditions using terminal electron acceptors such as nitrate, sulfate, or carbon dioxide, although not as much ATP is synthesized with these acceptors as with oxygen.

As a consequence of electron flow through the ETS, energy is released in a stepwise fashion and some of it is conserved in the high energy phosphate bonds of ATP. This process is called oxidative phosphorylation. The mechanism by which this occurs is unknown but many accept a theory called the chemiosmostic hypothesis proposed by Mitchell in 1961, which is based on the impermeability of the cytoplasmic membrane to either protons or electrons. It postulates that energy generating systems exist as loops within the prokaryotic cytoplasmic membrane. Flavoproteins are located at the inner surface and accept electrons and protons generated during substrate oxidation from NAD. Protons are extruded from the cell into the environment while the electrons are returned to the inner membrane surface. These electrons, with additional protons from substrate oxidation, are transferred to quinones, which also extrude protons from the cell. The electrons enter the cytochrome chain where they eventually are used to reduce the terminal acceptor. Proton extrusion creates an electrochemical gradient across the cytoplasmic membrane with the outside positive and the inside negative. This gradient is called the proton motive force and can be used to synthesize ATP, rotate flagella, and, as described previously, transport nutrients. ATP synthesis occurs as external protons reenter the cell through a multiprotein enzyme channel termed ATPase. As they flow into the cell, protons exhibit a drop in potential free energy that is captured by the ATPase and used to phosphorylate ADP to ATP. It is likewise possible for the enzyme to reverse the reaction and use ATP, synthesized by substrate level phosphorylation for example, to create a proton gradient that can be used for other kinds of work.

The ETS and oxidative phosphorylation make aerobes much more efficient than anaerobes at extracting energy from their environment. The net result is the complete oxidation of glucose to CO_2 and H_2O with the production of 36 molecules of ATP compared to a net gain of only 2 molecules under anaerobic conditions. Aerobes also are more versatile than anaerobes in use of substrates, since the terminal oxidation pathway is the same for all substrates. Anaerobes, on the other hand, must have the enzymatic machinery for substrate level phosphorylation of each substrate.

MACROMOLECULAR BIOSYNTHESIS

Energy produced by catabolism is used in several ways. Even the most efficient organism loses much of the energy available from a substrate as heat. Much of this loss is due to metabolic activity itself. The formation of an ester or amide bond, for example, requires about 3000 cal (12,600 J), but the organism expends 12,000 cal (50,400 J) to synthesize one. Chemical energy also is transformed into mechanical energy by flagella, thus providing a means of locomotion. The most common use of energy, however, is for bacterial growth—the uptake of nutrients and the synthesis of cellular constituents. Implied in this is maintenance of the physical integrity of the cell through the synthesis of structural and informational macromolecules.

Most cell structures are composed of four macromolecular classes: nucleic acids, proteins, polysaccharides, and complex lipids. Each are polymers of lower molecular weight precursors obtained from the environment or from catabolic or biosynthetic pathways. There are about 70 precursor molecules required to synthesize common macromolecules. Cells also require coenzymes and electron carriers that play catalytic roles. There are, in sum, about 150 molecules required to make and maintain a cell. All of these are derived by chemoheterotrophs either from the environment or as a result of cellular metabolism. Precursors, such as sugar phosphates, pyruvate, acetate, oxaloacetate, succinate, and α-ketoglutarate, are the starting points of biosynthesis from which cellular material is produced.

There are three principles that govern biosynthetic reactions. First, biosynthetic pathways are not simply the reverse of catabolic pathways. Even though many of the enzymes and intermediates may be similar, especially in such amphibolic pathways as glycolysis or the TCA cycle, there is usually at least one reaction in each direction that is unique. Second, ATP-yielding pathways are coupled with ATP-using or biosynthetic pathways so that the net reaction is exergonic. It is irreversible in the biosynthetic direction. Finally, biosynthesis and catabolism are independently regulated.

Biopolymer synthesis involves joining subunits via dehydration reactions. In an aqueous environment, dehydration is thermodynamically unfavorable. Breakdown via hydrolysis proceeds at a much faster rate than synthesis by dehydration. Therefore, synthesis must be coupled with ATP expenditure to drive the reaction in the proper direction. A subunit or precursor is chemically activated via ATP, which allows its attachment first to a carrier and then to a growing polymer chain. Following is a brief description of the synthesis of some important macromolecules.

Cell Wall Peptidoglycan Biosynthesis

Synthesis of the rigid backbone of bacterial cell walls occurs both in the cytoplasm and on the outside of the cell membrane (Fig 2–14). The subunits, N-acetylglucosamine (NAG) and N-acetylmuramic acid (NAM), are synthesized in the cytoplasm as esters of uridine diphosphate (UDP). NAM is then transferred from UDP to a 55-carbon isoprenoid lipid called bactoprenol that is located in the cytoplasmic membrane. NAG is added to complete the peptidoglycan subunit, which is then transported across the membrane and polymerized into the growing peptidoglycan polymer of the cell wall by enzymes associated with the outer membrane surface.

Lipopolysaccharide Synthesis

The lipopolysaccharide of gram-negative bacterial cell envelopes consists of a complex lipid called lipid A attached to a core polysaccharide containing several sugars including 2-keto-3-deoxyoctonate (KDO), which is unique to this molecule (Fig 2–15). Protruding from the lipid–sugar complex are polysaccharide strands called O-specific chains (O antigens) that confer strain-specific antigenic properties on some gram-negative cells. The complete molecule is called endotoxin. This molecule can cause severe, often life-threatening in-

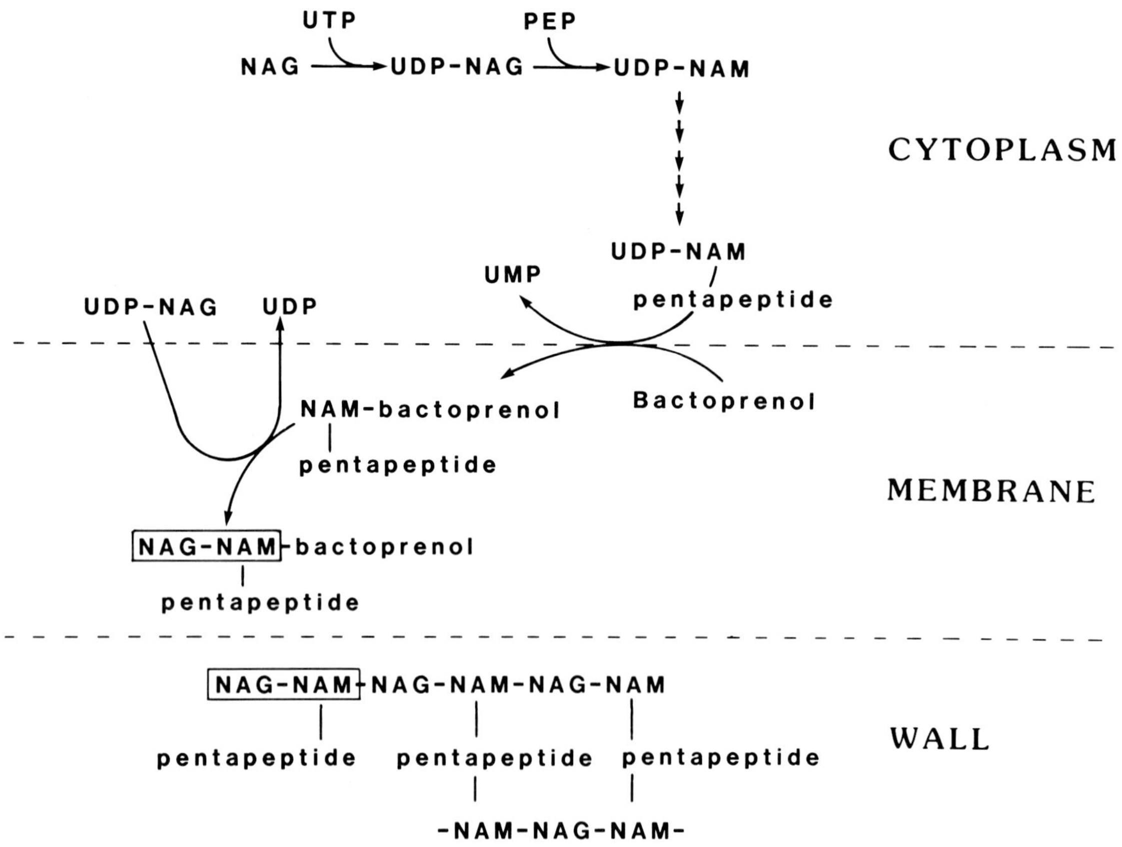

Figure 2–14. Biosynthesis of bacterial cell wall peptidoglycan.

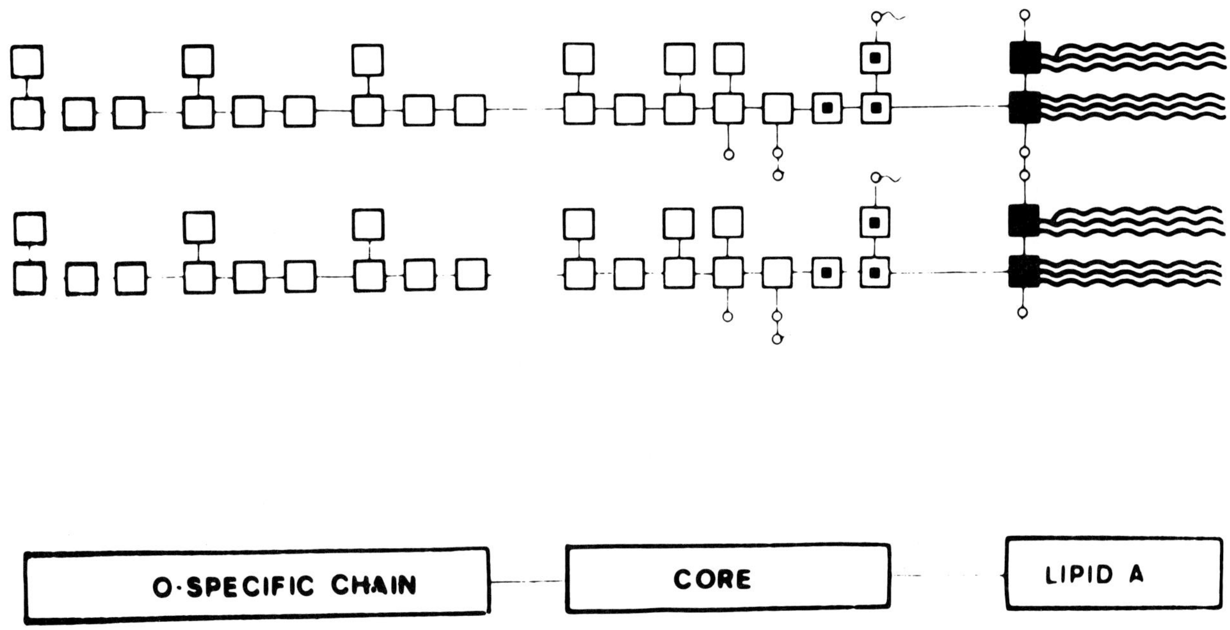

Figure 2–15. Schematic representation of a *Salmonella* lipopolysaccharide. The symbols represent monosaccharides (□), phosphate (○), phosphoethanolamine (○~), and fatty acids (heavy wavy lines). *(From Rietschel ET, Galanos C, Luderitz O. In: Schlessinger D, ed.* Microbiology—1975. *Washington, DC: American Society for Microbiology; 1975.)*

flammation in infected hosts. Synthesis of LPS is not well understood. It has been determined, however, that synthesis of the O-specific polysaccharides is similar to that of peptidoglycans.

Polysaccharide Biosynthesis

Most polysaccharide biosynthesis requires a primer, a short segment of the polymer being synthesized, to serve as acceptor for monomers that have been activated by coupling to UDP. Synthesis of capsular or cell wall polysaccharides takes place in the cell surface after monomers are transported across the membrane via bactoprenol.

Intracellular polysaccharides, such as glycogen, a (14) glucose polymer, are synthesized by addition of UDP-glucose to the growing chain. Many bacteria contain branching enzymes that cleave fragments from the end of the linear (1 → 4) chain and insert them at other places on the molecule by (1 → 6) bonds. The result is synthesis of polysaccharides with varying degrees of branching characteristic of the bacterium being examined. Intracellular polysaccharides are used as sources of carbon and energy during times of nutritional stress. They give plaque bacteria, for example, the substrates necessary to continue producing organic acids in the absence of dietary carbohydrates, thus exposing teeth to prolonged exposure to pH levels low enough to cause enamel dissolution.

Oral micoorganisms have been used widely to study extracellular polysaccharide biosynthesis. *Streptoccus mutans,* for example, produces two classes of extracellular polysaccharides from sucrose, glucans (glucose homopolymers) and fructans (fructose homopolymers). These polymers are synthesized by extracellular or cell-associated glucosyltransferases or fructosyltransferases, respectively. Their synthesis is dependent on the presence of sucrose, and the energy needed to add a monomer to the growing polysaccharide chain comes not from UDP but from hydrolysis of the sucrose glycosidic bond. One type of glucan produced by *S. mutans* is dextran, a water-soluble polymer with most of the glucose units linked by (1 → 6) bonds. Another type called mutan is water insoluble and contains more (1 → 3) linkages. This glucan is an important structural element in the dental plaque matrix. Levan, a common type of fructan, is produced from sucrose by the oral bacteria *S. mutans, S. sanguis, S. salivarius,* and *Actinomyces viscosus.*

Other types of polysaccharides also are produced by oral bacteria. These include cell wall constituents and heteropolysaccharides containing hexosamines, uronic acids, and other hexoses that are synthesized by actinomycetes and lactobacilli. Further details on the role of polysaccharides in oral disease can be found in Chapter 33.

DNA and Protein Synthesis

A detailed explanation of bacterial deoxyribonucleic acid (DNA) and protein synthesis is beyond the scope of this chapter. These remarks are intended to be an overview of the relationship between DNA and protein synthesis.

A bacterium can synthesize several thousand

proteins with an average length of 200 amino acids. The sequence of these amino acids and thus the functional significance of the proteins are genetically predetermined. The information necessary to direct the synthesis of all cellular components is passed from one generation to another by the nucleotide base pair sequence in DNA. As described in Chapter 1, bacterial DNA is contained in a membrane-associated circular chromosome that is precisely replicated so succeeding generations receive exact copies of parental DNA. Information contained in the DNA directs the amino acid sequence in proteins by transcription and translation.

METABOLIC REGULATION

For efficient bacterial growth and reproduction, all of the metabolic pathways leading to energy production and biosynthesis must be regulated carefully. Such regulation is achieved by controlling either the synthesis or activity of enzymes involved in metabolic pathways. Both mechanisms involve the interaction of small molecular weight compounds, called effectors, with either enzymatic or regulatory allosteric proteins. These interactions cause either a change in activity of preformed enzymes or a change in the amount of enzyme synthesized by the cell.

Regulation of Enzyme Activity

To achieve maximum metabolic efficiency, a bacterium must be able to balance the rate of energy and precursor synthesis with cellular needs. One way to achieve this balance is by feedback inhibition of an allosteric enzyme by an endproduct of the pathway in which it participates. An allosteric enzyme is one whose activity is changed by the binding of a small molecular weight molecule (in this case, an endproduct) to a specific site on the enzyme.

There are two kinds of binding sites on allosteric enzymes: one or more active sites where the substrate binds and an allosteric site where the inhibitor (negative effector) binds. Binding of the inhibitor causes a change in shape at the active site that decreases its substrate affinity. Because the substrate no longer binds as well to the enzyme, that reaction and ultimately the entire pathway slow down. As the endproduct concentration falls due to normal turnover or its use in biosynthesis, the amount bound to the allosteric enzyme decreases, enzyme activity increases, and the pathway speeds up again. Allosteric enzymes are very common in both catabolic and anabolic pathways, often at branchpoints or at the beginning of a pathway. They enable to bacterium to respond quickly to environmental conditions because there is no change in the amount of the enzyme, just in its activity. The Embden-Meyerhof-Parnas pathway contains two allosteric enzymes, phosphofructokinase (PKF) and pyruvate kinase (PK), that are important regulatory points for hexose metabolism (Fig 2–8). Both enzymes can be inhibited or activated by several small molecules. PFK, which catalyzes the phosphorylation of fructose 6-phosphate to fructose 1,6-diphosphate, is inhibited by ATP, a primary product of glycolysis. Conversely, it is activated by ADP and frucose 6-phosphate. Likewise, the affinity of PK for its substrate, phosphoenolpyruvate, is reduced at high ATP concentrations. PK is activated by AMP and fructose 1,6-diphosphate. Therefore, whenever cellular ATP levels are adequate, the carbon flow through this central, energy-yielding, catabolic pathway is reduced by the decreased activity of PFK or PK. Carbon can be diverted to other uses. As ATP is consumed, with the consequent accumulation of ADP and AMP as well as intermediates of the EMP, the affinity of PFK and PK for their substrates increases, enabling carbon to begin flowing again through this pathway, thus producing more energy and more metabolic intermediates.

Regulation of Enzyme Synthesis

Allosterism is probably sufficient to ensure balanced synthesis of precursors for cellular constituents. But if the product of a particular pathway is not needed, all of the carbon and energy used to synthesize the enzymes and cofactors of the pathway are wasted. Therefore, in addition to allosteric enzymes, bacteria contain mechanisms that regulate the enzymatic composition of the cell. These mechanisms control, at the gene level, the kinds and amounts of enzymes synthesized.

A bacterial cell is genetically capable of synthesizing many more enzymes than can be found in it at any particular time. The enzymatic complement is greatly influenced by the environment. If a precursor is available preformed, the enzymes necessary for its biosynthesis are not found in the cell. For example, if bacteria are growing in an artificial medium containing arginine, enzymes in the arginine biosynthetic pathway are not synthesized. Exogenous arginine represses synthesis of the enzymes required for arginine biosynthesis. Another example of this type of regulation is catabolite repression, which occurs in cells growing in an environment containing two or more energy sources that can be used at different rates. Bacteria growing in a medium containing glucose and lactose, for example, will preferentially use glucose. During glucose metabolism, none of the enzymes necessary to use lactose are synthesized. Only as glucose is depleted are β-galactosidase and galactose permease synthesized, with consequent lactose metabolism. Glucose specifically represses synthesis of enzymes necessary to metabolize lactose. This effect is not limited to glucose but applies to all situations in which substrates are available that differ in their ease of use. Repression is a common, specific method of bacterial metabolic regulation affecting enzymes involved in carbohydrate catabolism and in amino acid, purine, and pyrimidine synthesis.

Enzyme induction is a complement to repression. Only in the presence of the substrate (inducer) are the enzymes required for its metabolism synthesized. Inducible enzymes often are involved in the catabolism of carbohydrates and other carbon and energy sources. β-Galactosidase, which catalyzes the first step in lactose metabolism, is an example of an inducible enzyme. It cannot be detected in cells growing without lactose, but as soon as lactose is added to the medium, levels begin to rise. Remember, however, that catabolite repression also exerts control over this enzyme, so that it is not synthesized even in the presence of lactose as long as a more easily metabolized carbon and energy source, such as glucose, is available.

Both inducers and repressors exert their effects on protein synthesis at the level of mRNA transcription from the DNA template (Fig 2–16). They do so indirectly by combining with specific proteins that affect mRNA synthesis. Repressors such as arginine combine with allosteric repressor proteins that are then able to attach to the operator region of a structural gene and block mRNA synthesis. Consequently, synthesis of the protein specified by that gene region is prevented. In enzyme induction, the repressor protein is able to bind the operator gene only in the absence of the inducer. An inducer, such as lactose, binds to the repressor protein, inactivating it and permitting the transcription of the gene segment and subsequent synthesis of enzyme. A single inducer or repressor molecule often is able to control enzymes in an entire pathway because the genetic information necessary for their synthesis is under the control of a single operator gene.

Induction and repression give certain evolutionary advantages to bacteria. The energy and carbon conserved by these regulatory mechanisms can be diverted to synthesis of essential macromolecules, thus increasing efficiency and giving bacteria with such controls a competitive advantage over those without them. Induction and repression of enzymes can be regarded as coarse metabolic control, which, together with fine tuning of carbon and energy flow by feedback inhibition of enzyme activity, enables bacteria to channel their nutritional resources in the direction that leads to most efficient growth.

Regulation of DNA and RNA Synthesis

Regulation of DNA replication is essential so that each daughter cell receives a full genetic complement.

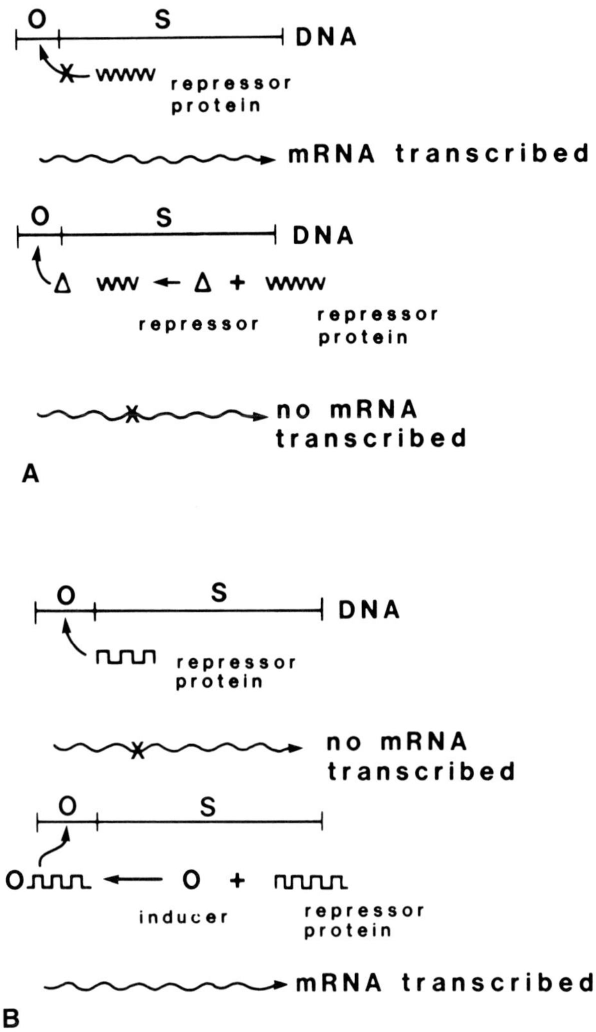

Figure 2–16. The role of repressors in enzyme repression and induction. **A.** Repression. **B.** Induction.

It is very closely integrated with cell division. For example, if DNA synthesis is inhibited, the cell grows and elongates but does not divide. Conversely, the segregation of DNA into daughter cells is a consequence of cell growth. Completion of DNA replication initiates a series of metabolic events resulting in segregation of daughter strands and, ultimately, cell division. The DNA copies, which are attached to the plasma membrane at adjacent sites, separate due to membrane growth. A transverse septum forms between the two DNA strands, causing their segregation into two still fused daughter cells.

Regulation of RNA synthesis is not fully understood, but evidence suggests that it is closely associated with protein synthesis. The binding of protein repressors to the operator regions of genes, with the consequent inhibition of mRNA synthesis, has been described. Little is known about the regulation of rRNA and tRNA synthesis except that intracytoplasmic concentrations of these compounds vary with environmental conditions and that the ratios of the two remain constant. There also appears to be a relationship with protein synthesis. As protein synthesis decreases so does that of rRNA and tRNA. In fact, evidence has been presented that continued synthesis of RNA in the absence of protein synthesis can be harmful to the cell.

ORAL ASPECTS

To colonize a particular site on the human body, bacteria must be able to adsorb to the surface and then use the available physical and chemical conditions to grow and reproduce. Oral bacteria, which are no exception, have the surface properties necessary to adhere to oral tissue, the transport mechanisms necessary to extract nutrients from the oral environment, and the metabolic pathways that ensure their survival in the mouth. Often, bacteria that have colonized a site coexist with the host without causing disease. Frequently, however, environmental changes or reduced host defenses allow these organisms to grow unchecked, and infectious disease results.

Oral bacteria such as *S. mutans* synthesize extracellular polysaccharides from dietary carbohydrates. These polymers serve as the intercellular matrix of dental plaque and facilitate retention of not only the organisms that produce them but a variety of microbes that become entrapped during synthesis. Many oral bacteria also synthesize intracellular storage polymers that are used as carbon and energy sources during times of nutritional stress or after the organisms become imbedded in the plaque matrix and are cut off from dietary carbohydrates in saliva as nutritional sources. The result is that oral bacteria can continue to grow and produce metabolic endproducts potentially toxic to host tissues under a variety of oral environmental conditions.

The endproducts of the pathways described in this chapter include a spectrum of compounds that can cause disease if they are not neutralized or inactivated by host defenses. Paramount among these, especially with respect to dental caries, are organic acid endproducts of carbohydrate metabolism. These acids rapidly demineralize tooth enamel, particularly if produced within the plaque matrix away from the diluting and neutralizing effects of saliva. Oral soft tissues also are susceptible to products of oral bacteria. Enzymes such as hyaluronidase and collagenase, which are synthesized and secreted by members of the periodontal microflora, contribute to the initiation and progression of periodontal disease by reducing the integrity of gingival tissues and by inducing hypersensitivities. These are but two examples of how the metabolic capabilities of oral microbes can predispose host tissues to disease if the delicate balance between the insult provided by microbial endproducts and oral host defenses is upset.

SUGGESTED READINGS

Anraku Y. Bacterial electron transport chains. *Annu Rev Biochem.* 1988;57:101–132.

Battley EH. *Energetics of Microbial Growth.* New York: Wiley, 1987.

Beaman L, Beaman BL. The role of oxygen and its derivatives in microbial pathogenesis and host defense. *Annu Rev Microbiol.* 1984;38:27–48.

Delwiche EA, Peska JJ, Tortorello ML. The Veillonellae: Gram-negative cocci with a unique physiology. *Annu Rev Microbiol.* 1985;39:175–193.

Gottschalk G. *Bacterial Metabolism,* 2nd ed. New York: Springer-Verlag; 1986.

Ingraham JL. Naale O, Neidhardt FC. *Growth of the Bacterial Cell.* Sunderland: Sinauer; 1983.

Kreig NR, Hoffman PS. Microaerophily and oxygen toxicity. *Am Rev Microbiol.* 1986;40:107–130.

Loesche WJ. Role of *Streptococcus mutans* in human dental decay. *Microbiol Rev.* 1986;50:353–380.

Mayrand D, Holt SC. Biology of asachorolytic black-pigmented *Bacteroides* species. *Microbiol Rev.* 1988;52:134–152.

Moat AG, Foster JW. *Microbial Physiology,* 2nd ed. New York: Wiley; 1988.

Neidhardt FC, ed. *Escherichia coli and Salmonella typhimurium: Cellular and Molecular Biology.* Washington: American Society for Microbiology; 1987.

Newbrun E. *Cariology,* 3rd ed. Chicago: Quintessence Publishing Co; 1989.

Newman MG, Nisengard R, eds. *Oral Microbiology and Immunology.* Philadelphia: WB Saunders Co; 1988.

Poolman B, Driessen AJM, Konings WN. Regulation of solute transport in streptococci by external and internal pH values. *Microbiol Rev.* 1987;51:498–508.

Randall LL, Hardy SJS. Export of protein in bacteria. *Microbiol Rev.* 1984;48:290–298.

Rosen BP. Recent advances in bacterial ion transport. *Annu Rev Microbiol.* 1986;40:263–286.

Stanier RY, Ingraham JL, Wheelis ML, Painter PR. *The Microbial World,* 5th ed. Englewood Cliffs, NJ: Prentice-Hall; 1986.

Sutherland IW. Biosynthesis of microbial exopolysaccharides. *Adv Microbiol Physiol.* 1982;23:80–142.

CHAPTER 3

Bacterial Genetics

John A. Mayo

INTRODUCTION

COMPOSITION STRUCTURE, FUNCTION, AND REPLICATION OF DNA

EXPRESSION OF INFORMATION STORED IN DNA

CONTROL OF EXPRESSION OF GENETIC INFORMATION
- **Mechanism of Transcriptional Control**
- **Operons**
- **Global Regulatory Networks**

GENETICS OF BACTERIA
- **Mutation**
- **Recombination**
- **Genetic Exchange**

ORAL ASPECTS

SUGGESTED READINGS

INTRODUCTION

Genetics deals with the characteristics of living things, the mechanisms controlling the expression of those characteristics, and the manner in which those characteristics are transmitted to following generations. All properties of bacteria, including those properties that cause disease, are specified by information carried in bacterial DNA. Thus, DNA directs all bacterial processes and controls all properties of bacteria. However, this control is mediated by enzymes and other proteins produced when information in DNA is expressed. It is therefore necessary to understand how genetic information is stored in DNA and how information stored in DNA is expressed in proteins that control and carry out cellular processes, how genetic information is exchanged among bacterial cells, how all of these processes determine the ability of pathogenic bacteria to cause disease, and how genetics determines the resistance of bacteria to antibiotics.

The genetically determined properties of pathogenic bacteria can have a major impact on the practice of dentistry and medicine. For instance, a dental patient might suffer from an acute oral infection that does not respond to the antibiotic the dentist usually prescribes for such cases. One of the greatest hazards of hospitalization may not be the disease that put the patient in the hospital, but acquisition while in the hospital of an infection with an antibiotic-resistant bacterium. These problems all are related to bacterial genetics, as are other aspects of bacterial pathogenicity. Thus, it has become important for dentists to have an understanding of the fundamentals of bacterial genetics.

COMPOSITION, STRUCTURE, FUNCTION, AND REPLICATION OF DNA

DNA is the cellular constituent that contains information for controlling activities of a cell during the present generation and for specifying the inheritance of the next generation; that is, DNA is the genetic material. DNA consists of deoxyribose, phosphate, the purines adenine and guanine, and the pyrimidines thymine and cytosine. The backbone of DNA is made of deoxyribose and phosphate. The ribose molecules are joined by 3′ −5′ phosphodiester linkages. The purines and pyrimidines also are attached to deoxyribose, one purine or pyrimidine to each deoxyribose, by means of an N-glycosidic linkage from C-1 of the deoxyribose to an N of the purine in pyrimidine. The combination of deoxyribose, phosphate, and purine or pyrimidine is a nucleotide, and a DNA chain is a polymer of nucleotide subunits. Each DNA molecule consists of two such chains coiled around each other so that the deoxyribose and phosphate are on the outside and the purines and pyrimidines are on the inside. The two strands are of opposite polarity; that is, one runs 3′ → 5′, and the other runs 5′ → 3′. The coiling is helical; that is, it resembles the threads on a screw. Thus, DNA is a double helix (Fig 3–1). The structure of the double helix is maintained by hydrogen bonds between the purine and pyrimidine bases of the opposing strands, (Fig 3–2). Hydrogen bonding between bases follows strict base pairing rules, and base pairing is specific—an adenine of one strand with a thymine of the opposing strand, and similarly guanine with cytosine. DNA structure and function are intimately related.

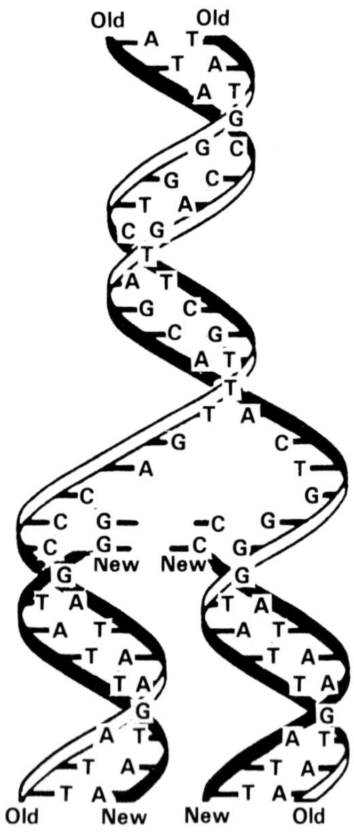

Figure 3–1. Structure and replication of DNA. The outer ribbons represent a backbone of alternating deoxyribose and phosphate, and the purine and pyrimidine bases are oriented to the inside. The two strands are coiled to make a double helix. When this molecule replicates, the two old strands separate, and each serves as template for formation of a new strand. Because the replication products each contain one old and one new strand, DNA replication is said to be semiconservative.

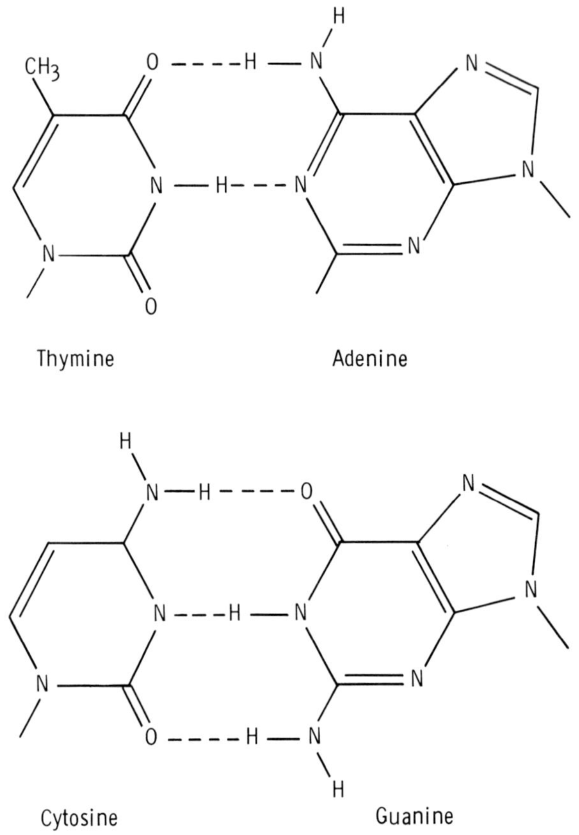

Figure 3–2. Pairing of DNA bases. Base pairing is specific, and base pairs are maintained by hydrogen bonding.

Genetic information is encoded in the sequence of bases along a DNA strand. A gene is such a sequence coding for a particular function or protein. For example, a gene on the DNA of the bacterium *Escherichia coli* codes for the enzyme *B*-galactosidase, which *E. coli* needs in order to metabolize the sugar lactose.

When DNA replicates, the strands separate, and each strand serves as the template for synthesis of a new opposite strand. DNA replication thus is semiconservative, since each new double helix is composed of one old and one new strand. This synthesis is mediated by a number of proteins, including the enzyme DNA polymerase, which uses the base-pairing rules to ensure that the proper bases are included in the new strand. A consequence of the double helical structure of DNA is a mechanism of replication that provides two identical copies of genetic information to be passed to the next generation of cells.

EXPRESSION OF INFORMATION STORED IN DNA

The information contained in the sequence of purine and pyrimidine bases in DNA is used to carry out and control cellular activities. This function of DNA is mediated by a second type of nucleic acid, ribonucleic acid or RNA. RNA differs from DNA in that it is single stranded, contains ribonucleotides rather than deoxyribonucleotides, and consequently uridine in place of thymidine. There are three classes of RNA, all of which are involved in expression of the information stored in DNA. They are messenger RNA (mRNA), which codes for enzymes and other proteins, ribosomal RNA (rRNA), a structural component of ribosomes, and transfer RNA (tRNA), which is used in the transfer of amino acids to growing polypeptides during protein synthesis. The three types of RNA are transcribed from DNA.

Transcription is the process in which information contained in DNA is copied to make RNA containing the same information (Fig 3–3). Transcription is mediated by RNA polymerase, which copies the information from one of the strands of DNA, using the same base-pairing rules as DNA with one exception. Because RNA contains uracil rather than thymine, uracil in RNA is specified by adenine in DNA. The three types of RNA are transcribed from DNA. Transcription of DNA sequences coding for enzymes and other proteins produces mRNA. rRNA is a structural component of ribosomes, and tRNA is used in the transfer of amino acids to growing polypeptides during protein synthesis.

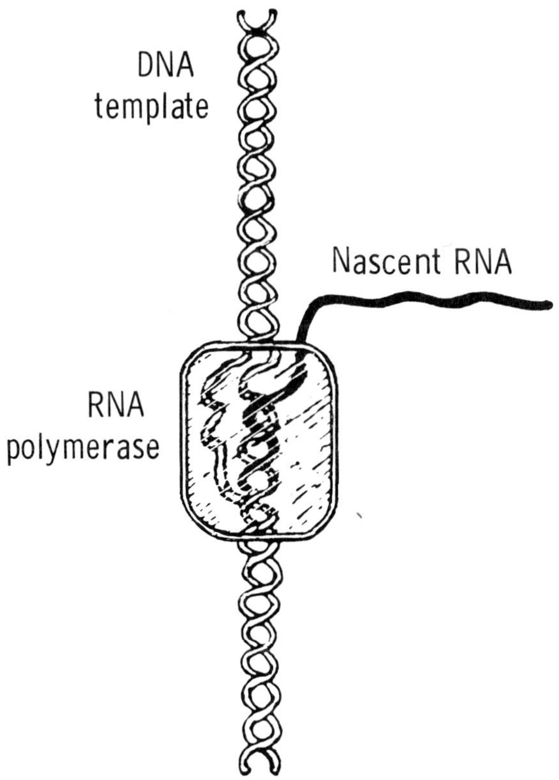

Figure 3–3. Transcription. The information encoded in the two DNA strands can be considered "sense" and "antisense." RNA polymerase copies the sense strand, and the nascent or newly synthesized molecule may be either messenger, ribosomal, or transfer RNA.

The final step in the expression of information stored in DNA is the translation of that information from the sequence of adenines, guanines, cytosines, and uracils of mRNA to the sequence of amino acids in proteins (Fig 3–4). The amino acid sequence of a protein is determined by the base sequence of an mRNA. The mRNA sequence is subdivided into units called codons, and each codon specifies one amino acid. A codon uses a sequence of three bases to code for one amino acid; for example, UUU codes for phenylalanine. Since there are four bases in mRNA and each codon uses three bases, there are 64 possible codons, more than enough to code for the 20 amino acids used in proteins and to serve as signals for terminating translation (Table 3–1).

Protein synthesis requires amino acids, tRNA, ATP, and ribosomes, in addition to mRNA. Ribosomes are composed of both rRNA and proteins. The ribosomal proteins catalyze the various reactions involved in formation of new peptide bonds during protein synthesis. Ribosomes function in protein synthesis by moving along mRNA codon by codon as amino acids are added to the growing peptide. However, amino acids are not added directly to proteins. Instead, each amino acid is activated with ATP, and the activated amino acid is attached to tRNA to make an aminoacyl-tRNA. The energy of the ATP is conserved in the process. Specific amino acids are joined to corresponding tRNAs; for example, alanine is attached to tRNA specific for alanine. Insertion of the proper amino acid is assured by the base-pairing rules. Each tRNA has a sequence of three bases, called an anticodon, that is specific for the particular amino acid and that recognizes the codon specifying that amino acid. Thus, addition of an amino acid at the proper place in a new protein is assured by basepairing. Through codon-anticodon interaction, an aminoacyl-tRNA is put at the proper place on a ribosome so that the amino acid can be added to the growing polypeptide chain. The ATP energy that was conserved in aminoacyl-tRNA provides the energy for peptide bond formation. When the ribosome reaches the end of the genetic message, a termination codon signals the ribosome to fall off the mRNA, releasing the new protein molecule.

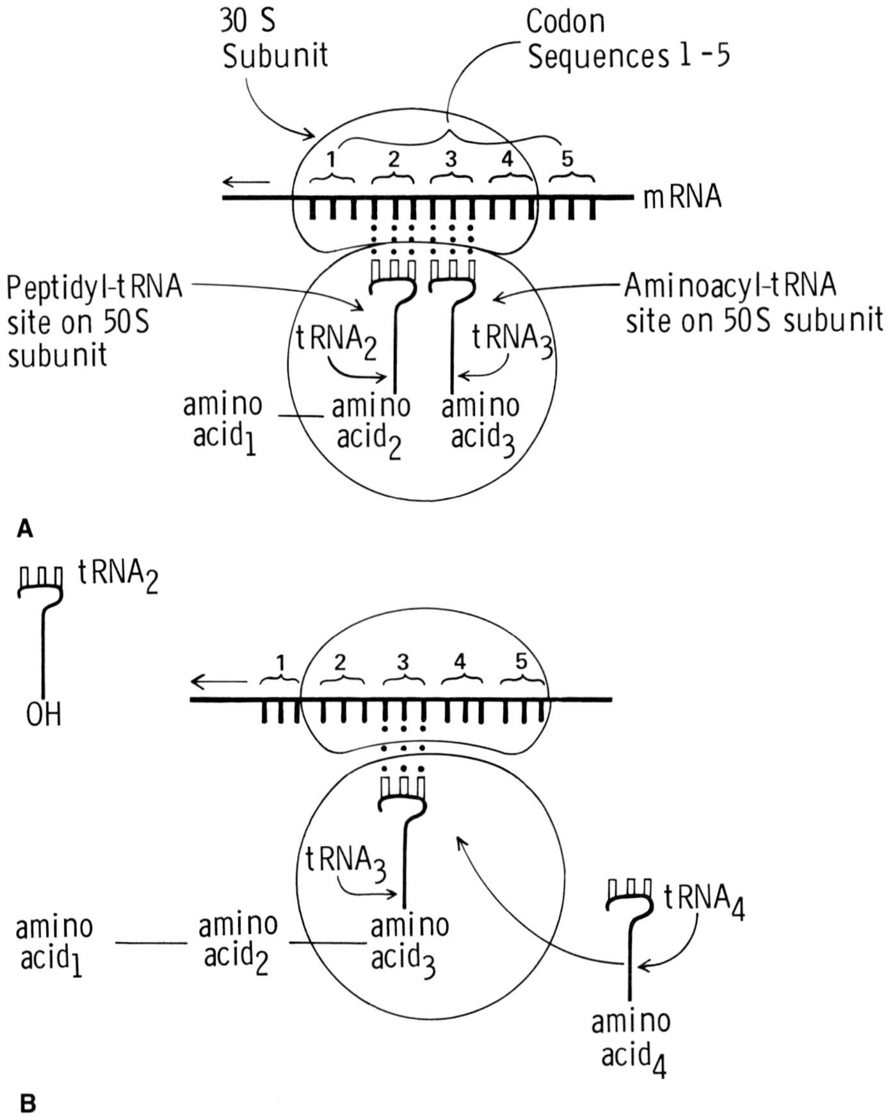

Figure 3–4. Translation. The messenger RNA is bound to the 30S ribosomal subunit, and five codons are indicated on the mRNA. Each codon can interact with an anticodon of a specific transfer RNA, which brings a particular amino acid to the growing polypeptide chain. **A.** The growing polypeptide and tRNA2 occupy the peptidyl site on the 50S ribosomal subunit. A third amino acid has been brought in on its tRNA and occupies the aminoacyl site. **B.** A new peptide bond is formed between amino acids 2 and 3, while tRNA2 is expelled and tRNA3 moves to the peptidyl site. Aminoacyl tRNA4 is ready to continue the process.

CONTROL OF EXPRESSION OF GENETIC INFORMATION

The bacterial DNA molecule has within it considerably more information than may be required at any one moment in the cell's lifetime. Cellular economy and need for rapid response to changes in the bacterium's environment dictate that expression of genetic information be controlled, for example, the genetic information that specifies the enzymes of lactose catabolism need not be expressed when bacterial cells are growing in medium without lactose, and expression of information coding for enzymes of histidine biosynthesis is not required when histidine is supplied. This control is carried out at the level of transcription.

Transcription of a gene may be constitutive, inducible, or repressible. Genes that are constitutive are transcribed all the time, and the products of these genes, therefore, are present all the time. For instance, genes encoding the enzymes of glycolysis are constitutive. Inducible genes are associated with catabolism, and in nature, their expression is induced by the substrate of the catabolic pathway. An example of an inducible system is that for lactose catabolism in *E. coli.* Galactoside permease and β-galactosidase are made when lactose is present in the growth medium but not in its absence. Repressible genes are associated with biosynthetic pathways, the end product of which turns off the transcription of the genes of that pathway. For instance, *E. coli* can synthesize amino acids such as histidine, and will do so if histidine is not supplied in the growth medium. However, if histidine is added to the medium, further transcription of the genes of the histidine pathway is repressed.

Mechanism of Transcriptional Control

The principles of transcriptional control will be illustrated by examining the control of lactose catabolism, and then those principles will be applied to several other systems.

TABLE 3–1. THE GENETIC CODE. CODONS SPECIFYING THE AMINO ACIDS ARE SHOWN, AND CODONS SIGNIFYING THE END OF THE GENETIC MESSAGE AND TERMINATION OF TRANSLATION ARE INDICATED BY TERM.

Codon	Amino acid	Codon	Amino acid	Codon	Amino acid	Codon	Amino acid
UUU	Phe	UCU	Ser	UAU	Tyr	UGU	Cys
UUC	Phe	UCC	Ser	UAC	Tyr	UGC	Cys
UUA	Leu	UCA	Ser	UAA	Term	UGA	Term
UUG	Leu	UCG	Ser	UAG	Term	UGG	Trp
CUU	Leu	CCU	Pro	CAU	His	CGU	Arg
CUC	Leu	CCC	Pro	CAC	His	CGC	Arg
CUA	Leu	CCA	Pro	CAA	Gln	CGA	Arg
CUG	Leu	CCG	Pro	CAG	Gln	CGG	Arg
AUU	Ile	ACU	Thr	AAU	Asn	AGU	Ser
AUC	Ile	ACC	Thr	AAC	Asn	AGC	Ser
AUA	Ile	ACA	Thr	AAA	Lys	AGA	Arg
AUG	Met	ACG	Thr	AAG	Lys	AGG	Arg
GUU	Val	GCU	Ala	GAU	Asp	GGU	Gly
GUC	Val	GCC	Ala	GAC	Asp	GGC	Gly
GUA	Val	GCA	Ala	GAA	Glu	GGA	Gly
GUG	Val	GCG	Ala	GAG	Glu	GGG	Gly

Consideration of control of lactose catabolism starts with the assumption that some genes code for regulatory proteins and others code for enzymes. First, start by considering a regulatory function carried out by a class of proteins called repressors. The function of repressors is to control the transcription of genes coding for various enzymes. The repressor for enzymes of lactose catabolism is called the lac repressor, lac being the genetic abbreviation for genes governing lactose catabolism. The lac repressor is encoded in a gene *I* separate from the other genes of lactose catabolism (Fig 3–5). Synthesis of the lac repressor (and, for that matter, all repressors) is constitutive; that is, lac repressor is made all the time. The lac repressor can recognize and bind to a specific DNA base sequence, called the operator (*O* in Fig 3–5). The operator is part of a larger sequence known as the promoter (Fig 3–5). The promoter is the site for binding of RNA polymerase and thus can be regarded as the place where transcription is initiated. The lac repressor normally is active and binds to the lac operator, blocking transcription. In this way, *E. coli* cells growing in the absence of lactose are prevented from making galactoside permease (product of the lac *Y* gene), which transports lactose into the cell, and β-galactosidase (product of the lac *Z* gene), which cleaves it into glucose and galactose.

When these same bacteria are grown on lactose rather than, for example, glucose, a few lactose molecules will get onto the cell by means of diffusion. These lactose molecules will bind to the lac repressor at a site distinct from the operator-binding region. The lac repressor is an allosteric protein, which changes conformation on binding lactose. A consequence of this conformational change is that the repressor can no longer bind to the operator region. The inactivated lac repressor detaches from DNA. RNA polymerase then can bind to the promoter and initiate transcription, beginning expression of the genes involved in lactose catabolism.

Operons

The genes coding for enzymes of lactose catabolism in *E. coli* are adjacent to each other and to their promoter and operator, and the simultaneous expression of all three genes is controlled by the binding of the lac repressor to the operator. This cluster of contiguous related genes all controlled by their own set of regulatory elements is called an operon. Operons are relatively common in prokaryotic organisms but very rare in eukaryotes.

Operons are transcribed as a unit; that is, transcription of the lac operon produces a single mRNA molecule with base sequences specifying all the enzymes. Such an mRNA is said to be polycistronic. Polycistronic mRNA is another unique characteristic of operons.

Operons may be under negative or positive control (Fig 3–6). Negative control is exerted by a repressor that binds to an operator and blocks transcription. The lac operon is under negative control. Many biosynthetic pathways also are under negative control. For example, *E. coli* is able to make its own histidine using an operon controlled in a way only slightly different from the way in which the lac operon is controlled. The his repressor is inactive in the absence of histidine and thus allows transcription of the operon and synthesis of histidine during growth on histidine-free medium. If histidine now is added to the growth medium, some of the exogenous histidine can bind to the regulatory site of the repressor, producing a conformational change in the repressor's operator-binding site so that it can bind to the operator and block transcription. When the exogenous histidine is exhausted, the process is reversed and the genes of the histidine operon again are expressed. This sort of control of biosynthetic operons is called end product repression.

Operons under positive control are regulated in a manner essentially opposite from the lac operon. The

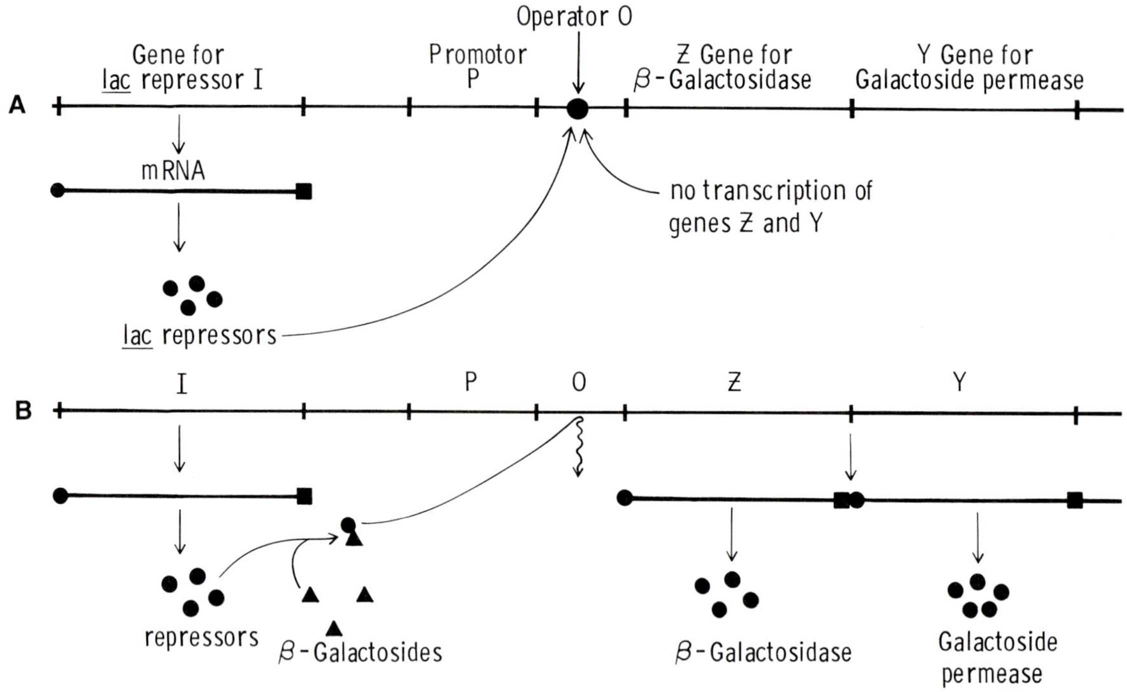

Figure 3–5. Mechanism of transcriptional control. Enzymes for the catabolism of β-galactosides, such as lactose, are made only when lactose or some other β-galactoside is present. **A.** In the absence of lactose, the lac repressor is active and can block transcription of the lac *Z* and *Y* genes. **B.** When lactose is present, it binds to the lac repressor, converting the repressor to a form that cannot block transcription.

regulatory protein allows rather than prevents transcription. Catabolism of the sugar arabinose by *E. coli* is under such control. Arabinose forms a complex with the regulatory protein, and this complex binds near the promoter for the arabinose operon. Only after this interaction will RNA polymerase bind to the promoter and transcribe the operon. When the arabinose is exhausted, the process is reversed, and transcription ceases.

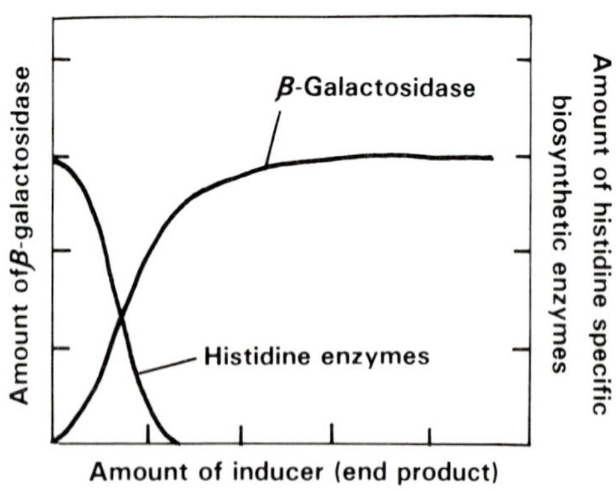

Figure 3–6. Comparison of induction and repression. As the amount of the inducer lactose in the growth medium increases, the amount of β-galactosidase per cell also increases to a constant level. As the amount of histidine (end product of the histidine biosynthetic pathway) increases, the amount per cell of histidine biosynthetic enzymes decreases to zero.

Global Regulatory Networks

The control mechanisms just described are specific controls activated by the presence of particular molecules involved in individual pathways. However, bacteria also can respond to higher-order controls, which are determined by the overall status of the cell. These are called global regulatory networks. Global regulatory networks consist of sets of two or more operons representing different functions and located in different parts of the bacterial chromosome. The operons of a global regulatory network are coordinately controlled. Global regulatory networks allow bacteria to respond to major changes in environment. Two of the best understood global regulatory networks are catabolite repression and the stringent response.

Catabolite repression comes into play when bacteria are faced with a choice of two or more substrates for energy-yielding metabolism (Fig 3–7). The substrate that can be degraded more efficiently is used first. For example, when *E. coli* cells are grown on a mixture of glucose and lactose, the glucose is used first. Only after the glucose is exhausted are lactose permease and β-galactosidase induced. The presence of glucose represses the lac operon even though the inducer of that operon is present. This phenomenon was studied in detail first by the French microbiologist, J. Monod, who observed that such a culture produced a biphasic growth curve. First, there was

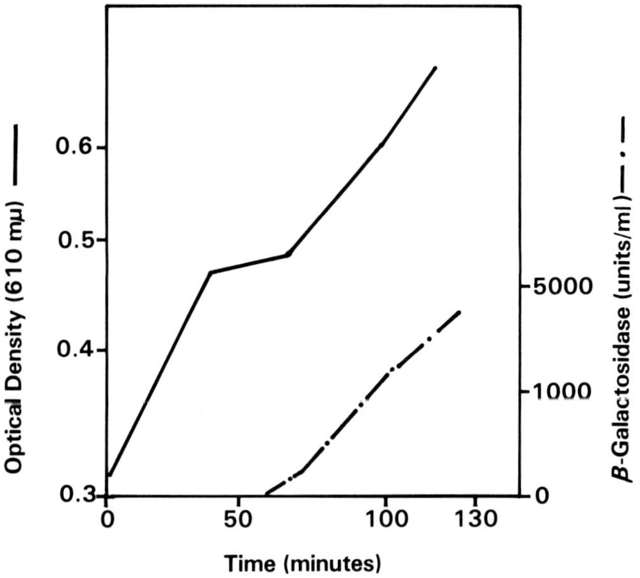

Figure 3–7. Catabolite repression, a global regulatory mechanism. *Escherichira coli* cells are grown on a mixture of glucose and lactose. Growth is monitored by measuring culture optical density, and the amount of β-galactosidase in the cells also is measured. Growth proceeds until the glucose is exhausted. After a pause, growth recommences using lactose. Synthesis of β-galactosidase is not seen until glucose has been consumed.

growth on glucose, then a lag during which enzymes unique to lactose catabolism were induced, then a second period of growth using lactose.

Catabolite repression controls catabolism of many other substrates besides lactose and controls other processes as well. Levels of ATP-synthesizing enzymes, synthesis of bacterial flagella, and synthesis of components of the electron transport chain all are controlled by catabolite repression.

Another global control is the stringent response. The stringent response is a mechanism used by bacteria to control synthesis of macromolecules, especially under starvation conditions. For example, during growth of a bacterium that requires histidine, it is expected that protein synthesis will stop when all the histidine in the growth medium had been consumed. However, not only does protein synthesis cease, but also synthesis of rRNA, tRNA, cell wall peptidoglycan, and membrane lipids ceases. In wild-type bacteria, this inhibition of macromolecular biosynthesis is tightly (ie, stringently) coordinated with cessation of protein synthesis. (Wild-type bacteria are not mutated in the gene under study and thus can express the function of that gene.) Bacteria using stringent control are able to avoid unbalanced growth during starvation, since unbalanced growth can be lethal.

Several other global controls are known. The SOS system is a global regulatory network induced by damage to DNA. It activates several metabolic pathways to repair that damage. Its name (the international distress signal) carries the implication of a response to a cellular emergency. The heat-shock response is a transient increase in synthesis of proteins coding for a battery of essential functions following a rise in environmental temperature. In *E. coli,* these proteins include the products of two DNA synthesis genes and a subunit of the enzyme RNA polymerase. Similarly, global regulatory mechanisms help bacteria to cope with shifts between aerobic and anaerobic environments and with environments limited in such nutrients as phosphate or nitrogen.

GENETICS OF BACTERIA

Bacteria are haploid (have single chromosomes), whereas most other familiar organisms are diploid (have duplicate chromosomes). Nevertheless, bacteria follow the same general concepts of genetics as do diploid organisms, such as fruit flies and humans. Some of those concepts will be reviewed and then applied to bacteria.

The aggregate of all genetic information possessed by an organism is its genotype. The genotype of a typical bacterium includes about 3000 genes, each coding for a single gene product. However, not all these genes are expressed all the time. For instance, the manner in which the lactose-catabolizing genes of *E. coli* are expressed only when lactose is present was described earlier.

The properties expressed in a particular environment are called the phenotype. Phenotype is limited by genotype, since an organism obviously cannot exhibit a property for which it lacks a gene. However, phenotype is not constant and can be modified in response to changes in environment, for example, by enzyme induction or repression.

Mutation

An organism's genotype represents the genetic information to be passed to succeeding generations. It is a common notion that a given species is pretty much the same from generation to generation and, therefore, that genotype must be stable. In general, this is true. However, it is possible for the genotype of a bacterium (or other organism) to be changed and for that change to be passed to following generations.

An abrupt change in structure of a gene is called a mutation, and organisms possessing that change are mutants. Mutated genes may be altered in function. The mutation may cause the gene or its product to work better, poorer, or not at all. Mutations are produced by a physical or chemical change in the structure of a gene. Change in gene structure can take

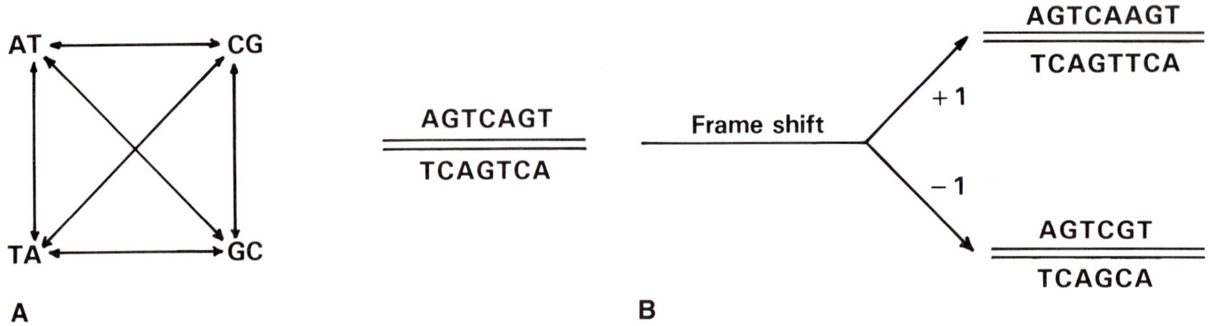

Figure 3–8. Types of mutations. Mutations involving changes in single bases are shown here. **A.** Base pair mutations. Transitions (replacement of a purine by the wrong purine or a pyrimidine by the wrong pyrimidine) are shown by horizontal and vertical lines, and transversions (replacement of a purine by a pyrimidine, or vice versa) are shown by diagonal lines. **B.** Frame-shift mutations, in which addition or deletion of a base puts the mechanisms for reading of genetic information out of phase.

several forms (Fig 3–8). A mistake during DNA replication could cause incorporation of a wrong base into a sequence of purines and pyrimidines, thus changing the information in that sequence. When the wrong purine or pyrimidine is incorporated in place of a correct purine or pyrimidine (eg, adenine in place of guanine or thymine in place of cytosine), the mutation is called a transition. In a similar change called a transversion, a purine is replaced by a pyrimidine, and vice versa. In another type of mutation, one or two DNA nucleotides might be deleted from or inserted into a gene. Either would put out of phase the mechanisms for reading the genetic information. These are called frame-shift mutations. If a longer piece of DNA is deleted from a gene, a deletion mutation results. The deleted DNA in such a mutation could include an entire gene or more. Finally, a piece of DNA might be put in backward (an inversion) or put in twice instead of once (a duplication). All of these sudden changes in the physical structure of a gene can lead to alteration in or loss of gene function.

Mutations can occur more or less randomly in any gene. Spontaneous mutations occur all the time but at very low frequencies. Typical spontaneous mutations rates in bacteria are 10^{-6} to 10^{-10} mutations per cell per generation. Mutation rates can be increased by physical or chemical agents that interact with and alter DNA. These agents are called mutagens. Ultraviolet light, x-rays, and alkylating agents, such as ethylmethane sulfonate are examples of mutagens. Mutagens have been valuable research tools because they increase mutation rates to experimentally convenient levels.

When mutagens are in the environment rather than confined to the laboratory, they are cause for concern. Environmental mutagens can interact with the DNA of organisms living in that environment, with consequent potential damage to that organism or its offspring.

Mutation has the effect of introducing genetic variation into the pooled genotype of a population of organisms. As noted previously, mutations occur all the time in bacteria but usually at very low frequency. They are spontaneous and random and can occur in any gene at any time. Once mutation has taken place, mutants can be selected by the environment. Thus, mutation provides one means by which bacteria respond to change in environment. These principles can be illustrated by an experiment known as replica plating, (Fig 3–9).

This experiment starts with a culture of a bacterium that is sensitive to the antibiotic streptomycin but has the ability to become streptomycin resistant. Samples of this culture are diluted and spread to produce

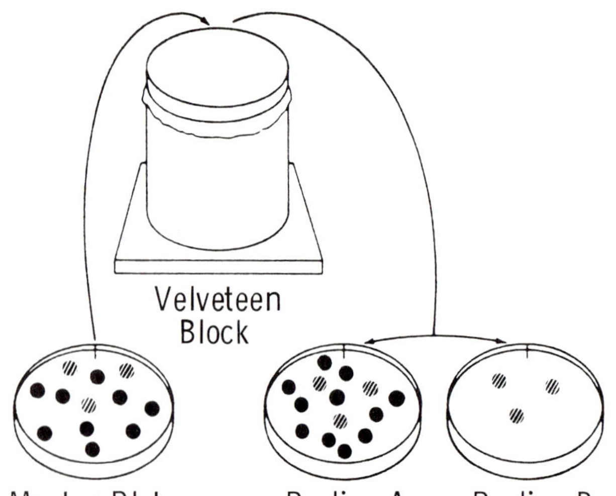

Figure 3–9. Replica plating. Colonies are allowed to grow on the master plate without streptomycin. The master plate is pressed gently onto the surface of a sterile velveteen block, and cells from each colony adhere to the cloth fibers. Fresh uninoculated plates then can be pressed onto the velveteen and incubated to make replicas of the master plate. Note that replica plate A (without streptomycin) has colonies in the same places as the master plate, whereas replica plate B (with streptomycin) has only three colonies, which grew from single streptomycin-resistant cells on the master plate.

isolated colonies on plates of streptomycin-free agar. These plates are the master plates. After incubation and colony formation, a master plate is pressed gently onto a piece of sterile velvet held in a stand. Cells from each colony will stick to the fibers of the velvet, forming an image of the colonies that were on the master plate. If a fresh plate now is pressed onto the velvet pad and then incubated, a replica of the master plate is produced. If the replica is made with a plate containing streptomycin agar, most of the colonies from the master plate will not grow. However, a few colonies might grow even in the presence of streptomycin. These streptomycin-resistant colonies arose from mutant bacteria present in the original culture that never had been exposed to streptomycin. They were selected out of the original population in response to an environment in which streptomycin was present. In theory, it is possible to find spontaneous mutations in any bacterial gene by application of these principles, along with an appropriate selection procedure.

Another important concept can be derived from this example. If there is a certain amount of genetic variation within a species, at least a few organisms of that species will be able to grow when exposed to selective pressure due to change in environment even if most members of the species are killed. Thus, the species will survive.

Mutation is one means of introducing genetic variation into a species and helps to ensure survival of the species in the face of selective pressure. Furthermore, it is important to note that to a bacterium an antibiotic is a form of selective pressure. This helps to explain why most bacteria that are recovered from hospital-acquired infections are resistant to at least one antibiotic. In the selective pressure of an antibiotic-rich environment (the hospital), only the antibiotic-resistant bacteria will survive. The emergence of large numbers of antibiotic-resistant strains of pathogenic bacteria is a consequence of a new kind of selective pressure in the bacteria's environment, namely antibiotics.

Recombination

Recombination is another means of introducing genetic variation into a population. Recombination is a process by which new combinations of genes are formed in an organism. Recombination in bacteria occurs after fragments of DNA are transferred from a donor cell to a recipient. This is different from higher organisms, in which recombination is a part of sexual reproduction in which both parents make equal contributions. In bacteria, the transfer of genes is unidirectional (from donor to recipient) and usually involves just a portion of the donor bacterium's chromosome. Once the gene transfer has taken place, recombination can occur. It can be imagined as follows.

- Recipient chromosome: *AB. . .LM. . .YZ*
- Donor DNA fragment: *. .lm. .*
- Recombinant chromosome: *AB. . .lm. . .YZ*

The newly formed chromosome has a new combination of genes and, therefore, is recombinant. In this example there was a bit of DNA (carrying the genes *L* and *M*) left over after the recombination. That DNA will be degraded by cell nucleases to deoxynucleotides, which then can be reused.

This type of recombination depends on extensive homology between donor and recipient DNA and is mediated by a set of recombination enzymes. These enzymes specialize in catalyzing recombination between identical or nearly identical pieces of DNA and have been purified and used in genetic engineering. This sort of recombination has been described as legitimate because it requires extensive homology between the pieces of recombining DNA. Legitimate recombination processes are the function of a family of bacterial genes called rec (for recombination).

In addition to the rec-dependent process, bacteria possess another, illegitimate mechanism for generating genetic diversity through recombination. This second type of recombination is not legitimate in that it takes place between nonidentical pieces of DNA. For example, there exists a bacterial virus called phage lambda that infects *E. coli*. It can replicate in one of two ways. First, it can make many new copies of itself in a process that kills the *E. coli* cell. Second, it can survive by integrating (that is, recombining) its DNA into the *E. coli* chromosome (Fig 3–10). In the integrated state (also called the prophage state), the lambda DNA is replicated during replication of the bacterial chromosome. *Escherichia coli* and phage lambda DNAs are not identical or even closely related, yet in the integration process, phage DNA is recombined into *E. coli* DNA. The recombination takes place between a specific site on the viral genome and another specific site on the bacterial genome. In contrast, homologous recombination can involve any gene in a genome. Integration of phage lambda DNA is rec independent. In fact, the necessary enzymes are encoded in the lambda genome rather than in the bacterial chromosome.

In recent years, a second type of rec-independent recombination has become important because of the problems it has given in the treatment of infectious diseases with antibiotics. The recombination process is called transposition after the ability of antibiotic-resistant genes to transpose or move from one site to another within a single chromosome or even to move from one chromosome to another. The genes are carried on DNA fragments called transposons, which can insert into other DNA molecules by a type of illegitimate recombination. Transposons carry genetic

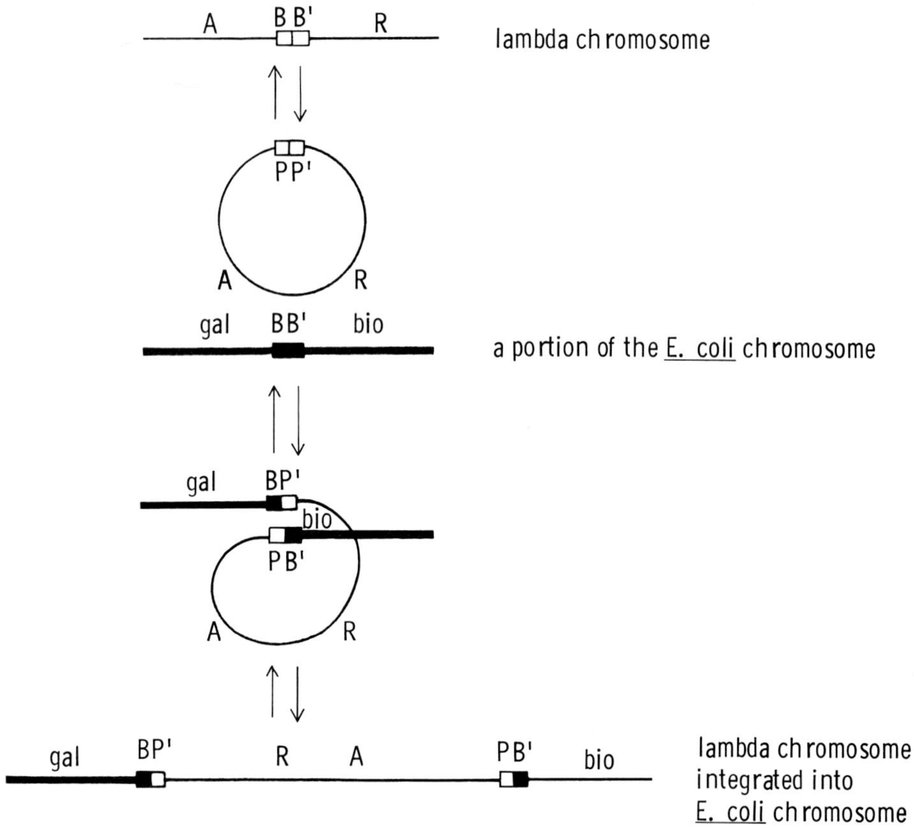

Figure 3–10. Recombination of bacteriophage lambda DNA into the *E. coli* chromosome. The specific recombination sites on the phage DNA are called P and P′, and the corresponding sites on the *E. coli* chromosome are called B and B′. The other genetic symbols mark various genes of the phage and bacterial chromosomes. The phage DNA converts from a linear to a circular form, and the recombination sites P, P′, B, and B′ come into proximity. The specific recombination event takes place, and lambda DNA is inserted into the *E. coli* chromosome between the *gal* and *bio* genes.

information coding for the enzymes needed for their insertion and, in addition, may carry genes for antibiotic resistance or for toxin production or may have no additional genes. Transposon-borne genes have been very important in the rapid spread of antibiotic resistance among bacteria.

Since integration of a transposon is rec independent and can take place between unrelated molecules, one would expect that transposition would be more or less random. In general, this is the case, although a few transposons show some specificity. The insertion process, however, depends absolutely on specialized sequences (called insertion sequences) at the end of the transposon.

A final important property of transposons is their inability to replicate autonomously. A transposon is not a replicon; a replicon is a genome having the capacity for self-replication. A transposon can survive and replicate only when integrated into a replicon—a bacterial chromosome, a phage genome, or a plasmid.

Genetic Exchange

Although recombination has been described in detail, little has been said about how gene-bearing pieces of DNA are moved from one bacterial cell to another. There are three such processes in bacteria: transformation, conjugation, and transduction.

Transformation. Transformation is gene transfer from donor to closely related recipient bacterium, using DNA molecules that have been released from the donor cell. The DNA may be released following death and lysis of the donor, or it may be chemically extracted and highly purified in a laboratory procedure. Regardless of the method, it is the donor DNA that is the active component. These DNA molecules actually are pieces of the broken-up donor chromosome, and each piece contains at most just a few genes. These pieces can be taken up by the recipient cells a few pieces per cell. The fragments of donor DNA are not replicons and cannot replicate autonomously or be expressed in the recipient cells until they are integrated into the recipient's chromosome. Donor and recipient DNAs are highly homologous, and the recombination is rec dependent.

It is entirely possible that transformation occurs in nature, and it may be that such recombination produces virulent organisms. In fact, the earliest studies of bacterial transformation, by Griffith in 1928, suggested such a conclusion. Griffith was concerned with *Streptococcus pneumoniae,* which causes lobar pneumonia. *Streptococcus pneumoniae* strains that produced smooth colonies on agar plates were highly virulent for mice and appeared encapsulated on microscopic examination. Strains that produced rough-appearing colonies were avirulent and had no capsules. Griffith heat-killed a smooth culture that had capsular serotype 1. He then obtained a rough strain that had been serotype 2 before it lost its ability to make a capsule. He mixed killed type 1 cells with living avirulent type 2 cells and injected susceptible mice with the mixture. Next day, the mice were sick or dying, and cultures from the sick mice yielded living encapsulated type 1 *S. pneumoniae*. Griffith reasoned that the killed type 1 bacteria released a substance that converted living type 2 cells into type 1. Subsequent work over many years by Avery, MacLeod, and McCarty showed that this substance was DNA. Transformation occurs in several bacterial genera, including medically and dentally important *Streptococcus, Neisseria,* and *Haemophilus.*

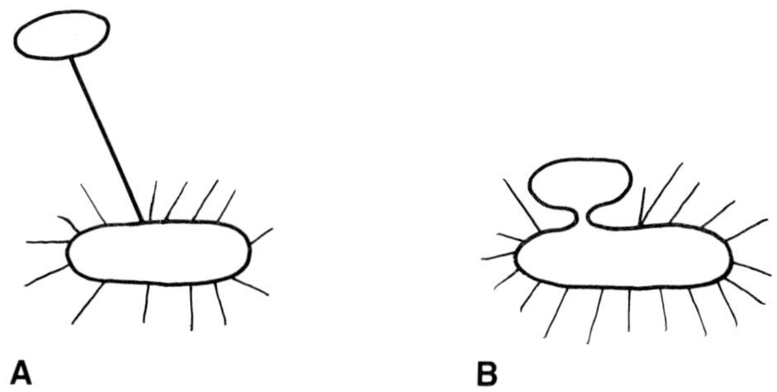

Figure 3–11. Bacterial conjugation. **A.** The lower male *E. coli* cell is covered with many short common pili and has one long F pilus that joins it to a female cell. Only the F pilus is involved in conjugation. **B.** A mating *E. coli* pair. The F pilus has retracted into the male cell, and the two cells are in direct contact.

Conjugation. The second gene transfer process in bacteria is conjugation. Bacterial conjugation was discovered in 1946 at Yale University by Lederberg, a medical student who was doing a research project in the laboratory of Tatum. Lederberg and Tatum observed bacterial conjugation in *E. coli* during a project designed to determine whether genetic recombination existed in bacteria.

Conjugation differs from other bacterial gene transfer processes in that direct contact between donor and recipient cells is required (Fig 3–11). Conjugation is common among gram-negative bacteria and can take place between unrelated as well as closely related strains, species, and genera. It is the most important mechanism for transfer of antibiotic resistance among gram-negative bacteria. Conjugation is observed in gram-positive bacteria, but it is rare.

In conjugation between two gram-negative bacterial cells, DNA is transferred from donor to recipient but only while the cells are in contact. Donor cells are able to transfer DNA because they contain genes coding for DNA transfer functions (tra genes). Recipient cells lack tra genes. Tra genes in the donor are not carried on the bacterial chromosome but are carried on an extra piece of DNA called a plasmid. Recipient cells lack tra genes.

Plasmids are extrachromosomal genetic elements; that is, they are pieces of DNA separate and distinct from the bacterial chromosome (Fig 3–12). In physical structure, they are circular, double stranded, and considerably smaller in size than the bacterial chromosome. The largest plasmids are about 5% of the size of the bacterial chromosome, and most are much smaller. Plasmids are autonomous and self-replicating. In other words, plasmids function as replicons. All plasmids encode for self-replication, and some have tra genes as well. Plasmids possessing tra genes are said to be conjugative because they can transfer DNA during conjugation. Many plasmids in addition code for functions that are not essential for cell growth and survival under normal conditions but are useful under unusual circumstances. For example, antibiotic resistance genes commonly are plasmid-borne.

Plasmids bearing tra genes can catalyze their own transfer. They also can catalyze the transfer of other genomes in the same cell. Thus, plasmids lacking tra genes can be transferred, and sometimes even the bacterial chromosome can be. Plasmid transfer can occur in a plasmid-containing gram-negative cell

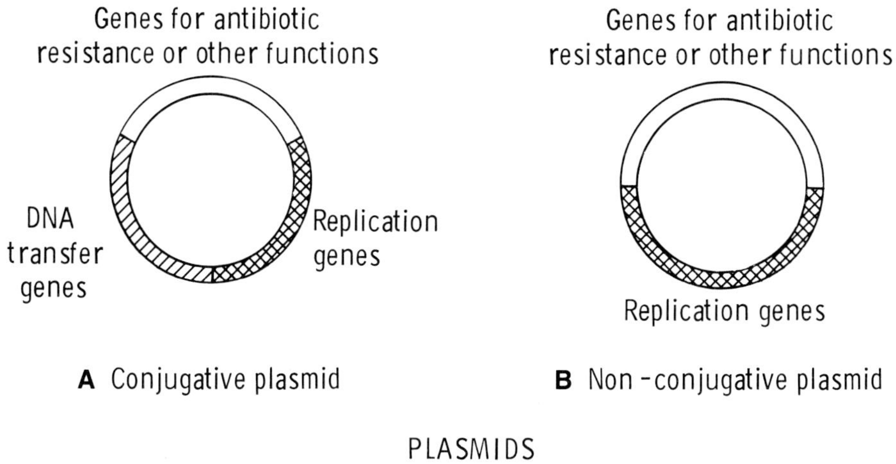

Figure 3–12. Plasmids. All plasmids have genes for their own replication and may or may not have genes for antibiotic resistance or other functions. **A.** Conjugative plasmids also have tra genes for DNA transfer. **B.** Nonconjugative genes lack tra genes.

when the tra genes are expressed. One of the most important tra genes codes for a bacterial surface structure called a sex pilus. This structure is filamentous and can make contact with a receptor on the surface of a recipient cell. On contact, the pilus withdraws into the donor cell, still in contact with the recipient. The two cells come into contact, a conjugation bridge is formed, and DNA transfer takes place.

It is important to note that the recipient cell now contains the conjugative plasmid and thus has been converted into a donor and that the donor still retains a copy of the plasmid. Thus, both cells now can serve as donors. Because plasmid transfer is rapid and can cross species and genus lines, the consequences of this process in the spread of antibiotic resistance through bacterial populations can be devastating and, in fact, can account for the presence of large numbers of antibiotic-resistant bacteria in hospitals.

Sometimes the bacterial chromosome can be transferred by conjugation (Fig 3–13). Conjugative transfer of bacterial chromosomal DNA had been studied extensively with *E. coli* and a conjugative plasmid called F (for fertility). Most of the time, the F plasmid is transferred as described and an F donor converts an F recipient into an F-bearing cell. However, on rare occasions, F can be integrated into the bacterial chromosome. In this state, F causes the transfer of the bacterial chromosome much more frequently than when F is not integrated. Therefore, such strains are called Hfr (high frequency of recombination). Hfr strains are capable of transferring the entire bacterial chromosome. This is a long process (about 2 hours), and the conjugation bridge usually breaks before then. Transferred DNA is integrated and expressed by means of rec-dependent recombination.

Plasmids as Accessory Chromosomes. Plasmids are found frequently in dentally and medically important bacteria isolated from patients. These plasmids often carry genes for antibiotic resistance, and it is not unusual for a single isolate to be resistant to six or more antibiotics. Since infections caused by antibiotic-resistant bacteria can be difficult to treat, plasmids and plasmid-mediated antibiotic resistance are very important in dentistry and medicine. In addition, plasmids can mediate several other activities of bacteria.

Plasmids can be regarded as accessory chromosomes. According to this line of reasoning, the bacterial chromosome is designated the euchromosome, and on it are the genes essential for bacterial growth under normal circumstances. Plasmids, in contrast, are accessory chromosomes and contain no genes that are unconditionally required for bacterial reproduction. As described earlier, plasmids contain genes for their own replication, and conjugative plasmids in addition have genes controlling conjugation. Some plasmids include genes that determine host traits, but traits that are needed by the bacterial host only intermittently. Already described is the trait of antibiotic resistance, in which the bacteria need only in an environment containing antibiotics. Among clinically important bacteria, plasmid genes are responsible for *E. coli* gastroenteritis toxin, as well as for various hemolytic and other hydrolytic enzymes. Thus, plasmids have great clinical significance.

Plasmid genes are important in the biology of other bacteria as well. Genes for a variety of auxiliary metabolic processes are carried on plasmids. These include resistance to toxic metals, such as mercury, resistance to ultraviolet irradiation, production of bacteriocins, and catabolism of hydrocarbons and other unusual substrates.

Genetic Engineering. Genetic engineering has been practiced ever since humans developed agrarian societies and began to practice selective breeding of plants and animals. The most recent practice of genetic engineering has been the use of gene cloning to obtain expression of foreign genes in microbial cells. By use of purified recombination enzymes, it is possible to isolate a gene from any organism and incorporate that gene into a plasmid. If the recombinant plasmid is put into a recipient bacterium by transformation, the foreign gene can be expressed in a bacterial cell. This methodology has been used to produce such useful substances as insulin, human growth hormone, and hepatitis B vaccine. Furthermore, this approach has great research value. For example, it is difficult or impossible to study genetics of the cariogenic bacterium *Streptococcus mutans* by transformation, transduction, or conjugation. Use of recombinant DNA technology has allowed the study of some *S. mutans* genes in *E. coli*, and there is beginning to be some understanding of the organization, function, and control of those *S. mutans* genes involved in caries formation.

Similar recombinant DNA experiments are being used to study virulence factors of suspected periodontal pathogens and to develop genetic probes for diagnosing and monitoring therapy of dental disease. However, despite its great potential for good, genetic engineering is not without its pitfalls. One can imagine cloning a potent toxin gene into an *E. coli* strain that could colonize the human gut. Accidental release of this recombinant strain could lead to an epidemic, with drastic consequences. For this reason, recombinant DNA experiments are done under guidelines designed to restrict the development of potentially pathogenic strains and to prevent the release of artificially recombinant organisms into the environment.

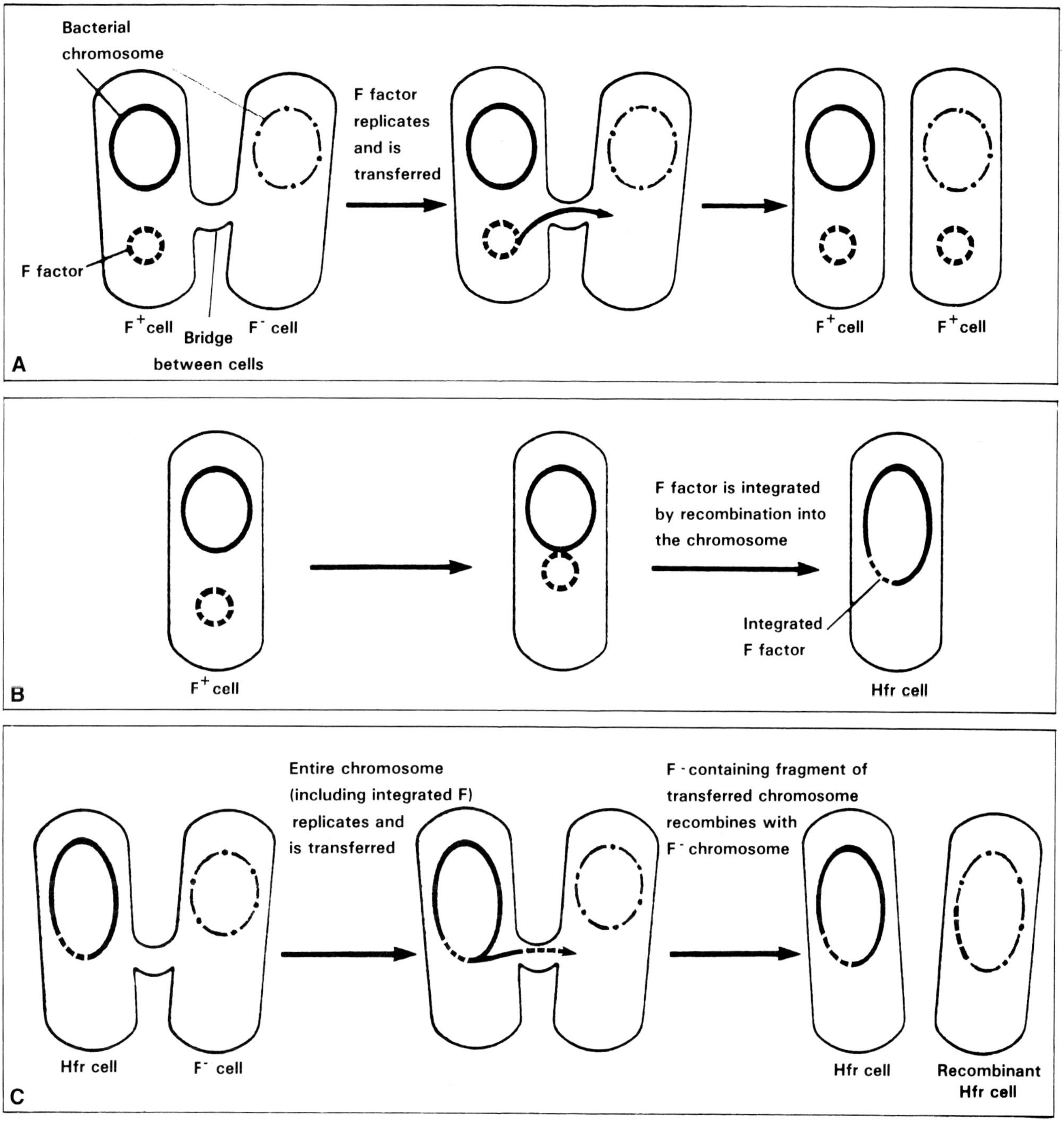

Figure 3–13. Transfer of the bacterial chromosome by conjugation. **A.** Conjugal transfer of F plasmid (also called F factor) from an F^+ to an F^- cell and conversion of the F^- to F^+. **B.** Production of an Hfr cell by integration of F into the bacterial chromosome. **C.** Conjugal transfer of the bacterial chromosome from an Hfr cell into an F^- cell.

Transduction. The third gene transfer process in bacteria is transduction. Transduction is the transfer of bacterial DNA from donor to recipient using a bacterial virus as a carrier. Transduction was discovered in 1951 by J. Lederberg and N. Zinder, working at the University of Wisconsin. There are two types of transduction, generalized and specialized.

Generalized transduction is a consequence of the assembly of particles of many types of bacterial viruses during the maturation phase of the bacteriophage infection process (Fig 3–14). During virus replication, some fragments of the bacterial chromosome are not destroyed. If these surviving fragments are of the right size, by mistake they might be incorporated

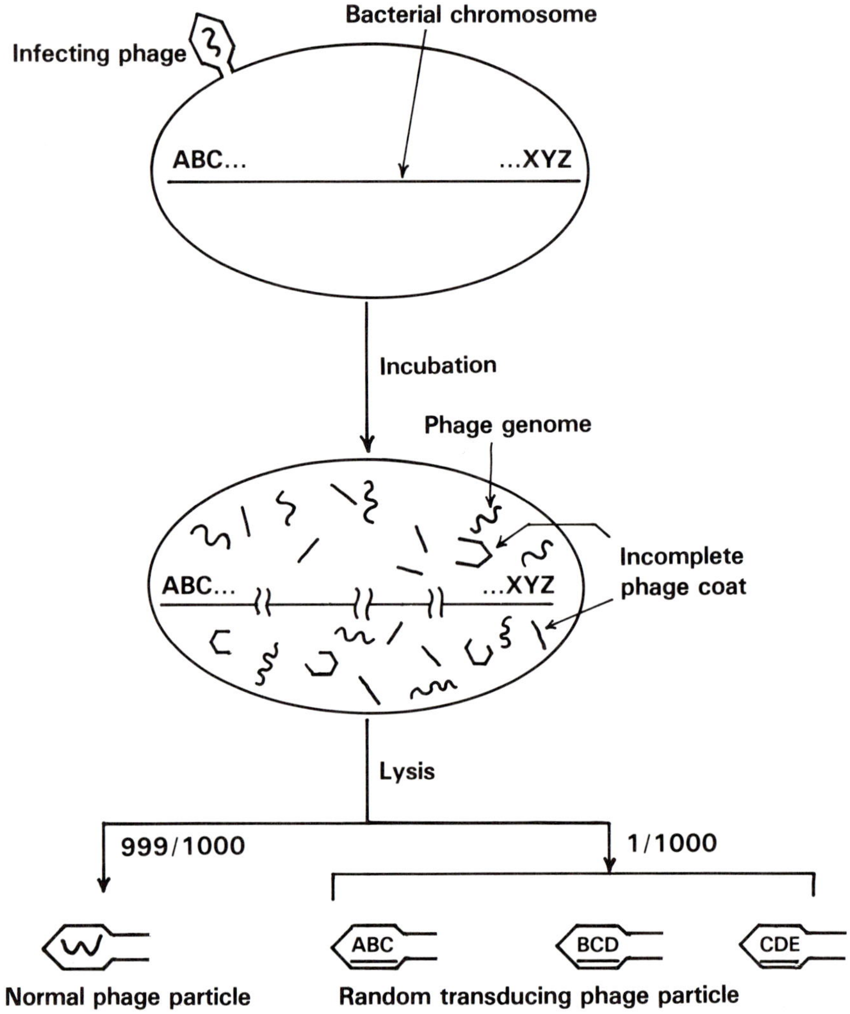

Figure 3–14. Generalized transduction. Most virus particles made in this infection are normal and contain viral DNA, but rarely a phage particle encloses a fragment of bacterial DNA. These rare particles can transfer bacterial DNA into a recipient cell. Since any bacterial gene at random might be enclosed, this transduction also is random or generalized.

into the virus particle in place of the viral DNA. These fraudulent viruses still can inject their DNA into another bacterial cell of the same species. The injected DNA is, of course, bacterial, and the recipient bacteria could acquire a new characteristic from that DNA. Any donor gene might be transferred and then recombined into the recipient bacterial chromosome by legitimate recombination.

To understand specialized transduction, first recall integration of phage lambda DNA into the *E. coli* chromosome by illegitimate site-specific recombination (Fig 3–15). Occasionally, that process is reversed, the lambda DNA is excised from the *E. coli* chromosome, and production of many new lambda particles ensues. Normally, this excision is very precise, and the lambda DNA is removed from the *E. coli* chromosome without error. Rarely, a mistake in excision happens, and at one end a bit of bacterial DNA adjacent to the integrated lambda DNA is excised, and at the other end a corresponding bit of lambda DNA is left behind. Since lambda DNA integrates between the *E. coli gal* (galactose catabolism) and *bio* (biotin synthesis) genes, these mistakes give rise to lambda particles carrying either *gal* or *bio*. Such phage can inject their DNA into a susceptible cell, and that DNA can be integrated (Fig 3–16). An *E. coli* that had lost the ability to grow on galactose or to make its own biotin could regain those abilities as a consequence of specialized transduction. However, note that specialized transduction can transfer only those bacterial genes adjacent to the site of integration of viral DNA.

Phage Conversion. The manner in which phage lambda DNA can be integrated into the *E. coli* chromosome has been described, as well as how during specialized transduction such integration can change the metabolic properties of the recipient cell. In a similar (but not identical) manner, the virulence properties of some medically important bacteria are changed on integration of a particular phage genome into the bacterial chromosome. To give an example, pathosis of the disease diphtheria is caused by a toxin produced

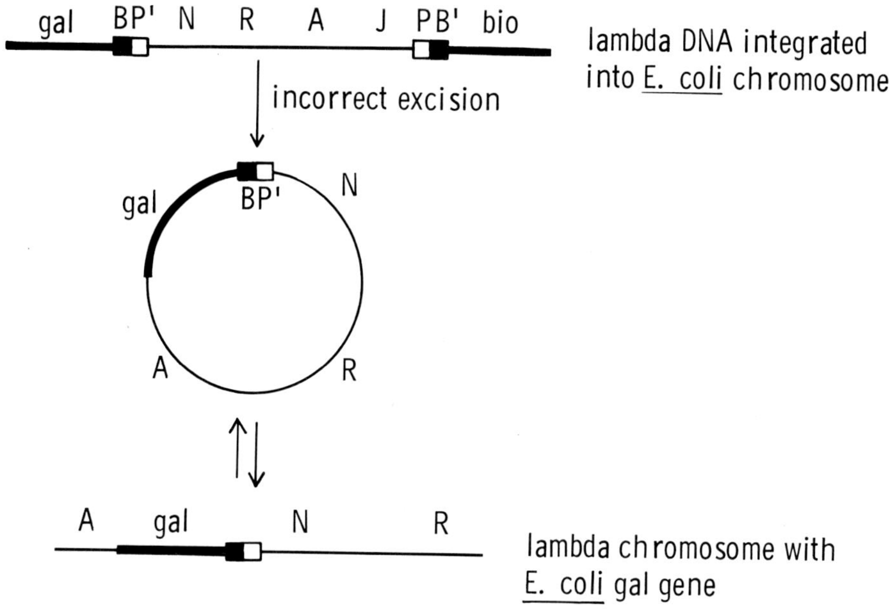

Figure 3–15. Specialized transduction: formation of transducing phage. A mistake in excision of lambda DNA from the *E. coli* chromosome leads to virus particles containing a bacterial gene, either gal or bio. This example shows formation of a gal-containing particle. Only gal or bio genes will be transduced.

by the bacterium *Corynebacterium diphtheriae.* However, a given strain of *C. diphtheriae* can produce toxin only if integrated into its chromosome is the DNA of phage β. If that DNA is absent, the bacteria cannot produce the toxin. Subsequent investigation has shown that the toxin is a product of a phage gene, the original source of which is unknown. The entire phenomenon is called phage conversion (also called lysogenic conversion), and there are numerous examples in medical bacteriology of toxin production or antigenic change after phage conversion. Note that in phage conversion, the properties of the recipient cell are changed by a phage gene, whereas in transduction, the properties of the recipient cell are changed after the phage carries in a new bacterial gene.

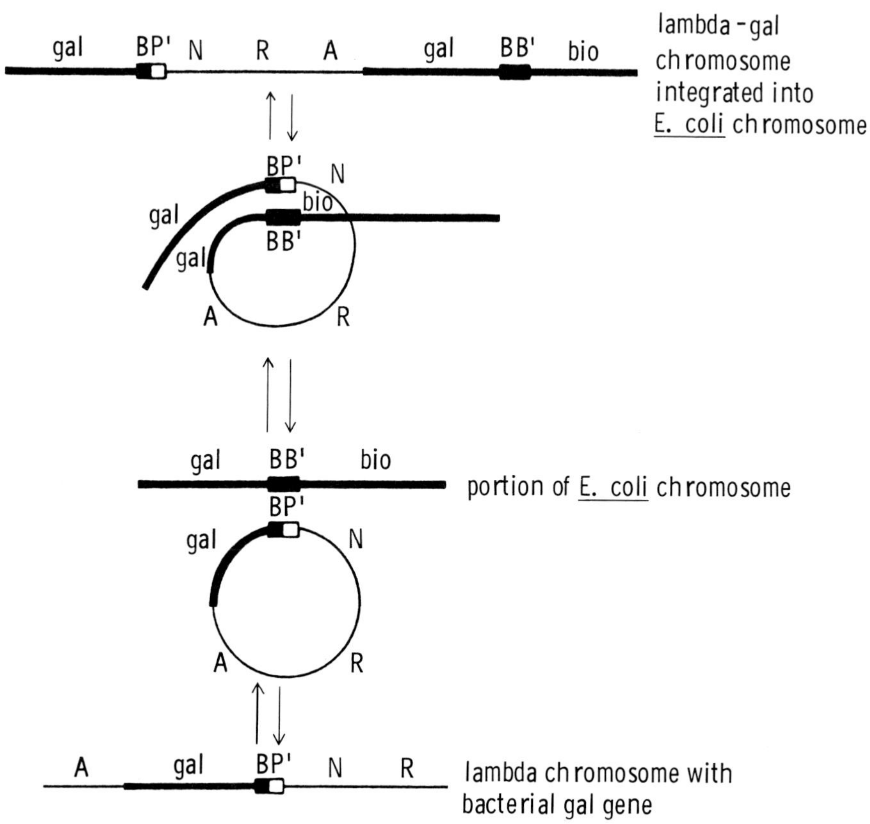

Figure 3–16. Specialized transduction. Insertion of a new *gal* gene from the transducing phage into the bacterial chromosome.

ORAL ASPECTS

Bacteria are able to respond rapidly to changes in environment. They do so by regulating their metabolism so that metabolic activities are expressed only when needed. The primary form of regulation is control of expression of genes. This regulation is exerted at the level of transcription. In addition, many gene products are allosteric proteins, the activities of which are controlled by low molecular weight compounds that accumulate or are consumed during metabolism.

Bacteria have access to a variety of ways to introduce genetic variation into populations of cells. When the population faces a new form of selective pressure, a few cells may have an altered gene, the altered function of which will allow those cells to survive. These altered genes can spread throughout a population by rapid growth and by genetic exchange. Some such genes are parts of transposons and, therefore, can hop from plasmid to plasmid, chromosome to plasmid, chromosome to transducing phage genome, and so on. Plasmid-borne genes can be spread by conjugation to different species or even genera. When one considers that bacteria can respond rapidly to environmental change both by genetic means and by growth rate, the evolutionary potential of bacterial populations is seen to be enormous. This has profound implications when we consider treatment of infectious diseases in our offices, clinics, and hospitals.

This rapid bacterial evolution, in fact, helps to explain the large numbers of antibiotic-resistant pathogenic bacteria with which clinicians must deal. Most hospital-acquired *Staphylococcus aureus* infections are caused by antibiotic-resistant strains, and penicillin-resistant *Neisseria gonorrheae* is increasingly prevalent.

The revolution in genetic engineering also has dental significance. The genetic engineering approach is valuable in understanding how pathogens, such as *S. mutans*, cause oral disease and probably will be important in developing a vaccine against dental caries. The value of genetic engineering to the dental professions already is apparent in the release of a new genetically engineered hepatitis B vaccine. This vaccine is made in yeast cells rather than from the serum of human patients and will likely be much more acceptable to those at risk of hepatitis B infection.

SUGGESTED READINGS

Campbell A. Evolutionary significance of accessory DNA elements in bacteria. *Annu Rev Microbiol.* 1981;35:55.

Clewell DB. Plasmids, drug resistance, and gene transfer in the genus *Streptococcus. Microbiol Rev.* 1981;45:409.

Cohen SN, Shapiro JA. Transposable genetic elements. *Sci Am.* 1980;242:40.

Curtiss R III. Genetic analysis of *Streptococcus mutans* virulence and prospects for an anticaries vaccine. *J Dent Res.* 1986;65:1034.

Dickinson DP, Kubiniec MA, Yoshimura F, Genco RJ. Molecular cloning and sequencing of the gene encoding the fimbrial subunit protein of *Bacteroides gingivalis. J Bacteriol.* 1988;170:1658.

Gottesman S. Bacterial regulation: Global regulatory networks. *Annu Rev Genet.* 1984;18:415.

Hanada N, Kuramitsu HK. Isolation and characterization of the *Streptococcus mutans gtfD* gene, coding for primer-dependent soluble glucan synthesis. *Infect Immun.* 1989;57:2079.

Helinski DR. Bacterial plasmids: Aulonomous replication and vehicles for gene cloning. *CRC Crit Rev Biochem.* 1979;7:83.

Kleckner N. Transposable elements in procaryotes. *Annu Rev Genet.* 1981;15:341.

Kolodrubetz D, Dailey T, Ebersole J, Kraig E. Cloning and expression of the leukotoxin gene from *Actinobacillus actinomycetemcomitans. Infect Immun.* 1989;57:1465.

Low KB, Porter RD. Modes of gene transfer and recombination in bacteria. *Annu Rev Genet.* 1978;12:249.

Neidhardt FC. Multigene systems and regulons. In: Neidhardt FC, ed. *Escherichia coli and Salmonella typhimurium: Cellular and Molecular Biology.* Washington, DC: American Society for Microbiology; 1987:1313–1317.

Quivey RG Jr. The use of DNA probes in dental diagnosis and therapy. *Adv Dent Res.* 1987;1:99.

Singer B, Kusmierek JT. Chemical mutagenesis. *Annu Rev Biochem.* 1982;52:655.

Smith HO, Danner DB, Reich RA. Genetic transformation. *Annu Rev Biochem.* 1981;50:41.

Weinberg R. The molecules of life. *Sci Am.* 1985;253:48.

CHAPTER 4

Disinfection and Sterilization

Robert Kolstad and Robert R. White

INTRODUCTION
- Terminology
- General Considerations

MECHANISMS OF ANTIMICROBIAL ACTION

ANTIMICROBIAL PHYSICAL AGENTS
- Steam
- Pasteurization
- Boiling Water
- Dry Heat
- Radiation
- Filtration
- Ultrasonic Vibrations

ANTIMICROBIAL CHEMICAL AGENTS
- Ethylene Oxide
- Aldehydes
- Chlorine
- Iodine
- Alcohol
- Phenols
- Biguanides
- Surface Active Agents
- Miscellaneous Agents

INFECTION CONTROL
- Infections in the Dental Operatory
- Universal Precautions
- Sterilization
- Operatory Asepsis
- Disinfection of Intraoral Devices

SUMMARY

SUGGESTED READINGS

INTRODUCTION

The control of microorganisms is essential to the study of microbiology and critical to the practice of good dentistry. Microbiology is based on information gained from study of pure cultures of microorganisms, the maintenance of which is dependent on sterilization of the instruments, vessels, and media used to manipulate and grow the microorganisms. Medical and industrial microbiology also rely on maintenance of a contaminant-free environment and the means of containment and subsequent destruction of microorganisms.

Dentists have their own professional concerns about antimicrobial agents. The clinician not only must know how to use antimicrobials properly but also must be aware of the concepts involved in the development and applications of these chemical or physical agents. The dental professional is exposed and may also expose patients to numerous pathogenic microorganisms. In addition, surgical procedures may compromise patients' resistance factors. Therefore, to prevent self-infection or cross-infection, the dentist should be aware of available antimicrobial agents and their potential advantages and disadvantages. The clinician, moreover, should undersand the basic considerations needed to make intelligent decisions concerning new antimicrobials yet to be developed. Finally, patients expect dental professionals to be able to give them valid recommendations concerning oral antiseptics and disinfectants. Knowledge of basic concepts allows one to better evaluate commercial agents and dispense accurate information to patients. The information in this chapter emphasizes the dental aspects of microbial control, but it is equally important in terms of medicine, industry, and our personal lives.

Terminology

Sterilizing refers to the killing of all microbial life. It applies equally to all microorganisms whether bacteria, viruses, or fungi. Sterilization is an absolute term. Items are either sterile or not sterile; there is no in between.

-static is a suffix that refers to the property of inhibiting microbial growth (reproduction) but not killing microorganisms. A bacteriostatic agent arrests the growth of bacteria. Generally, if the agent is inactivated or removed from the environment, the microorganisms may begin reproducing.

-cidal is a suffix that means to kill. A bactericide is an agent that kills bacteria; a fungicide kills fungi, and so on.

Sepsis or **septic** refers to the presence of infection, infectious material, or infectious agents.

Asepsis has two meanings. One is the opposite of sepsis, that is, freedom from infection, and the second is the prevention of contact with pathogens. The second definition is an umbrella term including not only sterilization and disinfection but other procedures as well. Examples of these other procedures in dental practice are the filtration of air via face masks, the use of safety glasses, and the scrubbing of hands and nails with a brush. Although the mechanics of sterilization and handwashing are different, their purpose is identical, that is, to prevent contact with microorganisms, or asepsis.

Disinfection is the destruction or inactivation of pathogenic microorganisms on inanimate objects. Disinfection often is incomplete, but the antimicrobial activity can range up to sterilization.

Disinfectant refers to an agent that kills most pathogens but not necessarily endospores on inanimate objects. The efficacy of disinfectants can be classified into three levels, high, intermediate, and low, as illustrated in Table 4–1. Disinfectants generally are more effective than antiseptics. In dental practice, liquid disinfectants are used on fixed surfaces and on some heat-sensitive instruments used in direct contact with the oral mucosa.

Antiseptic refers to a chemical agent that is used on or in living tissue to kill or prevent growth of microorganisms. The terms antiseptic and disinfectant are not absolute because an antimicrobial agent may fit both categories. For example, iodine, depending on how it is formulated, may be either or both. It is strong enough to kill nearly all, if not all, microbes but still can be used on living tissues.

General Considerations

Most antimicrobial agents function on the basis of chemical reactions and are subject to the various factors that affect the speed and efficiency of such reactions. When exposed to a chemical or physical antimicrobial agent, not all members of a population of microorganisms die simultaneously. The most sensitive die rapidly, whereas the more resistant will survive for longer exposures. Death of a uniform population is an extended event and usually proceeds by first order kinetics.

$$\text{Log survivors} = \text{log initial population} - K_t$$

During each unit of exposure time, the log of viable microorganisms at the end of that period divided by the number at the beginning is a constant value, *K*. This phenomenon is attributed to the probability per unit time of the agent's striking a single viable target per microbe. A delay in reaching such targets may be caused by the need for a disinfectant to first penetrate dried blood, or if dried, bacteria must first be wetted in order for a chemical to enter the cytoplasm. If delay occurs, the rate of death initially will be slower. The time required to destroy a population of microorganisms depends on the initial number of viable cells, on the particular type of cells, and on the agent (Fig 4–1).

TABLE 4–1. LEVELS OF DISINFECTION

	Bacteria					Viruses	
	Gram positive	*Gram negative*	Mycobacterium tuberculosis	*Spores*	Fungi	*Lipid*	*Nonlipid*
High	+	+	+	+	+	+	+
Intermediate	+	+	+	−	+	+	+
Low	+	+	−	−	±	+	−

Modified from Spaulding EH. Chemical disinfection and antisepsis in the hospital. J Hosp Res. *1972;9:5–31.*

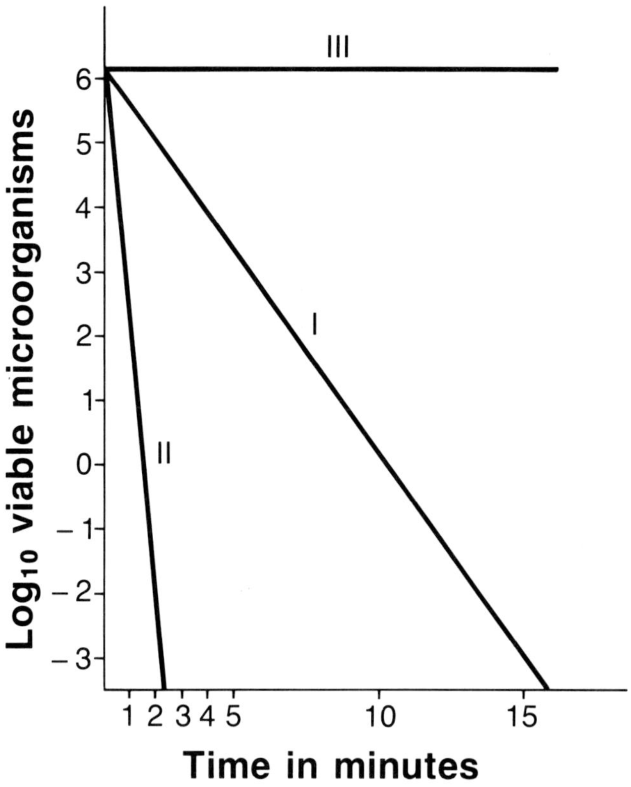

Figure 4–1. A sample of bacterial spores is reduced from 10^6 to 10^{-3} in 15 minutes by dry heat (I). These same spores are not affected by alcohol (III). In contrast, a culture of vegetative bacteria exposed 2 minutes to alcohol is reduced 9 logs. (II)

These conditions must be taken into consideration when evaluating antimicrobial agents, since the most resistant pathogens are no less dangerous than the most sensitive. Obviously, the time of exposure to an agent can be very critical.

A major influence on the effectiveness of an antimicrobial agent is the composition of the environment in or on which the agent is used, especially the presence of organic matter. Organic matter may (1) neutralize the agent or (2) shelter the microbe from the agent. Many chemical agents act by combining with organic components of the organisms, such as proteins. If extraneous organic material is present, it may react with the agent first, neutralizing it and reducing its effective concentration. This is especially a problem with -static agents. In addition, organisms embedded in organic masses, such as coagulated blood, tissues, or dental plaque, may be sheltered from both chemical and physical agents, since the agent cannot readily penetrate the organic mass to reach the microorganisms.

As with other chemical reactions, the antimicrobial process is affected by temperature and the physical state of the agent. The speed of the reaction increases with increasing temperature up to a point at which the heat destroys the antimicrobial agent. Liquids or gases energized with heat react faster with their microbial targets. Agents in the gaseous phase also have the advantage over liquids of ready exposure to some surfaces not accessible to liquids, for example, hinges of scissors.

In general, the more concentrated or intense the agent, the more effective it is. There are exceptions, such as alcohol, which is less effective at 100% than when diluted with water, or formalin-isopropanol, which is equally effective over a broad range of concentrations.

The effectiveness of an antimicrobial agent is determined not only by the factors mentioned but also by the kind of microbes that are to be killed. Bacterial endospores are much more resistant to heat and chemical agents than are other cellular forms. In general, resistance decreases in this order: hydrophilic viruses, fungal spores, bacterial vegetative cells, and lipophilic viruses. The killing of selected bacterial endospores is considered to be the index of sterilization.

MECHANISMS OF ANTIMICROBIAL ACTION

It is important to have some concept of how microorganisms are inhibited or killed, since knowledge of the mode of action of a particular agent may make it possible to decide how best to apply it. The various antimicrobial agents obstruct critical metabolic functions by inhibiting or destroying essential microbial components. Antimicrobial mechanisms include

- Protein denaturation: Proteins function as both structural units and enzymes, and agents such as alcohol and heat may denature them by disrupting the tertiary structure of these molecules.
- Damage to cell membranes: The cell membrane maintains the integrity of the cytoplasmic constituents and controls the selective transport of nutrients into the cell. Damage to the membrane by agents such as detergents usually results in death.
- Inhibition of enzymes: Enzymes may be inactivated without being denatured. Antimicrobial agents such as mercury may bind at or near the active site on an enzyme, rendering the enzyme inactive.
- Alteration of nucleic material: Much of the killing action of alkylation or radiation is due to the inhibition of replication of the nucleic acids that comprise the genetic material of the cell.

Although these various modes of action are presented as separate entities, any particular agent probably will act through a combination of these. For example, protein denaturation could affect structural components, membranes, and enzymes alike.

ANTIMICROBIAL PHYSICAL AGENTS

There is a broad variation in types of antimicrobial physical agents. Most involve heat, whereas others use the opposite extreme, cold. Filtration, radiation, and ultrasonic vibrations also are employed in controlling microorganisms. The most commonly used sterilizing agents are found among the antimicrobial physical agents.

Steam

The autoclave, or modifications of it, is the most commonly used method of sterilization in microbiology and dentistry. Basically, it is a pressure cooker in which the increased pressure allows the steam to attain the higher temperature needed to kill bacterial endospores. The sterilizing temperature and time of exposure can be varied (Table 4–2), but the most common standard conditions used with autoclaves are 121°C at 15 pounds pressure for at least 15 minutes. The time will vary depending on the bulk, nature, and packaging of the materials to be sterilized. The moist heat kills by denaturation of proteins.

Examples of items sterilized in the autoclave include microbial culture media and other heat-stable solutions, heavy duty rubber gloves, rust-resistant instruments, heat-resistant plastics, dressings, and some handpieces. Rust can be retarded by adding agents such as sodium nitrite, or by prepackaging in paper bags.

Chemiclave is a trade name for a dental office autoclave that uses chemical vapors rather than steam as the killing medium. The chemicals include alcohols, ketones, and formaldehyde. Standard conditions for use are given as 132°C for 20 minutes, but they may be varied over a limited range. The major advantage of the Chemiclave is that it is less corrosive to some instruments.

Pasteurization

Pasteurization is a disinfecting method. It is intended to kill the pathogenic bacteria that may be found in raw milk. Pasteurization does not sterilize, nor does it kill all of the vegetative forms in milk. The conditions for pasteurization of milk are 62.9°C for 30 minutes for vat-type pasteurization or 71.5°C for 15 seconds when thin layers of milk are treated. These conditions were established to kill the bacteria that cause Q fever, tuberculosis, and brucellosis. In addition to milk, other food products that are pasteurized include beer, juices, and wines.

Boiling Water

Boiling water is a method of disinfection, but it is not generally recommended for the modern dental operatory and should be used only in emergencies or in primitive areas. Vegetative bacteria and viruses are killed rapidly, but some spores are not affected. Boiling kills by denaturing proteins. The recommended conditions are 10 minutes exposure to actively boiling water.

Dry Heat

Hot air ovens also may be used as sterilizing devices. The standard conditions for sterilizing ovens without forced air are exposure for 1 hour at 170°C or 2 hours at 160°C. Forced air units operating at 191°C achieve sterilization within 6 minutes. It is possible to use higher temperature and reduce the time of exposure, but the increased temperatures also increase the chance of damaging some materials. This method kills microorganisms by coagulation or oxidation of

TABLE 4–2. American Dental Association-APPROVED STERILIZATION METHODS

Characteristic	Steam	Formalin-alcohol	Dry Heat	Ethylene Oxide	Glutaraldehye	Chlorine Dioxide
Activity	Protein denaturation	Alkylation and protein denaturation	Oxidation	Alkylation	Alkylation	Oxidation
Conditions	121°C (250°F) 15 minutes 132°C (270°F) 3–7 minutes	132°C (270°F) 20 minutes	160°C (320°F) 1 hour 191°C (375°F) 6 minutes	Ambient 12 hours	6–10 hours, depending on product	Bactericidal and virucidal 2 minutes; Sporicial 6 hours
Advantages	Speed, penetration	Speed, penetration	Low price, large capacity	No heat damage	No heat damage	Rapid acting, good for plastics
Limitations	Rust, corrosion, heat damage	Heat damage	Heat damage	Very slow	Postexposure handling	Corrosive, cannot be used for metals

Modified from Crawford JJ. Clinical Asepsis in Dentistry. *Mesquite, TX: 1989.*

proteins. Its advantages are that it does not affect many moisture-sensitive compounds and does not rust instruments. It is used to sterilize glassware, syringes, metal instruments, cotton pellets, some powdered chemicals and oil-based compounds, and some handpieces. Crucibles containing glass beads or salt granules heated to around 218°C also have been used to sterilize small dental instruments. The instruments must be immersed for at least 15 seconds.

Incineration. Burning of contaminated cloth, gauze, paper, and organic debris on instruments is an effective method of destroying microorganisms. Incineration, or flaming (oxidation), is used to sterilize bacterial inoculating loops and needles and dental broaches and burrs. The metal must be brought to red heat to insure sterilization.

Desiccation. Desiccation, or drying, cannot be relied on as a means of destroying microorganisms. Some microorganisms, such as those causing syphilis, are very sensitive to desiccation, but sporeformers can survive for years in the dried state. In addition, even microbes that are usually destroyed by desiccation may survive for weeks if they are embedded in tissue, pus, or other organic material.

Low Temperature. Low temperature (<4°C) is considered to be a -static agent. It usually is not microbicidal and often is used to preserve microbial cultures in the laboratory. Cold is used primarily to retard the growth of microorganisms in food or biologic products. Low temperature retards microbial metabolism.

Radiation

Ultraviolet rays and gamma rays are the two most commonly used forms of antimicrobial radiation. Ultraviolet rays (220 to 300 nm) have very low penetrating power. They cannot penetrate many materials, including glass, plastics, and cloth. They are effective against microorganisms in the air, in liquids, and on exposed surfaces. Their antimicrobial mechanism of action is a result of their ionizing activity. Ultraviolet rays produce linkages between adjacent pyrimidines of DNA, but their mechanism of action on RNA viruses is unknown. Exposure to visible light rays can reverse the -cidal effects of ultraviolet rays through a process called photoreactivation. Ultraviolet germicide lamps are used for disinfecting surfaces and for reducing airborne contamination in hospitals, nurseries, and laboratories.

Gamma rays and x-rays are extremely powerful and, depending on the dose, can penetrate several centimeters. They are sterilizing methods. Irradiation by these methods, however, is difficult to control and is too dangerous to use as an antimicrobial agent in the laboratory or the dental operatory. These forms of radiation kill by ionization of chromosomal materials and are used in industry to sterilize vaccines, heat-sensitive plastic items, pharmaceuticals, and foods.

Filtration

Filtration is a primary method of sterilizing heat-labile solutions. Cellulose acetate or other polymeric membranes are synthesized with special uniform pore sizes. Filters with pore sizes of 0.2 to 0.45 μm are used to remove bacteria. Most viruses can pass through these pores, but under the conditions of preparation and use, there is usually no chance of significant viral contamination.

Other filters also can be used to sterilize or at least reduce the numbers of microorganisms in the air or in gases. Surgical masks are used to block the passage of aerosol-borne bacteria and viruses. So-called clean rooms are maintained free of bacteria by circulating the air through high efficiency particulate air (HEPA) filters. Similar filters are used with laminar airflow laboratory hoods.

Ultrasonic Vibrations

Ultrasonic vibrations have limited antimicrobial activity, but they are useful to remove mechanically microbes or microbe-containing debris from surfaces exposed to the vibrations. The mechanism of action of ultrasonic vibrations is through cavitation. The formation of minute cavities or bubbles within the liquid exerts a disruptive action on the microorganisms or the debris attached. Many cells are resistant to ultrasonic vibrations, and, therefore, this method cannot be used for sterilization or even disinfection. Ultrasonic energy is useful in cleaning devices, and special ultrasonic tanks are available for cleaning instruments and prostheses. One can combine cleansing with disinfection by using a detergent–disinfectant as the sonication medium in the tank.

ANTIMICROBIAL CHEMICAL AGENTS

Antimicrobial chemical agents range from antiseptics to disinfectants to sterilizing agents. There is a wide variety of these agents, and new ones are appearing constantly because industry is trying constantly to produce the ultimate antimicrobial agent for medical and dental use, that is, a nontoxic, noncorrosive, long-lasting, inexpensive, and rapidly acting sterilizing agent. The agents to be described and summarized in Table 4–3 represent some of the more commonly used agents.

Ethylene Oxide

Several chemicals have been used for gaseous sterilization, but ethylene oxide is the only one that is widely used and the only one used in dentistry. This

TABLE 4–3. CHEMICAL AGENTS

Agent	Disinfectant Time (minutes)	Sterilant Time (hours)
Sodium hypochlorite (bleach)	10	—
Chlorine dioxide	2–3[a]	6
Iodophors	10	—
Combination synthetic phenolics	10	—
2% Glutaraldehydes (acidic, neutral, or alkaline)	10–90[a]	10
2% Glutaraldehyde (with phenolic buffer)	10	6

[a]Varies with formulation.

Adapted from ADA Council on Dental Materials, Instruments, and Equipment, ADA Council on Dental Practice, and ADA Council on Dental Therapeutics. J Am Dent Assoc. *1988;116:241.*

agent kills by alkylation of proteins and nucleic acids. The major advantages of ethylene oxide are low temperature, absence of significant moisture, and high penetrating power. Pure ethylene oxide is explosive but is safe when mixed with carbon dioxide. It requires a special chamber and proper ventilating facilities because it is toxic and carcinogenic. Sterilized items must be aerated for several hours before use to allow absorbed gases to escape. Sterilization with ethylene oxide calls for 12 hours exposure at room temperature or 3 hours at 60°C. This agent is used to sterilize instruments, heat-sensitive disposable plastic items, and biologics and drugs.

Aldehydes

Formaldehyde often is used as a preservative, but it is rarely used as a disinfectant because of its irritating and toxic nature. Formaldehyde kills by alkylating proteins and nucleic acids. It has been used for terminal disinfection of contaminated disposable materials and as a component of the chemical solution used in the Chemiclave.

Glutaraldehyde is an agent of choice for disinfecting metal-containing dental instruments, and it also may be used as a sterilizing agent. It kills by alkylation. Glutaraldehyde will disinfect in 10 minutes and will sterilize after 6 to 10 hours immersion at room temperature, depending on the particular formulation (Table 4–3). It has at least two disadvantages. One is that it is toxic and irritating and must be handled with caution, requiring the use of gloves and rinsing of instruments. The second disadvantage is the limited useful life of alkaline glutaraldehyde after activation. These solutions must be discarded within 1 day to 4 weeks after preparation. Glutaraldehyde is used principally for disinfecting and sterilizing instruments and heat-sensitive items.

Chlorine

Chlorine, either in the form of a gas or in certain aqueous formulations, represents one of the most widely used disinfectants. Some chlorine-containing agents are sterilizing. Sodium hypochlorite, chlorine dioxide, and chloramines are among the more commonly used agents in this group. The microbicidal actions of chlorine agents include disruption of the cell membrane and oxidation of critical enzymes. Sodium hypochlorite, the active component of household bleach, is a good disinfectant. Household bleach (5% hypochlorite) diluted 1:10 to 1:100 in water often is used as an antimicrobial and has been recommended for use as a dental surface disinfectant. It kills vegetative bacteria, viruses, and some, if not all, bacterial spores. Hypochlorite is caustic to tissues and to metals. In addition to its use as a surface disinfectant, it also is used to disinfect plastic items.

Chlorine dioxide is a disinfectant and a sterilizing agent. Chlorine dioxide disinfects instruments and surfaces within 3 minutes and sterilizes after 6 hours exposure. It is relatively nontoxic but is corrosive to some metals.

Chloramines are yet another group of chlorine compounds that are used as disinfectants and antiseptics. They do not sterilize. Chloramines are organic compounds in which chlorine replaces a hydrogen atom on an amino group. The chlorine is released slowly from the compound, and thus higher, nontoxic levels of chlorine may be used over a longer period.

Iodine

Iodine is effective against all forms of microorganisms, including spores, and has long been recognized as one of the best antiseptics. It has not yet been accepted as a sterilizing agent. It kills microorganisms rapidly, but its mechanism of action is uncertain. It may act as an oxidizing agent or bind to and inactivate enzymes or other proteins. Tinctures of iodine (2% iodine and 2% sodium iodide) and solutions of molecular iodine were once among the more popular antiseptics but have been replaced by iodophors. Iodophors are organic complexes containing iodine within micellar aggregates of nonionic surface active agents. The surface action improves wetting and aids in penetration through organic matter. Bound iodine is inactive. Water uncouples iodine from the detergent, activating it. At all dilutions, iodophors are less irritating than tinctures, because the concentration of free iodine is considerably less. Iodophors are good antiseptics and disinfectants and are being used increasingly as surface disinfectants and antiseptics in dentistry.

Alcohol

Ethyl and isopropyl alcohols are employed extensively as antiseptics. These agents coagulate proteins, a process that requires water. The most effective concentrations contain from 50% to 70% alcohol. Most commercial preparations are mixtures of approximately 70% alcohol and 30% water. Alcohol also is a lipid solvent, and much of its effectiveness as an antiseptic can be attributed to cleansing action. The antibacterial action of alcohols is very rapid, *Pseudomonas aeruginosa* being destroyed within 15 seconds and *Mycobacterium tuberculosis* within 1 minute. However, the rapid evaporation of alcohol reduces its effectiveness against some microorganisms, and alcohol is not recommended for disinfecting instruments and inanimate surfaces in dentistry.

Phenols

Phenols are strong antimicrobials, but they do not kill endospores. These compounds injure the cell membrane and denature proteins. Two to five percent phenol is used to disinfect sputum and fecal material, and previously this chemical was used to disinfect instruments. Many phenol derivatives have been produced, and the bis-phenols, consisting of two phenolic groups connected by various linkages, are among the more effective. Hexylresorcinol and hexachlorophene are two bis-phenols that have been used in antiseptics and antimicrobial soaps. Phenol and thymol, another phenolic compound, are used in oral antiseptics.

A mixture of *o*-phenylphenol and *o*-benzyl-*p*-chlorophenol has been accepted for use as a dental instrument disinfectant. The mixture is rapid acting and relatively nontoxic.

Biguanides

Chlorhexidine is the chemical name for the biguanide that has received the most attention in dentistry. It was and still is used as an antiseptic and surgical scrub, but its broad spectrum and low toxicity suggested that it would also be a good oral antiseptic. The mechanism of action is not known, but it may affect cell membranes at low concentrations and precipitate proteins at higher concentrations. It does not kill spores and is of limited use against viruses.

Chlorhexidine mouthwashes are effective in preventing gingivitis. This is primarily because of the compound's residual activity. Chlorhexidine adsorbs to enamel and the salivary pellicle on the tooth's surface, where it still retains antimicrobial activity. This residual effect is a major advantage over the active agents in other mouthwashes that are rapidly washed out of the oral cavity. Chlorhexidine has an unpleasant taste and may cause discoloration of the gingiva and the tooth's surface. However, biguanide analogs are being studied with the aim of developing an agent that retains the antimicrobial properties while reducing the adverse effects.

Surface Active Agents

There are several groups of surface active agents with varying degrees of antimicrobial activity. Soaps, sodium or potassium esters of fatty acids, possess only weak antimicrobial activity. They act primarily as cleansing agents that remove microorganisms from skin and inanimate surfaces by emulsifying the organisms and other organic debris. They are very effective cleansing agents, and, in some cases, their antimicrobial potential has been supplemented by addition of other antibacterial agents.

Nonionic and anionic detergents are weak antimicrobials, about as effective as soaps, but some cationic detergents possess strong antimicrobial properties. Quaternary ammonium compounds, the predominant cationic detergents, are used as antiseptics and disinfectants. Their mechanism of action is primarily disruption of lipoprotein membranes, and, therefore, they are effective against vegetative bacteria and enveloped viruses. The quaternary ammonium compounds do not kill tuberculosis bacteria and spores, and they are easily neutralized by extraneous organic matter. Therefore, although they may be used as disinfectants in other areas, quaternary ammonium compounds are not acceptable as dental disinfectants. They are, however, widely used in mouthwashes and antiseptics.

Miscellaneous Agents

Oxidizing Agents. Oxidizing agents were once popular as antimicrobial agents, and they are still used by some clinicians. Hydrogen peroxide and zinc peroxide are two of the latter. The peroxides exert their antimicrobial activity by reacting with sulfhydryl groups on enzymes.

Heavy Metals. Most of the heavy metals possess antimicrobial properties. Inorganic or organic mercury or silver compounds have been the most commonly used heavy metal agents. Although these compounds may precipitate proteins at high concentrations, the antimicrobial effect of mercury is primarily that of binding to sulfhydryl groups to inhibit enzyme activity. The bacteriostatic activity is easily reversed by organic compounds such as blood and other tissue fluids. Silver is a -cidal agent because it irreversibly denatures proteins. The use of heavy metals has been largely displaced by alcohols and iodine compounds.

Dyes. Many dyes have antibacterial activity. Crystal violet is effective against gram-positive bacteria at very low concentrations, and for this reason, it has been incorporated into selective media used to isolate gram-negative bacteria (especially enteric bacteria). Trypan blue and crystal violet are used as inhibitory agents in mitis-salivarius agar, a selective medium used for isolating oral streptococci. The mechanisms of action of these dyes are not known.

INFECTION CONTROL

As noted previously, the dental practitioner must have a good understanding of antimicrobial agents and their uses because both dental personnel and their patients are at risk of contracting infectious diseases in the operatory. The application of this knowledge comes under the heading of infection control. Although infection control has been practiced in dentistry to some extent for many years, the need for it has been emphasized dramatically by two recent events.

The first event was the recognition that hepatitis B is a significant occupational hazard for dental personnel. Not only can the disease itself be very debilitating, but also, if the dentist becomes a carrier, it may prevent the dentist from practicing dentistry. The second event was the tremendous public and professional reaction to the hazards of AIDS, both real and perceived. This has resulted in the formulation by the Centers for Disease Control and the American Dental Association of even stricter infection control guidelines.

Infections in the Dental Operatory

Dental procedures can sometimes result in disease. These diseases may be autogenous infections or cross-infections. Autogenous infections are those caused by the microorganisms that the patient carries on or in his or her own body. Many of the procedures in dentistry are invasive and open the tissues to infection by oral organisms. These microbes usually are harmless within the oral cavity but may cause disease if they enter the tissues. Examples of autogenous infections include bacterial endocarditis and some oral abscesses. Many autogenous infections can be prevented by peroperative prophylactic therapy. Endocarditis is prevented by the use of antibiotics, whereas the frequency of abscesses may be reduced by applying an antiseptic, such as iodophor, to the mucous membranes that might be punctured or cut. These are relatively simple but effective infection control procedures.

Cross-infections are caused by infectious agents that are transmitted among dental personnel, patients, and the environment. The transfer of disease may be from patient to dentist or from dentist to patient. For example, hepatitis B is an occupational hazard for dental personnel. On the other hand, there are several documented cases of dentists transmitting hepatitis B to patients, sometimes with fatal results. However, *M. tuberculosis* is more resistant to chemicals than hepatitis B virus, and this pathogen serves as the benchmark for disinfection.

The most important route of transmission from the patient to the dentist is the exposure of the practitioner's unprotected broken or abraded skin or mucous membranes to blood or saliva contaminated with occult blood or gingival fluid. Needlesticks or cuts with sharp instruments are common occurrences among dental health professionals. Salivary or spatter transmission of many blood-borne diseases, for example, hepatitis B, herpes, or respiratory diseases, such as influenza, to unprotected mucous membranes of the eyes and mouth is another important route of infection of these diseases. Dentist to patient transfer via the same routes as described also occurs. Still another route of transmission can occur via inanimate objects (fomites) touched before, during, or after appointments. Patient to patient transmission occurs largely due to improper recirculation of instruments and inadequate operatory hygiene.

A number of variables affect cross-infection. Included among these are the etiologic agent, the routes of infection, and survival time in the environment. A summary of these variables is shown in Table 4–4. Other important variables include the use of appropriate barrier techniques, such as gloves, masks, and glasses, and application of proper sterilization and disinfection procedures. A last set of variables that affect cross-infection, and which must be considered, is contamination from environmental sources, such as water lines and defective air conditioning systems, especially the filters. The important concept is that cross-infection from all etiologic agents can be reduced or eliminated by blocking the routes of transmission with barrier techniques and appropriate disinfection and sterilization procedures.

Universal Precautions

The unreliability of medical histories and physical examinations to identify patients infected with blood-borne pathogens, such as human immunodeficiency virus (HIV) or hepatitis B virus, stimulated the Centers for Disease Control in 1985 to formulate a series of guidelines termed Universal Precautions. These were further expanded and amplified in 1986 and 1987. Under this concept, body fluids, for example, blood, amniotic, pericardial, pleural, synovial, cerebrospinal, semen, and vaginal fluids, or any body fluids visibly contaminated with blood, are considered infectious even when the infectious state of the patient is un-

TABLE 4–4. ROUTES OF TRANSMISSION OF CROSS-INFECTION

Agent	Sources	Estimated Survival at Ambient Temperature
Respiratory viruses	Secretions, saliva	Hours
Varicella-Zoster virus	Saliva, vesicles	Hours
Mumps virus	Saliva, secretions	Hours
Herpes simplex viruses 1, 2	Saliva, vesicles	Minutes
Hepatitis virus A	Saliva, feces, blood	Weeks
Hepatitis virus B	Saliva, blood	Weeks
Hepatitis virus non A/non B	Saliva, blood	Weeks
Epstein-Barr virus	Saliva	Seconds
Cytomegalovirus	Saliva, blood	Seconds or minutes
Human immunodeficiency viruses (HIV)	Blood	Seconds
Mycobacterium tuberculosis	Saliva, sputum	Days to weeks
Staphylococcus aureus	Exudates, skin, saliva	Days
Streptococcus pyogenes	Saliva, secretions	Hours to days
Mycoplasma pnuemoniae	Saliva, secretions	Seconds or minutes
Treponema pallidum	Contact with lesions	Seconds
Streptococcus mutans	Saliva	Hours(?)

Modified from Crawford JJ. Clinical Asepsis in Dentistry. *Mesquite, TX: 1989.*

known. Appropriate barrier techniques must be used by all health care personnel who might come in contact with those body fluids. In the case of dental personnel, blood, saliva, and gingival fluid from all patients must be considered infectious. Appropriate barrier techniques are discussed later in this chapter.

Sterilization

The American Dental Association approves six sterilants: steam, chemical vapor, dry heat, chlorine dioxide ethylene oxide, and glutaraldehyde-containing liquid (Table 4–2). Each has its own set of advantages and disadvantages, a fact that accounts for the use of multiple agents in numerous large institutions. In private practice, steam, chemical vapor, or dry heat frequently is supplemented by glutaraldehyde-containing liquid. The specified times for procedures involving heat are the stated number of minutes at the cited temperature of the least accessible part of the load. Thus, for example, it will take longer for the center of a heavy load of instruments in an office model autoclave to reach a sterilizing temperature than the surface of that load. Sterilization or disinfection of reusable items can occur only if the agent has free access to all surfaces. Blood, saliva, and other debris act as barriers to the penetration of a sterilant, and these must be removed before the sterilization cycle is initiated. Water, too, must be removed because its evaporation tends to cool instrument surfaces. Water protects spores from the lethal effects of dry heat. In the case of ethylene oxide sterilization, water converts that chemical to the harmless ethylene glycol.

Sterilization Monitoring. In order to determine that the requisite conditions for sterilization are present, that is, that the sterilization equipment is operating properly and the sterilant is reaching all parts of the load in an adequate amount of time, biologic indicators (BIs) are included on a regular basis. These consist of paper strips onto which spores of *Bacillus subtilis* or *Bacillus stearothermophilus* have been adsorbed. Sterilization conditions are considered to be met when all spores on a BI fail to germinate and proliferate in recovery medium. Commercially available BIs carrying *B. subtilis* are used to monitor dry heat and ethylene oxide. BIs containing *B. stearothermophilus* are used for steam and formalin-alcohol vapor. The rationale for using different species is to match that organism most resistant to a particular process.

Packaging. Instruments can be packaged in paper, nylon, cloth, or metal cassettes. However, each material has its own advantages and disadvantages. As an example, tightly closed metal containers are useful only for dry heat sterilization, because of the transmission of the energy through metal. Only a few modern-age plastics can withstand dry heat. The most important principle in packaging is that the material to be used allow free access of the agent. The advantages of packaging sets of instruments are both organizational and hygienic. Practitioners usually work with defined sets of instruments, and packaging as a unit maintains the aseptic integrity of these sets.

Operatory Asepsis

Barriers and Surface Disinfection. Viruses and microbes on exposed surfaces of nontransportable items can be eliminated or reduced in number in two ways: inactivation by chemicals or removal by wiping. The two can be combined, whereby surfaces are wiped vigorously with a disinfectant-soaked sponge or towel. Alternatively, surfaces may be sprayed with the disinfectant, using a manual spray bottle, followed by wiping. All surfaces that must be contacted directly or indirectly must be disinfected. A sample list of these is shown in Table 4–5.

Special care should be taken with critical surfaces that come into direct or close contact with the mouth but that are not sterilized. Three-way syringes, hose couplings, and heat-sensitive handpieces fall into this category. In addition, bench surfaces should be disinfected. If possible, all surfaces to be contacted should be covered with transparent plastic wrap.

Ideally, agents for surface disinfection kill all vegetative bacteria and viruses (including *M. tuberculosis* and HBV). Moreover, such agents must be nonirritating, nonallergenic, harmless to cloth, and noncorrosive. In addition, the ideal surface germicide should have a long shelf life and be relatively inexpensive. From the standpoint of microbial destruction, four agents are effective: formaldehyde, glutaraldehyde, chlorine, and iodine (Table 4–3). On consideration of other criteria, however, only iodine approaches the ideal. It should be noted that alcohol, aqueous phenol, and quaternary ammonium compounds are not recommended for surface disinfection.

Barrier Techniques

Handcleaning. The transmission of pathogens via contaminated hands is a major route of cross-infection in dentistry. Skin cracks and abrasions can harbor or allow entrance of many pathogens. Blood or other infectious materials can be harbored under the fingernails for several days.

Efficient handcleaning with an acceptable antiseptic is the initial procedure and one of the most important techniques that dental personnel must use to prevent cross-infection. This will eliminate transient microbial flora and reduce the permanent flora. Effective agents include iodine surgical scrubs and such agents as chlorhexidine. The latter is more effective against gram-positive and gram-negative bacteria. Its activity against mycobacteria and hepatitis B is negligible. Antiseptics must be nontoxic, nonallergenic, and preferably germicidal rather than bacteriostatic. Hands should be washed thoroughly before patient treatment, between patients, and before putting on gloves.

TABLE 4–5. EXAMPLES OF OPERATORY SURFACES THAT SHOULD BE DISINFECTED

Drawer pulls
Hose ends
Couplings to saliva evacuator and ejector tips
Handheld cuspidor
Lamp switch and handles
Chair armrests
Supports for handpieces and air-water syringes

Gloving. Gloves should be worn for all procedures. This is underscored by the fact that hepatitis B not only is an occupational hazard to dental health care personnel but also can be transmitted to patient populations. A common factor in each of the several outbreaks of hepatitis B in dental patients was the lack of gloving by the dental practitioners.

Only two guidelines are suggested.

1. The practitioner may choose the type of glove best suited to his or her own needs and practice.
2. Gloves should be discarded after each patient and not reused.

Masks and Protective Eyewear. Masks provide filtration of aerosol and spatter-borne bacteria and viruses. They should be worn at any time when an aerosol generating procedure is used, for example, the high speed drill. In addition, they should be worn at times when respiratory type diseases are prevalent in the community or when either the patient or the dentist may have symptoms of a communicable disease—sore throat, sneezing, or cough.

Glasses should be worn to protect from infectious organisms that are carried in aerosols or spatter. They also provide a barrier against physical injury by solid particles.

Disinfection of Intraoral Devices

Dental laboratory technicians are subject to the same infectious hazards as are dental personnel in the operatory. Impressions made in the operatory are transported to the laboratory for casting. Following this, they are returned to the dentist for fitting. Thus, the possibility of cross-infection exists at several points. Initially, they can be contaminated with saliva from the patient. At the laboratory, the appliances may become cross-contaminated from other oral devices present in the laboratory that came from other dentists. This may, in turn, provide a focus of cross-infection to dental personnel in the original setting. In view of this, special precautions must be taken, with the underlying strategy being physical isolation of a device, coupled with disinfection.

Alginate and reversible hydrocolloid impressions may be distorted by prolonged immersion in the disinfectant. The recommended disinfectant in most cases for such devices is an iodophore in water. Other devices, for example, removable prosthodontic and orthodontic appliances, also can be treated with an iodophore.

SUMMARY

Infection control is critical to good dental practice. To this end, it is essential that the practitioner not only understand the concepts involved in the development and applications of antimicrobial physical and chemical agents but also know how to use them properly in the dental operatory. Practical applications of infection control are more fully described in several of the Suggested Readings.

SUGGESTED READINGS

ADA Council on Dental Therapeutics. Section I: General principles of sterilization and disinfection of dental interest. Section II: Therapeutic agents. In: *Accepted Dental Therapeutics*, 40th ed. Chicago: American Dental Association, 1984.

ADA Council on Dental Materials, Instruments, and Equipment, ADA Council on Dental Practice, and ADA Council on Dental Therapeutics. Infection control recommendations for the dental office and the dental laboratory. *J Am Dent Assoc.* 1988;116:241.

Block S. *Disinfection, Sterilization & Preservation*, 3rd ed. Philadelphia: Lea & Febiger; 1983.

Centers for Disease Control. Guidelines for prevention of transmission of human immunodeficiency virus and hepatitis B virus to health care and public safety workers. *MMWR.* 1989;38:S-6.

Centers for Disease Control. Hepatitis B among dental patients in Indiana. *MMWR.* 1985;34:73.

Centers for Disease Control. ACIP: Update on hepatitis B prevention. *MMWR.* 1987;36:253.

Crawford JJ. *Clinical Asepsis in Dentistry.* Mesquite, TX: 1989.

Mitchell R, et al. The use (and re-use) of operatory gloves in dental practice: Decreasing the risk of infection. *Oral Surg.* 1985;75:25.

Petit H, Kolstad R. Disinfection of removable appliances. *J Clin Orthodont.* 1985;19:293–295.

Runnells RR. *Infection Control in the Former Wet Finger Environment.* Salt Lake City: IC Publications; 1987.

CHAPTER 5

Antibiotics and Chemotherapy

Norman P. Willett and James Crawford

INTRODUCTION

CELL WALL INHIBITORS
- Penicillins
- Extended Spectrum Penicillins
- Cephalosporins
- Other Cell Wall Inhibitors

INHIBITORS OF PROTEIN SYNTHESIS
- Macrolide Antibiotics
- Lincomycin and Clindamycin
- Aminoglycosides
- Tetracyclines
- Chloramphenicol

ANTIBIOTICS WITH OTHER MODES OF ACTION
- Rifampin
- Synthetic Antimicrobials: Sulfonamides, Isoniazid, Nitrofurans, and Nalidixic Acid

ANTIFUNGAL AGENTS

RESISTANCE
- Nongenetic Resistance
- Genetic Resistance
- Biochemical Mechanisms of Resistance

USE OF ANTIBIOTICS FOR ORAL INFECTIONS

DANGERS OF INDISCRIMINATE USE OF ANTIBIOTICS

MEASUREMENT OF MICROBIAL SUSCEPTIBILITY TO ANTIBIOTICS

ORAL ASPECTS

SUGGESTED READINGS

INTRODUCTION

The selective inhibition of microorganisms by chemotherapeutic agents ranks among the greatest discoveries in medicine and follows as a logical consequence of the germ theory of disease. The clinical usefulness of chemotherapeutic agents is directly related to selective toxicity. Selective toxicity is based on certain unique features or structures of the microbe that set it apart from the host cell. Thus, the antibiotic must act selectively on these unique microbial factors while not affecting host cells. This contrasts with the action of disinfectants, which may harm the host as much as the microbe.

The significance of antibiotic use for the dental profession is manifested by the increasing evidence of antibiotic-resistant orofacial infections and appropriate use of antimicrobials as prophylactic measures when treating patients with heart valve abnormalities. The continued proliferation of new antimicrobial agents, each of which claims to be more effective, adds to the confusion of the medical and dental practitioner as to the best agent to use. The ever increasing menace of multiple drug resistance and the various adverse immunologic manifestations caused by antibiotics have become some of the most important public health problems facing medicine and dentistry today.

Chemotherapeutic agents may be broadly divided into three categories; antibiotics, semisynthetic antibiotics, and synthetic antimicrobial chemotherapeutic agents. Although a number of definitions of the term antibiotic have been suggested, the most commonly accepted is that an antibiotic is a chemical compound usually produced by or derived from microorganisms, which is capable in small concentrations of inhibiting the life processes of some microbes.

It is useful to examine each section of this definition as a basis for discussion later in the chapter. Chemical compound implies that antibiotics have a definite organic chemical structure, and, indeed, we shall see as we progress that they can be classified according to their structures, which in turn have significance in regard to their biologic properties. The fact that it is produced by or derived from microorganisms excludes natural substances of plant or animal origin that, although they may have antimicrobial effects, are not true antibiotics. Although three quarters of the antibiotics are produced by members of the bacterial order Actinomycetes, other bacteria and fungi produce clinically useful antibiotics as well. In fact, perhaps the best known of all antibiotics, Penicillin G, is produced by a fungus, *Penicillium chrysogenum,* which is related to the green molds that grow commonly on the foods in our refrigerators. Activity in small concentrations eliminates the primary metabolites, such as organic acids or alcohol, that are active in high concentrations. The inhibition of life processes, such as protein synthesis or cell wall metabolism, represents the original antagonistic effects of these compounds. In order for an antibiotic to be clinically useful, it obviously must be selectively toxic for the suspected pathogen without injuring the host cell.

Synthetic antimicrobial chemotherapeutic agents are similar to antibiotics, but they are manufactured from other chemicals rather than being produced by microorganisms. The term semisynthetic is usually applied to penicillins and cephalosporins and refers to those antibiotics that may be produced by living organisms but are then modified chemically. The development of semisynthetic penicillins and cephalosporins has led to improved modified biologic and chemical properties, such as expanded spectra, stability to acid or β-lactamases, and improved pharmacokinetic properties, for example, absorption and decreased binding to blood proteins.

The ideal antibiotic should also possess a number of other biologic, chemical, and physical properties. These are listed in Table 5–1. It should be noted that over the 40 years that span the antibiotic era, although approximately 3000 antibiotics have been isolated and described, only 300 to 350 have been potentially useful. Of these, 100 to 150 are in active use, and 15 to 20 of these have achieved the greatest clinical success.

The mechanism of action of chemotherapeutic agents on microbial cells can affect a number of widely divergent processes important to cell metabolism and integrity. These are listed in Table 5–2, along with examples of chemotherapeutic agents that produce their antimicrobial effect by that particular action. These are grouped and discussed subsequently according to their mode of action.

TABLE 5–1. IDEAL PROPERTIES OF AN ANTIBIOTIC FROM A MEDICAL POINT OF VIEW

Water Soluble
Selectively toxic for microorganisms without injuring host
Active at physiologic pH
Nonallergenic
Susceptible organisms should not develop resistance
Administration in large doses without producing undesirable side effects
Bactericidal rather than bacteriostatic
Should remain stable and active at bactericidal levels when present in body
Activity should not be reduced by serum or pus

CELL WALL INHIBITORS

Penicillins

Penicillin is not a single substance but a family of closely related entities that share a common nucleus and ring structure but differ in the nature of the side chain that is attached to the nucleus (Fig 5–1). The nucleus of the molecule (6-aminopenicillanic acid) consists of a β-lactam and a thiazolidine ring. Derivatives, both natural and semisynthetic, are made by substitution of the 6-amino group of the β-lactam

TABLE 5–2. MODE OF ACTION OF CHEMOTHERAPEUTIC AGENTS

Mode of Action	Examples of Chemotherapeutic Agents
Inhibitors of cell wall synthesis	Penicillins, cephalosporins, vancomycin, bacitracin
Inhibitors of protein synthesis	
Affect transduction, bind to 30S ribosome subunit of 70S ribosome	Streptomycin, kanamycin, neomycin, gentamicin
Inhibits aminoacyl RNA binding	Tetracycline
Affect translocation, bind to 50S ribosome subunit of 70S ribosome	Chloramphenicol, erythromycin, lincomycin
Inhibitors of transcription and replication and transcription of genetic material	Rifampicin, nalidixic acid
Inhibitors of cell membrane function	Amphotericin B, nystatin, colistin
Antimetabolites	Sulfonamides, trimethoprim, 5-fluocytosine

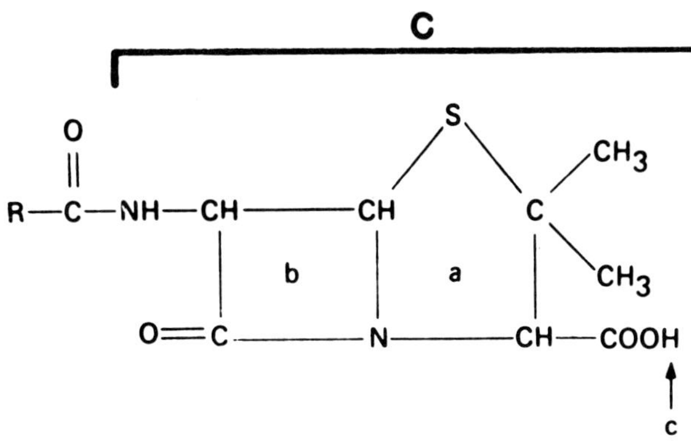

a thiazolidine ring
b β-lactam ring
c 6-amino penicillanic acid nucleus (6 APA)
R side chain

Figure 5–1. Structure of a typical penicillin.

ring, usually via the amide group. In the case of penicillin G, the side chain is a benzyl group. Modification or substitution of this group for other side chains will lead to changes in the biologic or clinical properties of the antibiotic.

The spectrum of an antibiotic refers to its range of activity against different species of microorganisms. Pencillin G is generally accepted to have a narrow spectrum. However, it should be remembered that the descriptions narrow and wide are used only in a comparative sense.

Penicillin G is generally active against most gram-positive cocci, such as staphylococci, streptococci, and pneumococci, but not against enterococci or β-lactamase-producing staphylococci. In addition, it is active against certain gram-negative cocci, such as gonococci and meningococci. Other organisms sensitive to penicillin G include gram-positive rods, such as *Corynebacteria* and *Clostridia,* spirochetes, and actinomycetes. Although penicillin G is effective against many bacteria, it still possesses several disadvantages. It cannot be taken orally because gastric acid inactivates it by hydrolyzing the β-lactam linkage. Second, the emergence of staphylococci that produced hydrolytic enzymes (penicillinases or β-lactamases) to attack the β-lactam linkage rendered penicillin G useless for treating such staphylococcal infections. A third disadvantage to penicillin G is that a small percentage of the population, approximately 5%, is extremely hypersensitive to the action of the antibiotic. Finally, with the exception of certain oropharyngeal strains of *Bacteroides,* penicillin G has little or no activity against gram-negative rods, the main etiologic agents for a number of serious gastrointestinal and urinary tract infections. All of these disadvantages stimulated the search for newer penicillins or β-lactam antibiotics.

Substitution of a phenoxymethyl group for the benzyl group led to the development of penicillin V. Because the addition of this group stabilized the β-lactam linkage in the presence of acid, this penicillin could be taken orally. However, the other disadvantages persisted, including sensitivity to β-lactamases. In addition, although the spectrum of penicillin V was the same as that of penicillin G, the phenoxymethyl group decreased the relative biologic potency of the antibiotic as compared to penicillin G.

Isolation of the penicillin nucleus 6-aminopenicillanic acid in 1959 provided the impetus for development of numerous semisynthetic penicillins that minimized the disadvantages of penicillins G and V. Six-aminopenicillanic acid is produced by hydrolytic enzymes that remove the side chain from penicillin G. Different side chains could then be substituted chemically on the nucleus, modifying the biologic, chemical, and physiologic properties of the original antibiotic. Examples of these semisynthetic penicillins and their biologic and chemical properties are shown in Table 5–3.

The prototype of these semisynthetic penicillins was methicillin, which is resistant to β-lactamase and, therefore, useful in the treatment of life-threatening staphylococcal infections. Acid lability of methicillin, however, necessitates parenteral administration. In addition, its overall antibacterial activity was reduced drastically as compared to penicillin G.

Substitution of isoxazolyl derivatives as side chains on the 6 APA nucleus led to the development

TABLE 5–3. SEMISYNTHETIC PENICILLINS AND SELECTED BIOLOGIC AND CHEMICAL PROPERTIES

	Generic name	Biologic/Chemical Properties
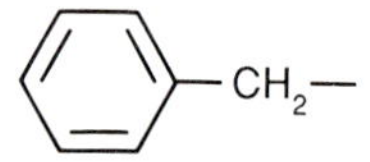	Benzylpenicillin (penicillin G)	Narrow spectrum, acid labile, β-lactamase labile
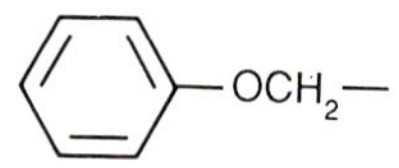	Phenoxymethylpenicillin (penicillin V)	Narrow spectrum, acid stable, β-lactamase labile
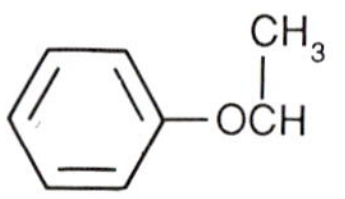	Phenethicillin	Narrow spectrum, acid stable, β-lactamase labile
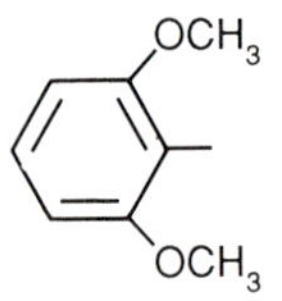	Methicillin	Narrow spectrum, acid labile, β-lactamase stable
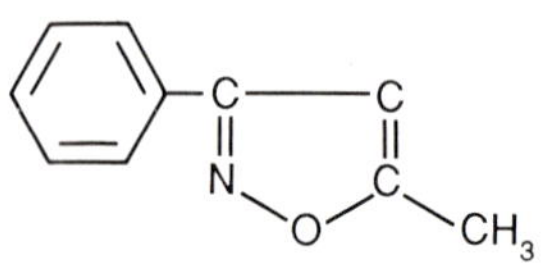	Oxacillin	Narrow spectrum, acid stable, β-lactamase stable
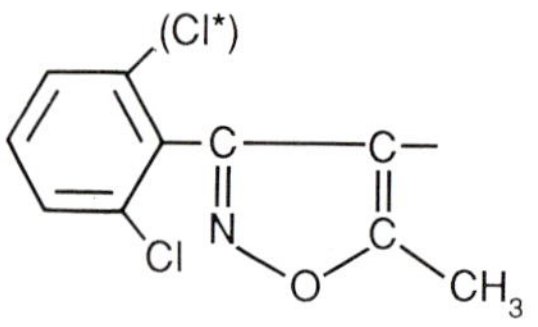	Cloxacillin (*dicloxacillin)	Narrow spectrum, acid stable, β-lactamase stable
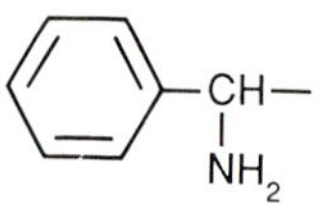	Ampicillin	Extended spectrum, acid stable, β-lactamase labile
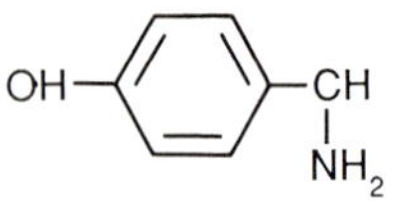	Amoxicillin	Extended spectrum, acid stable, β-lactamase labile
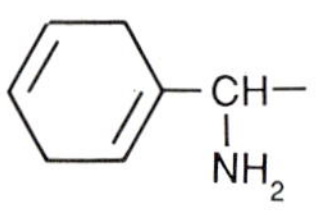	Epicillin	Extended spectrum, acid stable, β-lactamase labile
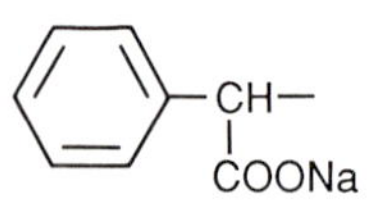	Carbenicillin	Active against *Pseudomonas* and other gram-negative bacilli, acid labile, β-lactamase labile

of oxacillin, cloxacillin, and dicloxacillin, which are stable to acid and to β-lactamase.

Extended Spectrum Penicillins. The increasing public health importance of urinary and gastrointestinal tract infections led scientists to attempt to develop penicillins with activity against gram-negative bacilli. This was accomplished by the addition of an amino group to the benzyl ring of penicillin G, resulting in ampicillin. Ampicillin has the distinct advantages that it can be given orally, that is, it is stable to acid, it has an extended spectrum against the gram-negative etiologic agents causing the diseases mentioned, and its antibacterial activity approaches that of penicillin G. Additional aminopenicillins include amoxycillin and hetacillin.

The disadvantage for these antibiotics is that they are susceptible to attack by β-lactamases and they are not active against *Pseudomonas,* an important nosocomial (hospital-acquired) pathogen and a colonizer of burn tissue.

Although carbenicillin, the carboxy derivative of benzylpenicillin, is active against *Pseudomonas* and selected strains of *Proteus* and *Serratia*, it is less active against most other gram-negative and gram-positive organisms normally included in the spectrum of ampicillin. It is acid labile, and must be given parenterally. It is also destroyed by β-lactamases of gram-positive and gram-negative organisms.

Additional expanded spectrum penicillins active against *Pseudomonas* and other gram-negative infections include piperacillin, mezlocillin, and ticarcillin. Piperacillin, which is a derivative of ampicillin, has increased activity over ampicillin against *Pseudomonas* and *Klebsiella pneumoniae*, which is most likely due to its greater ability to penetrate the outer membrane of these organisms and bind to their characteristic penicillin-binding proteins (PBPs). However, reports of the emergence of resistance against these antibiotics already have appeared in the literature.

Hypersensitivity. Penicillins are the least toxic among the antibiotics. However, because of their allergenic properties, 5 to 10% of the population are subject to hypersensitivity reactions. These range from very severe reactions, such as anaphylactic shock, which has been estimated to cause as much as 300 deaths per year, to less severe reactions, such as fever and hives.

Penicillins are not immunogenic in themselves because their molecular weight is less than 1000. However, the degradation products of penicillins act as haptens and form firm covalent bonds with plasma proteins. The most important of these degradation products include penicillanic acid and its derivatives and penicillamine. A typical reaction illustrating the formation of one of these complexes is shown in Fig. 5–2.

The 6-aminopenicillanic (6 APA) nucleus common to all penicillins is the portion of the molecule involved with immunologic reactivity. Therefore, modifications in the side chain do not significantly decrease hypersensitivity, and complete cross-reactivity between all penicillins is observed. Individuals may become sensitized by penicillins in food or milk or by previous administration of the drug. Parenteral administration is more likely to induce a severe hypersensitivity reaction than is oral administration. Detection of hypersensitivity to penicillins can be carried out using the reagent, penicilloyl poly-D-lysine. Use of this nonimmunogenic compound has eliminated the risks associated with previous skin tests, which used either penicillin or one of its degradation products.

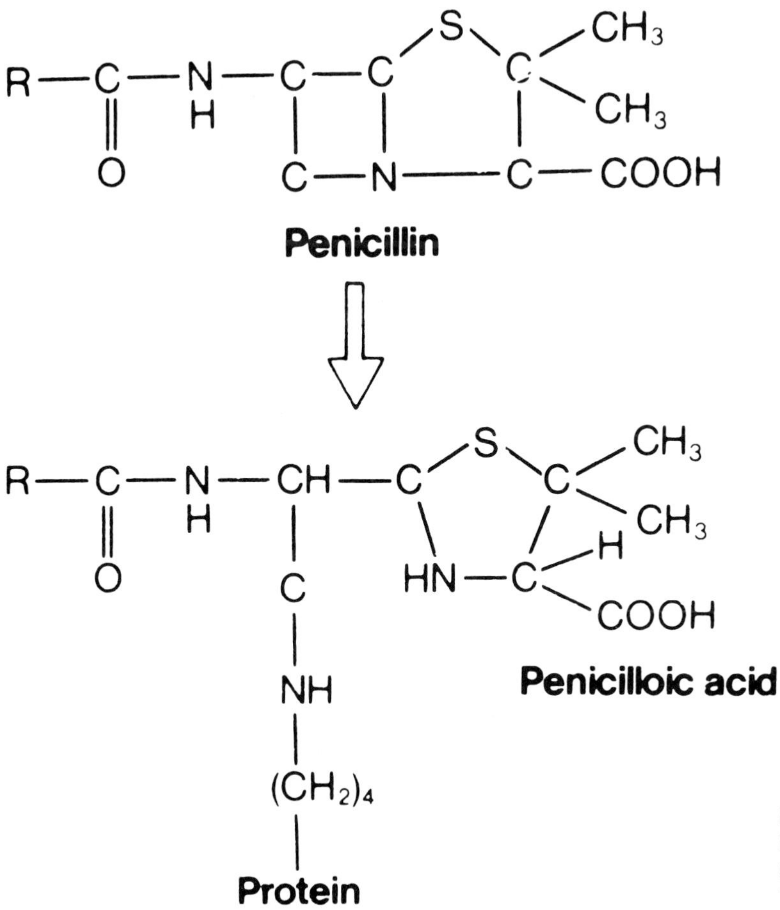

Figure 5–2. Penicilloyl-protein complex, the cause of allergic reactions to penicillins. *(From Kagan B.* Antimicrobial Therapy, *3rd ed. Philadelphia: WB Saunders; 1980.)*

Mode of Action. Penicillin affects growing but not metabolically inactive cells by inhibition of cell wall synthesis. The inhibitory processes involved are enormously more complex than initially thought and may involve different mechanisms for different bacteria by identical β-lactam antibiotics or other actions by different β-lactam compounds. The presence of peptidoglycans in bacterial cell walls, and in particular D-alanyl D-alanine in the carboxyterminal portion of the murein subunit, accounts for the selective toxicity of the penicillins and cephalosporins. A critical step in transpeptidation, that is, loss of D-alanine, is interfered with due to structural similarity of the nucleus of β-lactam antibiotics to D-alanyl D-alanine. Penicillins also reversibly inhibit D-alanine carboxypeptidase, which is of special importance in cell wall synthesis in gram-negative bacteria. In addition to inhibition of cell wall biosynthesis reactions, morphologic abnormalities in the shape of bacterial cells occur. These are thought to be due to binding of β-lactam antibiotics to characteristic proteins in bacterial cell membranes of individual species. These penicillin-binding proteins vary in number and function. However, the mechanism of how they interfere with growth, viability, and eventual lysis of the organism is not completely understood at this point. Current evidence suggests that the lytic effect of the β-lactam antibiotics results from the release of endogenous enzymes called autolysins, which hydrolyze peptidoglycan. These enzymes, which are usually tightly controlled, become activated in the presence of penicillin.

Cephalosporins

In the early days of the search for new β-lactam antibiotics, a penicillin-like antibiotic was isolated from a fungus of the genus *Cephalosporium.* Differences between this antibiotic and the penicillins included a D-α-amino adipic acid side chain and a 6-membered ring, a dihydrothiazine fused to the β-lactam nucleus. The basic structure of a typical cephalosporin is shown in Fig 5–3. Isolation of the nucleus of the cephalosporin molecule, 7 α-amino cephalosporanic acid (7 ACA), which is analogous to the 6 APA nucleus of penicillin, opened the way to production of semisynthetic derivatives of the cephalosporins. In addition, substitutions could be carried out on the 6-membered ring fused to the β-lactam grouping, thus, making possible at least two times as many derivatives as the penicillin nucleus.

The first semisynthetic cephalosporins, such as cephalothin and cephazolin, were stable to the action of β-lactamases and were effective against a number of gram-negative bacilli. However, both of these had to be given parenterally, because although acid stable, they were poorly absorbed from the gut.

Further modification of the side chain or the fused ring led to the development of derivatives that are acid stable and readily absorbed from the gut and possess a broader gram-negative spectrum than the older cephalosporins. They are also active against some nosocomially acquired strains that are resistant. The terminology first, second, and third generation cephalosporins is sometimes used to classify these antibiotics. This is based on the broader activity against gram-negative organisms of the later cephalosporins. Examples of some typical cephalosporins, their uses, and disadvantages are shown in Table 5–4.

Hypersensitivity occurs with cephalosporins, because they are structurally similar to penicillins, but these reactions are of a local nature and usually milder than those produced by penicillin.

Cephalosporins and penicillins have similar action on peptidoglycan synthesis but may differ in the selectivity of their binding to particular penicillin-binding proteins.

Other Cell Wall Inhibitors

Bacitracin. Bacitracin is a bactericidal, polypeptide antibiotic that is active primarily against gram-positive cocci and pathogenic *Neisseria.* Its nephrotoxic properties limit its clinical applications to topical applications in combination with neomycin and polymyxins for superficial infections of the skin and mucous membranes. Its mode of action differs from the

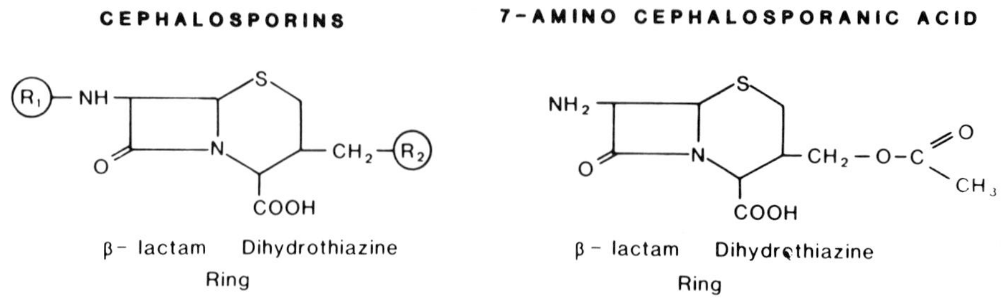

Figure 5–3. Structure of a typical cephalosporin and its nucleus. *(Modified from Waldvogel F.* Rev Infect Dis. *1982;4:S491.)*

TABLE 5–4. PROPERTIES OF TYPICAL CEPHALOSPORINS

Drug	Resistance to β-Lactamase	Biologic/Medical Properties
First generation		
Cephalothin sodium	+	Active against gram-positive cocci except enterococci or methicillin-resistant *Streptococcus aureus*
Cefazolin sodium	+	Active against gram-negative bacilli except *Bacteroides fragilis, Pseudomonas,* indole-positive *Proteus* sp., *Enterobacter,* and *Haemophilus influenzae*
Cephalexin	+	Active against actinomycetes and black-pigmented *Bacteroides*
Second generation		
Cefoxitin	+	More active against *Bacteroides fragilis,* some gram-negative bacilli, and *Neisseria gonorrhoeae*
Cefaclor	+	Greater activity against *Haemophilus influenzae,* may be useful in otitis media
Third generation		
Cefotaxime sodium	+	Increased activity against gram-negative bacilli, good CSF penetration
Cefoperazone	+	Increased activity against *Pseudomonas aeruginosa,* no accumulation in renal failure

penicillins in the particular stages of peptidoglycan biosynthesis with which it interferes.

Vancomycin. Vancomycin is a bactericidal glycopeptide antibiotic that interferes with cell wall biosynthesis but with mechanisms that differ from the penicillins and bacitracin. Its principal use has been as an alternative antibiotic in serious gram-positive infections in patients allergic to penicillin or where β-lactamase-producing organisms are present. It also is useful in patients who are on clindamycin therapy to prevent colitis produced by clindamycin-resistant *Clostridia.* Its side effects include ototoxicity, tissue irritability, and nephrotoxicity, and it may cause necrosis when injected.

INHIBITORS OF PROTEIN SYNTHESIS

Macrolide Antibiotics

A group of antibiotics were isolated from streptomyces fermentation broths in the early 1950s. These were divided into two groups, one of which had a spectrum similar to that of penicillin G and inhibited protein synthesis, whereas the second group possessed antifungal activity and a different mode of action. These antibiotics are called macrolides because their molecular structure contains large alphatic lactones (Fig 5–4). The antifungal macrolides are termed polyene macrolides because of their conjugated double-bond system. Antifungal activity increases with the number of double bonds. The biologic activity and other properties of these agents are discussed in the section on antifungal agents.

The most widely used of the antibacterial group is erythromycin, which has activity against gram-positive cocci, including β-lactamase-producing staphylococci. Erythromycin is considered to be a drug of initial choice in the treatment of infections caused by *Legionella, Bordetella pertussis* (whooping cough), *Mycoplasma pneumoniae,* and *Chlamydia trachomitis.* Many aerobic and anaerobic bacteria found in oral infections are susceptible to erythromycin, although more are susceptible to penicillin. Erythromycin, cephalosporins, vancomycin, or clindamycin may be used as alternatives to penicillin in the treatment of streptococcal infections, syphilis, and some infections caused by gram-negative cocci, with the exception of penicillin-resistant strains of *Neisseria gonorrhoeae.*

Erythromycin inhibits protein synthesis by binding selectively to the 70S ribosome and, in particular, the 50S subunit. It interferes with the shift of ribosomes along the messenger RNA chain. Erythromycin has few side effects, but nausea or diarrhea occur in about 2 to 3% of the cases.

Lincomycin and Clindamycin

Lincomycin and its derivative clindamycin have a spectrum that includes gram-positive and gram-negative cocci and some gram-positive rods, such as *Clostridium, Actinomyces,* and *Nocardia.* In addition, they are active against certain gram-negative bacilli, such as *Bacteroides fragilis* and *Bacteroides melaninogenicus.*

Its most effective clinical use is against penicillin-resistant anaerobes, such as *Bacteroides fragilis.* It also is useful in treating staphylococcal cellulitis or osteomyelitis in patients allergic to penicillin.

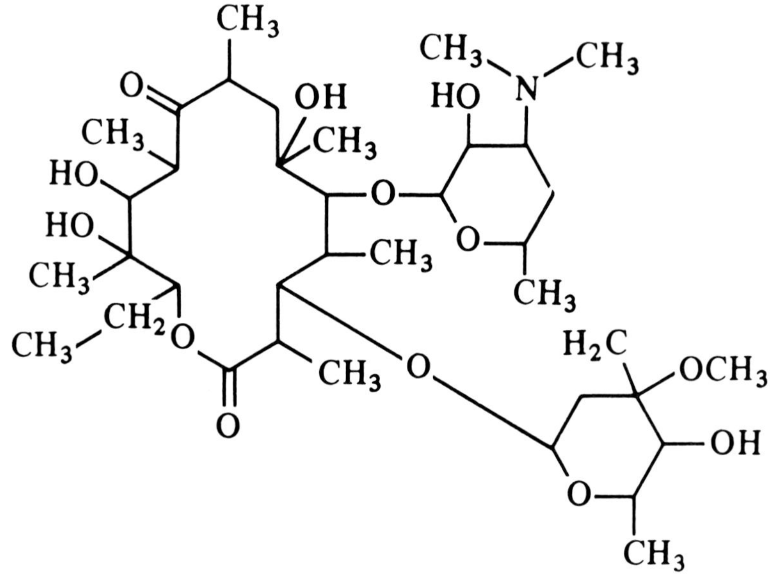

Figure 5–4. Structure of macrolide, erythromycin A.

Clindamycin inhibits protein synthesis by binding to the 50S ribosomal subunit. Clindamycin has been associated with pseudomembranous colitis, which is caused by *Clostridium difficile* toxin. More recent evidence suggests that many other antibiotics, including ampicillin, also are associated with this serious side effect. This may be prevented by the administration of oral vancomycin. There is a more extensive discussion of this disorder in Chapter 14.

Aminoglycosides

The prototype of these antibiotics was streptomycin. Other aminoglycosides include neomycin, kanamycin, gentamicin, tobramycin, and amikacin.

Initially, streptomycin was the agent of choice for tuberculosis, either by itself or in conjunction with other synthetic antimicrobials, such as para-aminosalicylic acid, isoniazid, or ethambutol. Although it is still widely used in this manner, many clinicians have preferred to use the newer, less toxic agents for the treatment of tuberculosis. In addition to tuberculosis, streptomycin is used to treat infections caused by aerobic gram-negative bacilli, such as *Franciscella tularensis* (tularemia) and *Yersinia pestis* (bubonic plague). Streptomycin and most of the other aminoglycosides may cause deafness or severe vestibular problems as a result of injury to the eighth cranial nerve. An additional problem associated with the aminoglycosides is the high frequency with which resistant mutants occur. Aminoglycoside antibiotics are highly stable to biodegradation and soluble in water and body fluids.

Kanamycin and Neomycin. Kanamycin is useful in the treatment of certain gram-negative urinary tract and enteric infections, but its influence has been limited by its ototoxic properties and the increasing number of plasmid-mediated resistance occurring in gram-negative organisms of hospital origin.

Neomycin has an antibacterial spectrum similar to that of streptomycin. However, its extreme ototoxicity and nephrotoxicity limit clinical usefulness to the treatment of topical infections. Because it is absorbed poorly from the gut, it is also used as a preoperative bowel sterilant.

Amikacin, Tobramycin, and Gentamicin. Amikacin and tobramycin are derivatives of the kanamycin molecule. Gentamicin is, in reality, a mixture of several compounds that differ only slightly in their structure.

These aminoglycoside antibiotics are active in vitro against aerobic gram-negative bacilli, such as *Escherichia coli, Klebsiella,* and *Proteus* and, consequently, are valuable for treating bacteremias and pneumonias caused by these organisms. Gentamicin and tobramycin have increased activity against *Pseudomonas,* and they are useful in combination with other antibiotic agents in topical treatment of burns infected with *Pseudomonas* or *Staphylococcus.* Amikacin is active against organisms that have developed resistance to tobramycin and gentamicin and usually is reserved for those cases. These aminoglycosides also are ototoxic and nephrotoxic.

Mode of Action. These antibiotics, which are all bactericidal, inhibit protein synthesis by binding to the 30S subunit of the 70S ribosome. This binding causes specific misreadings of the genetic code, which results in formation of defective proteins and peptides.

Tetracyclines

Tetracycline and its analogs are considered to be broad-spectrum antibiotics that have in common a 4-

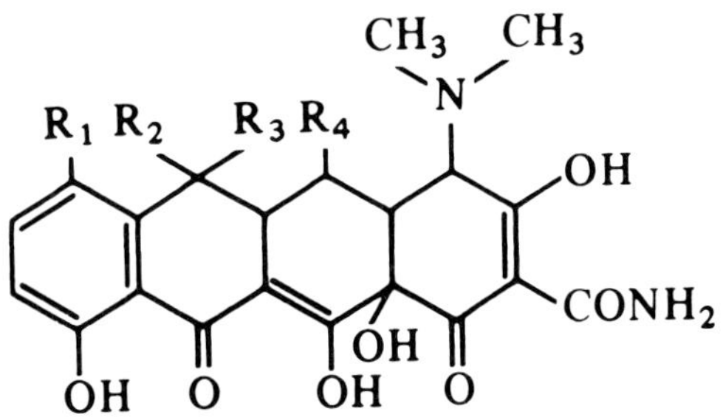

R_1	R_2	R_3	R_4	Name
Cl	H	OH	H	Demethylchlortetracycline
H		$=CH_2$	OH	Methacycline
H	CH_3	H	OH	Doxycycline
$N(CH_3)_2$	H	H	H	Minocycline

Figure 5–5. Tetracycline and its analogs. *(Modified from Lancini G, Parenti F.* Antibiotics: An Integrated View. *New York: Springer-Verlag; 1982.)*

membered ring structure (Fig 5–5). The spectrum of activity not only includes most gram-positive and gram-negative cocci and rods, but mycoplasma, rickettsiae, and chlamydia. They are usually the drug of first choice for diseases caused by gram-negative organisms, such as cholera and brucellosis. Infections due to *M. pneumoniae* also respond excellently to the tetracyclines. Chlamydial diseases in which the tetracyclines are usually the most effective antibiotic, include psittacosis, trachoma, pelvic inflammatory disease, and lymphogranuloma venereum. Almost all the rickettsial diseases, including Rocky Mountain spotted fever and typhus, respond excellently to the tetracyclines.

Other clinical uses for tetracycline include the prophylactic use of doxycycline for travelers' diarrhea and the use of low doses of tetracycline for treatment of acne. Two of the most widely used derivatives include doxycycline and minocycline.

Tetracycline acts by inhibiting protein synthesis by blocking the binding of the transfer RNA-amino acid complex to the ribosome. Thus, polypeptides cannot be produced because amino acids are not available. Tetracycline and all of its analogs are bacteriostatic.

Adverse reactions include gastric disturbances predisposing to the overgrowth of other organisms in the oral cavity, vagina, and intestinal tract. The best example of this latter phenomenon is the appearance of oral or vaginal candidiasis following the administration of tetracycline. Tetracyclines also form chelates with calcium and related cations and can bind firmly to bone and teeth. Residues of tetracycline localize and persist in these tissues long after the drug is cleared from the body. As a result, severe permanent staining can occur in developing teeth. Staining of developing incisors in the fetus may be avoided by not using tetracycline after the fourth month of gestation. To prevent staining of permanent teeth, tetracycline should not be administered to children less than 8 years of age.

Finally, tetracycline, once one of the most widely used antibiotics, has the disadvantage that many resistant strains of microorganisms have emerged over the past few years.

Chloramphenicol

Chloramphenicol is a bacteriostatic, broad-spectrum antibiotic and is active against a wide variety of gram-positive and gram-negative cocci and bacilli, as well as rickettsiae and chlamydia. Chloramphenicol is the antibiotic of choice for typhoid fever and a preferred agent in enteric fevers or bacteremias caused by other salmonellae. Because chloramphenicol has the ability to penetrate the blood–brain barrier, it is active against bacterial pathogens within the central nervous system. In this regard, it is the preferred antibiotic either by itself or in combination with ampicillin for bacterial meningitis.

Chloramphenicol inhibits protein synthesis. However, the particular sites are different than those affected by tetracycline. Chloramphenicol inhibits peptidyl transferase activity by binding to the 50S subunit of the 70S ribosome. Chloramphenicol, erythromycin, and clindamycin compete for the same or neighboring sites and, therefore, are antagonistic. Chloramphenicol may cause bone marrow toxicity due to the similarity of mitochondrial ribosomes and 70S ribosomes. Because of its extreme toxicity, use of chloramphenicol should be reserved for serious infections of the type indicated. The most serious side effect of the antibiotic is an aplastic anemia, which is usually irreversible. Symptoms may develop for days to months after therapy is discontinued. The patient usually hemorrhages and develops other infections.

ANTIBIOTICS WITH OTHER MODES OF ACTION

Rifampin

Rifampin is a semisynthetic derivative of rifamycin, which is produced by *Nocardia*. Although it has a wide spectrum of bactericidal activity against gram-positive and gram-negative bacteria, its most important clinical use has been primarily for tuberculosis. When used in conjunction with isoniazid, it made possible the first short-term therapy of the disease. Resistant strains, however, develop rapidly if rifampin is used alone. A second valuable clinical activity of rifampin is its ability to eliminate nasal carriage of meningococci, thus preventing outbreaks of meningococcal meningitis, as well as treating close contacts of patients with meningitis. The antibiotic is used in the same manner for prevention of disease due to *Haemophilus influenzae*. Rifampin serves as an excellent alternative against methicillin-resistant staphylococci, as well as being useful in eliminating staphylococci from nasal carriers.

Rifampin has a number of unusual biochemical and pharmaceutical properties. It is highly lipid soluble, which enables it to penetrate abscesses, cavities, and bone. It also has high intraphagocytic activity. Rifampin also has a unique mode of action based on the ability to bind and inactivate specific bacterial DNA-dependent RNA polymerase. This enzyme polymerizes RNA triphosphates on a DNA template and catalyzes the transcription of DNA to RNA. The antibiotic has the distinct advantage of inactivating the enzyme at extremely low levels. The corresponding mammalian enzymes are affected only at much higher levels. Thus, toxic effects of the antibiotic on the host are minimized.

The specificity of the mode of action in relation to the target enzyme may actually be a disadvantage, since any slight modification will alter binding of the antibiotic and produce resistance.

Synthetic Antimicrobials: Sulfonamides, Isoniazid, Nitrofurans, and Nalidixic Acid

The chemotherapeutic antimicrobial agents discussed in this section are grouped together primarily because they are all produced by chemical synthesis, as opposed to being produced by or extracted from microorganisms by a combination of microbiologic and chemical synthesis.

Sulfonamides. The antibacterial activity of the sulfonamides has been recognized since the mid-1930s, when Domagk demonstrated that the dye Prontosil had antibacterial activity against streptococci. He soon identified sulfanilamide as the active portion of the dye molecule.

Originally active against a great number of gram-positive and gram-negative organisms, the sulfa drugs and their derivatives have had their clinical usefulness limited because of the development of resistance, their primarily bacteriostatic effect, and their side effects. However, a combination of sulfamethoxazole and trimethoprim is still very useful for some infectious diseases. This compound is effective against *Shigella* infections that do not respond to ampicillin. It is still used for urinary tract infections. However, the increasing number of resistant strains of *E. coli* and *Proteus* and others are rapidly decreasing the usefulness of this agent. Sulfaisoxasole is useful in certain sexually transmitted diseases, such as lymphogranuloma venerum, nongonococcal urethritis caused by *C. trachomatis*, and chancroid, caused by *Haemophilus ducreyi*.

Sulfa drugs are antimetabolites that act by competitive inhibition of folic acid metabolism. Figure 5–6 illustrates the structural similarity between sulfanilamide and *p*-aminobenzoic acid. The sulfonamides act by inhibiting the incorporation of *p*-aminobenzoic acid into folic acid by inhibiting dihydrofolate synthetase. Because mammalian cells, in contrast to bacteria, are unable to synthesize folic acid and require an

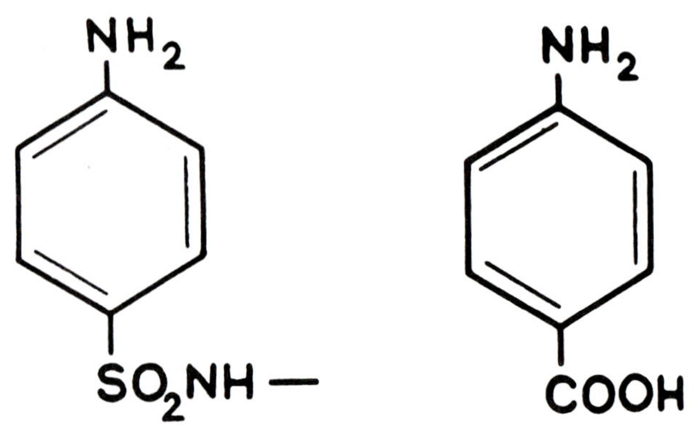

Figure 5–6. Structure of *p*-aminobenzoic acid (*right*) and sulfonamides (*left*). Note similarity.

exogenous source, sulfa compounds have no effect on these cells. Thus, the action of the sulfa compounds exploits the difference between the metabolic pathways of mammalian and bacterial cells. Trimethoprim inhibits biochemical use of folic acid by inhibiting dihydrofolic reductase, which catalyzes the reduction of dihydrofolate to tetrahydrofolate. Although the enzyme is present in many groups of organisms from bacteria to mammals, structural differences in the enzyme favor a selective inhibition of the bacterial enzyme but not the mammalian enzyme. As shown in equations 1 and 2, the combination of the two compounds, sulfamethoxazole and trimethoprim, acts on the bacterial cell, first by inhibiting the synthesis of folic acid and second by preventing the proper use of folic acid.

Pteridine-pyrophosphate + para-aminobenzoic acid —synthetase (↓ sulfonamides)→ dihydropteroate [Eq. 1]

Dihydropteroate → dihydrofolate —reductase (↑ trimethoprim)→ tetrahydrofolate [Eq. 2]

The chief contraindication for trimethoprim-sulfamethoxazole is in patients with impaired folate metabolism, such as pregnant women, alcoholics, and those people who suffer from malnutrition.

Isoniazid. Isoniazid, or isonicotinic acid hydrazide, is an excellent agent for use in treating tuberculosis. It usually is used in combination with one or more other drugs, such as streptomycin, rifampin, ethambutol, or para-aminosalicylic acid, to prevent the emergence of resistant bacteria. The mechanism of action is uncertain but is related to mycobacterial peroxidase and nicotinamide adenine dinucleotide (NAD). It is possible that these enyzmatic systems generate radicals, such as superoxide and free hydroxide, that inhibit mycolic acid synthesis.

The chief side effects appear to be hepatoxicity and depletion of pyridoxine, resulting in peripheral neuritis.

Nitrofurans and Nalidixic Acid. Nitrofurantoin is active against urinary tract pathogens, such as *E. coli* and some strains of *Proteus* and *Klebsiella*. The chief side effect of nitrofurantoin is gastrointestinal upset. Nalidixic acid is active against most gram-negative organisms, with the exception of *Pseudomonas* and *Bacteroides*. Nalidixic acid acts by blocking DNA-gyrase, thus inhibiting DNA synthesis.

Quinolones. The quinolones are a new class of antimicrobial agents that are structurally related to nalidixic acid, usually as a fluoroderivative. The best known of these are ciprofloxacin and norfloxacin. They differ in their spectra from nalidixic acid in that they are active against staphylococci, including resistant strains, as well as gram-negative pathogens, such as *H. influenzae* and *N. gonorrhoeae*. In addition, they are active against many of the gram-negative bacteria involved in urinary and gastrointestinal tract infections.

These antimicrobial agents inhibit DNAgyrase, an enzyme involved in a number of critical DNA reactions. The most common adverse reactions are gastrointestinal.

ANTIFUNGAL AGENTS

The antimicrobial agents responsible for treating fungal infections may be classified according to the type of infection they act against.

1. Superficial *Candida* infections: *Candida* exist as saprophytes on cutaneous and mucosal surfaces and involve adjacent organs when environmental conditions change.
2. Systemic or deep mycoses: These affect primarily internal organs.
3. Dermatophytes: These proliferate within the epidermis or hair shafts.

Antibiotics Useful in Treating Superficial* Candida *Infections. Nystatin is produced by a streptomycete and is water soluble. It consists of a large ring containing a lactone group and a region consisting of four conjugated double bonds. As a result of the numerous double bonds, it is called a polyene agent.

Nystatin is active against superficial and localized *Candida* infections of the oropharyngeal region, vagina, or intestinal tract. Because it is not absorbed from the gut, it is not used for systemic fungal infections. It binds to sterols in fungal cell membranes. This results in injury to the membranes and resulting loss of vital cellular constituents, such as K^+, NH_4^+, and low molecular weight sugars. Since bacterial cells do not contain sterols, they are not affected by nystatin.

Antibiotics Useful in Treating Deep Mycoses. Amphotericin B is also a polyene antifungal agent. It also contains the lactone group characteristic of macrolides but contains seven conjugated double bonds. It differs from nystatin also in that it is active against a number of systemic fungal infections. It usually is the drug of choice for systemic fungal infections caused by yeasts (eg, *Cryptococcus neoformans*), dimorphic fungi (eg, *Histoplasma capsulatum*), or mold infections (eg, aspergillosis).

Amphotericin B is administered intravenously or intrathecally as an aqueous colloidal suspension because it is insoluble in water. The methyl ester of the antibiotic is less toxic than the parent compound. Renal toxicity is the most important side effect of the drug. Despite these drawbacks, it is one of the most effective antifungal drugs, especially in the case of immunocompromised patients.

Its mode of action is on the cell membrane. The relative specificity of the drug for fungi as opposed to mammalian cells is probably related to the drug's greater avidity for ergosterol, which is found in fungi, than for cholesterol, found in mammalian cells.

Recent information has shown that the lytic effect of the antibiotic on the cell membrane may be separated out from the permeability-producing effect. Evidence points to the role of toxic oxygen intermediates, which will result in these lytic effects.

5-Flucytosine is a synthetic antifungal agent that also is useful for treating systemic infections, especially cryptococcal meningitis. Its chief advantages are that it is less toxic than amphotericin B and that it can be administered orally. The chief side effects are hematologic and hepatic in nature. The mode of action is thought to result from the conversion of 5-flucytosine to 5-flurouracil, an antimetabolite that inhibits RNA and DNA synthesis by inhibiting the action of thymidylate synthetase.

Imidazoles. The imidazoles have a wide spectrum of antifungal activity. The best known of these are miconazole and ketoconazole.

Miconazole has been shown to be effective against coccidioidomycosis and paracoccidioidomycosis. Long periods of treatment are required, and there is a high rate of relapse. Side effects include anaphylaxis and arrythmia that may occur during intravenous administration. For these reasons, it should be used primarily on patients who cannot tolerate or who have not responded to amphotericin B. Miconazole acts by changing the permeability of the cell membrane, in addition to inhibition of sterol demethylase.

Ketoconazole has a similar spectrum to that of miconazole but appears to have more action against *Coccidioides* infections. It has limited activity against histoplasmosis and oropharyngeal candidiasis. Ketoconazole can be taken orally, is well absorbed from the gastrointestinal tract, and has few side effects. There is a high rate of recurrence of the fungal disease once treatment is stopped, and the drug is ineffective in immunocompromised patients. Ketoconazole also alters permeability of cell membrane, resulting in leakage of K^+, NH_4^+, and adenine nucleotides, with resultant loss of fungal viability.

Other imidazole derivatives include chlortrimazole and terconozole, which are active against a wide variety of dermatophytic fungi, as well as cutaneous *Candida* infections.

Antibiotics Useful Against Dermatophytic Infections. Griseofulvin is an antifungal agent that is useful for treatment of superficial dermatophytic infections, such as ringworm. It can be taken orally and is concentrated in the stratum corneum or the keratinocytes. It is selectively toxic for fungi that contain chitin, such as the dermatophytes. Griseofulvin binds to proteins involved in tubulin assembly. This inhibits the mitotic process through prevention of assembly of microtubules, which govern chromosomal movement during meiosis.

RESISTANCE

Shortly after the advent of the age of antibiotics, the miracle of these chemotherapeutic agents was tempered by the emergence of resistant strains of microorganisms. The resistance usually was manifested by therapeutic failure of the agent that had formerly been effective. The resistance usually was confirmed by in vitro susceptibility testing, which demonstrated the resistant isolate was no longer inhibited by the minimal inhibitory concentration that usually inhibited a standardized control strain of that same species. As each new antibiotic or antibiotic derivative was introduced into the patient population, the pattern was, for the most part, similar. There was an initial period of excellent activity, followed by an increasing number of reports of resistance, which in many cases led to the abandonment of a particular antibiotic for use in the treatment of an infectious disease.

Examples of clinical implications of some of these mechanisms include the emergence of methicillin-resistant staphylococci and the rise in hospitals of drug-resistant infections caused by *Enterobacter, Proteus, Klebsiella*, and *Pseudomonas.*

Nongenetic Resistance

Resistance may have either a nongenetic or a genetic origin. Nongenetic or intrinsic resistance can be due to the inability of the antibiotic to diffuse through the pores of the outer membrane because of complexity of the cell membrane, or it can be due to lack of a particular target structure, such as a cell wall, as in mycoplasma. Another form of nongenetic resistance is the inability of antibiotics, such as the penicillins, to kill or inhibit bacterial cells that are not actively reproducing.

Genetic Resistance

The origin of acquired resistance generally is accepted as being due to mutation and selection and is based on genetic changes that alter or induce specific proteins, such as enzymes or binding sites. These genetic changes can be either chromosomal or extrachromosomal in origin.

Chromosomal Resistance. Changes of chromosomal origin occur spontaneously as a result of mutations independent of the various biochemical mechanisms of the antibiotic. These mutations occur at an extremely low frequency, 10^{-7} or 10^{-9}. However, the antibiotic acts as a selective agent, killing or inhibiting the susceptible organisms and allowing the resistant organisms to multiply and eventually predominate. Chromosomal resistance can be transferred from one bacterium to another by at least three mechanisms. These include conjugation, that is, physical contact between bacterial cells with consequent transfer of genetic material, transduction, that is, transfer of fragments of the genome from a donor organism to a recipient by means of bacteriophage, and transformation, that is, uptake from the environment of DNA fragments liberated by a donor bacterium. The details of these mechanisms are discussed in Chapter 3.

Extrachromosomal Resistance. The genetic loci controlling drug resistance often occur on extrachromosomal pieces of DNA called plasmids. Plasmids are extremely important because resistance factors, or R factors, to several antibiotics can be transferred from one organism to another simultaneously by a number of genetic mechanisms. Thus, nonpathogens or susceptible pathogens can acquire plasmid-mediated resistance and become clinically significant.

Conjugation is probably the most important mechanism for transfer of R factors in gram-negative organisms, with resultant survival of antibiotic-resistant intestinal flora that present great hazards not only to hospitalized patients with normal immune systems but especially to those who are immunocompromised.

Other genetic mechanisms of plasmid transfer, such as transduction, transformation, and transposons, can occur between species in either gram-positive or gram-negative organisms. In the case of transformation, which occurs in gram-positive bacteria, transfer can occur either between species or between genera.

Biochemical Mechanisms of Resistance

Probably the most common and widely studied mechanisms of resistance are those that involve some type of interaction of the organism and the antibiotic. These are due to the production of an enzyme either induced or constitutively produced that will partially or completely inactivate the antibiotic.

β-Lactamases, which hydrolyze the β-lactam group of penicillins and the cephalosporins, can be either plasmid-mediated or chromosomal in origin. A new approach to the problem of β-lactamases has been the development of inhibitors, such as clavulinic acid, that inactivate those enzymes, thus affording protection for β-lactam substrates.

Another example of an enzyme that acts on an antibiotic is chloramphenicol acetyltransferase. The chloramphenicol derivative produced by the enzyme is inactive because it is unable to bind to the bacterial ribosome, thus blocking the mode of action. This mechanism is important in both gram-negative and gram-positive bacteria. Plasmid-specified enzymes also are responsible for bacterial resistance to aminoglycoside antibiotics. Bacterial phosphotransferase, acetyltransferase, and adenyltransferase all produce derivatives of these antibiotics that no longer bind to ribosomes and, therefore, cannot inhibit protein synthesis.

A second group of resistant mechanisms are those that cause resistance when the organism is able to bypass the antibiotic-sensitive stage and proceed on with the normal metabolism, thus negating any inhibitory effect. An example of this is shown by the sulfonamides. The sulfonamide-sensitive step, that is, interference with the reaction of para-aminobenzoic acid and the pteridine pyrophosphate intermediate, is bypassed because of the increased production of para-aminobenzoic acid by plasmid-coded enzymes. This reduces the inhibitory action of the drug.

A third mechanism of resistance is a change in permeability of the bacterial cell. This is exemplified by tetracycline resistance. These changes result in a decreased drug accumulation and an increased release of the drug from the bacterial cell. Tetracycline resistance is usually plasmid regulated.

Another resistance mechanism involves the alteration of the antibiotic target site. This occurs with erythromycin and clindamycin. Bacterial enzymes methylate adenine residues of RNA, thus preventing the antibiotic from binding to the site of action. Alterations in penicillin-binding proteins may cause resistance due to changes in target sites or permeability changes.

USE OF ANTIBIOTICS FOR ORAL INFECTION

Most oral infections are caused by gram-positive bacteria and gram-negative anaerobes. Penicillins, erythromycin, cephalosporins, tetracyclines, and clindamycin are the usual drugs of choice. In minor oral infections, penicillin V (phenoxymethyl penicillin) is the drug of choice, since oral administration has a lower risk of hypersensitivity than has parenteral administration. In the case of serious oral infections, for example, cellulitis, parenteral penicillin or an equivalent alternative is used. Clindamycin, with a special affinity for bone, has good activity against gram-positive cocci. However, it has the drawback of sometimes causing pseudomembranous colitis. For anaerobes, especially black-pigmented *Bacteroides,* penicillin, ampicillin, erythromycin, and doxycycline are used.

Recently, investigators have shown that *B. melaninogenicus* isolated from orofacial infections refractory to treatment by penicillins commonly produce β-lactamase. Because *Bacteroides* are a predominant organism in orofacial infections, these observations have great clinical significance. Clindamycin usually was effective against these resistant strains and is used most frequently in hospitalized patients.

For facultative gram-negative rods (coliforms, *Klebsiella-Enterobacter, Proteus,* or *Pseudomonas* spp.), doxycycline, ampicillin, and aminoglycosides, such as gentamycin and tobramycin, usually are used.

Minocycline and doxycycline (tetracycline derivatives) have been used for treatment of periodontal disease. They concentrate in gingival crevicular fluid at levels much higher than in serum. Metronidazole is another agent used in the treatment of periodontal disease and in refractile maxillofacial infections involving anaerobes. Both the metronizadole and the tetracycline derivatives suppress the growth of facultative and anaerobic organisms believed to be specific pathogens in periodontal pockets. Recently, investigators have shown that minocycline inhibits tissue collagenolytic activity by a mechanism independent of the drug's known antibacterial properties.

Bacterial endocarditis (discussed in Chapter 11) remains one of the most serious complications of valvular disease in individuals undergoing medical or dental invasive procedures. Antibiotic prophylaxis is recommended with all dental procedures, including routine professional cleanings, that are likely to cause gingival bleeding.

Most clinicians believe that immediate antibiotic therapy must be instituted along with the appropriate supportive and therapeutic measures for severe infections of the head and neck because of the risks of infection spreading to the cavernous sinus, brain, pharyngeal, endocardial, or pericardial tissues or to other vital organs. Severe infections usually are considered to be those with cellulitis or that are progressive or accompanied by signs of systemic response or involvement, such as fever and localized lymphadenopathy. Patients with compound fractures of the mandible also are considered in need of immediate antibiotic therapy. Patients with well-localized minor infections are not ordinarily medicated with antibiotics, despite the presence of an exudate, swelling, pain, or loss of function, unless they have a high risk of endocardial or systemic infection or other reasons of systemic impairment. Unnecessary use of antibiotics for every patient with minor abscesses is considered an abuse and unnecessary risk of sensitizing patients or creating resistant flora.

DANGERS OF INDISCRIMINATE USE OF ANTIBIOTICS

The use and abuse of antibiotics has been discussed ever since the first side effects of these agents were noticed, and the implications of resistant strains of organisms have been discussed in relation to each agent. However, the effect of antibiotics on normal flora and the danger of inducing secondary infections must be addressed. One of the most common problems is an overgrowth of *Candida albicans* and related species that result in candidiasis of the colon, oral cavity, and vagina. This is less frequently seen as pharyngitis or esophagitis.

Tetracycline antibiotics were found to suppress the bacterial flora that kept *Candida* in check. They also tend to create a leukopenia that reduces white cell defenses, which regulate *Candida* populations. Fatal *Candida* periocarditis is seen as a sudden resurgence in fever in patients convalescing from a febrile bacterial infection.

Selective inhibition of intestinal flora can be caused by a number of antibiotics, most commonly clindamycin. Resultant overgrowth by *C. difficile* can cause severe or fatal pseudomembranous colitis. Depression of coliforms and enterococci can lead to overgrowth of *Proteus* and *Pseudomonas* species in the intestines that can infect the urinary tract and kidneys.

Overgrowth of resistant *Staphylococcus aureus* caused by therapy can result in staphylococcal pharyngitis.

MEASUREMENT OF MICROBIAL SUSCEPTIBILITY TO ANTIBIOTICS

In choosing the appropriate antibiotic to treat a particular infection, the physician or dentist must consider a number of parameters. Included among these are the pharmacologic characteristics of the drug and the particular site infection. Two of the most important, however, are identification of the correct etiologic agent and the determination of the microbial susceptibility of that agent to a battery of antibiotics. These tests are critical for a number of reasons.

1. If a clinical response is not satisfactory, the treatment can be modified using the sensitivity results.
2. Both the host and parasite are in a constant state of change before, during, and after therapy, and microbial susceptibility may change via different mechanisms of resistance.
3. Some pathogens vary greatly in response to the same agent.

Antimicrobial activity is measured in vitro in order to determine (1) the potency of the antibacterial agent in solution, (2) its concentration in body fluids or tissues, and (3) the sensitivity of a given microorganism to known concentrations of the drug. Two general types of tests are used.

1. Dilution tests: Increasing amounts of antimicrobial substances are incorporated into liquid or solid bacteriologic media. The media are subsequently inoculated with test bacteria and incubated. The end point is taken as that amount of antimicrobial substance required to inhibit the growth of or to kill the test bacteria. Tube dilution tests usually are more accurate than any of the diffusion tests but are not done routinely because of time and expense.
2. Diffusion method: A filter paper disk, a porous cup, or an open-ended cylinder containing measured quantities of drug is placed on a solid medium that has been heavily seeded with the test organisms. Most laboratories use disks of antibiotic-impregnated filter paper. A concentration gradient of antibiotic is produced in the medium by diffusion from the disk. After incubation, the diameter of the clear zone of inhibition surrounding the deposit of drug is taken as a measure of the inhibitory power of the drug against the particular test organism. The size of the zone of growth varies with the molecular characteristics of different antibiotics. Therefore, the zone sites for different antibiotics acting on an organism cannot be compared directly. However, they can be compared to standard zone sizes, as done in the Bauer-Kirby procedure, if all conditions of media, incubation, and inoculation are standardized. Results of a disk diffusion assay similar to a typical Bauer-Kirby test are shown in Fig 5–7. The disk diffusion test measures the ability of an agent to inhibit rather than kill. The concentration at which the antibiotic produces a zone size equivalent to that obtained with a standardized strain under standard conditions is termed the minimal inhibitory concentration (MIC). The concentration in the disks is used to determine the susceptibility of the particular bacterial strain to the level of antibiotic obtainable in the blood. An organism usually is considered susceptible when the peak serum concentration is at least 4 times the MIC.

An MBC (minimal bactericidal concentration) may be determined using a tube test. Samples are removed from those tubes that show no growth as the antibiotic is serially diluted and plated out on antibiotic-free medium. The amount of antibiotic in the first tube from which the organism does not grow is the MBC.

Susceptibility testing of anaerobic bacteria presents its own unique problems. Most anaerobic infections involve a mixed aerobic-anaerobic flora, which makes it difficult to obtain accurate values to manage the infection. Other complicating factors that may influence the choice of an appropriate chemotherapeutic agent for anaerobic infections include whether or not surgical intervention took place, the general state of the patient, and the pharmacology of the drug. For these reasons, testing of individual isolates usually should be limited to such infections as endocarditis, osteomyelitis, joint infections, or infections of prosthetic devices.

Because of the slow growth of anaerobes, disk diffusion tests are useless in testing the susceptibility patterns of etiologic agents involved in anaerobic infections. However, the broth disk dilution test has proved to be a useful alternative. In this test, antimicrobial agents on commercial disks are eluted into prereduced broth medium in order to obtain a specific concentration. Susceptibility is defined as either the absence of turbidity or turbidity less than 50% of a growth control.

Whether performed on agar plates or in broth, sensitivity tests may be affected by a number of variables, including the pH of the medium, the stability of the drug, components of the medium that may antagonize the drug, the size of the inoculum, the length of incubation, and the metabolic state of the organism. These must be controlled in order to ensure accurate values.

ORAL ASPECTS

The problem of antimicrobial resistance present since the birth of the antibiotic era has still not been solved and, in fact, continues to increase in scope and intensity. This is compounded by the emergence of new

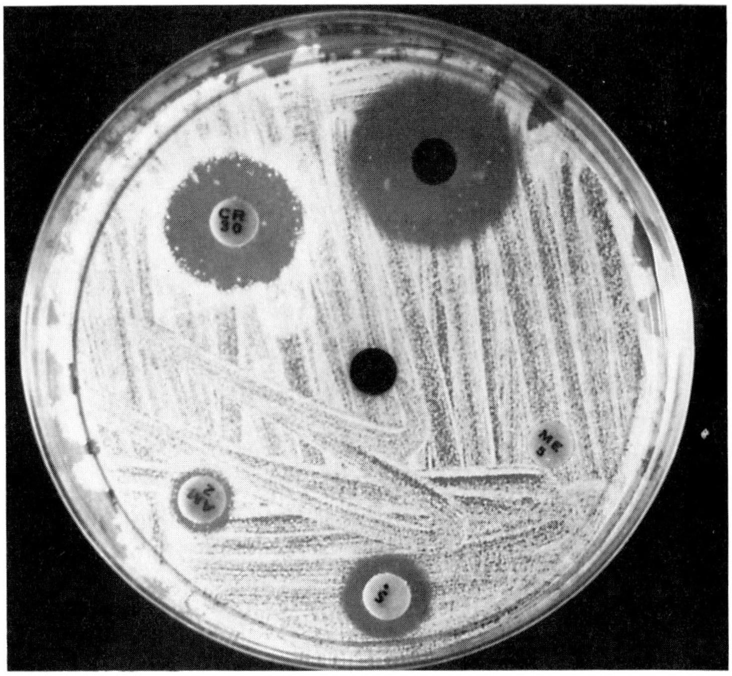

CR 30	Cephalothin	30 MCG
AM 2	Streptomycin	5 MCG
S	Streptomycin	5 MCG
ME 5	Methicillin	5 MCG
TE •	Tetracycline	10 MCG
E •	Middle disk erythromycin	5 MCG

Figure 5–7. Typical zones of inhibition produced by selected antibiotics when used in a disk diffusion technique.

pathogens and the changing status of older etiologic agents. This is of special importance to the dentist because of the increasing importance of anaerobic bacteria in the pathogenesis of orofacial infection and the reports of clinical failures of antibiotics due to the presence of β-lactamase-producing organisms. The dentist must be aware of the appropriate prophylactic use of antimicrobial agents, even for the simplest dental procedure, when there is a medical history of heart or valve damage. It is critical to remember that antibiotics are a two-edged sword. If they are used properly, they represent a huge advance in the never ending battle against infectious disease. On the other hand, side effects and the development of resistant strains of organisms make a strong case for continuous monitoring of patients receiving these chemotherapeutic agents.

Another area of investigation has opened new frontiers in the area of the effect of antibiotics on host-parasite relationships. These include the effects of antibiotics on both the cellular and humoral immune response, on phagocytosis, and on such parameters of virulence as adherence and the production of toxins. These effects can modulate the complex dynamic ecologic relationships of the oral flora and have a strong influence on the regulation of both oral and systemic infection.

SUGGESTED READINGS

Abraham EP. The beta-lactam antibiotics. *Sci Am.* 1981; June: 76–86.

Drouhet E, Dupont B. Evolution of antifungal agents: Past, present, and future. *Rev Infect Dis.* 1987;9:S4–S14.

Foster TJ. Plasmid-determined resistance to antimicrobial drugs and toxic metal ions in bacteria. *Microbiol Rev.* 1983;47:361–409.

Franklin TJ, Snow EA. *Biochemistry of Antimicrobial Action*, 4th ed. London: Chapman and Hall; 1989.

Georgiv V. Antifungal drugs. *Ann NY Acad Sci.* 1988;544:1–610.

Greenwood D, O'Grady F, ed. *The Scientific Basis of Antimicrobial Chemotherapy, Society for General Microbiology, Symposium 38.* Cambridge: Cambridge University Press; 1985.

Jackson GG. The key role of aminoglycosides in antibacterial therapy and Prophylaxis. *J Antimicrob Ther.* 1984;13:1–5, 47–49.

Kagan B. *Antimicrobial Therapy,* 3rd ed. Philadelphia: WB Saunders; 1980.

Koch A. Evolution of antibiotic resistance: Gene function. *Microbiol Rev.* 1981;45:355–378.

Lancini G, Parenti F. *Antibiotics: An Integrated View.* New York: Springer-Verlag; 1982.

Lorian V. *Antibiotics in Laboratory Medicine.* Baltimore: Williams & Wilkins; 1986.

Newman M, Goodman A. *Guide to Antibiotic Use in Dental Practice.* Chicago: Quintessence Publishing Co: 1984.

Ogawara H. Antibiotic resistance in pathogenic and producing bacteria with special reference to beta-lactam antibiotics. *Microbiol Rev.* 1981;45:591–619.

Tomasz A. The mechanism of the irreversible antimicrobial effects of penicillin: How the beta-lactam antibiotics kill and lyse bacteria. *Annu Rev Microbiol.* 1979;33:113–138.

Valdes MV, Lobbins PM, Slots J. Beta-lactamase-producing bacteria in human oral cavity. *J Oral Pathol.* 1982;11:58.

CHAPTER 6

Antigens, Antibodies, and Complement

Robert R. White and Peggy A. O'Neill

INTRODUCTION

ANTIGENS
- Properties of Antigens
- Antigenic Determinants
- Haptens
- Specificity
- Sources of Antigens
- Terminology

ANTIBODIES
- Antibody Structure
- Immunoglobulin Domains
- Fab and Fc Fragments
- Antigenic Variations in Immunoglobulins
- Properties of Each Class
- Antibody in the Oral Cavity

COMPLEMENT
- Complement Activation
- Biologic Activities of Complement
- Complement in the Oral Cavity

SEROLOGY
- The Immune Complex
- The Precipitation Reaction
- Precipitation Tests
- Agglutination Tests
- Complement-Fixation Tests
- Labeled Antibodies
- Fluorescent Antibody Tests
- Radioimmunoassays
- Enzyme-Linked Immunosorbent Assays
- Immunodot Assays
- Monoclonal Antibodies

ORAL ASPECTS

SUGGESTED READINGS

INTRODUCTION

The immune response is concerned with recognition and rejection of foreign substances by the immune system in order to maintain the integrity of the body. If the material that stimulates the immune response is an infectious agent, the rejection may be beneficial. However, this rejection process is inflammatory, and surrounding tissues may be injured during the process. Thus, the immune response can also be harmful. The beneficial and harmful effects coexist, and the extent of the resultant protection or injury is determined by the particular stimulant and the interaction of the various immune factors recruited in the response.

Manifestations of the immune response occur in the oral cavity. Oral effects of systemic immunologic processes, such as systemic allergies or protective immunity against systemic pathogens that produce oral disease, are readily apparent. In addition, immunity may have direct oral implications. Immunologic factors are evident in periodontal disease, dental caries, and oral abscesses.

There are three major components in the immune response, antigens, antibodies, and lymphocytes. The antigen is the material, foreign to the body or at least to the immune system, that induces the immune response. Lymphocytes are stimulated, activated, or otherwise modified by the antigen and will react with the antigen on reexposure. These activated or antigen-reactive lymphocytes are responsible for cell-mediated immunity. Antibodies are specific proteins produced by certain of the stimulated lymphocytes and are capable of reacting with the antigen that caused their production. Antibodies are the mediators of humoral immunity. This chapter and Chapters 7 and 8 describe these components, the reactions they mediate, and the results of these reactions, both protective and harmful.

ANTIGENS

Antigens may be defined as compounds that can induce the formation of antibodies and antigen-reactive lymphocytes and that will react specifically with these antibodies or antigen-reactive lymphocytes. This definition recognizes the two major properties of antigens. One is the ability to stimulate the immune system to produce immune components, and the second is the ability to react specifically with the immune components produced by the immune system.

There are, however, some substances, called haptens, that possess only the second property associated with antigens, the ability to react with immune components. Therefore, in order to define better the terminology used in speaking of antigens, immunologists coined two new words, immunogen and immunogenicity. An immunogen is a compound that evokes an immune response, and immunogenicity refers to the ability to evoke a response. Antigenicity refers to the ability to react with antibodies or antigen-reactive cells. These definitions have not been applied universally, and in practice, the terms antigen and antigenicity are still often used to designate both properties of antigens.

Properties of Antigens

All substances are not antigens, nor are all antigens equally immunogenic. There are several properties that characterize antigens and that may determine not only if a compound is an antigen but also the degree of immunogenicity. Antigens are usually foreign to the host that responds to them. Except for a few substances such as the red blood cell (RBC) typing and histocompatibility antigens, antigens are derived from another species. Although an animal's tissues are composed of potentially antigenic materials, the animal does not normally react to its own tissues because the immune system is capable of differentiating its antigens from those of another species or even antigens of another individual of the same species. One's own antigens are called self antigens, whereas those from another source are nonself antigens. The immune system will not respond against self antigens but will respond to nonself antigens. This ability to differentiate self from nonself antigens is critical, since it prevents the development of potentially harmful autoimmune reactions.

Generally, the degree of unrelatedness determines the immunogenicity of an antigen. For example, a human's response to a microbial antigen would be expected to be much stronger than the response to antigens derived from a lower primate. As noted previously, foreignness also exists within species, and this serves as the basis for the immune rejection of transplanted organs and blood transfusion reactions.

Antigens are relatively large molecular weight compounds. The lower size limits of antigens are around 5000 to 10,000 MW, and these are usually weak immunogens. Even smaller compounds have been shown to be immunogenic, but they are the exception. The relationship between immunogenicity and molecular weight is a function of the antigen's chemical composition. Most proteins greater than 20,000 MW are good immunogens, whereas the lower limit for polysaccharides is from 75,000 to 100,000 MW. In general, the greater the molecular weight of an antigen, the greater its immunogenicity.

The chemical nature of a compound also can determine its immunogenicity. Proteins are excellent immunogens. Polysaccharides also are immunogenic, but less so than proteins. Nucleic acids alone do not induce an immune response, but when they are injected as part of a nucleoprotein, antibodies reactive with the nucleic acid moiety are produced. Lipids also are not immunogenic alone but may become so when incorporated into lipoproteins or lipopolysaccharides.

It was long believed that substances must be biodegradable in order to evoke an immune response, but there is at least one exception to this. The synthetic polymer, polystyrene, is not biodegradable, but it has been shown to induce an immune response in some species.

Antigenic Determinants

Although antigens are large molecules, only a small part of the molecule is involved in determining the specificity of the molecule and its subsequent reactions with immune components. These small reactive sites that are responsible for specificity are called antigenic determinants, or epitopes. Antigenic determinants protrude from the surface of the antigenic molecule and range in size from 8 to 12 amino acids in a protein to 2 to 6 sugar residues in a polysaccharide. The numbers of antigenic determinants on a molecule increase with increasing size of the antigen. For example, ovalbumin with a molecular weight of 50,000 has 5 determinants, whereas thyroglobulin, 700,000 MW, has about 40 determinants. The antigenic determinants on an antigen are not identical unless the molecule is symmetrical or composed of repeating subunits. Theoretically, each antigenic determinant should induce the production of an antibody of a different specificity. Thus, a single antigen will evoke the production of several populations of antibodies with different specificities.

Haptens

Much of what has been learned about antigens and about the immune response in general has resulted from the use of compounds called haptens. Haptens can react with antibodies but cannot stimulate an immune response; that is, they are antigenic but not immunogenic. Haptens can be made immunogenic by covalently binding them to molecules called carriers. Carriers are large molecular weight compounds that usually are antigenic by themselves. The combined hapten and carrier, called a conjugated antigen, can evoke an immune response against the hapten, which serves as an antigenic determinant on the conjugated antigen. Immune components resulting from immunization with a conjugated antigen will react with the conjugated antigen or the unbound hapten. Haptens are quite varied. They may be single atoms, such as nickel or mercury, they may be simple organic radicals, such as aniline or penicilloic acid, or they may be larger compounds, such as lipids.

Artificially produced conjugated antigens have been very useful in immunology. Haptens have been used to prepare conjugated antigens with a known single determinant or with limited numbers of known determinants or with known mixtures of determinants. These synthetic conjugated antigens serve as excellent tools to study the immune response.

Of even more importance from a clinical point is that spontaneous formation of conjugated antigens can occur naturally. After entering the tissues, some haptenic compounds can bind to the body's proteins. The immune system recognizes such conjugated antigens as nonself, and they may induce an allergic reaction. Penicillin, mercury, and methyl methacrylate monomer are examples of clinically significant haptens that may induce harmful reactions.

Specificity

The hallmark of the immune response is its remarkable specificity. Antibodies and lymphocytes react in a highly selective manner with the antigen that induced their formation. They will not react with the multitude of other antigens that they may encounter unless these other antigens have an identical or very similar determinant. Landsteiner demonstrated that specificity is a function of the antigenic determinants and that variations on specificity may result from very minor differences in the structure of a determinant. He did this by preparing conjugated antigens composed of a common carrier and haptens that varied only in very minor respects. Figure 6–1 illustrates the results of one of Landsteiner's studies in which he analyzed the reactivity of antibodies directed against stereoisomers of tartaric acid. Note that a change in the position of a small hydroxyl group on the hapten can change drastically the specificity of the antigen. In other studies, Landsteiner showed that the immune system could recognize variables as simple as the position of a double bond or the length of aliphatic chains. The antigenic determinants in natural antigens exhibit equal specificity. Even minor physical or chemical alterations may be sufficient to change the conformation of the determinant enough to reader it unable to react with the original antibody or to render self antigens nonself.

Sources of Antigens

All living things are antigenic. Tissue fluids, such as blood and lymph, contain antigens such as enzymes,

	Antigens from:		
	1-Tartaric acid	d-Tartaric acid	m-Tartaric acid
Immune Sera:	COOH | HOCH | HCOH | COOH	COOH | HCOH | HOCH | COOH	COOH | HCOH | HCOH | COOH
l-Tartaric acid	+++	±	+
d-Tartaric acid	⊖	+++	+
m-Tartaric acid	±	⊖	+++

Figure 6–1. Specificity of the reaction between antibody and hapten (ie, an antigenic determinant). Antisera raised against conjugated antigens containing stereoisomers of tartaric acid were tested against the conjugated antigens. + and − indicate the relative reactivity. *(From Landsteiner K.* The Specificity of Serological Reactions. *New York: Dover Publications; 1962.)*

globulins, albumin, and polypeptide hormones. In animal and plant cells, the cytoplasmic contents, the cell membranes, and the nuclear components are composed of antigens. Similar components in bacteria and fungi also are antigenic, as are toxins, cell walls, capsules, and flagella. Antigens in the virion include components of the capsid and the envelope and the enzymes present in the viral particle. One can better appreciate the immensity of the antigen load that confronts the immune system if one considers that every different cell is composed of a number of different antigens, each of which possesses several antigenic determinants.

Antigens also can be synthesized in the laboratory. Synthetic polypeptide antigens have been used extensively to study the immune response. Finally, as noted previously, natural antigens can be converted to conjugated antigens with haptens to produce what might be considered to be a semisynthetic antigen.

Terminology

Antigens may be grouped according to distinctive properties. Heterophilic antigens are antigens with identical or similar specificities derived from different species. The antigenic molecules need not be identical, but they must share at least one antigenic determinant. Several of these antigens, also called cross-reacting antigens, are of medical importance. For example, the Epstein-Barr virus and sheep RBCs share a heterophilic antigen that makes it possible to use the RBCs in the diagnosis of infectious mononucleosis, a disease caused by the virus. In addition, one of the theories concerning the autoimmune etiology of recurrent aphthous ulcers involves a cross-reacting antigen shared by oral mucosa and *Streptococcus sanguis*.

Alloantigens are antigens found in some members of a species but not in others. Those members of the species that do not possess the antigen will treat it as nonself. Examples in humans include the RBC typing antigens and the histocompatibility antigens, which are responsible for the rejection of organ transplants. Another important group of alloantigens is the serotype antigens in bacteria, which are of diagnostic use. Different strains of a species of bacterium may possess alloantigens that can be used to subclassify the bacteria for epidemiologic purposes. Thus, *Streptococcus mutans*, the bacterium implicated in human dental caries, has been shown to consist of at least eight serotypes.

Allergen is a term used to designate compounds that evoke allergic or hypersensitivity reactions. These may be true antigens, such as the proteins found in pollen, or they may be haptens, such as penicilloic acid or mercury.

ANTIBODIES

Antibodies are a heterogeneous group of glycoproteins found in plasma, lymph, other tissue fluids, and exocrine secretions. These mediators of humoral immunity occur in the globulin fraction of plasma and have been given the name immunoglobulins, a term used interchangeably with antibody. Immunoglobulins are divided into five major classes, A, G, M, D, and E, based on differences in physical and biologic properties (Table 6–1). They are designated immunoglobulin A, immunoglobulin G, and so on, and are abbreviated to IgA, IgG, and so on. Several of the classes have been divided further into subclasses.

Antibody Structure

All antibodies have a similar fundamental molecular structure. Variations on this basic structure allow differentiation into classes and subclasses. Beyond this, there is a more complex variation that is reflected in the antigenic specificity associated with each antibody. In order to understand the structural and func-

TABLE 6–1. PROPERTIES OF THE HUMAN IMMUNOGLOBULIN CLASSES

	IgG	IgA	IgM	IgD	IgE
Molecular weight	150,000	160,000	900,000	185,000	200,000
% Carbohydrate	3	8	12	13	12
Valence	2	2[a]	5	?	2
Serum concentration (mg/mL)	8–16	1.4–4	0.5–2	0–0.4	17–450 (ng/ml)
% Total immunoglobulin	80	13	6	1	0.002
Complement activation	+	–	+	–	–
Placental transfer	+	–	–	–	–
Fix to mast cells	–	–	–	–	+
Opsonin activity	+	–	–	–	–

[a]Secretory IgA and other polymers have a valence of 4 or more.

tional relationships among immunoglubulins, one first must understand the fundamental molecular structure.

The basic molecular unit is a symmetrical glycoprotein composed of four polypeptide chains and a carbohydrate moiety (Fig 6–2). The carbohydrate comprises 3% to 13% of the molecule depending on the class. The function of the carbohydrate is unknown, but it may be involved in secretion of the immunoglobulin from the plasma cell that produced it. The molecule contains two identical light polypeptide chains with a molecular weight of 22,000 each and two identical heavy chains of 50,000 to 75,000 MW, depending on the class. The light chains are of two types designated by the Greek letters κ and λ. These two types are shared by all immunoglobulin classes, but any one immunoglobulin molecule contains only κ or λ chains. There are five major types of heavy chains corresponding to the five classes of antibody. They are designated by the Greek letter that corresponds to the English letter used to name the class. Thus, α, γ, μ, δ, and ϵ refer to the heavy chains of IgA, IgG, IgM, IgD, and IgE, respectively. The differences in chemical, biologic, and antigenic properties that are unique to each class of antibody are the result of differences in the heavy chains. The polypeptide chains are arranged in pairs composed of a light and heavy chain held together by disulfide bonds, as shown in Fig 6–2. Immunoglobulins are large molecular weight proteins and, therefore, are themselves excellent antigens. Thus, it is possible to produce antiantibodies or antiglobulins. This antigenicity has been a useful aid in studying these molecules.

One of the paradoxes of immunology was that despite the fact that antibodies shared many physical and chemical properties, they showed an exquisite variation in terms of specificity for their antigens. This paradox was resolved when amino acid sequence studies of the polypeptide chains were carried out. It was noted that each peptide could be divided into constant and variable regions based on their amino acid sequences. For example, all κ chains possess a similar, or constant, 110 amino acid sequence at their carboxyl terminal end, with the remaining part of each peptide (also 110 amino acids) being composed of varying sequences of amino acids (Fig 6–2). A similar division into constant and variable regions is found in the λ chains. Heavy chains also are divided into constant and variable regions, but rather than being of equal length, the variable region encompasses only one fourth, again about 110 amino acids, of the peptide chain. The constant regions of heavy chains are similar within each class but vary from class to class.

As shown in Fig 6–2, the peptides are arranged in pairs, and the variable regions of each of the chains in a pair are aligned next to each other. The variable regions form the reactive site, the antigen-binding site, that is specific for a particular antigenic determinant. This variability provides for the vast number of different antibodies necessary to react with the multiplicity of antigenic determinants to which the immune system is exposed. On the other hand, the constant regions of the heavy chains are responsible for the properties (eg, complement activation) that characterize each class of immunoglobulin. In addition, the constant regions of both the heavy and light chains give antibodies those common properties that make them all globulins.

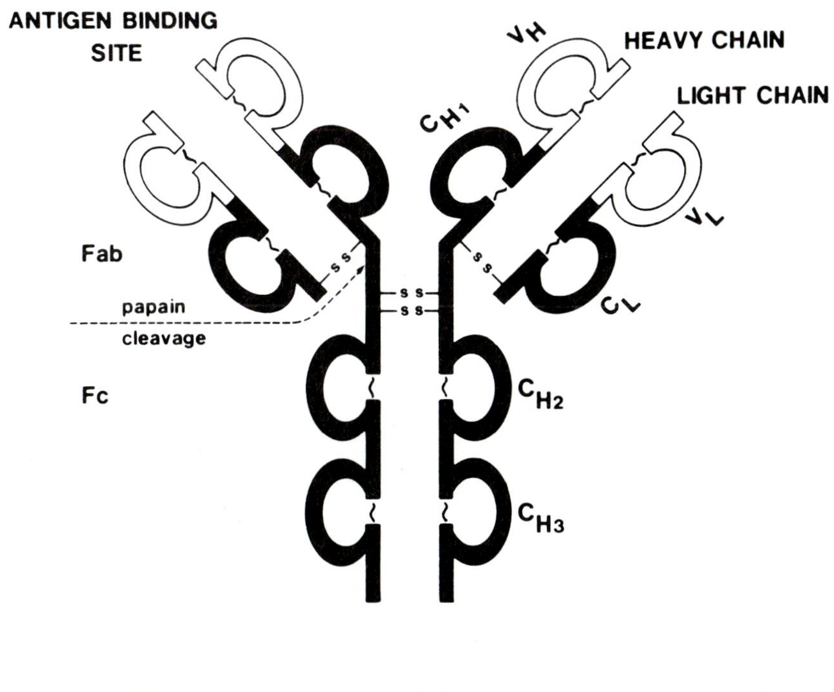

Figure 6–2. Schematic representation of the basic immunoglobulin unit. C_H represents domain on constant sequence of heavy chain; V_L represents domain on variable amino acid sequence of light chain.

Immunoglobulin Domains

Sulfhydryl groups on the different chains form interchain disulfide bonds that hold the peptides together. Other sulfhydryl groups within the same chain form intrachain disulfide bonds that, in association with other intermolecular forces, cause each peptide to fold into globular formations called domains (Fig 6–2). The variable region on each chain constitutes a domain (V_L and V_H), and the constant region of the light chain also constitutes a single domain (C_L). The constant regions of the heavy chains contain three or four domains (C_H1, C_H2, C_H3, and C_H4), depending on the class. Antigen binding is a function of the variable domains, and the constant domains of the heavy chains contain the sites responsible for the different biologic activities associated with each class.

Fab and Fc Fragments

Initial studies of antibody molecules included enzymatic degradation analyses. The results obtained when immunoglobulins are treated with papain are especially significant because these studies resulted in terminology that is in use today. When exposed to papain, the molecule is split into three fragments (Fig 6–2). Two of the fragments, which are identical, each possess a single antigen-binding site. These are designated Fab. The third fragment is designated the Fc fragment. The Fc fragment, composed of C_H2, C_H3, and C_H4 (if present) domains, carries the antigenic and biologic activities of the particular immunoglobulin class.

Antigenic Variations in Immunoglobulins

Immunoglobulins may be characterized further by their antigenicity. The antigenic variation between classes was noted previously. Subclasses also display unique antigenic determinants. The classes and subclasses are designated as isotypes based on these particular antigenic determinants that are found on the constant parts of the heavy or light chains.

There also are antigenic differences in the same immunoglobulin classes in different humans. That is, the IgG of one individual may possess determinants that are different from those of the IgG from another individual. Thus, immunoglobulins from different individuals may be alloantigens and are designated allotypes. As with the isotypes, the allotypic antigenic determinants are found on the constant part of the heavy or light chains.

Finally, each antibody molecule possesses a unique moiety, the antigen-binding site. These sites vary structurally from antibody to antibody depending on their specificity and contain antigenic determinants that are unique to the specific antibody molecule. Each different antibody will possess different determinants at the antigen-binding site. These antigenic variations are called idiotypes and, as will be described, appear to play a role in regulation of the immune response in a system called the idiotypic network.

Properties of Each Class

IgG consists of the basic divalent four-chain structure with a molecular weight of 160,000 (Fig 6–3). The plasma concentration of IgG ranges from 8 to 16 mg/mL, about 80% of the total plasma antibody (Table 6–1). There are four subclasses of IgG, which differ to varying degrees with regard to the properties associated with the class as a whole. IgG is the only antibody actively transported across the placenta to the fetus. This transported antibody, which in the fetus reaches levels comparable to maternal concentrations, is extremely important to the health of the neonate. IgG can fix or activate complement by the classic pathway. Through sites on its Fc fragment, IgG also can bind to Fc receptors on phagocytes and facilitate phagocytosis (opsonization). IgG plays a major role in

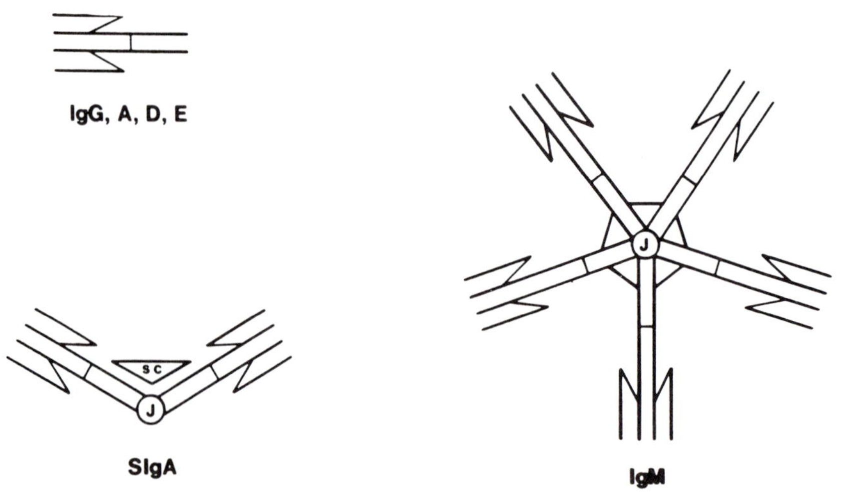

Figure 6–3. Schematic representations of the structures of the different immunoglobulin classes.

immune protection, since, in addition to complement fixation and opsonization, most antiviral, antibacterial, and antitoxic antibodies are found in this class. Conversely, as a result of its many biologic activities, IgG also plays a major role in several allergic reactions. IgG is second highest in concentration of all immunoglobulins in whole saliva. The major source of this salivary IgG is gingival fluid.

IgA is a polymorphic immunoglobulin. In serum, it occurs primarily as a divalent four-chain unit, but it also may be a polymer of two, three, or four of the basic structural units. The polymers possess an additional 15,000 MW polypeptide, the J-chain, which is thought to be involved in polymerization. The monomer is approximately 160,000 MW. Plasma concentrations of IgA range from 1.4 to 4 mg/mL, about 13% of the plasma antibody. IgA is the predominant immunoglobulin in exocrine secretions, including saliva, tears, colostrum, and gastrointestinal and mucosal secretions (see Table 7–16).

Secretory IgA (SIgA) is usually a dimer with a J-chain and an additional 75,000 MW peptide called secretory component. Secretory component's function is uncertain, but it is believed that it facilitates transport of the immunoglobulin through the epithelium by serving as a receptor site through which the IgA dimer can recognize and enter the epithelial cell. In addition, it is known that SIgA is much more resistant to proteolysis than are IgA and other immunoglobulins. Secretory component apparently protects SIgA from proteolysis. This resistance to proteolysis probably is significant in the adverse environments of the oral cavity, the gut, and other areas bathed by SIgA-containing secretions.

SIgA is of primary importance on the tissues bathed by exocrine secretions, where it may neutralize pathogens before they enter the tissues. SIgA is the predominant immunoglobulin in salivary gland secretions and in whole saliva. It also is passed from the mother to the newborn in the mother's milk and protects the infant from intestinal pathogens.

IgM is a pentamer composed of five of the four-chain units bound through their Fc fragments with a J-chain similar to that of SIgA. As a result of its large size, 900,000 MW, IgM has been called the macroglobulin. Although it would be expected to have a valence of 10, only 5 of the potential binding sites usually are reactive. The loss of the 5 other antigen-binding sites is thought to result from steric hindrance. IgM, which comprises about 6% of the plasma antibody, ranges in concentration from 0.5 to 2 mg/mL. IgM can activate complement by the classic pathway and does so much more efficiently than does IgG. On initial exposure to an antigen, it is the first antibody formed, but its production is limited, and its concentration is rapidly exceeded by IgG. Its multiple valency makes IgM a superior activitor of complement, and this, coupled with its early formation, suggests that IgM may be of importance in the initial defense against an infectious process. There is very little IgM present in whole saliva. This is because of its relatively low concentration in the plasma from which gingival fluid is derived.

IgD is a divalent four-chain molecule of 185,000 MW. Its concentration ranges from 0 to 0.4 mg/mL, and it comprises about 1% of the plasma antibody. No antibody activity, harmful or protective, has been associated with IgD. There is evidence that IgD may function as an antigen-specific receptor on lymphocyte membranes, where it may serve as a triggering site that stimulates or suppresses lymphocytes.

IgE is a divalent four-chain molecule of 190,000 MW. Serum concentrations of IgE are very low, ranging from 17 to 450 ng/mL. This represents only about 0.002% of the plasma antibody. It also is found in secretions, but its concentrations do not approach those of SIgA. IgE mediates allergic reactions through its ability to bind to mast cells and basophils and cause degranulation of these cells. IgE, which also is called reagin, may be markedly increased in the serum and secretions of allergic individuals. Although it is best known for mediating anaphylaxis, IgE plays a protective role in helminthic infestations and respiratory infections.

Antibody in the Oral Cavity

The soft tissues lining the buccal cavity, the periodontium, and the dental pulp are vascularized, and antibody found within these tissues, when they are healthy, is similar to that in the circulation and in other areas of the body. Gingival fluid is derived from plasma, and its immunoglobulin composition resembles that of dilute plasma; that is, IgG predominates. With increasing severity of gingivitis, there is an increase in the antibody in gingival fluid. The specificity of the antibody present in gingival fluid from a healthy gingival crevice is similar to that of peripheral blood. However, as a result of local immune responses to dental plaque antigens infiltrating gingival tissues, the specificity of the antibody in gingival fluid and gingival tissues of patients with periodontal disease may vary from that of peripheral blood. Gingival fluid will contain higher concentrations of antibody directed against subgingival bacteria.

The concentration of antibody in saliva is only a small percentage of that found in the plasma, but it is generally accepted that this antibody is sufficient to be immunologically effective. Whole saliva within the oral cavity receives antibody from three sources: the salivary glands, the gingival crevice, and antibody-forming plasma cells in the oral mucosa. IgA, predominantly SIgA from the salivary glands, is present in highest concentrations in whole saliva. Concentra-

TABLE 6–2. IMMUNOGLOBULINS IN ORAL FLUIDS

	IgG	IgA	IgM	IgD	IgE
Whole saliva (unstimulated)	1.4[a]	19.4	0.2	?	?
Parotid saliva (stimulated)	0.04	4.0	0.04	?	?
Gingival fluid (periodontitis)	350.0	110.0	25.0	?	?[b]

[a]Values are mg/100 mL.
[b]Subgingival plaque bacteria have been reported to be coated with IgE, indicating the presence of IgE in gingival fluid.
Adapted from Roitt IM, Lehner T. Immunology of Oral Diseases. *London: Blackwell Scientific Publications; 1980.*

tions from 20 to 40 mg/100 mL of saliva have been reported. Most of this is from the major salivary glands, but as much as 30% of this SIgA originates in the minor salivary glands throughout the oral cavity. The major salivary glands supply only minute amounts of IgG and IgM to the total salivary antibody (Table 6–2). The major source of IgG and IgM in whole saliva is gingival fluid. As noted previously, the quantity and specificity of gingival antibody will vary with the state of oral hygiene of the individual.

Antibody-forming cells have been shown to be present in the oral mucosa, and it is probable that the antibody produced by these cells can reach the oral cavity by intercellular diffusion. These isolated cells contribute only a very small proportion of the antibody found in saliva.

COMPLEMENT

Complement is a group of at least 20 different plasma proteins whose activities are closely associated with the immune system. These proteins circulate as inactive precursors that, when activated, potentiate, or complement, many immune reactions. Complement is essential to homeostasis, and any deviation from the normal complement status, either qualitative or quantitative, can result in disease. It plays a critical role in both beneficial and harmful aspects of immunity and in the inflammatory response throughout the body.

The complement proteins are activated in a sequence of reactions called the complement cascade. The initial activating reactions are characterized by a common pattern. An inactive precursor is hydrolized through limited proteolysis, which produces biologically active cleavage products. At least one of the products possesses proteolytic activity, and it cleaves the next protein in the sequence, which then repeats the procedure. The later components in the sequence are activated by complexing with complement proteins activated earlier in the cascade.

A key factor in the complement cascade is that certain of the activated products can cleave several of the complement proteins that serve as their substrates. This amplification mechanism is such that the initial activation of a single molecule can lead to the production of several thousand active molecules at the distal end of the cascade. Amplification greatly magnifies the effects of complement on immune reactions.

To facilitate discussions concerning the numerous complement components and products, a shorthand system has been devised. Complement is designated as C′, and the individual components are indicated by the letter C followed by the component's number (eg, C1, C2, C3). The cleavage products are assigned lower case letters. Thus, C2 is split into C2a and C2b. During the sequence, several active complexes are formed, and these are designated by a bar over the complex (eg, $\overline{\text{C4a2b}}$). Finally, it should be noted that C4 is activated before C2 in the cascade. This occurs because the complement factors were given numerical designations based on the time of their discovery, and C2 was discovered before C4.

Complement Activation

The complement cascade may be activated by two mechanisms. The classic pathway of complement activation usually is initiated by immune complexes acting on C1. The alternative pathway is a nonimmunologic mechanism that activates the cascade through C3, skipping C1, C2, and C4. Both pathways are of importance in health and disease. The final biologic activity resulting from the complement cascade is membranolysis, and the complement cascade usually is demonstrated using RBCs exposed to anti-RBC antibodies as the initiating immune complex. The formation of an immune complex between the antibody (hemolysin) and the cell's membrane in the presence of complement culminates in lysis of the cell. The descriptions that follow are based on this model system.

The classic pathway is activated by immune complexes containing IgG or IgM (Fig 6–4). These immunoglobulins possess a complement-activating site on their C_H2 domain that is inactive on unbound immunoglobulins but is activated when the molecules complex with their antigens. C1, which is composed of three subunits, C1q, C1r, and C1s, binds to the activiating site. The binding of C1 to the immune complex through C1q activates C1r, which in turn activates C1s, an esterase. C1 esterase cleaves C4 into C4a and C4b. C4a goes into solution, and C4b attaches to the cell membrane in the vicinity of the immune complex. The presence of C4b enables C1 to cleave C2. C2a binds to C4b, and C2b is released into the surrounding medium.

The $\overline{\text{C4b2a}}$ complex, called C3 convertase, is a protease that splits C3. C3a diffuses into the surround-

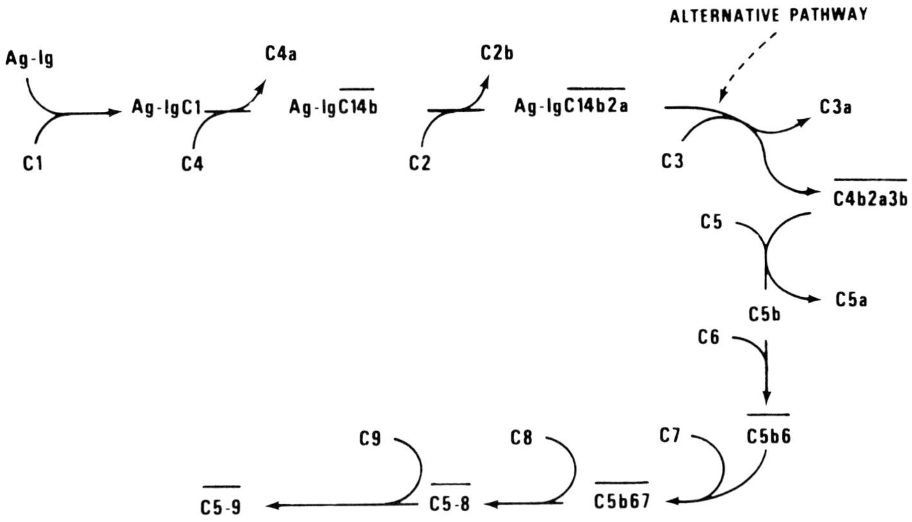

Figure 6–4. The classic pathway of complement activation.

ing medium, and C3b combines with C4b2a to form yet another proteolytic complex C4b2a3b.

From this point on, C5 through C9, the sequence is called the membrane attack system and is similar for both classic and alternative pathways. C5 may be activated by C4b2a3b or by a product of the alternative pathway that will be described later. C5a is released into the fluid phase, and C5b binds to the cell membrane at the site of the original reaction. C6 and C7 then form a complex with C5b. The C5b67 complex may remain on the original membrane, or it may be released into the surrounding medium and attach to another cell. The latter phenomenon, which may result in membranolysis of the second cell (reactive lysis), is of significance in certain allergic reactions.

C8 attaches to the C567 complex, and at this point, the membrane allows fluids to leak into the cell. Several molecules of C9 then attach to the complex to complete the cascade, and cytolysis proceeds rapidly.

Although the classic pathway is activated primarily by immune complexes containing IgG and IgM, other nonimmunologic compounds may initiate the reaction. These include thrombin, plasmin, and other trypsinlike enzymes, DNA, and C-reative protein.

The alternative pathway (Fig 6–5) is activated by bacterial and fungal polysaccharides, gram-negative bacterial lipopolysaccharides, trypsinlike enzymes, and many bacteria, including those found in the oral cavity. This pathway was first called the properdin system, and one of the components is still called properdin. The other components have been given many names, but the currently accepted ones are factor B and factor D.

In order to explain the alternative pathway, it was first postulated and then proven that there is a continuous low level conversion of C3 to C3a and C3b in body fluids. The C3b is labile and rapidly inactivated in the fluid stage but is stabilized by adsorption to the polysaccharides and compounds similar to those listed previously. This stable C3b is then able to interact with the components of the alternative pathway. C3b and factor B unite, and this complex is acted on by factor D to form C3bBb, an unstable group. Properdin (P) attaches to C3bBb to form the stable complex C3bPBb, which possesses proteolytic properties. Each molecule of C3bPBb is able to split many molecules of C3 and C5. C5 products set off the membrane attack mechanisms that continue the cascade through the activation of C9. Newly formed C3b is fed back into the alternative pathway in a cyclic amplifying mechanism that potentiates the initial reaction.

Biologic Activities of Complement

Activated complement factors possess many biologic activities (Table 6–3). Some of the more significant include

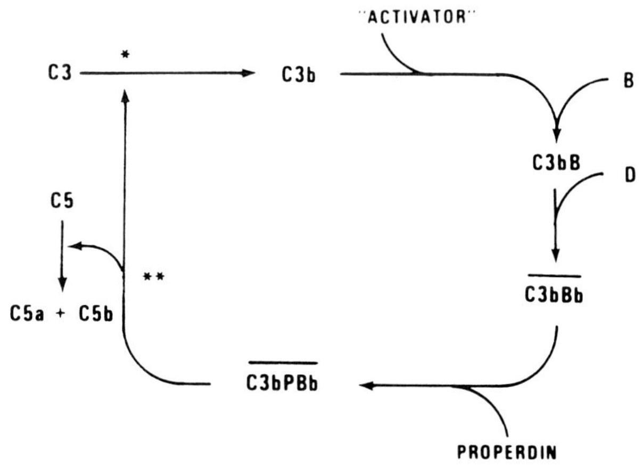

Figure 6–5. The alternative pathway of complement activation. Activator represents compounds such as bacterial lipopolysaccharides. *Initially C3b is formed spontaneously. ** C3bPBb may cleave C3 or C5.

TABLE 6–3. BIOLOGIC ACTIVITIES OF COMPLEMENT COMPONENTS

Component	Activity
C4a	Kinin activity
C4b	Virus neutralization
	Adheres to lymphocytes and phagocytes
C2	Kinin activity
C3a	Histamine release
	Induces release of lysosomal enzymes
C3b	Opsonic activity
	Adheres to lymphocytes and phagocytes
	Activates alternative pathway
	Activates B cell production of lymphokines
C5a	Chemotactic activity
	Histamine release
	Induces release of lysosomal enzymes
$\overline{\text{C5b67}}$	Chemotactic activity
	Reactive lysis
C6	Induces prostaglandin synthesis
C8	Slow membrane damage
C9	Rapid membrane damage

- Membranolysis: Activation of the cascade at the surface of a biologic membrane results in lysis of the membrane. This occurs with bacteria, mammalian cells, and some viruses possessing envelopes.
- Chemotaxis: At least two activated complement factors are chemotactic—that is, they attract leukocytes to the area in which complement is activated.
- Anaphylatoxins: Several activated complement factors cause degranulation of mast cells, with accompanying release of histamine and other pharmacologically active compounds. They are called anaphylatoxins because they mimic the effects seen in the allergic reaction, anaphylaxis.
- Opsonization: Some complement products enhance phagocytosis by leukocytes. They aid phagocytic cells in capturing and ingesting bacteria and immune complexes.
- Lysosomal enzyme release: Interaction of some activated complement factors with macrophages and PMNs results in the release of hydrolytic lysosomal enzymes.
- Lymphokine release: Interaction of some activated complement factors with lymphocytes induces lymphokine production by these lymphocytes.

Like most of the components associated with the immune response, complement is involved in both protective and harmful reactions. C4a has been shown to neutralize viruses in the presence of specific antibody. The increase in vascular permeability caused by C2b, C4a, C3a, and C5a facilitates the movement of antimicrobial factors into the area of an infection, and the fluid entering the lesion dilutes and assists in carrying away toxic products. The chemotactic factors, C5a, and $\overline{\text{C567}}$, attract polymorphonuclear leukocytes and macrophages. C3b and C5b also are opsonins, which enhance the phagocytic activity of the inflammatory cells. The membranolytic action of complement protects against bacterial diseases, especially those caused by gram-negative bacteria. B lymphocyte release of lymphokines, mediated by C3b, also may serve a protective function. Finally, the alternative pathway serves as a resistance mechanism through which the body can neutralize toxins and kill bacteria in the absence of adequate immunity.

Unfortunately, complement also mediates pathologic processes. It is involved in type II and type III hypersensitivity reactions and in some rejections of transplanted organs. As noted, complement also mediates lymphocyte release of lymphokines, which are thought to mediate inflammatory diseases, such as periodontal disease. There also are some nonimmunologic pathologic processes, such as the Shwartzman reaction, that are mediated by complement.

Complement in the Oral Cavity

Gingival tissues, the oral mucosa, and the dental pulp are vascularized and contain complement in concentrations comparable to those found in other tissues. Because gingival fluid is derived from plasma, complement would be expected to be present, and, indeed, several complement components, including C3, C4, and C5, have been identified in gingival fluid, as has factor B of the alternative pathway. Analysis of this fluid, however, is complicated by the fact that bacteria found in the gingival crevice or pocket are able to activate complement. This is apparent not only from in vitro studies but also from the fact that bacteria in subgingival plaque have been shown to have complement on their surfaces and that a complement degradation product, C3d, has been identified in gingival fluid. Although the complement present in the gingival crevice has been suspected of being involved in periodontal disease, its significance is uncertain.

SEROLOGY

Serology is the study of the interaction of antigens and antibodies. It encompasses not only the nature of the reactions between these two molecules but also the application of this knowledge to diagnosis and research. Serologic tests can be used to identify and quantitate antigen or antibody in solutions, they can be used to identify clinical specimens isolated from infectious disease processes, and they can be used to identify antigenic molecules or cells in histologic sections.

Serum from an animal that has produced antibodies to an antigen is called an immune serum or an antiserum. One may indicate the antigen by including it in the designation for the serum, for example, antiinfluenza serum, anti-RBC serum, and so on.

Antibodies exhibit a number of different serologic activities and may be designated according to the activity. Antibodies that are involved in the precipitation reaction are called precipitins. Precipitins form immune complexes with soluble antigens to form precipitates. Other names used to describe the serologic activities of antibodies include

- Agglutinins: Antibodies that form complexes with cellular or particulate antigens in suspensions.
- Antitoxins: Antibodies that neutralize antigenic toxins.
- Antiadherence antibodies: Antibodies that prevent antigen-bearing cells from adhering to tissues or other surfaces.
- Lysins: Antibodies that, together with complement, dissolve antigen-bearing cell membranes.
- Opsonins: Antibodies that enhance phagocytosis by leukocytes.

A single antibody molecule may mediate any of these activities. For example, an antibody reactive with an RBC membrane antigen could agglutinate the RBCs, could facilitate phagocytosis of the cells as an opsonin, or could, in association with complement, lyse the cells. The determining factor would be the conditions under which the antigen and antibody are allowed to react.

Serologic tests can be made semiquantitative. The concentration of antigen or antibody in a particular specimen can be determined by mixing known antigen- or antibody-containing reagents with dilutions of the specimen and determining at what dilution one no longer gets a demonstrable serologic reaction, such as agglutination. This is called the endpoint. To simplify discussions, the end point concentration is usually referred to in terms of titer. The titer of a specimen is the reciprocal of the endpoint. For example, if the endpoint dilution is 1/10, the titer will be 10, and if the endpoint is 1/100, the titer will be 100.

The Immune Complex

The union of an antigen and an antibody to form an immune complex is not simply two molecules adhering to each other at their surfaces. It is a specific reaction between two relatively small areas on the two molecules. The reactive site on the antigen, the antigenic determinant or epitope, may be composed of only a few amino acids or sugar residues, and only 10 or 12 amino acids in the antibody-binding site of the immunoglobulin actually take part in the formation of the complex. The antigenic determinant projects from the surface of the antigen, and the binding site on the antibody resembles a slot or a pocket into which the determinant fits. Thus, rather than simply being two surfaces in contact with each other, the union of the two reactive sites is three dimensional, with the projecting determinant fitting into the antibody's binding site.

The specificity of the reaction between antigen and antibody is determined by the steric configurations of these active sites. Specificity is proportional to the degree of steric complementarity between the determinant and the binding site. In other words, the better the fit, the greater the specificity. Steric configuration is of such importance because the bonds involved in the formation of the complex consist of coulombic forces, polar forces, and van der Waals forces. All of these bonds are very weak, and the strength of each is proportional to the distance between reacting groups—the greater the distance, the weaker the bond. In order to get a stable union between antigen and antibody, multiple bonds in close proximity to each other are required. Antigens and antibodies specific for each other share a high degree of complementarity and can form a stable complex as a result of the many bonds formed. Thus, as illustrated in Fig 6–6, B would represent a stable, highly specific complex, C would be less so, and A would be nonreactive.

The initial reaction of an antigen with its antibody is called the primary stage. This reaction results in a firm but reversible bond between the two molecules. If conditions are correct, the initial reaction is followed by a secondary stage in which a visible, or otherwise demonstrable, reaction is manifested.

The Precipitation Reaction

The simplest example of the secondary stage is the precipitation reaction, which can be demonstrated by adding increasing concentrations of antigen to a series of tubes containing a constant amount of antibody. After the compounds are mixed and incubated, precipitates will appear in some of the tubes (Fig 6–7). The first tubes, which contain the least antigen, will have little if any precipitate. As the antigen in the series of tubes increases, precipitates will appear and will increase in volume up to a point. However, as the concentration of antigen in the tubes continues to increase, the precipitates will begin to decrease. This semiquantitative precipitation reaction is useful in explaining some of the characteristics of serologic reactions.

If the precipitates are removed from each tube and the supernatants are analyzed, the first tubes will be found to contain free antibody in their supernatants, whereas the last tubes will contain free

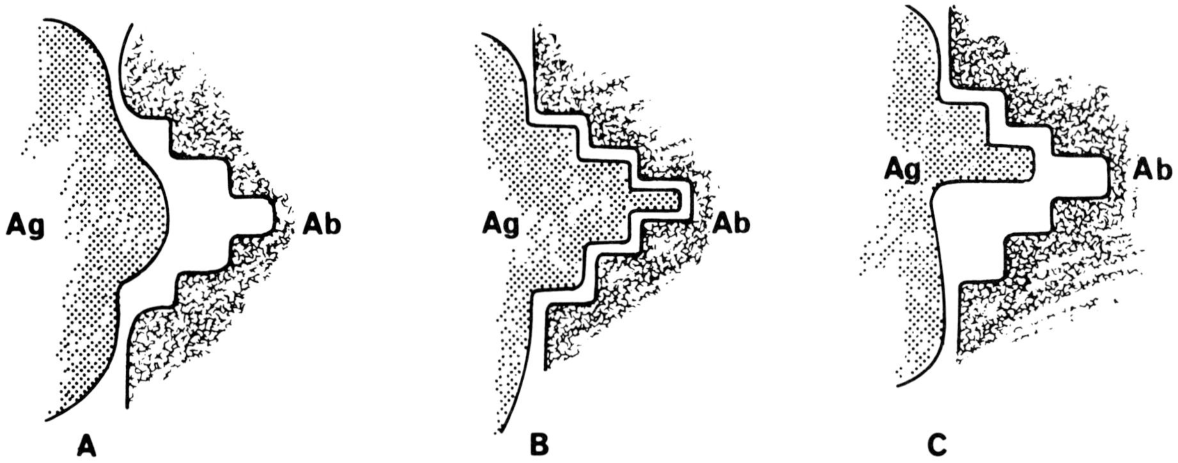

Figure 6–6. Schematic representation of the reactions between antigenic determinants and the antigen binding site on an antibody. **B** would form the most stable union and exhibit the greatest specificity. AG, antigenic determinant; Ab, antigen-binding site.

antigen. As the central tubes of the series are approached, there will be less of either free antibody or free antigen in the tubes, until at some point, that is, the tube with the largest amount of precipitate, neither free antigen nor free antibody will be present in the supernatant fluid.

This phenomenon has been explained by the lattice theory (Fig 6–7). The initial immune complexes aggregate into larger complexes resembling three-dimensional lattices composed of alternating antigen and antibody molecules. As long as the ratio of antigen/antibody is correct, the lattice will increase in size and eventually will precipitate out of solution. In the initial tubes, however, there is an excess of antibody, and lattice formation is inhibited because of this excess. In the last tubes, lattice formation is inhibited as a result of antigen excess. In the central tubes of the series, the proportions of antigen/antibody are more conducive to lattice formation, and maximal precipitation occurs. This area of maximal precipitation is called the zone of equivalence or zone of optimal proportions.

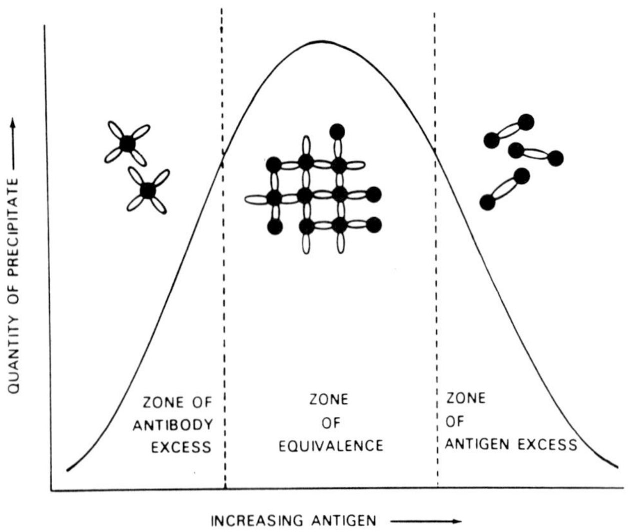

Figure 6–7. The quantitative precipitation reaction. ○, antibody; ●, antigen.

Precipitation Tests

The concept of immunoprecipitation has been applied to numerous serologic tests. The simplest is the ring test, in which a solution containing the antigen is layered carefully over antiserum in a test tube. A precipitate resembling a ring will form at the interface of the two solutions. This test gives qualitative evidence of the presence of an antigen or its specific antibody. The test may be made semiquantitative by mixing a constant concentration of antibody with serial dilutions of antigen. The last dilution in which a precipitate is detectable is considered to be the titer of the antigen. One can determine the antibody content of an antiserum by reversing the procedure and mixing a constant concentration of antigen with serial dilutions of antiserum.

The ring test cannot differentiate between multiple antigen–antibody systems within a tube. If multiple reactants are present, they will appear as one precipitate as a result of diffusion and convection. This deficiency can be overcome by preparing the antigen and antibody in a semisolid medium (eg, agar gel) before placing them in the tube. As the compounds diffuse toward each other, each antigen–antibody system will precipitate at its zone of optimal proportions, and the semisolid medium locks the precipitates in place. Since the location of the zone of optimal proportions will vary as a function of the diffusibility and concen-

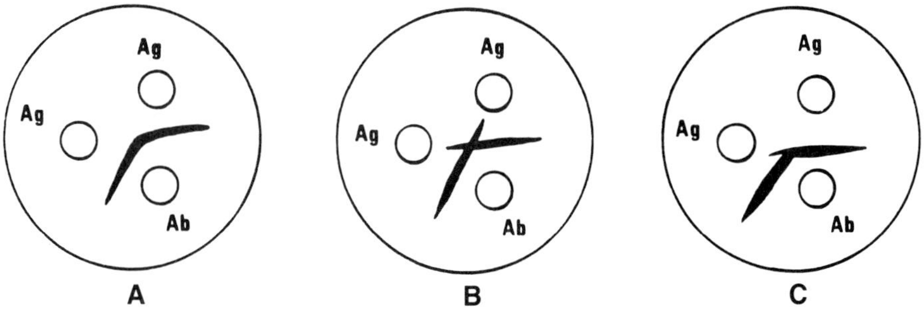

Figure 6–8. Schematic representation of three precipitation patterns that may be produced in a double diffusion in gel test. A, line of identity; B, line of nonidentity; C, line of partial identity.

tration of the reactants, these precipitates will occur at different points, and multiple antigen–antibody reactions can be detected.

This method, double diffusion in agar, has been modified further to enable the analysis of yet another parameter, the relationship between antigens in different preparations. In this test, called the Ouchterlony test, an agar plate in which wells have been punched is used. The wells are filled with antigen or antibody, the compounds diffuse from the wells through the gel, and precipitates appear at the zones of optimal proportions. Precipitates formed between an antibody well and two or more adjacent antigen wells can reveal if the antigens in each well are similar or different (Figs 6–8, 6–9). If the antigens in adjacent wells are identical, the lines of precipitate will fuse. If the antigens are completely different, the ends of the precipitate lines will cross. If the antigens are not identical but do share at least one antigenic determinant, the ends of the precipitate lines will fuse, but an extension of the precipitate line, called a spur, will form. These precipitate lines are referred to as lines of identity, lines of nonidentity, and lines of partial identity, respectively.

Radial immunodiffusion is a quantitative application of immunoprecipitation in semisolid media. Antibody is incorporated in the agar before the plate is poured, and wells are punched in it. Antigen placed in the wells will diffuse into the agar, and a ring of precipitate will form around the well (Fig 6–10). The diameter of the precipitate ring is a function of the concentration of the antigen. Using known antigen concentrations, a standard curve can be produced, and the concentrations of the antigen in other preparations can be determined from the curve.

The concepts in radial immunodiffusion have been extended further by the addition of electrophoresis. Antigen is placed in wells punched at the edge of a sheet of agar or cellulose acetate containing antibody. An electric field is generated across the sheet,

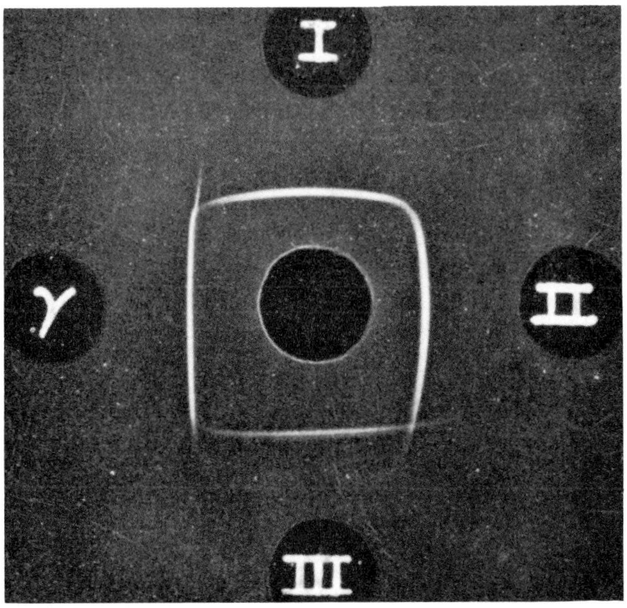

Figure 6–9 Double diffusion in gel test. RGG, rabbit gamma globulin (antibody); 1 and 2, Fab fragment; 3, Fc fragment. Note reaction of identity between 1 and 2, nonidentity between 1 and 3, and partial identity between RGG and 2 and RGG and 3. *(From Putnam FW, et al. The cleavage of rabbit gamma globulin by papain.* J Biol Chem. *1962;237:717.)*

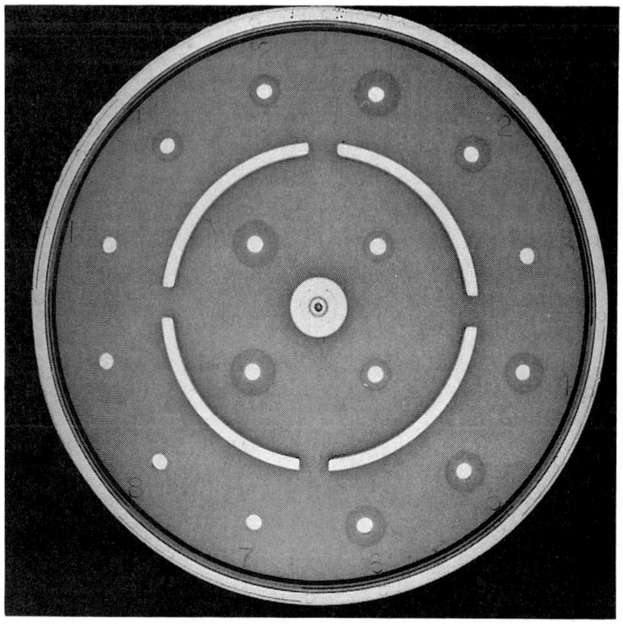

Figure 6–10. Radial immunodiffusion. The precipitates appear as darker rings surrounding the white well in which the antigen is placed. *(Courtesy of Helena Laboratories, Beaumont, TX.)*

and the electric current carries the charged antigens through the semisolid medium by a process called electrophoresis. An immunoprecipitate resembling a spike forms. The distance from the edge of the well to the point of the spike is proportional to the concentration of antigen placed in the well. The spike also has been described as a rocket, and the common name for this quantitative technique is rocket immunoelectrophoresis.

Agglutination Tests

The antigen in agglutination tests is particulate and commonly consists of suspensions of microorganisms, RBCs, or other particles. When mixed with specific antibody, the particulate antigens aggregate. This continues until large, visible aggregates are formed. Agglutination tests are used for RBC typing and to identify microorganisms cultured from clinical specimens. Agglutination tests also are used to determine the titer of antibacterial antibody in a serum.

In passive agglutination tests, soluble antigen molecules are adsorbed to the surface of particles such as RBCs or latex beads. When antibody is mixed with these antigen-coated particles, they will agglutinate. It is called passive, or indirect, agglutination because the particle acts as an inert carrier of the antigen and does not take part in the actual antigen–antibody reaction. Specific antibodies also may be adsorbed to similar particles, which can then be used to detect antigens. Latex passive agglutination assays are used in several commercial diagnostic kits.

The slide agglutination test is performed by mixing antiserum and microorganisms on a slide and viewing them either macroscopically or microscopically. This slide test, which is qualitative, is used for identification of unknown bacteria and for RBC typing. The tube agglutination test is a semiquantitative test used to estimate the titer of antibody in a solution. A constant amount of particulate antigen is added to each tube of a series of antiserum dilutions, and the titer is determined by observing the sedimented aggregates.

Complement-fixation Tests

Complement-fixation tests, which are among the more sensitive serologic techniques, incorporate the ability of complement to lyse RBCs in the presence of their specific antibodies (ie, hemolysins). Complement-fixation tests depend on two distinct reactions. The first involves antigen and antibody, of which one is known and the other unknown, and complement. If the antigen and antibody are specific for each other, they will react, and the immune complex formed will activate or consume (fix) the complement. The second reaction involves testing for the presence of complement to determine if the initial reaction has occurred. This is done by adding RBCs and hemolysin to the tube. If complement has been fixed by an immune complex, none will be available to react with the RBC–hemolysin complex, and the RBCs will not lyse. Conversely, if an immune complex was not formed in the first reaction, complement was not fixed, and it is free to react with the RBC–hemolysin complex, and the cells will lyse. Thus, a positive complement-fixation test results in no hemolysis, whereas a negative test is indicated by hemolysis. Complement-fixation tests have been used in diagnosis of viral and bacterial infections and in research.

Labeled Antibodies

Compounds such as radioactive isotopes, fluorescent dyes, and enzymes can be covalently attached to immunoglobulins without interfering with their antigen-binding capacity. These labeled antibodies have greatly expanded the scope of serology and are rapidly replacing many of the older techniques. Isotope-labeled antibody in an immune complex can be quantitated with a scintillation counter, and ultraviolet light microscopes can detect fluorescent antibodies. The addition of appropriate enzyme substrates to enzyme-labeled antibody systems and subsequent spectrophotometric quantitation of the enzyme product is the most rapidly developing field in serology.

Fluorescent Antibody Tests

Fluorescent antibodies can be used to locate and identify antigens in tissue sections and cell suspensions and to identify bacteria in clinical specimens. The direct fluorescent antibody test involves the use of labeled antibody specific for the antigen being studied. The specimen on a slide is flooded with the antibody, the unbound antibody is washed off, and the slide is viewed under an ultraviolet light microscope. Antibody that has bound to antigens in the specimen will fluoresce (Figs 6–11, 6–12).

The indirect fluorescent antibody test uses labeled antiglobulin antibody, that is, antibody directed against other antibody molecules. In the indirect test (Fig 6–13), the specimen on a slide is first flooded with specific but unlabeled antibody. This is followed by labeled antiglobulin antibody. The labeled antiglobulin will react with any immunoglobulins that were bound to the antigens in the specimen in the first step of the procedure. A major advantage of the indirect test is the need for only one labeled antibody reagent. Rather than having a large group labeled antibodies, a single labeled antiglobulin is all that is necessary.

Similar methodology can be used with antibodies labeled with enzymes, such as peroxidase. After the labeled antibody reacts with its antigen, the slide is flooded with substrate, and the enzymatic products

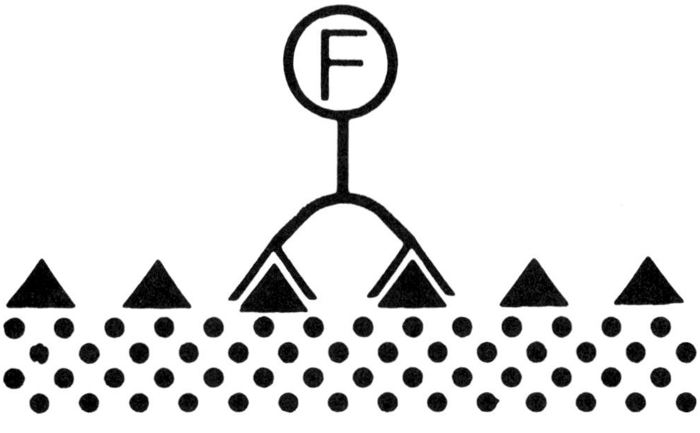

Figure 6–11. Direct fluorescent antibody test. Specific antibody labeled with a fluorescent dye (F) reacts with its antigenic determinant (▶). *(From Jennette JC.* Immunohistology in Diagnostic Pathology. *Boca Raton, Fla: CRC Press; 1989.)*

form a colored precipitate that can be seen with a brightfield microscope.

Radioimmunoassays

Radioimmunoassays (RIA) can detect picogram quantities of a substance using radioisotope-labeled antibodies or antigens. RIA can be run in either a liquid or a solid phase. In the liquid phase test, an isotope-labeled compound and a similar unlabeled compound to be quantitated in the specimen being analyzed compete for antigen-binding sites on a known quantity of antibody. Constant quantities of antibody and labeled antigen or hapten are mixed with the sample to be analyzed. The immune complexes formed are separated from the unbound reagents, and the amount of labeled compound in the complexes is determined in a scintillation counter. The competition for antigen-binding sites on the antibody is presumed to be equal, and, therefore, as the concentration of the unlabeled compound in the specimen increases, the concentration of labeled compound in the immune complex will decrease. Using known standards, a curve can be prepared, and the concentrations of the antigen or hapten in clinical or research specimens can be determined from the standard curve.

Solid phase RIA tests use test tubes or similar containers coated with a known antibody or antigen. To quantitate antigens, the antigen-containing specimen is added to a tube coated with antibody and allowed to bind to the antibody. The unbound specimen is then washed out of the tube. Isotope-labeled secondary antibody is added to the tube to react with antigen bound to the initial antibody. Unbound secondary antibody is then washed out. The amount of secondary antibody, or radioactivity bound in the tube, is a measure of the antigen present in the specimen.

RIA, which is one of the most sensitive serologic tests available (Table 6–4), can be used to measure haptens, since antibodies to the hapten can be produced by immunization with conjugated antigens containing the hapten. Most RIA tests have been replaced by the enzyme-linked assays to be described, but RIA is still used extensively to measure nonimmunogenic substances, such as hormones, antibiotics, and other drugs.

Enzyme-linked Immunosorbent Assays

Enzyme-linked immunosorbent assays (ELISA) use antibody labeled with an enzyme. In order to

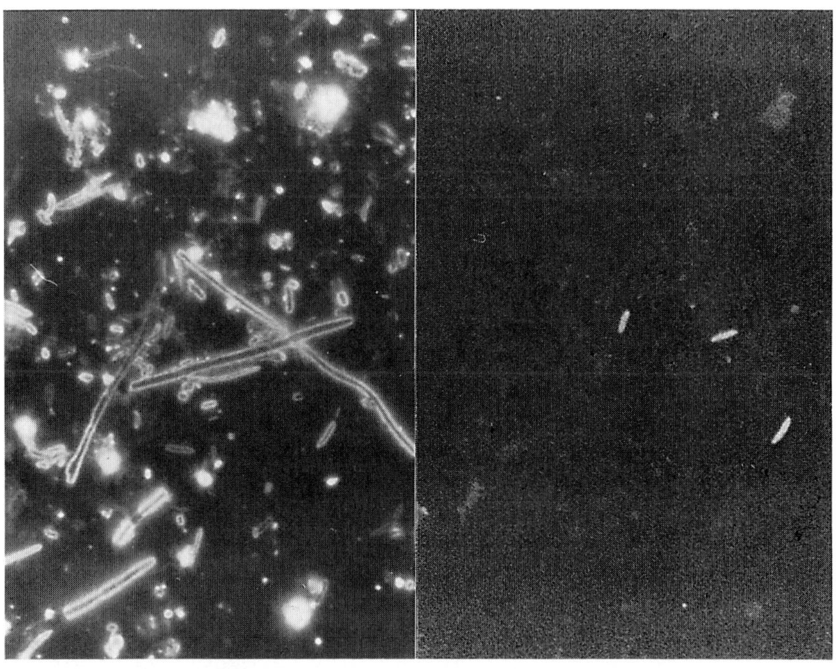

Figure 6–12. Fluorescent antibody assay. Subgingival plaque smear was stained with fluorescent anti-*Bacteroides forsythus* antibody and then viewed under darkfield (left) and ultraviolet microscope (right). Note three *B. forsythus* cells on right. *(Courtesy of Dr. C. H. Lai, School of Dental Medicine, University of Pennsylvania.)*

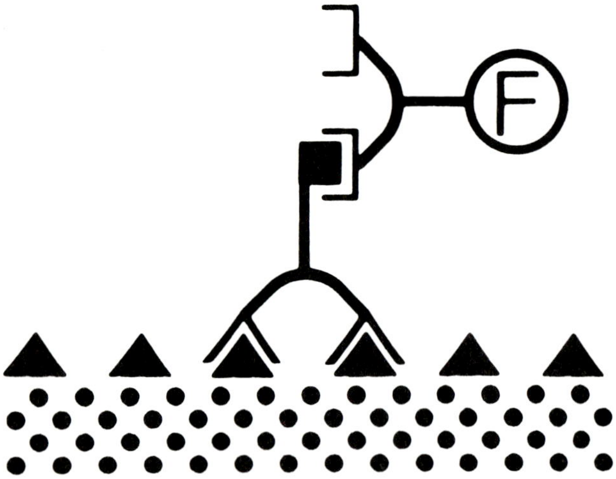

Figure 6–13. Indirect fluorescent antibody test. Anti-antibody (secondary antibody) labeled with a fluorescent dye (F) reacts with specific antibody (primary antibody), which previously has reacted with its antigenic determinant (▲). *(From Jennette JC.* Immunohistology in Diagnostic Pathology. *Boca Raton, Fla: CRC Press; 1989).*

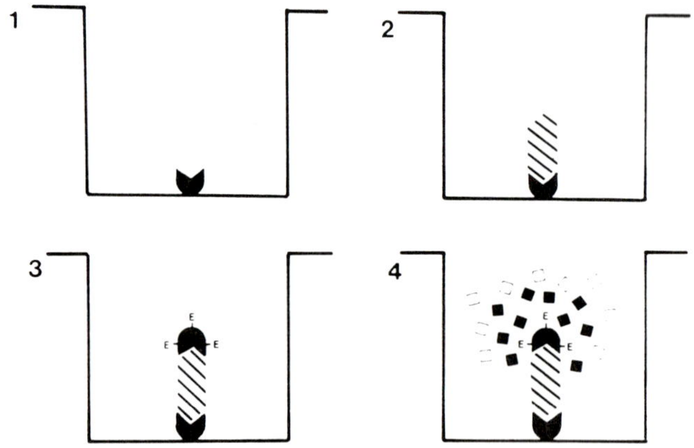

Figure 6–14. Enzyme-linked immunosorbent assay. 1. Antibody is adsorbed to the walls of the tube. 2. Specimen containing antigen is reacted with the antibody. 3. Enzyme-linked antibody is reacted with antigen that has bound to the initial antibody. 4. Enzyme substrate is added, and the product of the enzymatic reaction is measured. The amount of product is proportional to the amount of antigen present in the specimen. *(From Voller A, et al.* Bull WHO. *1976;53:55–65.)*

quantitate antigens, unlabeled antibody is bound to the walls of a tube, and the antigen-containing specimen is then placed in the tube and allowed to complex (Fig 6–14). Enzyme-linked antibody specific for the antigen is then put in the tube and allowed to react, after which excess antibody is removed. Finally, the enzyme's substrate is added to the tube, and enzymatic activity is recorded. The amount of enzymatic activity is proportional to the concentration of enzyme-linked antibody bound to the antigen, which in turn is determined by the concentration of antigen present in the original specimen. ELISA also can be used to quantitate specific antibody by binding antigen onto the walls of the tube, adding the antibody-containing specimens, and measuring the bound antibody with an enzyme-linked antiglobulin antibody. ELISA is used in analyses similar to those for which RIA has been used. It is as sensitive as RIA and has the advantage that it does not require radioisotopes.

TABLE 6–4. APPROXIMATE SENSITIVITY OF SEROLOGIC TESTS

TEST	Mg AB N/mL or TEST[a]
Precipitin reactions	1–10
Double diffusion in agar	0.1–1.0
Complement fixation	0.01–0.1
Radial immunodiffusion	0.01–0.025
Bacterial agglutination	0.01–0.1
Radioimmunoassay	0.0001–0.001
Enzyme-linked assays	0.0001–0.001

[a]Milligrams of antibody nitrogen per milliliter or per test.

Immunoblot Assays

Immunoblot assays are another group of tests that use enzyme-labeled compounds. For example, to detect a specific antigen, antibody is first adsorbed to a nitrocellulose membrane, and the membrane is flooded with the suspected antigen-containing specimen. If the specific antigen is present, it will bind to the antibody. To detect the bound antigen, the membrane is flooded with enzyme-labeled antibody, which will react with the antigen. Finally, enzyme substrate is added, and the enzymatic products form a colored precipitate that appears as a dot on the membrane.

Monoclonal Antibodies

The serologic techniques described have been enhanced greatly as a result of the development of monoclonal antibodies. The immune response to an antigen usually results in the appearance of several different plasma cell populations, each of which produces an immunoglobulin specific for a different antigenic determinant on the antigen. Normally, therefore, there are many different antigenic specificities represented among the immunoglobulins produced in response to an antigen. Using antisera containing this multiplicity of immunoglobulins can be a problem, and methods have been developed to produce antibodies derived from a single (monoclonal) plasma cell line. These antibodies, called monoclonal antibodies, are chemically, physically, and immunologically homogeneous; that is, they all react with the same antigenic determinant. Monoclonal antibodies are highly specific tools for research, diagnosis, and therapy.

Monoclonal plasma cell lines are produced in vitro

by mixing lymphocytes from an immunized animal and neoplastic cells from a myeloma cell line in the presence of a fusing agent, polyethylene glycol. The cells will fuse, and the hybridomas formed possess the antibody-forming capacity of the lymphocyte and the immortality of the myeloma cell and are able to produce antibody continuously in large quantities. Individual hybridomas are cloned in tissue culture, and the specificity of the antibody they produce is determined. The clones that produce the desired antibody are grown in large numbers in tissue cultures, which have been described as antibody factories. Purified preparations of these identical immunoglobulins may be used to differentiate molecules, or even whole cells, that vary by as little as one antigenic determinant.

ORAL ASPECTS

This chapter gives only brief descriptions of the methodology involved with each of the tests. Many variations, some routine and some very specialized, have been developed for each of the tests. In addition, there are other, less commonly used serologic techniques. Many of these tests have been used to study the tissues and fluids of the oral cavity. Precipitation tests, RIA, complement fixation, and ELISA have been used to quantitate immunoglobulins, complement factors, and bacterial and viral antigens in saliva, gingival fluid, and the soft and hard tissues of the oral cavity. Labeled antibodies have been used to study the cells and bacteria in the pulp, periodontium, and enamel.

SUGGESTED READINGS

Gazi MI. Monoclonal antibodies in dentistry. *Br Dent J.* 1986;161:399.

Matthews JB. Immunocytochemical methods: A technical overview. *J Oral Pathol.* 1987;16:185.

Mestecky J, McGhee JR, Bienenstock J, Ogra PL, eds. *Recent Advances in Mucosal Immunology,* New York: Plenum; 1987.

Roitt IM, Lehner T. *Immunology of Oral Diseases,* 2nd ed. London: Blackwell; 1983.

Rose NR, Friedman H, Fahey JL, eds. *Manual of Clinical Immunology,* 3rd ed. Washington, DC: American Society for Microbiology; 1986.

Sell S. *Immunology, Immunopathology, and Immunity,* 4th ed. New York: Elsevier; 1987.

Stites DP, Stobo JD, Wells JV, eds. *Basic and Clinical Immunology,* 6th ed. E Norwalk, Conn: Appleton & Lange; 1987.

Towbin H, Gordon J. Immunoblotting and dot immunoblotting—Current status and outlook. *J Immunol Methods.* 1984;72:313.

Voller A, Bartlett A, Bidwell D. *Immunoassays for the '80s.* Baltimore: University Press; 1981.

CHAPTER 7

The Immune Response

Robert R. White and Peggy A. O'Neill

INTRODUCTION

ORGANS AND TISSUES IN THE IMMUNE RESPONSE

MOLECULES AND CELLS IN THE IMMUNE RESPONSE
- Major Histocompatibility Complex Molecules
- CD Antigens
- Cytokines
- T Lymphocytes
- B Lymphocytes
- Plasma Cells
- Memory Cells
- Other Leukocytes
- Macrophages

THE IMMUNE RESPONSE
- Clonal Selection
- Cellular Interactions in the Immune Response
- Control of the Immune Response
- T-Dependent Antigens
- Mitogens

THE HUMORAL IMMUNE RESPONSE
- The Secretory IgA Response

THE CELL-MEDIATED IMMUNE RESPONSE

IMMUNIZATION
- Adjuvants

IN VITRO CORRELATES OF IMMUNITY
- Lymphocyte Transformation
- Lymphokine Assays
- Cytotoxic Cell Assays

IMMUNOLOGIC UNRESPONSIVENESS
- Self Recognition
- Immunologic Tolerance
- Immunodeficiency Diseases
- Immunosuppression

SUGGESTED READINGS

INTRODUCTION

Immunity is a function of the lymphoid tissues and cells of the body. The response to an antigen includes several different cells and molecules interacting with each other in a complex series of events. Much is known about the response, but there are still many questions unanswered. The discussion in this chapter is not inclusive but is meant to present the major events in the immune response. Detailed accounts of the immune response may be found in the citations in the Suggested Readings.

The immune response is divided into two branches mediated by different groups of lymphocytes. One branch, called cell-mediated immunity (CMI), is mediated primarily by lymphocytes (T lymphocytes) that become immunologically competent through exposure to the thymus gland. The second branch of the immune response, humoral immunity, is mediated by antibodies produced by plasma cells descended from a second population of lymphocytes called B lymphocytes. Although these two branches may be readily distinguished in print, the activities of the two are not so easily differentiated in the normal individual. There are several reasons for this. One is that several important functions are shared by both groups of lymphocytes. A second is that one group of cells may influence or regulate the actions of the other. Finally, when the immune system responds to an immunogenic stimulus, both branches usually respond. Only rarely is there a purely CMI or humoral immune response to an antigen. Although one branch may predominate, the immune response of an individual is the summation of the actions of both of these branches. The discussions that follow are presented in terms of these two branches, but one should always be aware of the simultaneous presence and interdependence of the two.

ORGANS AND TISSUES IN THE IMMUNE RESPONSE

Lymphoid tissues supply the cells and soluble factors necessary for the immune response and also store these cells until they are needed to respond to an immunogen. These tissues are divided into two categories based on their role in the immune response. The primary tissues are responsible for the development of immunocompetence, that is, the ability to mount an immune response. These tissues supply the cells that mediate the immune response, or they furnish substances needed for the maturation of these cells. The secondary tissues are sites in which the immunocompetent cells await and respond to antigenic stimulation. This classification of lymphoid tissues is not strict. As will be noted, some tissues carry out both primary and secondary functions.

In humans, the primary, or central, lymphoid tissues include the fetal liver, bone marrow, thymus, and gastrointestinal lymphoid tissues. The liver in early fetal life and the bone marrow later supply pleuripotent stem cells from which the cells of the immune response are derived. The progeny of these stem cells eventually populate other primary and secondary lymphoid tissues. The marrow also produces factors responsible for the maturation of some of these cells (Fig 7–1).

The thymus is an organ located in the midline of the upper thorax. During embryonic development, stem cells from the bone marrow migrate to the thymus. In the thymus, these cells, called thymocytes, are induced to differentiate into mature, immunocompetent lymphocytes by peptide hormones secreted by the epithelial cells of the thymus. The mature, immunocompetent lymphocytes, called T lymphocytes or T cells to designate that they are of thymic derivation, are responsible for CMI.

The existence of the primary lymphoid tissue responsible for maturation of the humoral immune response was discovered first in chickens in which humoral immunocompetence was found to be controlled by a lymphoid organ, the bursa of Fabricius, located at the lower end of the gastrointestinal tract. The lymphocytes were called B lymphocytes or B cells because they were of bursal derivation. Mammals do not possess a bursa, and the lymphoid tissue responsible for B cell maturation in humans is uncertain. The fetal liver, the bone marrow, and gastrointestinal tissues have been

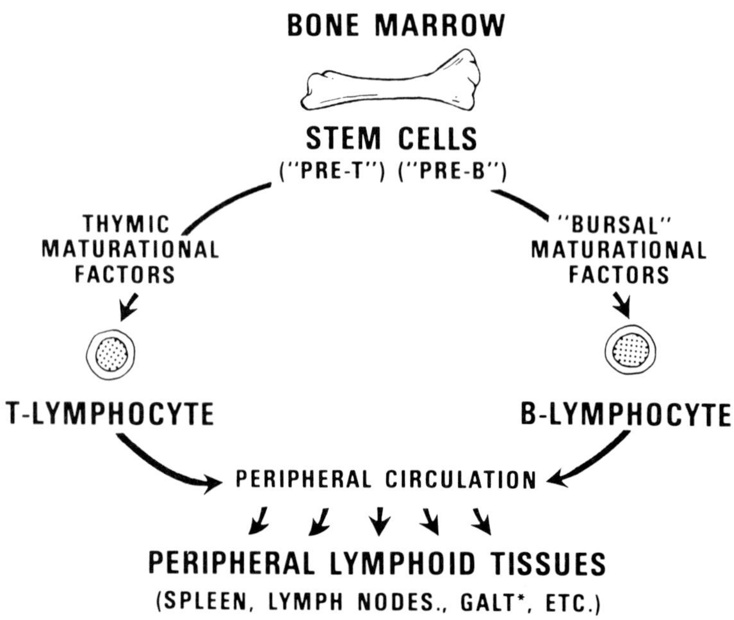

Figure 7–1. Maturation of the two branches of the immune response. Stem cells from the bone marrow are induced by thymic or bursal factors to become mature, immunocompetent lymphocytes that eventually populate the peripheral lymphoid tissues. GALT, gastrointestinal-associated lymphoid tissues.

suggested as bursal equivalents in humans and other mammals.

Localized collections of lymphoid cells can be found lining the submucosal tissue of the gut and the respiratory tract. The gastrointestinal-associated lymphoid tissues (GALT) include the tonsils, Peyer's patches, lymphoid nodules in the colon, and the appendix, whereas bronchus-associated lymphoid tissues (BALT) underlie the epithelium of the bronchi. These tissues may serve both primary and secondary functions. They play the major role in secretory and mucosal immunity, which is so important in the oral cavity.

Mature, immunocompetent T and B cells populate the secondary, or peripheral, lymphoid tissues. These tissues include the lymph nodes, spleen, and GALT. Lymph nodes throughout the body are major sites of the immune response to immunogens. Antigens that gain entrance to the tissues but do not enter the bloodstream are carried in the lymph to the regional lymph nodes, where they stimulate the resident lymphocytes. B lymphocytes selectively populate the cortex of a node. They form the primary follicles, which develop into germinal centers when the cells respond to an immunogen. The paracortex region of the node is populated with T lymphocytes. This compartmentalization of the lymphocytes responsible for humoral and cellular immunity is apparent in animals responding to different immunogens. When animals are exposed to immunogens that stimulate only humoral immunity, the cortical areas will be reactive. Exposure to an immunogen known to stimulate only CMI will induce a predominantly paracortical response. Immune components produced in the lymph nodes may react with antigens in the lymph node, or they may be carried via the efferent lymph to the thoracic duct and the bloodstream to other areas of the body.

The spleen shows similar T and B lymphocyte compartmentalization. B cells are localized in the follicles in the white pulp, and T cells populate the periarteriolar sheaths. Immunogens entering the bloodstream are trapped in the spleen, where they stimulate an immune response. The specific immune components produced as a result of the response are carried throughout the body in the blood.

In addition to GALT and BALT, there are collections of other mucosal-associated lymphoid tissues in the genitourinary tract and conjunctiva that serve secondary functions. Some of these lymphocytes, such as those in the Peyer's patches and the appendix, occur as well-defined concentrations of cells. Others occur as diffuse aggregates of lymphoid cells in the subepithelial regions. These, as well as lymphoid tissues in the lactating breast, are especially important in secretory and mucosal immunity.

MOLECULES AND CELLS IN THE IMMUNE RESPONSE

There are many cellular and molecular components in the immune response. Immunoglobulins and complement are described in Chapter 6. Some of the other major components are described here.

Major Histocompatibility Complex Molecules

The major histocompatibility complex (MHC) refers to a cluster of genes on human chromosome 6 whose protein products mediate several key functions of the immune response. The products of the MHC were recognized first as membrane antigens involved in the rejection of tissues transplanted from one individual to another. Thus, the term histocompatibility. However, it is known now that these molecules, and others coded in the MHC, play even more significant roles in immunity. These genes and their products are divided into three groups designated class I, class II, and class III. The products are interchangeably referred to as MHC molecules, antigens, or proteins.

Class I and class II genes and their products are those originally associated with graft rejection. Their products comprise a large group of the cell surface antigens, the human leukocyte antigens (HLA), that serve as target antigens (alloantigens) in the rejection process. Class I molecules are carried by all nucleated cells. Three genes in the MHC code for class I molecules represented by the HLA-A, HLA-B, and HLA-C groups of histocompatibility antigens.

Class II molecules are found on macrophages, B cells, and other antigen-presenting cells. These molecules, represented by the HLA-D, HLA-DR, HLA-DQ, and HLA-DP histocompatibility antigens, are coded for by four other genes in the MHC.

The products of class III genes include several components of the complement cascade, including C2 and C4 and factor B of the alternative pathway.

There is a great degree of polymorphism in the class I and class II genes, giving rise to multiple alleles that produce the many different alloantigens responsible for graft rejection. Among class I antigens, at least 23 A, 50 B, and 8 C specificities have been identified. The different specificities are assigned numerical designations, for example, HLA-A1, HLA-A2, HLA-A3, and so on. There also are numerous alleles among the class II genes. At least 19 D, 16 DR, 3 DQ, and 6 DP specificities have been noted among the class II antigens. This large number of varying antigenic specificities is the main reason for the difficulty in successful organ transplantation.

Although the HLA antigens were first recognized in the graft rejection process, tissue transplantation is, of itself, a highly artificial, unnatural event, and the part that these MHC molecules play in rejec-

TABLE 7–1. EXAMPLES OF HLA DISEASE ASSOCIATIONS

Disease	HLA Antigen	Relative Risk[a] (%)
Ankylosing spondylitis	B27	88
Reiter's disease	B27	46
Psoriasis	Bw17	5
Celiac disease	B8	10
Graves' disease	B8	4
Chronic hepatitis	DR3	14
Sjögren's syndrome	DR3	10

[a]Relative risk is the chance an individual bearing the HLA antigen has of developing the disease compared to an individual who lacks the antigen.

tion is only incidental to their natural role in immunity. They play much more significant roles as cell surface recognition molecules in immune responses. Some of the areas of immunology in which molecules of the MHC are involved include the following.

1. The class I and class II molecules are involved in antigen processing and presentation by macrophages and other antigen-presenting cells and in subsequent antigen recognition by T cells. As will be noted, T cells will not respond to an isolated antigen. The antigenic determinant must be associated with a class I molecule (in the case of cytotoxic T cells) or a class II molecule (in the case of helper T cells) and presented to the T cell in this associated form.
2. In graft rejection, the HLA antigens on the cell membranes of the grafted tissues are recognized as foreign antigens against which the recipient's immune system will respond. As discussed in Chapter 8, the HLA antigens of donor and recipient must be identical or very similar for an organ transplant to succeed.
3. Correlations have been found between the incidence of a number of diseases and the presence of certain HLA antigens. Individuals who express these HLA antigens on their cells are at higher risk of developing certain diseases (Table 7–1). The relationship between a particular HLA antigen and the disease is unknown. There is no evidence that the presence of the antigen might cause the disease, nor has its presence been shown to predispose to the disease. It may be significant, however, that many of the diseases are immunologic in nature and that the genes coding for the MHC and the immune response genes are located in close proximity on the same chromosome. It has been suggested that some periodontal diseases may have an HLA association, but there is no definitive evidence of this.
4. The HLA antigens are also of significance in forensic medicine. The number of different possible HLA antigen combinations is so great that the probability that any two randomly selected unrelated individuals might carry identical HLA antigen is one in tens of thousands. Therefore, in several judicial courts, HLA matching has been accepted as a means of legally establishing the relationship, or the lack thereof, of one individual to another or to match blood or tissue specimens to a specific individual. HLA tests are replacing AB blood group antigen analyses in paternity testing and other areas in which matching of blood cells or other tissues might be of forensic interest.

CD Antigens

Laboratories throughout the world have produced many monoclonal antibodies directed against T cell membrane antigens. In order to establish uniformity, an international committee arranged these antibodies and their respective antigens into clusters of differentiation. The antigens are designated as cluster differentiating (CD) antigens. Many of these were previously designated as T antigens. Some CD antigens are found on all T cells, whereas others are unique to T cell subsets (Table 7–2). CD antigens are useful in identifying and isolating T cells. Some are known to have specific functions. For example, CD3 (T3) is found on all T cells and is associated with the T cell antigen receptor. CD4 (T4) is found on helper T cells, and CD8 (T8) occurs on suppressor and cytotoxic T cells. Both antigens are involved in the antigen presentation process in that they appear to stabilize the association between the reacting cells.

Cytokines

Cytokines is a general term for another large group of molecules involved in induction of the immune response and mediation of immune reactions. A cytokine is a biologically active molecule produced and secreted by a cell. Cytokines are very important as signal molecules in immunity. The cytokines may act on other cells, or it may act on the cell that pro-

TABLE 7–2. CD ANTIGENS ON T CELLS

Marker	Found on	Function/Association
CD2	All T cells	Sheep red blood cell receptor
CD3	All T cells	Associated with antigen receptor
CD4	Helper T cells	Associated with MHC class II recognition
CD8	Suppressor/cytotoxic T cells	Associated with MHC class I recognition

duced it. Cytokines may be designated according to the cells that produce them. Thus, lymphokines are produced by lymphocytes, and monokines are produced by mononuclear cells or macrophages. These are not definitive classifications. Several cytokines were designated as lymphokines or monokines because they were initially associated with lymphocytes and monocytes, respectively. Subsequently, it was discovered that other cells also produce them. For example, interleukin I, a monokine, is produced by several other cells. Table 7–3 lists several cytokines involved in the induction of the immune response.

T Lymphocytes

T lymphocytes are derived from bone marrow stem cells (pre-T cells) that are genetically programmed to become T cells and that mature to immunocompetence under the influence of thymic hormones. If the thymus is lacking as a result of a congenital deficiency or early postnatal removal, mature T lymphocytes will not develop. An extract of thymus tissues, thymosin, has been used to induce T cell maturation in humans and other animals lacking a thymus. Thymosin consists of several peptide hormones that appear to be involved in different stages of T cell maturation.

T cells comprise about 60 to 70% of the circulating lymphocytes (Table 7–4). These cells may be identified by their distinctive membrane antigens. T cells also possess a receptor for sheep red blood cells. When incubated with sheep erythrocytes, the red blood cells spontaneously form a rosette (Fig 7–2) around the lymphocyte. This distinctive property, called E-rosetting, is used to identify, count, and isolate T lymphocytes. For the most part, monoclonal antibodies have replaced E-rosetting as a tool for identifying T cells.

The major functions of T lymphocytes include mediation of cellular immunity and regulation of other cells in the immune response. These functions are carried out by several different subsets of T lymphocytes. Helper T cells (T-h) and suppressor T cells (T-s) regulate the immune response. T-h cells and their products play a dual role in the immune response. They initiate all T cell and most B cell responses to antigens. T-h cells also produce several lymphokines that are involved in immune reactions. T-h cells can respond only to antigenic determinants

TABLE 7–4. SOME PROPERTIES OF T AND B LYMPHOCYTES

Property	T	B
E-rosette	+	–
EAC-rosette	–	+
Surface immunoglobulins	–	+
Fc receptor	+	+
C3 receptor	–	+
Cell-specific antigens	+	+
Frequency in blood	70%	20%
Frequency in lymph nodes	75%	25%
Frequency in spleen	50%	50%
Frequency in bone marrow	25%	75%

TABLE 7–3. CYTOKINES INVOLVED IN INDUCTION OF THE IMMUNE RESPONSE

Name	Partial List of Activities
Macrophage	
Interleukin 1 (IL-1)	Activates T-h cells and induces IL-2 production; displays many other biologic activities
T Lymphocytes	
Interleukin 2 (IL-2)	Induces proliferation of T cells and B cells; activates T-c cells; induces other lymphokines
B cell growth factor I (IL-4)[a]	Stimulates B and cell proliferation and expression of MHC class II molecules; enhances T-c cell activity
B cell growth factor II (IL-5)	Induces B cell differentiation into Ig-secreting cells
B cell differentiation factor (IL-6)	Induces B cell differentiation and T cell activation
Gamma interferon	Activates macrophages; enhances T-c and NK cell activity; augments other lymphokines

[a]Many of these factors have been designated as interleukins.

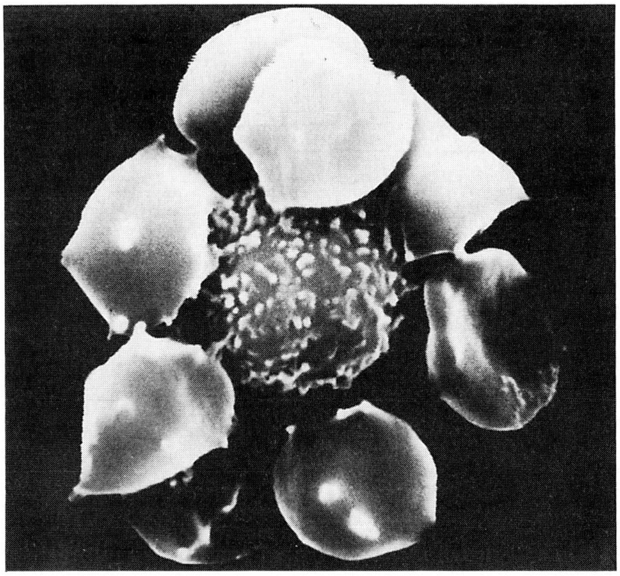

Figure 7–2. Scanning electron micrograph of an E-rosette, erythrocytes adhering to T cell membrane through CD2. *(Courtesy of C.L. Burek, School of Hygiene and Public Health, Johns Hopkins University.)*

presented in association with an MHC class II molecule. Inducer T cell is another name given to T-h cells. T-h cells also mediate delayed-type hypersensitivity (DTH) reactions. It has been suggested that the DTH cells actually form yet another subset that should be designated T-dth. T-h cells carry the CD4 antigen.

Suppressor T cells limit the activities of other T and B cells. They provide a negative feedback that limits the immune response to an antigen. This prevents the continued production of immune factors when antigen is cleared from the tissues. T-s cells also maintain immunologic tolerance and self-recognition. An abnormality in T-s cells may result in autoimmunity. T-s cells carry the CD8 antigen.

Cytotoxic T lymphocytes (T-c or CTL cells) lyse cells that carry antigens that appear to be foreign to the host. These include virus-infected cells, transplanted cells with incompatible MHC antigens, and cancer cells. T-c cells also possess the CD8 antigen on their membranes. T-c cells can respond only to an antigen that is presented in association with an MHC class I molecule.

B Lymphocytes

B lymphocytes are derived from bone marrow stem cells, pre-B cells, but the tissues that control the maturation of these cells are unknown. The presence of a bursa-equivalent tissue has been postulated, but as previously noted, it has not been definitively identified in humans. A B cell maturational hormone similar to thymosin has not been identified. The major function of mature B lymphocytes is antibody production, but B cells can mediate some activities previously associated only with T cells.

B cells comprise about 15 to 20% of the circulating lymphocytes (Table 7–4). These cells also have distinctive antigens and carry immunoglobulin molecules on their membranes. These immunoglobulins are considered to be identifying markers of B lymphocytes. B lymphocytes possess membrane receptors for the Fc portion of the IgG molecule and for the activation products of the third component of complement, C3. Sheep erythrocytes bearing an immunoglobulin or complement will bind B cells to form rosettes. EAC (erythrocyte-antibody-complement) rosetting is used for identification, counting, and isolation of B lymphocytes. However, as with T cells, monoclonal antibodies are more commonly used for these purposes today.

Plasma Cells

The plasma cell is one of the terminal cells in the B cell lineage. In response to antigenic stimulation, the B cell will eventually differentiate into a plasma cell, the primary antibody-producing cell. It has been estimated that plasma cells produce and secrete hundreds of antibody molecules per minute.

Memory Cells

Memory cells are terminal effector cells of both T and B lymphocytes. During the primary immune response, part of the progeny of the responding clone will differentiate into memory cells that will replace the original clone of cells. On subsequent exposure to the same antigen, the memory cell will proliferate and differentiate, as did the original T or B cell, and will, in turn, produce new memory cells. As a result of the primary response, the memory cell population is much larger than the original clone, and, therefore, the secondary or booster response is more intense and enduring. These cells also are called primed antigen-reactive cells.

Other Leukocytes

There is a third, smaller population of leukocytes that cannot be classified as T or B cells. Some of these lymphocytes will form EAC rosettes, but they do not have immunoglobulins on their membranes. Some, but not all, possess T cell markers. As a result of these discrepancies, they were designated as null cells. Others display monocytic characteristics. These leukocytes probably represent several subpopulations of cells. Other names given to cells within this group include L cells, killer cells, and natural killer (NK) cells, or large granular lymphocytes. Killer cells are part of a large group of Fc-receptor bearing cells that mediate antibody-dependent cell-mediated cytotoxicity (ADCC). When IgG binds to a membrane antigen on a target cell, the killer cell will attach to the cell, using the IgG molecule as an attachment bridge. It will then kill the target cell.

NK cells are cytotoxic against tumor cells. They are called natural because they do not require prior exposure and immunologic sensitization to the tumor cell antigens. These cells are not antigen specific; they can kill many different tumor cells. Their cytotoxic effects are increased by lymphokines, such as interferon and interleukin 2.

Macrophages

Macrophages are derived from monocytes, which evolve from undifferentiated bone marrow stem cells. Macrophages are found in circulating blood and lymph and in lymphoid and other tissues. Unlike T and B cells, macrophages are not immunologically specific in their actions. However, these cells serve two important roles in immune reactions. First, they are phagocytic cells that can engulf and destroy microorganisms. Lymphokines can enhance these antimicrobial activities. Second, macrophages are involved in the initiation of immune responses. Most antigens must be processed by a macrophage before T or B lymphocytes can respond to them.

Several cells other than macrophages may process and present antigens in the immune response. These include B cells, dendritic cells in the lymph nodes, Kupffer cells in the liver, Langerhans cells in the skin and gingiva, and astrocytes in the central nervous system.

THE IMMUNE RESPONSE

The components that mediate humoral and cellular immunity differ, but the general patterns of the responses to an immunogen are similar. Antigen stimulation of a lymphocyte induces proliferation of the lymphocyte, leading to an increase in the number of antigen-reactive cells. These proliferating cells then differentiate into effector cells, which mediate immune reactions or produce effector molecules. The first encounter with an antigen is called the primary immunization, and it is said to stimulate a primary response. All subsequent encounters with the same antigen are secondary or booster immunizations, and they stimulate secondary, memory, or anamnestic (Gr. *to remember*) responses. Primary and secondary responses vary in many respects, which will be described. Finally, although we speak of a lymphocyte's response to an antigen, it should be understood that lymphocytes do not respond to the whole antigen but rather to specific antigenic determinants on the antigen molecule.

Clonal Selection

A lymphocyte will not respond to just any antigen that it might encounter in the body. Lymphocyte specificity is genetically programmed; that is, a lymphocyte can respond only to a specific antigenic determinant. This is the basis for the clonal selection theory. According to this theory, an individual can produce antibodies of many different specificities because his or her total population of lymphocytes is composed of a correspondingly large number of different lymphocyte clones, each able to synthesize antibodies of one specificity. Each clone is presumed to have the genetic capacity to respond to an antigenic determinant of a particular specificity. Before exposure to the antigen, the clone is made up of few cells. When the antigen enters the body, it reacts selectively with the cells of its corresponding clone, stimulating their proliferation and differentiation. Thus, an individual possesses the potential to respond to all possible antigenic determinants, but only certain lymphocytes are capable of being stimulated by a particular antigenic determinant. These lymphocytes will produce antibody or antigen-sensitive cells reactive only with that specific determinant.

Members of each clone possess specific receptors on their membranes that will recognize the antigenic determinant against which the clone is genetically destined to respond. B lymphocytes have membrane-bound immunoglobulins (about 10^6 per cell) that serve as specific recognition and triggering sites on the lymphocyte membrane. An antigen will encounter many different lymphocytes when it enters the body, but it can react only with the cells of the clone carrying a specific immunoglobulin. When antigens bind to these membrane-bound antibodies, they induce an immune response by the specific clone. Other clones with different specificities are unaffected.

T lymphocytes do not produce immunoglobulins, but they possess other antigen-specific receptors on their membranes. The T cell receptor is composed of two polypeptide chains that are similar but not identical to the polypeptide chains of immunoglobulins. These two chains contain regions with constant and variable amino acid sequences formed into domains bound by disulfide bonds. The variable domains project from the membrane to form the specific antigen-binding site on the receptor.

B lymphocyte antigen receptors, immunoglobulins, can react directly with an antigenic determinant. T cell receptors cannot. The T cell receptor can only bind to an antigenic determinant associated with an MHC class I or class II molecule, depending on the particular T cell. The antigen must be processed by an antigen-presenting cell, and the antigenic determinant must be presented complexed to an MHC molecule.

Cellular Interactions in the Immune Response

When an antigen enters the body, it may be ingested by a macrophage and carried to a lymph node, or it may be carried in the lymph or blood to a lymph node or the spleen, the organs in which most immune responses occur. The subsequent immune response to the antigen is not simply the result of the actions of one cell or one clone. It is, rather, the result of several different cell types acting in concert.

Macrophages and other antigen-presenting cells (APC) are responsible for the initial steps in the primary immune response. In order to respond to most antigens, T and B cells require that the antigen be processed and presented by an APC. That is, the antigen first must be ingested and partially degraded, after which the remaining antigenic determinant is complexed to an MHC class I or II molecule. This complex (AG/MHC) is then returned to the membrane of the APC, where a specific lymphocyte can react with it (Fig 7–3). The macrophage also secretes interleukin 1 (IL-1), a monokine that activates T helper cells. The IL-1 and the binding of the T lymphocyte antigen receptor to the AG/MHC complex provide activating signals for the lymphocytes (Fig 7–4).

With most antigens, the T-h cell is the initial lymphocyte activated in both humoral and cell-mediated

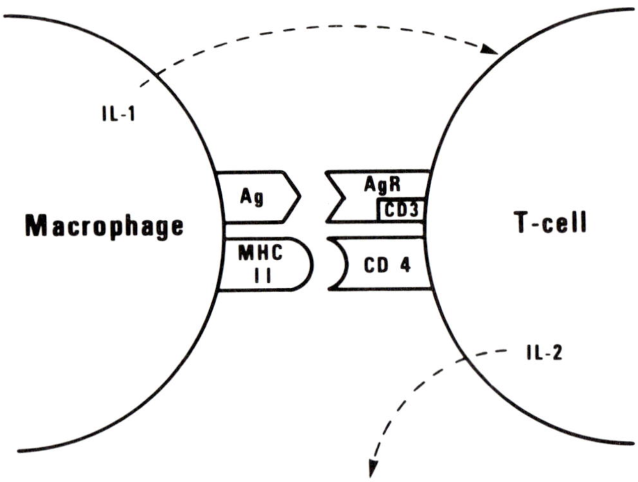

Figure 7–3. Macrophage antigen presentation to T cell. As indicated, the CD4 molecule stabilizes this union with T-h cells. The CD8 molecule serves a similar function with T-c cells.

immunity. Specific T-h cells bind to the Ag/MHCII on the macrophage membrane and this, with IL-1, activates the T cell. These activated T-h cells proliferate and secrete interleukin 2 (IL-2) and several other lymphocyte growth promoting and differentiating factors (Table 7–3). IL-2 is critical to proliferation and activation of T cell subsets and B cells.

At this point, the activation of T and B cells follows different pathways. In the case of T cells, the specific clones of T-h cells will themselves be activated and will activate other T cell subsets to proliferate and differentiate. The differentiated subsets resulting from this include T-dth, T-s, T-c cells, and T memory cells. The activating signals include lymphokines from the T-h cells and antigen presented by macrophages. T-c cells will recognize and respond only to a specific AG/MHC complex containing a class I molecule. It is unclear whether T-s cells are restricted to responding only to AG/MHC class I molecule complexes.

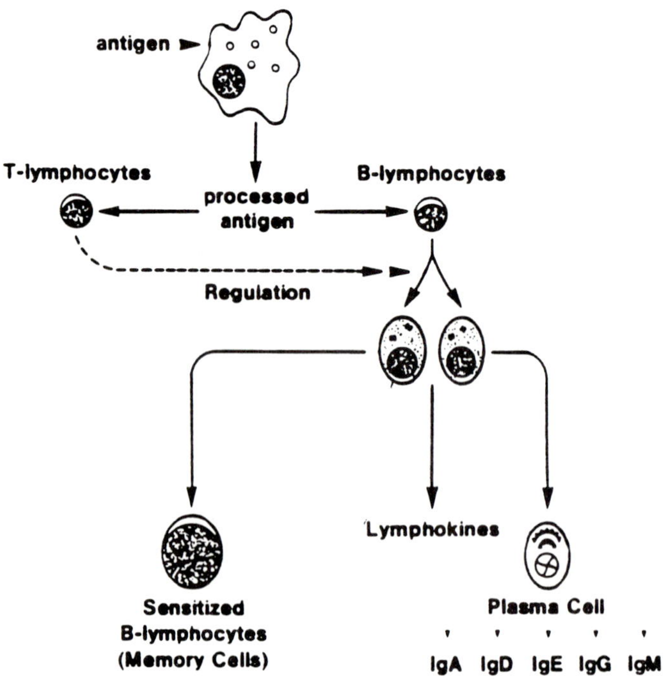

Figure 7–4. The B cell response. Regulation refers to the actions of T-h and T-s cells.

Complete activation of the B cell response to most antigens requires assistance of activated T-h cells. These antigens are called T-dependent antigens. The response to a second, smaller group, called T-independent antigens, is described later. B cell membrane-bound immunoglobulins bind the T-dependent antigen. It is not clear whether direct binding by native antigen is sufficient or if an antigen must be presented by the macrophage. The B cell, which is also an APC, processes the antigen and presents it, again associated with an appropriate MHC class II molecule, to the activated T-h cell. The T-h cell reacts with the B cell AG/MHC complex and induces the final activation of the B cell. At least three signals may be necessary for this initial B cell activation: (1) the stimulus the B cell receives from the macrophage, (2) the stimulus provided when the T-h cell binds to the B cell AG/MHC complex, and (3) stimuli from monokines and lymphokines produced by these cells.

Activated T cells produce several lymphokines that drive the B cell through proliferative and differentiating stages. Some of these lymphokines are listed in Table 7–3. Others are known to exist but have not been adequately characterized. The rapidly proliferating B cells will expand the clone, which will differentiate into antigen-reactive memory cells and immunoglobulin-producing plasma cells.

Control of the Immune Response

The immune system must be regulated to prevent excessive or prolonged production of immune factors when they are no longer needed. The proliferation of cells and production of antibody abates as the antigenic stimulus recedes and disappears from the body. At least three mechanisms that may regulate the extent and duration of the immune response have been proposed. These are specific antibody, T-s cells, and the idiotypic network.

It has been shown experimentally that passsive administration of specific antibody will suppress or curtail the immune response to an antigen. Similar negative feedback mediated by antibody produced during an immune response may naturally suppress the immune system. T-s cells also limit the immune response. Again, there is experimental evidence of their suppressor activity. The mechanisms are uncertain, but T-s cells are known to produce soluble suppressor molecules that act on T-h cells.

Each antibody molecule possesses a segment, the specific antigen-binding site, that makes it different from antibodies directed against other antigens. The unique molecular structure of the antigen-binding site is in itself antigenic and endows each antibody with unique antigenic determinants. These are referred to as idiotypic determinants (Chapter 6).

Although the immune system usually does not respond to self antigens, it does respond to its own idiotypic determinants. That is, if the immune system produces antibody (anti-A) directed against antigen A, for example, it also will subsequently produce antibody directed against the antigen A-binding site on the anti-A antibody. That is, the idiotypic determinants of the anti-A antibody will stimulate the autoimmune response. Thus, a second antibody, anti-anti-A, will be produced. Since anti-anti-A has its own unique binding site, yet a third antibody, anti-anti-antiA, will be formed. It is unclear just how far the immune system will extend this idiotypic network.

Although this idiotypic response may seem strange and wasteful, there is evidence that this network may be a regulatory system. That is, the purpose of the anti-anti-A may be to react with the anti-A immunoglobulin receptors on remaining B cells and turn them off. Similar idiotypic responses have been noted with T cell receptors, and they may function in a similar idiotypic control system. There are, however, still many questions concerning the nature and role of the idiotypic network.

T-Independent Antigens

T-independent antigens require neither T cells nor macrophages to initiate a B lymphocyte response. The B cell response, however, is incomplete because only IgM-forming plasma cells are produced. T-independent antigens do not stimulate B cell differentiation into memory cells and other immunoglobulin-forming plasma cells. Thus, the only product of a response to a T-independent antigen is IgM, and on subsequent exposure to the same antigen, the immune system will respond, as in the case of a primary immunization.

T-independent antigens include bacterial lipopolysaccharides, capsular polysaccharides, and other polymeric molecules. These antigens possess several properties that may induce B cell stimulation in the absence of T cells and macrophages. Some are polymers composed of multiple, repeating antigenic determinants. The polymeric structure may fulfill the presentation role of the macrophage (eg, proper spatial arrangement of the antigenic determinants?). Other T-independent antigens are mitogenic. The polymeric presentation or mitogenicity may replace the helper T cell function needed to induce proliferation of the B cell. However, these antigens apparently do not possess the capacity to induce the last step, differentiation, and thus only IgM is produced.

Mitogens

A number of natural compounds have been shown to nonspecifically activate lymphocytes. Originally, these substances were called mitogens because they induced lymphocyte proliferation. Now it is known that mitogens also induce other cellular activities. For example, some mitogens stimulate T lymphocytes not only to proliferate but also to differentiate into cytotoxic and lymphokine-producing cells. Other mitogens induce B cell proliferation, differentiation, and antibody production. Mitogens do not act on specific clones of lymphocytes. They activate clones directed against many different antigenic specificities. Therefore, they are called polyclonal activators to differentiate them from antigens (monoclonal activators) that activate lymphocytes of a single antigenic specificity.

Some mitogens activate only T lymphocytes. These include the plant lectins, phytohemagglutinin (PHA), and conconavalin A (Con A). Others, such as bacterial lipopolysaccharides and pokeweed mitogen (PWM), activate B lymphocytes. Mitogens have been used extensively to study the roles of lymphocytes in the immune response. Polyclonal B cell activators also play a role in oral disease. It has been reported that polyclonal B cell activation of gingival lymphocytes by bacterial mitogens in the gingival tissues may contribute to inflammatory periodontal disease.

THE HUMORAL IMMUNE RESPONSE

Following primary exposure to an antigen, B lymphocytes will transform into blast cells, proliferate, and differentiate into two effector cells, antibody-forming plasma cells, and memory cells (Fig 7–4). Antibodies are the major effector molecules of humoral immunity. In addition, although lymphokine production usually is considered to be a function of T lymphocytes, B cells also produce several of these effector molecules (Table 7–5).

Following primary immunization, circulating antibody will appear in the blood after 5 to 7 days, and the levels of antibody will peak at 14 to 21 days (Fig 7–5). The period between immunization and the appearance of antibody is called the lag period. Antibody synthesis begins within hours after immunization. The lag period represents the time necessary for induction of the B cell response and the production of measurable levels of circulating antibody. IgM is the first immunoglobulin to appear, but its production falls off

TABLE 7–5. T CELL LYMPHOKINES INVOLVED IN CELL-MEDIATED IMMUNITY REACTIONS

Name	Activities
Skin reactive factor	Causes increased vascular permeability
Chemotactic factor[a]	Attracts macrophages, neutrophils, and lymphocytes to site of the reaction
Macrophage-activating factor	Activates macrophage, enhancing their antimicrobial activities
Macrophage migration inhibition factor[a]	Inhibits migration of macrophages, causing them to accumulate at reaction site
Mitogenic factor	Increases the proliferation of lymphocytes at reaction site
Lymphotoxin	Kills cells, including normal tissue cells, at reaction site
Transfer factor	Converts normal, nonsensitized lymphocytes into specific antigen-sensitized lymphocytes
γ-Interferon[a]	Activates cells, prevents virus replication
Osteoclast-activating factor[a]	Activates osteoclasts, leading to bone resorption

[a]Also produced by B cells.

rapidly. IgG may be detected soon after and is usually the predominant immunoglobulin class formed. IgA is produced in smaller quantities. The lag period, the class and concentration of immunoglobulin produced, and the duration of antibody production vary with the antigen, the dosage, the immunization route, and the physical state of the antigen. As a result of individual physiologic differences, the response also varies with the individual being immunized. After reaching a peak, the levels of circulating antibody gradually will diminish. This is a result of suppression of the immune response by the previously mentioned regulatory mechanisms, the death of plasma cells, and the catabolism of circulating antibodies.

If, after the primary response subsides and for years thereafter, the same antigen is injected into a primed individual, the secondary response, mediated by memory cells, will be rapidly induced. As a result of the expanded clone of memory cells, the response will be of greater magnitude and duration (Fig 7–5). IgG will appear more rapidly and will comprise a much greater proportion of the antibody produced. In addition, the IgG will have a stronger and more specific antigen-binding capacity. New memory cells also will be produced. The same variables that affect the primary response also affect secondary responses.

The Secretory IgA Response

Secretory immunoglobulin A (SIgA) is of special interest in dental medicine. SIgA is the predominant immunoglobulin found in oral secretions. However, it is of equal extraoral importance because it is the major mediator of secretory or mucosal immunity throughout the body (Table 7–6). The mucosal immune system is not simply an extension of systemic immunity. It is dissociated from the systemic response and varies from it in terms of induction of the response, the predominance of SIgA, and the synthesis and secretion of this molecule.

The lymphoid tissues lining the gut (GALT) and those in the respiratory tract (BALT) are critical to the mucosal immune system. These tissues, which are the major source of IgA-forming lymphocytes in the body, contribute to mucosal immunity in several ways. First, they can respond to antigens that pass through the epithelial tissues in the gut or respiratory tract. These tissues contain not only IgA-forming cells, but also a complete set of T cells needed for induction of the IgA response. There is some evidence that these cells are separate from those that mediate systemic immunity. Second, GALT and BALT serve as the primary source of IgA-forming lymphocytes that populate secretory and mucosal lymphoid tissues throughout the body. They pass from the GALT through the draining lymph vessels into the general circulation and selectively localize in secretory and mucosal tissues. Once having reached these areas, they remain as immunocom-

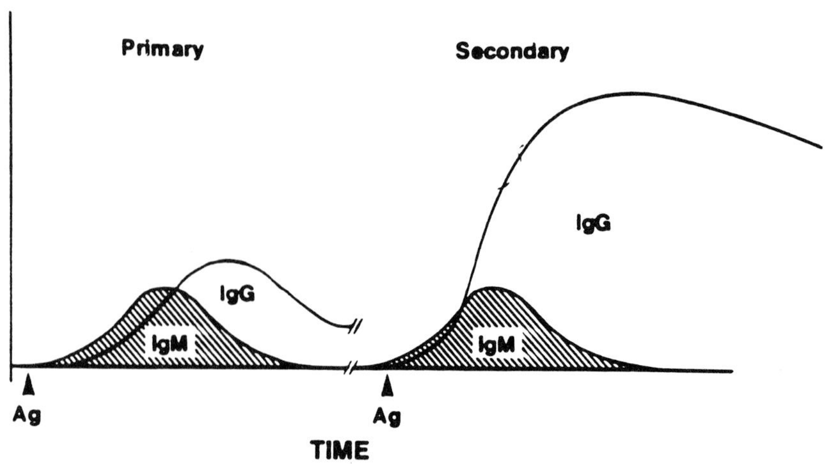

Figure 7–5. Immunoglobulin production in the primary and secondary immune responses.

TABLE 7–6. IMMUNOGLOBULIN CONCENTRATIONS (MG/100 ML) OF SECRETIONS FROM THE MUCOSAL IMMUNE SYSTEM

Source	IgA	IgG	IgA/IgG
Normal serum	290	1477	0.2
Nasal washings	26	6	4.3
Sputum	27	11	2.5
Parotid salivary fluid	4	0.04	100.0
Whole saliva	30	5	6.0
Jejunal aspirate	28	34	0.8

Modified from Knight V. Viral and Mycoplasmal Infections of the Respiratory Tract. *Philadelphia: Lea & Febiger; 1973.*

petent IgA-forming lymphocytes awaiting local stimulation by antigens entering these tissues. IgA-forming lymphocytes derived from the GALT and BALT have been found in the mammary, salivary, lacrimal, and uterine cervical glands and in the connective tissues underlying mucosal membranes throughout the body. Finally, the gut and respiratory tract can supply activated lymphocytes to other secretory and mucosal tissues. When some IgA-forming cells in the GALT and BALT are stimulated by antigens, they differentiate into the proliferative stage, and some of these blast cells migrate through the lymph and systemic circulation to secretory and mucosal tissues throughout the body. The activation of the blast cells continues, and IgA-forming plasma cells are produced. Thus, ingestion of an antigen my induce the eventual production of SIgA in secretory tissues distant from the gastrointestinal tract. Specific SIgA has been demonstrated in saliva, tears, and breast milk after oral administration of an antigen.

Only a very small amount of systemic or serum-derived IgA appears as SIgA. Almost all SIgA is produced locally in the tissues from which it is secreted. Plasma cells in the submucosa of the secretory tissues or glands produce dimers of IgA united with a J-chain and release these polymers into the intercellular subepithelial spaces (Fig 7–6). Epithelial cells lining the mucosal tissues or ducts of exocrine glands produce secretory component, which is localized on the lateral and basal membranes of the epithelial cells. The IgA polymers bind to the membrane-bound secretory component, and the complex, which is now SIgA, is transported into the cell. It is carried through the cytoplasm and secreted into the lumen of the secretory duct or onto the mucous membrane.

There are several points about the mucosal response that need further study. Two of these are the IgA memory response and oral tolerance. It is not clear if there is a secondary IgA response. Although some investigators have presented evidence that there is a secondary response, others have reported that there is no such immunologic memory. This question remains to be answered. Oral tolerance refers to the phenomenon that oral immunization may not only stimulate a local mucosal SIgA response but also induce systemic tolerance to the antigen. That is, if the same antigen is later injected parenterally, there will be no circulating IgG or IgM produced. Conversely, if antigen is first given parenterally to induce a systemic immune response, this may inhibit subsequent immunization through the mucosal route. There is evidence that these forms of tolerance are mediated by T-s cells, but many questions remain to be answered about oral tolerance.

A specific SIgA response may be stimulated by several methods. A local response in a particular gland or tissue may be induced by topical application of the antigen to the mucosal tissues or by injection of the antigen into the submucosa of the secretory gland or tissue. For example, SIgA has been induced in the salivary glands of laboratory animals by injecting the antigen directly into the glands or the vicinity of the glands and by perfusing the salivary gland ducts with

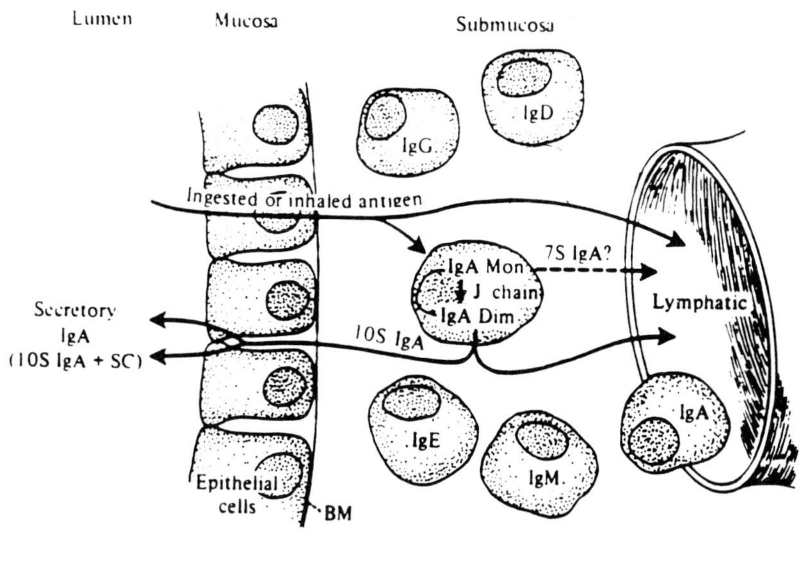

Figure 7–6. Synthesis and secretion of SIgA. Secretory component (SC) combines with the IgA dimer (10S IgA) at the lateral or basal membranes of the epithelial membranes to form SIgA. SIgA is then transported through the epithelial cell and into the lumen of the secretory duct. Some of the IgA dimer may enter the systemic circulation. *(From Tomasi TB.* The Immune System of Secretions. *Englewood Cliffs, NJ: Prentice-Hall, Inc.; 1976.)*

the antigen. Inhalation of an antigen will induce an SIgA response in the respiratory tract, and ingestion of an antigen, if it is not digested, may stimulate production and secretion of SIgA in the gastrointestinal tract. The latter also will induce immunity throughout the mucosal immune system. It should be obvious that because of the ease of administration of oral vaccines and the protective potential of such local immune responses, oral immunization is receiving a great deal of study. Several experimental caries vaccines are based on oral immunization.

THE CELL-MEDIATED IMMUNE RESPONSE

The induction of T cell-mediated immunity (CMI) is similar in many respects to that of the humoral response, but the effector cells and effector molecules are different. The effector cells include helper, suppressor, cytotoxic, and memory T cells, and the effector molecules are lymphokines (Fig 7–7). Lymphokines are involved in induction of the immune response, as noted previously, and in CMI reactions.

Following primary immunization, CMI activity is detectable more rapidly than humoral immunity, usually within 4 or 5 days. There is only limited production of cytotoxic cells and lymphokines in the primary CMI response. Therefore, the memory cell is the key effector cell produced in the primary CMI response because it sets the stage for the more rapid and intense secondary response. Most of the clinically apparent reactions in CMI are initiated by memory cells responding to a secondary immunization or an extended primary stimulus, such as a chronic infection.

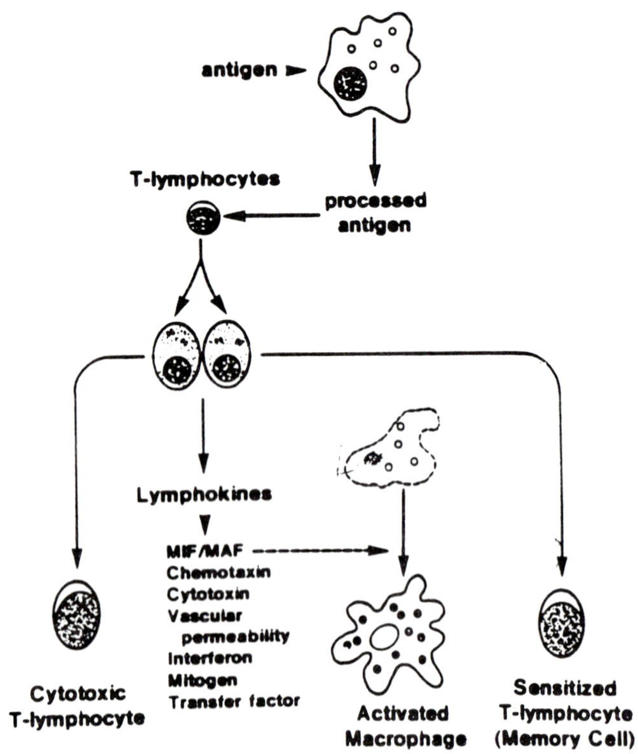

Figure 7–7. The T cell response. The T-s cell, another effector cell, is represented by the T-c cell.

The secondary response is more rapid, more intense, and of longer duration than the primary response. Lymphokines are produced in much higher concentrations, the various T cell subsets proliferate, and new memory cells are generated.

CMI functions may be divided into those involved in lymphocyte activation and the CMI reactions associated with immune protection and injury. CMI reactions may be divided into two branches, one mediated by lymphokines and the other mediated by cytotoxic T cells. Since the classic lymphokine-mediated reaction is delayed-type hypersensitivity (DTH), the T cell responsible for these reactions has been designated as the T-dth cell. It is not clear if the T-dth cell is a separate T cell subset, a memory cell, a T-h cell, or some derivative of these. It is considered to be the major producer of the lymphokines that mediate CMI reactions.

Some of the lymphokines associated with CMI reactions are listed in Table 7–5. These proteins regulate and potentiate the activities of the various cells involved in CMI reactions. Unlike immunoglobulins, lymphokines are nonspecific in their induction and their reactivity. All antigens stimulate the production of the same lymphokines, and lymphokine-mediated reactions affect all antigens present, regardless of which antigen induced lymphokine production.

Lymphokines intensify the normal inflammatory response directed against the antigen that stimulated their production. Skin reactive factor increases vascular permeability so that inflammatory cells and antimicrobial molecules can move into the site more rapidly. Chemotactic factor attracts other cells, particularly neutrophils and macrophages, to the area, and the macrophages are activated and prevented from leaving by other lymphokines. Mitogenic factor increases the numbers of cells, and transfer factor converts nonsensitized cells into antigen-specific cells that can then participate in the reaction. Cytotoxic factors and interferon exert protective effects in the presence of infectious processes. However, this amplification of what is essentially an inflammatory response can be both beneficial and harmful. These same lymphokines mediate allergic reactions.

Cytotoxic, or killer, T lymphocytes (CTL) kill other cells by a specific interaction between the cytotoxic lymphocyte and the antigen-bearing target cell. Target cells include virus-infected cells in which viral antigens are expressed on the host cell membrane, tumor cells, and cells of tissues or organs transplanted from one individual to another. The

CTL antigen receptor will react with the MHC class I molecules on allograft cells or the viral antigenic determinant associated with an MHC class I molecule on virus-infected cells and kill the cells. The lethal mechanism is uncertain but is thought to involve lymphotoxins and perforins. A single cytotoxic cell can kill many target cells.

Lawrence's dialyzable transfer factor (DTF) is another biologically active molecule associated with CMI. DTF is not a lymphokine. It differs from the lymphokine transfer factor in that it is a preexisting entity in memory T cells and does not require a secondary antigenic stimulus to induce its synthesis. DTF can be extracted from T lymphocytes and has the capacity to transfer specific CMI, but not humoral immunity, from a sensitized lymphocyte to a nonsensitized lymphocyte. For example, if an individual has CMI against tuberculosis, an extract of that individual's T cells will confer CMI against *Mycobacterium tuberculosis* on the recipient. DTF currently is being used as therapy in individuals with defects in their CMI and cancer patients. Unfortunately, the effects are not permanent, and the procedure must be repeated to maintain immunity in the recipient.

IMMUNIZATION

As noted previously, the response to an immunogen is a function of many variables. These include the route of immunization, the dose of immunogen, the number of immunizations, the form in which antigen is given, and the genetic and physiologic condition of the recipient.

Almost any route that gets the immunogen into the tissues will serve as an immunizing route. Natural exposure through inhalation, ingestion, injection, or mucous membrane and skin contact may evoke an immune response to an antigen. Deliberate induction of an immune response has been accomplished through the routes mentioned and with intradermal, subcutaneous, intravenous, intramuscular, and intraperitoneal injections of antigens. The route of immunization can affect the response. An antigen injected subcutaneously may induce a greater response than it will if injected intravenously. In addition, an antigen entering the gastric mucosa may induce an SIgA response rather than a systemic response in which IgG predominates.

The minimum dose necessary to induce an immune response may be only a few micrograms. Generally, increasing amounts of antigen result in increasing, but usually less than proportionate, immune responses. If too little or too much antigen is given, immune tolerance, a specific immunologic unresponsiveness, may occur. As noted, the dose needed to evoke a secondary response is much less than that necessary for a primary response.

The number of immunizations also affects the response. The immune response to a second immunization is usually greater than the response to the first. As even more injections are given, the response may increase, but it soon will reach a plateau beyond which additional injections will not further increase the response.

The ability to mount an immune response is under genetic control. Different strains of mice, for example, will show significantly different immune responses to the same antigen. In addition, the physiologic state of the individual can affect the immune response. Very old and very young people will not respond as strongly as others, and malnutrition, disease, and stress can depress the immune response in any age group.

Adjuvants

The immune response to antigen can be increased severalfold by administering the antigen in conjunction with compounds called adjuvants. Adjuvants may potentiate immunogenicity by at least three mechanisms. The adjuvant may be absorbed into or incorporated in a compound that will retard destruction and excretion of the antigen and permit prolonged exposure (antigen depot effect) in the tissues. Second, the adjuvant may provoke an inflammatory response that attracts more immunologically reactive cells into the area. Finally, the adjuvant may hyperactivate T or B lymphocytes and evoke a greater response from these cells.

Only one adjuvant is used routinely in humans. Alum, a potassium aluminum phosphate gel, is incorporated into the tetanus and diphtheria toxoid vaccines. The antigens are adsorbed to the alum, and after injection, the antigen is slowly released from the gel. In addition to this antigen depot effect, an intense inflammatory response occurs at the injection site.

Freund's adjuvant is a water-in-oil mixture that is one of the most effective adjuvants available. A very strong immune response may continue for months after immunization with an antigen emulsified in the adjuvant. Freund's adjuvant is not used in humans because it induces severe granulomas. It has been used extensively in animal research, including oral research.

IN VITRO CORRELATES OF IMMUNITY

Methods used to assay humoral immune response (ie, quantifying specific antibody) are described in Chapter 6. Several methods used for assessing specific CMI responses are described here.

Lymphocyte Transformation

Lymphocyte transformation tests are based on the proliferative stage of the immune response and measure the blastogenic activity of antigen-stimulated lymphocytes. The production of new DNA is used as an indicator of blastogenesis. The test is performed by mixing antigen, lymphocytes, and radioisotope-labeled thymidine (tritiated thymidine) and incubating the mixture. The cells then are separated from the culture fluid, and the amount of tritiated thymidine incorporated into new DNA is measured in a scintillation counter. The amount of new DNA is a measure of blastogenesis, which in turn is a measure of specific lymphocyte reactivity to the antigen, that is, specific CMI.

Lymphokine Assays

CMI can be detected by measuring the production of lymphokines by antigen-stimulated lymphocyte tissue cultures. Lymphokine production may be assessed using lymphokine-mediated cell function tests or by serologic methods using antibody directed against the lymphokine. For example, osteoclast-activating factor (OAF), the lymphokine that induces bone adsorption and destruction, can be assayed by adding lymphocytes and specific antigen to a tissue culture of fetal rat bone containing isotope-labeled calcium. If the lymphocytes are sensitized to the antigen, they will produce OAF. The lymphokine will induce osteoclasts to break down the fetal bone and release the radioactive calcium. The concentration of released calcium compared to the concentration of calcium released in an antigen-free tissue culture is a relative measure of the OAF produced by the sensitized lymphocytes. Lymphokine-mediated cell function assays also are available for chemotactic factor, migration-inhibition factor, and cytotoxic factor.

Cytotoxic Cell Assays

Cytotoxic cell assays are used to evaluate the cell killing potential of cytotoxic T lymphocytes. When sensitized T cells are incubated with their specific antigen-bearing target cells, the lymphocytes will kill the target cells. The degree of CMI of the lymphocytes can be quantitated by counting the live target cells before and after exposure to the lymphocytes being tested or by labeling the target cells with a radioactive isotope and measuring the release of the isotope from killed cells. Similar assays are used to evaluate ADCC and other cytotoxic activities.

IMMUNOLOGIC UNRESPONSIVENESS

An individual may not respond to an antigenic stimulus. This is called immunologic unresponsiveness, and it can be divided into four categories: self recognition, tolerance, immunodeficiencies, and immunosuppression.

Self Recognition

Self recognition refers to the mechanism by which the immune system is able to recognize self antigens and prevent an immune response to these antigens. The mechanism of self recognition is not clear, but somehow the body rids itself of (clonal deletion) or inactivates (clonal anergy) those clones of lymphocytes that would react against its own antigens; that is, it prevents autoimmunity.

Induction of self recognition has been demonstrated to take place in the fetus or in early neonatal life. If nonself antigens are presented in the body during the self recognition period and are maintained in the body, they are treated as self antigens later in life. The immune system will not mount a response against them. What appeared as self in early life continues to be recognized as such in the mature immunocompetent animal. This phenomenon, called fetal tolerance, has been demonstrated to occur both naturally and in laboratory experiments. Since fetal tolerance can only be induced in utero or in the neonate, it is apparent that self recognition is established in this early period of life. Since self recognition resembles artificially induced immunologic tolerance, it also has been called self tolerance.

Immunologic Tolerance

Immunologic tolerance is a form of specific unresponsiveness that can be induced in immunologically mature animals. It may be induced in two ways. One is by repeated injections of very small doses of soluble antigen. The animal will not respond to these injections or to subsequent, larger doses of the same antigen. This is called low dose tolerance. The other form of tolerance, high dose tolerance, is induced by injecting massive doses of antigen into an animal. The animal's immune system will not respond to the initial massive dose or to subsequent, normally immunogenic doses. Both high and low dose tolerance are immunologically specific. The animal tolerates only that specific antigen or, more precisely, the specific antigenic determinant.

Low dose tolerance is mediated by T suppressor cells. The tolerizing dose of antigen induces excessive suppressor cell activity, which blocks the normal immune response by other specific T cells and B cells. In high dose tolerance, the antigen tolerizes both T and B cells. Clonal deletion and clonal anergy have been proposed as mechanisms responsible for high dose tolerance. The clone of T or B cells specific for the tolerizing antigen may be eliminated, or it may be inactivated when subjected to the massive antigenic dose. However, the molecular mechanisms that result in excessive T suppressor cell activity in low dose tolerance or clonal elimination or inactivation in high dose tolerance have not been established.

Both forms of tolerance are the center of much interest because elucidation of the mechanisms of these phenomena could lead to solutions to some critical immunologic problems, such as autoimmunity, graft rejection, allergy, and cancer. Self recognition is thought to be a form of self tolerance, and, therefore, understanding tolerance could aid in correcting the defects resulting in autoimmunity. Induction of tolerance to organ transplant antigens or to allergens could alleviate the problems associated with these medical problems. Finally, there is evidence that tolerance to tumor antigens might be the reason the immune system does not reject tumors.

Immunodeficiency Diseases

Individuals may be born with a defective or deficient immune system, or they may lose all or part of it during life. These immunodeficiencies predispose to infectious diseases and tumors. If the defect is mild, there may be little or no apparent disease. As the defects increase in severity, however, the patient may suffer from increasing complications often caused by normally avirulent, opportunistic pathogens.

These immunodeficiency diseases may be either congenital or acquired. Congenital, or primary, immunodeficiencies occur when an individual is born without the ability to develop a normal immune response. Acquired, or secondary, immunodeficiencies occur when an individual born with the ability to respond normally loses immunocompetence later in life. Immunodeficiencies may include either or both CMI and humoral immunity, and they may involve all or only part of the CMI or humoral responses. For example, CMI deficiencies may result from the absence of pre-T stem cells, from inactivity of the thymus, which produces T cell maturational factors, or from the inability of T cells to mature even in the presence of a normal thymus.

Humoral immunodeficiencies are referred to as agammaglobulinemias or hypogammaglobulinemias, the absence of or depressed levels of immunoglobulins, respectively. X-linked infantile hypogammaglobulinemia (Bruton's agammaglobulinemia) is a congenital humoral immunodeficiency found in male infants. It is characterized by low levels of circulating antibody and B lymphocytes. B cell areas in the lymph nodes and spleen are devoid of B cells and plasma cells, and little or no antibody is formed in response to immunization with vaccines. T cell responses are normal. This disease has been attributed to a defect in pre-B cell maturation. Patients with this deficiency suffer from chronic pyogenic bacterial infections and must be maintained on antibiotic and γ-globulin therapy.

Selective immunoglobulin deficiencies also occur. Any class of immunoglobulin may be involved, but it is interesting from a dental viewpoint that before the appearance of AIDS, selective IgA deficiency was the most common immunodeficiency. The incidence varied between 1:800 and 1:600. The absence of IgA would be expected to predispose to diseases of the mucous membranes and other tissues usually protected by secretory IgA, and in fact, patients with this deficiency often suffer from repeated infections of the respiratory and alimentary tracts. In addition, studies of patients with selective IgA deficiency suggest that it may predispose to dental caries, but the evidence for this is not definitive. Fortunately, many patients with selective IgA deficiencies do not have problems in part because the immune system often compensates for the lack of secretory IgA by producing IgM in the exocrine secretions in which SIgA is usually found. IgA-deficient patients are treated with antibiotics. They cannot be given γ-globulins because these preparations contain IgA, which the patient's IgA-deficient immune system might recognize as immunologically foreign.

Congenital thymic aplasia (DiGeorge syndrome) is the classic congenital CMI deficiency. This disease is characterized by thymic aplasia or hypoplasia and the absence of T cells and CMI functions. Humoral immunity is present, but, probably as a result of the absence of T-h cells, the B cell response to T-dependent antigens is depressed. Patients with DiGeorge syndrome have recurrent infections by microbes against which CMI usually protects, that is, fungal, viral, and intracellular bacterial infections. Treatment consists of transplantation of fetal thymus cells. These cells are immunologically immature and have not completed the self recognition process. Thymosin treatments have been partially successful, but they must be given repeatedly.

Severe combined immunodeficiency disease (SCID) is a congenital bone marrow stem cell defect. Both T and B cells are absent, and neither humoral immunity nor CMI activities can be demonstrated. Infants with SCID rarely survive beyond 1 year without intensive medical care. Bone marrow transplants are dangerous because unless the transplant is closely matched, a graft-versus-host reaction (Chapter 8) may occur. Bone marrow transplants from distantly related donors, in association with the monoclonal antibody directed against the donor's T cells (anti-CD3 monoclonal antibody), have been successful in some SCID patients, and as a result, the prognosis for this immunodeficiency may be improving.

Acquired humoral immunodeficiencies are of multiple etiologies. The most common are those associated with neoplasias, such as leukemias and myelomas. These malignancies often result in a selective proliferation of clones of lymphocytes or plasma cells that produce antibodies of only one or a very few specificities. There also is a spontaneously developing hypogammaglobulinemia that may develop at any age. In addition, transient hypogammaglobulinemias may accompany some infectious diseases, and a gradually developing humoral deficiency may occur with age.

Acquired immunodeficiencies are more common in CMI than in humoral immunity. Malignancies, such as lymphomas and leukemias, often affect the CMI response. Infections, especially chronic granulomatous diseases and viral infections, often induce transient deficiencies. Aging affects the immune response in general, but it appears to exert a more pronounced effect on CMI than on humoral immunity.

The most widespread immunodeficiency disease is acquired immunodeficiency syndrome (AIDS), which is discussed in detail in Chapter 31. The human immunodeficiency virus (HIV) invades helper T cells using the CD4 molecule as virus receptor. This infection results in a depletion of T-h cells, leading to the characteristic inversion of the normal T-h:T-s cell or CD4:CD8 ratio (Table 7–7). HIV also infects monocytes, macrophages, and several other cells, because the destruction of T-h cells that are so necessary to activation of all lymphocytes is the critical effect. The resulting immunodeficiency leaves the patient susceptible to many opportunistic infections and tumors. There is no cure for AIDS. Therapy is directed primarily against opportunistic infections. Azidothymidine (AZT), a compound that blocks the reverse transcriptase enzyme of HIV, may delay the progression of the disease, but it is not a cure.

Immunosuppression

Immunosuppression is an artificially induced form of immunologic unresponsiveness. Immunosuppressive agents primarily are used to prevent organ transplant rejection and as therapy for autoimmune diseases. Some of the more commonly used immunosuppressive agents include antithymocyte sera, corticosteroids, azathioprine, cyclophosphamide, and cyclosporine.

Antithymocyte sera were produced in rabbits and horses by immunization with human thymus cells. Because these antisera are selective for T cells, they are especially useful in preventing graft rejection mediated by cellular immunity. Since these animal sera are composed of many foreign antigens, however, extended use often resulted in allergic reactions. Such sera are being replaced with monoclonal antibodies (anti-CD3) that, although still foreign, carry fewer extraneous antigens and are less allergenic.

TABLE 7–7. COMPARISON OF T LYMPHOCYTE SUBSETS OF PATIENTS WITH AIDS AND NORMAL CONTROLS

	Normal controls	AIDS patients
Helper T cells/mm^3	468–1433	12–96
Suppressor T cells/mm^3	192–726	58–320
Helper/suppressor ratio	1.1–3.5	0.04–0.66

Adapted from Pitchenik AE, et al. Ann Intern Med. *1983;98:277.*

Corticosteroids appear to exert several effects on the immune response. Initially, steroids interfere with the induction of the immune response, and later, they function at the effector level through their anti-inflammatory action. Azathioprine and cyclophosphamide are cytotoxic immunosuppressive agents. Azathioprine kills actively proliferating cells, that is, immunoblasts. It is a purine antagonist that inhibits nucleic acid synthesis. Cyclophosphamide is an alkylating agent that forms crosslinks on DNA and RNA molecules and prevents replication of lymphocyte nucleic acids.

Cyclosporine, a fungal peptide, is now the most commonly used immunosuppressant. It appears to suppress helper T cells and inhibit IL-2 production, but the complete mechanism of action has not been determined. Cyclosporine has been used successfully with all types of organ transplants. Side effects include kidney and liver toxicities and, although certainly not as critical, gingival hyperplasia.

Despite the fact that immunosuppressive agents are effective and used extensively, they must be used with care. All are somewhat toxic, and patients must be closely monitored. An even greater problem is that they are nonspecific in their actions and suppress the immune response to all antigens. This leaves the patient immunologically defenseless against infectious agents. Therefore, the patient is in constant danger of life-threatening infectious diseases, many of which are caused by the normal microbial flora of the body.

SUGGESTED READINGS

Mestecky J, McGhee JR, Bienenstock J, Ogra PL, eds. *Recent Advances in Mucosal Immunity.* New York: Plenum; 1987.

Oppenheim JJ, Cohen S. *Interleukins, Lymphokines and Cytokines.* New York: Academic Press; 1983.

Roitt IM, Lehner T. *Immunology of Oral Diseases,* 2nd ed. London: Blackwell; 1983.

Sell S. *Immunology, Immunopathology, and Immunity.* New York: Elsevier; 1987.

Stites DP, Stobo JD, Wells JV, eds. *Basic and Clinical Immunology,* 6th ed. E. Norwalk, Conn: Appleton & Lange; 1987.

Strober W, Lamm ME, McGhee JR, James SP, eds. *Mucosal Immunity and Infections at Mucosal Surfaces.* New York: Oxford University Press; 1988.

CHAPTER 8

Immune Protection and Injury

Robert R. White and Peggy A. O'Neill

INTRODUCTION

ACQUISITION OF IMMUNITY
- Vaccines

PROTECTIVE IMMUNITY
- Protective Immunity Mediated by Antibody
- Protective Immunity Mediated by Lymphocytes

IMMUNOLOGIC INJURY
- Anaphylactic Reactions
- Cytotoxic Reactions
- Immune Complex Reactions
- Type IV Reactions
- Transplantation Immunity
- Autoimmunity
- Tumor Immunology

SUGGESTED READINGS

INTRODUCTION

Immunity often is described as a two-edged sword. One edge is beneficial, as noted in the protective responses to infectious diseases. The other edge, however, may be very detrimental. Allergies and graft rejection are both mediated by the immune system. The same basic mechanisms are involved in both protection and injury, and at times they may occur simultaneously. The beneficial and harmful effects of immunity are observed readily in the oral cavity. Protective immunity is constantly active against the microorganisms that reside in or pass through the mouth, and any significant systemic or oral immune deficiency almost always is accompanied by an oral pathologic condition. The harmful effects of immunity are manifest in allergies to dental medicaments and hypersensitivity reactions against oral microbial antigens, such as those associated with periodontal disease.

ACQUISITION OF IMMUNITY

An individual may become immune by several means. Immune responses to natural antigen exposures are the most frequent means of acquiring antibodies and antigen-sensitive lymphocytes, but there are several other means as well. The immunity induced by any of these methods may mediate the protective or injurious reactions that are described later in this chapter.

Natural active immunity occurs as a response to natural exposure to an antigenic stimulus; that is, the host is naturally stimulated to produce immune factors as a result of infection, either clinical or subclinical, or from ingestion, inhalation, or topical application of antigens or haptens. This immunity usually is very strong and long-lasting. Memory cells or their progeny may survive for the life of the host. Natural active immunity may be beneficial, as in the protective immunity that follows an infection, or it may be harmful, such as occurs with allergic conditions.

Artificial active immunity is a result of an immune response to antigens administered by humans. The immune response is considered to be artificial because it is induced by humans but active because the host actively produces antibodies and sensitized cells. Vaccines are used to produce artificial active immunity. Although the primary purpose of a vaccine is to induce protective immunity, some individuals may become allergic to components in the vaccine, and injurious hypersensitivity reactions may occur. Since memory cells are formed, artificial active immunity may be as strong and long-lasting as natural active immunity.

Natural passive immunity refers to the passage of antibodies from the mother to the fetus or the neonate. The acquisition of antibodies is natural, but the host does not produce its own antibodies or sensitized cells. Therefore, there is no secondary response. In humans, IgG is actively transported through the placenta to the fetus, whereas both IgG and IgA are passed to the neonate in the mother's milk. Both sources of antibody are extremely important in protecting the immunologically immature infant from infectious diseases. Natural passive immunity also may be harmful. Hemolytic disease of the newborn, or Rh disease, is mediated by maternal IgG directed against the newborn's red blood cells. Effective levels of maternal antibody are maintained in the infant for 5 to 6 months after birth.

Artificial passive immunity involves the transfer, by humans, of antibody from one individual to another. γ-Globulins extracted from the plasma of a number of donors may be used as a prophylactic in people exposed to common diseases, such as infectious hepatitis and measles. Use of these pooled γ-globulins is based on the assumption that most adults will have been exposed to these common infectious organisms and will carry antibody against them. With less common diseases (eg, tetanus, diphtheria, serum hepatitis), antisera from recent convalescents, or from hyperimmunized human volunteers or domestic animals are used as the source of preformed antibody to be transferred to a nonimmune individual. Artificial passive immunity lasts only about 4 to 6 weeks because the immunoglobulins are more rapidly catabolized by the adult recipient. Since sensitized cells are not produced, there is no secondary response. Allergic reactions to the immunoglobulin antigens can occur and are especially a problem when immune globulins from domestic animals are used.

Vaccines

Vaccines used to stimulate artificial active immunity consist of the disease-producing microorganism or its antigenic products. These are administered for the purpose of evoking a protective immune response, that is, immunity that can neutralize the factors that cause disease. These immunizing agents may be killed microorganisms, avirulent live microorganisms, or noncellular preparations of pure or semipure antigens. Most vaccines that are used routinely are very effective in disease prevention and play an extremely important role in preventive medicine. The common childhood vaccines and their schedule of immunizations are shown in Table 8–1.

Ideally, a vaccine should consist only of the protective antigen, that is, the antigen or antigens that will stimulate protective immunity in the recipient. Currently, there are three types of these vaccines. Toxoids are bacterial exotoxins that have been treated with formalin to inactivate the toxic part of the molecule without affecting its immunogenicity. When injected, toxoids are innocuous but still able to evoke the formation of antibodies that can neutralize the natural toxin. Toxoids are used as vaccines against tetanus, diphtheria, and botulism. Another purified protective antigen vaccine is that used to prevent pneumonia caused by *Streptococcus pneumoniae.* The virulence factor of the pneumococcus is its capsule, and, therefore, the vaccine is composed of purified capsular antigens from the pneumococcal types that most frequently are involved in the disease. The third vaccine in this group is the hepatitis type B vaccine. This vaccine consists of the viral surface antigen (HBsAg) purified from the plasma of carriers of the disease or produced through genetic engineering. In addition to these, it is worth noting that an anticaries vaccine, consisting of a purified cell wall protein from *Streptococcus mutans,* has been tested successfully in animals.

It is expected that the numbers of purified antigen vaccines will increase as a result of genetic engineering. The gene coding for the protective antigen can be taken from a pathogen and inserted into an organism, such as *Escherichia coli,* and the antigen can

TABLE 8–1. GUIDELINES FOR CHILDHOOD IMMUNIZATIONS

		Schedule of Doses				
Disease	**Vaccine**	***1st***	***2nd***	***3rd***	***4th***	***5th***
Diptheria-tetanus-pertussis	DPT	2 months	4 months	6 months	15 months	4–6 years[a]
Poliovirus type I, II, III	Trivalent oral	2 months	4 months	15 months	4–6 years	—
Measles, mumps, rubella	Combined or singly	15 months	—	—	—	—
Haemophilus meningitis	*Haemophilus* B	24 months	—	—	—	—

From MMWR. *1986;35:577–579. New recommended schedule for active immunization of normal infants and children.*

[a]Adult type DT vaccine at 10-year intervals thereafter.

then be produced and purified in large quantities. The HBsAg recombinant vaccine produced in yeast cells was one of the first of what will eventually be many such vaccines.

Killed, whole cell vaccines consist of suspensions of bacteria or viruses exposed to lethal heat, chemicals, or radiation treatments. The whooping cough, typhoid fever, influenza, rabies, and Salk polio vaccines consist of suspensions of killed microorganisms. These vaccines are of varying efficacy, but they are or have been used routinely.

Live vaccines must be attenuated. In some cases, antigenically related avirulent species are used as vaccine strains. In fact, the first vaccine, Jenner's smallpox vaccine, was not variola, the virus that causes smallpox, but rather the antigenically related cowpox virus, vaccinia. Other live vaccines contain avirulent mutants that were induced by culturing under adverse or unnatural conditions. The BCG (bacille Calmette-Guérin) tuberculosis vaccine was rendered avirulent by passage through suboptimal culture media, and the Sabin poliovaccine was attenuated by repeated passage through tissue cultures. Other live attenuated vaccines include the rubella, rubeola, and mumps vaccines.

Avirulent live vaccines generally are more effective than killed vaccines. This has been ascribed to several factors, including the facts that (1) the killed microbes are grown in vitro where they do not produce all of the antigens necessary for protective immunity, (2) essential antigens may be denatured during the killing process, and (3) microbial reproduction in the body may be necessary to induce a persistent immunogenic stimulus in the specific tissues in which the natural infection occurs. The major disadvantage of live vaccines is the possibility that the attenuated strain might revert to virulence and cause disease.

PROTECTIVE IMMUNITY

The importance of immunity in resistance to disease is readily observed in individuals with immunodeficiencies or in patients who are immunosuppressed. These individuals are highly susceptible to repeated and chronic infections, often by microorganisms that cannot infect normal subjects. Protective immunity, or its absence, is extremely important in the oral cavity. Immunodeficient and immunosuppressed patients are at high risk of developing oral infections by opportunistic pathogens. Systemic or local immunodeficiencies also may result in increased dental caries or more severe periodontal disease and dental pulp infections.

Protective Immunity Mediated by Antibody

IgG, IgM, and IgA are the most important antibodies in protective humoral immunity—IgG and IgM within the tissues and IgA (SIgA) on the mucous membranes. In addition to these immunoglobulins, complement also plays a very important role in humoral protection against infectious diseases. These immunoglobulins can protect by several different mechanisms.

The protective nature of antitoxins is readily apparent in diseases in which toxemia is the determinant of the pathologic process. Tetanus, diphtheria, and botulism are toxemias that can be prevented by immunization with toxoids or cured with antitoxic sera. Toxin-neutralizing antibodies are the only effective treatment, and antibodies directed against other antigens are useless. Toxin neutralization may occur through steric hindrance by the immunoglobulin bound to the toxin or allosteric conformational changes in the toxin molecule induced by the binding of antibody to toxin. IgG comprises the bulk of the circulating antitoxins, and IgM and IgA are involved to a lesser extent.

Agglutination, another antibody-mediated protective mechanism, may function in two ways. In a nonimmune animal, proliferation of invading bacteria can lead to a rapid spread of the organisms. In the immune animal, agglutination localizes the microorganisms at the site of initial invasion. Agglutination also can augment phagocytosis. By aggregating bacteria, agglutination enables the leukocyte to engulf many organisms with a single phagocytic process rather than having to engulf each organism individually. Again, because it is present in the highest concentration, IgG is the most important immunoglobulin class among the agglutinins, followed by IgA and IgM.

Phagocytosis is the most important means of clearing microorganisms from the body. Opsonins are antibodies that facilitate phagocytosis, and they are absolutely critical to immune protection. There are several opsonizing mechanisms in the body. After IgG reacts with a microbial surface antigen, the Fc portion can bind to Fc receptor sites on the membranes of polymorphonuclear neutrophils and macrophages. This enhances the phagocyte's ability to grasp and engulf the microorganism. In addition, IgG and IgM also activate complement, which produces C3b and C5b, both of which also are opsonic because phagocytes possess receptors for these molecules on their membranes.

Opsonins are especially important in protection against encapsulated bacteria, whose capsules inhibit phagocytosis. Antibodies directed against capsular antigens neutralize the antiphagocytic effect of the capsule and thus enhance phagocytosis. An outstanding example is seen in protective immunity against pneumococcal pneumonia. Opsonins directed against the capsular antigens of *S. pneumoniae* are all that is necessary for protection against the disease, and, therefore, the vaccine for this pneumonia consists of purified capsular antigens.

Lysins are antibodies that damage cell membranes and cause osmotic lysis. Lysis by IgG and IgM acting in concert with complement is effective against some gram-negative bacteria, spirochetes, and viruses. In addition, endotoxin-bearing gram-negative bacteria may activate complement through the alternative pathway. This activation of complement on the cell membrane may result in lysis of the bacterial cell.

In order to infect certain tissues, many pathogens first must adhere to the tissues. This is dependent on specific sites that bind to receptors on the host's cells. Antibodies that react with or near these binding sites can block adherence and prevent infection. The oral cavity, the respiratory tract, the gut, and the genitourinary tract are protected by antiadherence antibody, usually SIgA, which bathes the mucous membranes and prevents attachment and subsequent invasion of pathogens. The microorganisms are washed away in the secretions. Immunity to enteric infections, strep throat, and gonorrhea is mediated by antiadherence activity of SIgA. Caries immunity is thought to be dependent in part on antibody inhibition of bacterial adherence to and colonization of tooth enamel. Antiadherence immunity also occurs within the tissues. Viruses first must adhere to the cell they are going to infect before they can invade it. Antibody within the body can prevent infection by blocking viral adherence to susceptible cells.

Antibodies can inhibit critical extracellular microbial enzymes by binding on or near the active site of the enzyme. Antibody to the influenza virus enzyme, neuraminidase, inhibits replication and spread of this virus. Caries in laboratory animals has been shown to be inhibited by antibody against the *S. mutans* glycosyl transferases and glycolytic hydrolases involved in the carbohydrate metabolism associated with the disease. Externally, SIgA is most important in enzyme neutralization, whereas IgG is dominant within the tissues.

Protective Immunity Mediated by Lymphocytes

CMI is especially important in protection against intracellular pathogens that are isolated from antibody and can survive within phagocytes. These microbes include bacteria that grow and multiply within the host's cells, viruses that pass from cell to cell without an extracellular stage, and most fungi. Protective cell-mediated responses are carried out by sensitized lymphocytes and lymphokines.

Lymphokines released by T lymphocytes stimulated by the antigens of the invading microorganisms mediate this protective response. Skin reactive factor increases vascular permeability, which, in association with chemotactic factors, enhances the ingress of protective inflammatory cells. Migration inhibition factors hold the cells in the tissues, and macrophage activation factor increases the antimicrobial capacity of the macrophages in the lesion. These events amplify the initial immunologic reaction and intensify the inflammatory response to the pathogen.

The activated macrophage is the major effector of cell-mediated protection. Macrophage activating factor causes normal macrophages to enlarge and become hyperactive and increases their antimicrobial and antitumor activity. Activated macrophages have an increased metabolic rate, increased numbers of lysosomes and hydrolytic enzymes, and increased glucose oxidase, phagocytic, and bactericidal activity. Whereas normal macrophages would be overcome by the intracellular pathogens they ingest, the activated macrophage can phagocytize the organisms more efficiently and can kill the ingested microbes.

Although macrophage activation is the result of a specific immune response, that is, the specific interaction between an antigen and a sensitized T lymphocyte, the actions of the activated macrophage are not specific. For example, macrophages activated by lymphokines produced by a T lymphocyte sensitive to tuberculosis are able to kill other intracellular pathogens, such as *Listeria* and *Brucella*.

The antiviral substance interferon is another mediator of CMI protection. Interferon, which is produced by sensitized lymphocytes and activated macrophages, is taken up by uninfected host cells in the surrounding tissues and prevents viral replication within these cells (Chapter 24).

Viral infections characterized by the appearance of viral antigens on the membranes of infected cells are susceptible to attack by specific cytotoxic T lymphocytes. These viral diseases include influenza, measles, mumps, and herpes infections. The T-c cells recognize the viral antigens on the membrane and kill the cell. Killing the infected cell prevents replication of the virus and the subsequent infection of many other cells.

Although discussed separately, these protective activities may take place simultaneously in the immune host. For example, if an intracellular pathogen enters an immune individual, it may encounter multiple protective mechanisms. Antibodies will react with surface binding sites to prevent adherence, and the antibodies will agglutinate the bacteria and, in conjunction with complement, opsonize the pathogen. Activated macrophages may then rapidly ingest and destroy the microbe. Depending on the invading microorganism, one or more of these protective actions may play a dominant role in resistance, but all can occur. Often, it is difficult to assess the significance of each in prophylaxis against, or recovery from, an infection.

IMMUNOLOGIC INJURY

The reaction between an antigen and the body's specific immune components can be harmful to the body. These injurious immune reactions are called allergy or hypersensitivity. The basic immune mechanisms of allergies are identical to those of protective immunity. However, in the former, it is the host's own cells and tissues that are injured as a result of the immune reactions. The antigens that induce hypersensitivities are called allergens, and they can be found throughout our environment. They include not only virulent microbial antigens but also allergens, such as mercury or pollen, and even medicaments, such as penicillin.

Allergies are important in dentistry. On the one hand, hypersensitivity reactions are known to be involved in many diseases with oral manifestations, including periodontal diseases and pulpitis. On the other, both the clinician and the patient can become allergic to the various dental materials, anesthetics, and therapeutics commonly used in dental practice.

Allergic reactions initially were divided into two types, immediate hypersensitivity and delayed hypersensitivity, based on the time of occurrence of the immunologic reactions after the entry of the antigen into the tissues. Immediate allergies occurred within minutes, whereas delayed reactions took days to develop. The two terms are still in use, but the differences in the allergies now are recognized as resulting from the immunologic components that mediate the reactions. Immediate reactions are mediated by antibodies, that is, humoral immunity, and delayed hypersensitivities are mediated by CMI.

Another classification of the hypersensitivity reactions that more closely reflects the differences in the mechanisms of the reactions has been devised. This classification divides the hypersensitivity reactions into the four types shown in Table 8–2. Types I, II, and III are humoral immune hypersensitivities, mediated by antibodies, and type IV reactions are CMI responses. Type IV may be further subdivided into reactions mediated by lymphokines and those mediated by cytotoxic cells.

TABLE 8–2. TYPES, NAMES, AND MAJOR MEDIATORS OF THE HYPERSENSITIVITY REACTIONS

Type	Name	Mediator
I	Anaphylaxis Atopy	IgE
II	Cytotoxic Antitissue	IgG, IgM
III	Immune complex Arthus Serum sickness	IgG, IgM
IV	Cell-mediated delayed hypersensitivity	Lymphocytes

Anaphylactic Reactions

Anaphylactic, or type I, reactions may be systemic or local. Anaphylaxis, the classic immediate hypersensitivity reaction, is the systemic type I reaction. Atopy is the local reaction commonly manifested as hay fever or asthma. The basic mechanisms of anaphylaxis and atopy are similar. The differences lie in the relative dissemination of the reaction and the accompanying severity.

Type I reactions are mediated by IgE (Table 8–3). Having been formed as a result of a sensitizing antigenic stimulus, IgE is secreted from the plasma cell and circulates until it attaches to a tissue mast cell or blood basophil through special receptors on the Fc area of the heavy chain. The IgE may remain bound to the cell for weeks.

On subsequent exposure to the antigen, the formation of an immune complex between the antigen and the cell-bound IgE initiates a chain of reactions that result in degranulation of the cell, release of pharmacologically active agents from the granules, and stimulation of synthetic processes in cells nearby. The major compounds released from the mast cells or formed as a result of mast cell degranulation include the following.

Histamine, which originates in mast cell granules, is considered to be the major mediator of type I reactions. Histamine increases capillary permeability, is a vasodilator and smooth muscle constrictor, and stimulates nasal and bronchial mucosal secretions.

Platelet-activating factor (PAF) induces aggregation and degranulation of platelets, which release serotonin.

Slow reacting substance of anaphylaxis (SRS-A) is produced by mast cells and lung tissue. SRS-A is a mixture of leukotrienes (LTC4, LTD4, and LTE4) that cause smooth muscle contraction and broncho-

TABLE 8–3. CELLULAR AND MOLECULAR FACTORS IN TYPE I REACTIONS

IgE
Mast cells
Basophils
Histamine
Slow reacting substance of anaphylaxis
Platelet-activating factor
Prostaglandins
Kinins
Eosinophil chemotactic factor of anaphylaxis

spasms. Unlike the rapid, short-lived effects of histamine, SRS-A causes a slow, long-lasting spasm. It appears to be especially significant in asthma.

Two other groups of vasoactive substances are involved in type I reactions. Mast cell degranulation results in the direct release of mast cell prostaglandins and also stimulates formation of prostaglandins by other leukocytes in the area. Kinin-generating proteases act on Hageman factor, which generates plasma and tissue kinins.

The vasoactive, secretion-enhancing and smooth muscle-contracting properties of these compounds produce the symptoms of type I reactions. There is a marked vasodilatation and loss of fluids to the extravascular spaces, intense smooth muscle contraction, especially in the respiratory tract, and an increase in secretory activity by nasal and bronchial mucosal glands.

The reactions are usually short-lived because the pharmacologic mediators are degraded rapidly by enzymes and inhibitors in tissue fluids. In addition, when the mast cell degranulates, it releases another compound, eosinophil chemotactic factor of anaphylaxis (ECF-A), which attracts eosinophils that mediate a negative feedback control mechanism on type I reactions. Eosinophils produce three enzymes, histaminase, arylsulfatase, and phospholipase, which degrade histamine, SRS-A, and PAF, respectively.

Systemic Anaphylaxis. A systemic anaphylactic reaction begins within minutes after the allergen enters the tissues. Flushing, urticaria, and respiratory and gastrointestinal distress often precede the more severe symptoms, which include generalized shock and asphyxia. The shock is the result of circulatory collapse induced by systemic vasodilatation and extravasation of fluids. The asphyxia results from bronchial and laryngeal obstruction brought on by smooth muscle contraction, edema, and mucosal secretions. Death may be caused by laryngeal edema, respiratory failure, shock, or cardiac arrhythmia.

Atopic Reactions. Atopy, the localized form of anaphlyaxis, occurs in about 10% of the population. The most common forms are allergic rhinitis (hay fever) and asthma. Hay fever symptoms include irritation and hypersecretion in the nasal mucosa and conjunctiva. These occur as a result of local mast cell degranulation following exposure to aerosolized environmental allergens, such as plant pollens.

Asthma is a more severe atopic allergy involving the bronchial tree. It is characterized by intense bronchoconstriction and hypersecretion of mucus and ranges from a mild to a life-threatening disease. Atopic dermatitis, angioedema, and atopic gastroenteritis are other atopic diseases.

There appears to be a genetic predisposition to the development of atopy. Children of parents with such allergies have a much greater tendency to become atopic than do others. If one parent is atopic, there is about a 30% chance that the child will develop an atopic allergy. If both parents are allergic, there is a 50% to 60% chance that the child will become allergic. The child will not necessarily become allergic to the same antigen but simply will have a greater tendency to develop atopy.

Allergens. Clinically administered allergens that frequently evoke systemic anaphylactic reactions include penicillin, cephalosporin, and immune sera. Type I reactions to penicillin, the leading cause of iatrogenic anaphylaxis, are directed against the haptenic metabolic degradation products of the antibiotic, especially penicilloic acid. Natural antigens that most frequently cause systemic reactions include the venoms of stinging insects, such as honeybees, hornets, and fire ants. In addition, foods, such as egg albumin and seafoods, may induce systemic anaphylaxis.

The allergens that evoke respiratory atopic reactions usually are environmental antigens, such as pollens, animal dander, house dust, and fungal spores. Various drugs, milk, fish, corn, and other grains have been implicated as allergens causing angioedema, atopic dermatitis, and atopic food allergies.

Therapy. Pharmacologic management of anaphylactic reactions depends on the stage of the reaction. Inhibition of mast cell degranulation may be accomplished with drugs, such as methylxanthines and cromolyn sodium. If mast cell degranulation is not possible, the pharmacologically active agents may be neutralized. Since histamine is responsible for most of the injury occurring in anaphylactic reactions, inhibition of histamine activity with antihistamines may be all that is necessary to prevent a type I reaction. Finally, epinephrine is used to reverse the effects after an anaphylactic reaction has commenced. Administration of epinephrine may be a life-saving measure for systemic shock reactions.

Desensitization is used to prevent severe hay fever or asthma reactions and for individuals with severe allergies to insect venoms. Desensitization is accomplished by multiple subcutaneous injections of very small quantities of the allergen. These small doses evoke the release of relatively harmless quantities of histamine while apparently modifying the immune status of the patient. The basis for desensitization is not clear. One hypothesis is that the many small injections stimulate the formation of IgG, which reacts with the allergen before it can reach the mast cell-bound IgE. These competitive IgG molecules, called blocking antibodies, have not been demonstrated in all cases, however, and this leaves the hypothesis in doubt. Low dose tolerance also has been proposed as a possible desensitizing mechanism.

Oral Aspects. Drug-induced anaphylactic reactions are always a potential office emergency. This is especially so in the case of penicillin, but there are reports of type I reactions to almost all pharmacologic agents used in dental medicine. Many of the materials used in dentistry, including mercury, acrylic monomer, and impression materials, also may be type I allergens. In addition, type I reactions to oral microorganisms have been implicated in the inflammatory reactions occuring in periodontal disease, pulp and periapical lesions, and other orofacial infections.

Cytotoxic Reactions

Type II reactions are called cytotoxic or antitissue hypersensitivities because there is direct injury to circulating or fixed cells in the body. Cytotoxic hypersensitivities differ from the other humoral hypersensitivities in that the major tissue injury occurs as a result of immune complex formation on the tissue; that is, antibodies are directed against antigenic determinants on the target cell that is injured. In type I and III reactions, immune complexes induce the release of nonspecific molecular mediators, which subsequently injure the target cells. Cytotoxic hypersensitivities include transfusion reactions, drug-induced reactions, and several autoimmune diseases.

Mechanisms of Injury. Type II reactions are mediated by IgG and IgM. The formation of an immune complex between these immunoglobulins and antigens in the cell membrane results in destruction of the cell. The injury-producing mechanisms are complement-dependent lysis, opsonization and phagocytosis, and another cytolytic process, antibody-dependent cell-mediated cytotoxicity (ADCC).

Complement-dependent lysis is mediated by IgG and IgM (Table 8–4). The activation of complement by the immune complex on the target cell membrane results in membranolysis and death of the cell. Both fixed and circulating cells are susceptible to this injury.

The IgG in the immune complex also is an opsonin that, usually in association with the activated complement components C3b and C5b, makes the target cell susceptible to phagocytosis by polymorphonuclear leukocytes and macrophages. Phagocytosis acts on circulating elements, such as red blood cells, leukocytes, and platelets.

ADCC is a mechanism through which several different types of leukocytes react with the Fc portion of IgG molecules in the immune complex on the target cell membrane. The leukocyte then kills the target cell by an unknown mechanism. The leukocytes may be polymorphonuclear neutrophils, macrophages, or lymphoreticular cells, called killer, or K, cells. ADCC can kill both fixed and circulating cells.

TABLE 8–4. CELLULAR AND MOLECULAR FACTORS IN TYPE II REACTIONS

IgG
IgM
Complement (opsonic, membranolytic)
Polymorphonuclear neutrophils
Macrophages
Killer cells (ADCC)

Blood Group Reactions Blood group antigens, especially the A and B and Rh antigenic systems, are responsible for many type II reactions. A person with B antigens on the red blood cells has preformed antitype A antibodies, called isoagglutinins, in his or her plasma. Therefore, if type A blood is transfused into this individual, the anti-A isoagglutinins will lyse the type A cells. Since previous exposure to type A blood is not necessary for the reaction to occur, it has been postulated that these isoagglutinins, called natural antibody, are produced in response to natural exposure to heterophile (cross-reacting) antigens carried by microorganisms in the gastrointestinal tract. As noted in Table 8–5, the isoagglutinins an individual possesses are determined by the antigens present in his or her red blood cells. Thus, individuals with type A blood carry anti-B isoagglutinins, those with type O blood, carry anti-A and anti-B isoagglutinins, and those with type AB blood have no isoagglutinins.

Hemolytic disease of the newborn involves the Rh antigenic system and also is called Rh disease. When an Rh-negative mother carries an Rh-positive fetus, the possiblity exists that the mother may become sensitized to the Rh antigenic determinants and produce anti-Rh antibody. This antibody is IgG, which can cross the placenta and lyse the fetal red blood cells, releasing toxic amounts of bilirubin.

Drug-Induced Reactions. Drug-induced cytotoxic reactions can be caused by several mechanisms. The drug may adsorb to the cell membrane and form a conjugated antigen, which serves as the target for a cytotoxic reaction. Second, the drug may adsorb to the cell and modify the membrane so that hidden determinants are exposed. The immune system then produces cytotoxic antibodies directed against these exposed determinants. Finally, the drug can react with circulating antibody, and the immune complex formed may spontaneously attach to a cell membrane and initiate a lytic complement cascade (reactive lysis). Drug-induced cytotoxic reactions, which often are life-threatening, have been demonstrated against

TABLE 8–5. SEROLOGIC RELATIONSHIPS OF HUMAN BLOOD GROUPS

Blood group	RBC antigen	Isoagglutinins	Serum reaction with RBC from group			
			A	*B*	*AB*	*O*
A	A	Anti-B	−	+	+	−
B	B	Anti-A	+	−	+	−
AB	A and B		−	−	−	−
O		Anti-A+B	+	+	+	−

red blood cells, polymorphonuclear leukocytes, and platelets. Table 8–6 lists several of the drugs that have been implicated in type II reactions.

Cytotoxic reactions also are involved in autoimmune diseases and organ transplant rejections, which are discussed subsequently.

Therapy. Treatment of cytotoxic hypersensitivities varies with the etiology of the disease. Drug-induced reactions may be alleviated by ceasing administration of the drug and treating with anti-inflammatory agents. Severe type II reactions may be treated with immunosuppressive drugs that suppress antibody formation.

Oral Aspects. Type II reactions are of primary regard to dentistry as a result of their role in drug-induced reactions. All of the drugs listed in Table 8–6 that have been shown to cause cytotoxic reactions are used in dentistry. In addition, there is evidence that several oral diseases, such as recurrent aphthous ulcers, Behcet's syndrome, and Sjogren's syndrome, are autoimmune diseases mediated, at least in part, by type II reactions.

Immune Complex Reactions

Immune complex reactions, or type III hypersensitivities, may be local or systemic. The local reaction is called the Arthus reaction, and the systemic reaction is called serum sickness. The mechanisms of both are similar, but there are differences in the events leading to these injurious inflammatory reactions. Type III reactions occur in microbial infections, malignancies, autoimmune diseases, and as a consequence of drug therapy.

Mechanisms of Type III Reactions. Type III reactions are initiated by immune complexes containing the complement-activating immunoglobulins, IgG and IgM (Table 8–7). When complement reacts with the immune complexes, chemotactic, vasoactive, and opsonic compounds are produced. The immune complexes also stimulate release of vasoactive amines from platelets. Polymorphonuclear neutrophils (PMNs) are attracted to the area by the chemotactic stimuli and attempt to phagocytize the immune complexes. Normally, this would be considered a protective response, but during the phagocytic process, lysosomes release their contents into the surrounding area. The lysosomes contain many biologically active compounds, including potent hydrolytic enzymes (Table 8–8), and it is these enzymes that damage the surrounding cells and tissues and are responsible for the injury occurring in type III reactions.

The Arthus Reaction. The local immune complex reaction can be demonstrated by intradermally injecting an antigen into an animal possessing a high antibody titer. Immune complexes form precipitates in the perivascular areas and are deposited within blood vessel walls. The immune complexes activate complement, PMNs infiltrate the area, and lysosomal enzymes are released. The basement membrane and endothelium of the vessels are injured by the enzymes, causing a focal vasculitis. The injury ranges from local hemorrhage and thrombosis to necrosis in a strong response. The reaction becomes apparent about 2 hours after the antigen is injected, peaks at 3 to 6 hours, and disappears within 9 to 12 hours after injection. The intensity and duration of the reaction are proportional to the antibody titer.

Although Arthus reactions occur infrequently in humans, there are several allergic pneumonitides, caused by inhalation of microbial antigens, that are considered to be intrapulmonary immune complex re-

TABLE 8–6. SOME COMPOUNDS OF DENTAL INTEREST IMPLICATED IN DRUG-INDUCED CYTOTOXIC REACTIONS

Antihistamines	Meprobamate
Aspirin	Novobiocin
Carbamazepine	Penicillins
Chlorpromazine	Sulfamethazine
Mefenamic acid	Tetracycline

TABLE 8–7. CELLULAR AND MOLECULAR FACTORS IN TYPE III REACTIONS

IgG
IgM
Complement (anaphylatoxic, chemotactic, opsonic)
Polymorphonuclear neutrophils
Lysosomal enzymes

TABLE 8–8. REPRESENTATIVE CONSTITUENTS OF POLYMORPHONUCLEAR NEUTROPHIL LYSOSOMES

Enzymes	Miscellaneous
Acid RNAse	Cationic polypeptides and proteins
Acid DNAse	Mucopolysaccharides
Acid phosphatase	Glycoproteins
Alkaline phosphatase	Endogenous pyrogen
β-Glucuronidase	Phagocytin
5-Nucleotidase	Slow reacting substance of anaphylaxis
Cathepsins A, B, C, D, E	
Lysozyme	
NADP-oxidase	
Kinin-forming enzymes	
Kinin-destroying enzymes	
Peroxidase	
Arylsulfatase A and B	
Phospholipase	
Plasminogen activator	
Collagenase	
Vascular permeability-promoting proteases	
Hyaluronidase	

Adapted from Taichman NS. J Periodontol. *1970;41:228–231.*

actions. In addition, there is evidence suggesting that local type III reactions may play a role in periodontal disease.

Serum Sickness. Systemic type III reactions were named serum sickness because the syndrome was first noted in patients receiving immune animal antisera for treatment of diphtheria and other bacterial toxemias. The reactions, which usually occur 1 or 2 weeks after injection of the serum, are characterized by fever, enlarged lymph nodes and spleen, a generalized urticarial rash, and painful swollen joints. Histologic analysis reveals disseminated vascular lesions similar to those of an Arthus reaction.

The reaction is initiated when the foreign serum proteins circulating in the blood stimulate an immune response, and the new antibody forms complexes with remaining foreign proteins. The first immune complexes formed are soluble because there is excess antigen (Fig 6–7). The soluble complexes circulate until they are deposited in the vascular endothelium throughout the body, and minute vascular lesions occur wherever the immune complexes are trapped. There is a predilection for deposition of immune complexes in the vessel walls of the renal glomeruli and synovial joints, and, therefore, glomerulonephritis and arthralgia are frequent symptoms of the disease. Serum sickness rarely is fatal, and except in those cases in which there is a chronic exposure to the offending antigen, symptoms disappear within 2 weeks after onset.

Animal sera are used less frequently today, but systemic immune complex reactions still occur as a result of exposure to other allergens. The reactions may occur when patients are given large or repeated doses of drugs. Many therapeutic agents may induce immune complex reactions, but as with most iatrogenic hypersensitivity reactions, penicillin is the most frequently involved. In addition, serum sickness often is a complication of microbial diseases, such as chronic type B viral hepatitis, malaria, and streptococcal infections. It also occurs in autoimmune diseases, such as systemic lupus erythematosus and rheumatoid arthritis, in which circulating antibodies react with self antigens, and in malignancies, such as leukemia or carcinomas, in which immune complexes are formed with antigens shed from tumor cells.

Therapy. The initial step in therapy is to attempt to remove the offending antigen. In drug-induced reactions, the drug should be discontinued. If the immune stimulus is of an infectious nature, the microorganisms should be eradicated. Anti-inflammatory drugs may be given to relieve the symptoms of the reaction, and if the disease is severe, as in autoimmune diseases, immunosuppressive drugs may be administered to block production of antibody.

Oral Aspects. Penicillin is the most common agent for type III reactions in medicine and probably ranks in the same position in dentistry. Several other antimicrobials and anti-inflammatory agents also have been implicated in immune complex reactions. In addition, there is evidence that type III reactions contribute to the inflammatory injury occurring in pulp and periapical infections and in periodontal disease.

Type IV Reactions

Type IV hypersensitivities are cell-mediated reactions. They are divided into two groups. One group is mediated by lymphokines produced by sensitized T lymphocytes, and the second is mediated by cytotoxic T lymphocytes (T-c or CTL) (Table 8–9). Lymphokine-mediated reactions include delayed-type hypersensitivity (DTH) reactions, such as infection allergy and contact dermatitis. Cytotoxic cells are responsible for some organ transplant rejections and autoimmune diseases.

TABLE 8–9. CELLULAR AND MOLECULAR FACTORS IN TYPE IV REACTIONS

Lymphocytes (T-dth)
Lymphokines
Activated macrophages
Lysosomal enzymes
Cytotoxic T lymphocytes

Delayed-Type Hypersensitivity. The tuberculin reaction is the classic DTH reaction and can be demonstrated in an animal or human who has been sensitized, either artificially or through infection, to the tubercle bacillus, *Mycobacterium tuberculosis*. If tuberculin, a proteinaceous extract of the bacterium, is injected into the skin of a sensitized individual, the injection site becomes inflamed and indurated in about 8 hours, with the reaction peaking at 24 to 48 hours after the injection. In very sensitive individuals, the site may hemorrhage and necrose. Histologically, the lesion is characterized by an intense mononuclear cell infiltrate, predominantly macrophages. Following a single antigen injection, the reaction will subside within days, but the mononuclear cell infiltrate may remain for weeks. In the presence of a persistent exposure to an antigen, such as an infectious process, a chronic granuloma will develop.

The DTH reaction is the result of lymphokines released by T-dth lymphocytes responding to the tuberculin antigens (Table 7–5A). Skin reactive factor increases vascular permeability, causing erythema and edema. Chemotactic factors attract lymphocytes and macrophages into the site, and mitogenic factors further increase the numbers of leukocytes present. Migration inhibition factors hold the cells in the tissue, and macrophage activating factor increases the metabolic and phagocytic activity of the macrophages in the lesion. Injury results primarily from lysosomal enzymes released by the macrophages. These include collagenase, hyaluronidase, and others similar to the PMN enzymes listed in Table 8–8. In addition, lymphotoxin, the nonspecific cytotoxic lymphokine, kills cells in the area. Cytotoxic T cells also may be involved in some DTH reactions.

DTH is associated with several infectious diseases and has been called infection allergy. It is responsible for much of the injury occurring in tuberculosis, leprosy, syphilis, other bacterial infections, and almost all fungal infections. These diseases are characterized by chronic, often necrotic, granulomas. DTH reactions also occur in viral infections. The rash seen in measles is the result of DTH reactions against viral antigens that have localized in the skin, and the pox, or skin lesion, in smallpox is caused by DTH to the virus that proliferates in the skin.

Contact Dermatitis. Contact dermatitis is a form of DTH in which sensitization and the subsequent hypersensitivity reaction are elicited by lipid-soluble haptens that penetrate the skin. These haptens are usually highly reactive compounds that bind covalently to proteins in the skin to form conjugated antigens. Langerhans cells in the skin may replace macrophages as antigen-processing and presenting cells in contact dermatitis. Sensitization may occur after the first exposure to the conjugated antigen, but often it takes repeated exposures to sensitize the tissues sufficiently. On subsequent skin contact with the hapten, T-dth cells in the skin release lymphokines, and a DTH reaction ensues. The reaction is evident about 24 hours after contact with the hapten and peaks at 48 to 72 hours. The time course of contact dermatitis is slower than the tuberculin reaction because the hapten first must penetrate the skin. Initially, the reaction will appear similar to the tuberculin reaction, but eventually, vesicles containing serous fluid and leukocytes will form at the reaction site. The sensitivity may last for years, even in the absence of the allergen. Chronic exposure to a contact allergen will cause thickening, crusting, and scaling of the skin. Allergens that cause contact dermatitis include many drugs, dyes, metals, and plant resins, such as those of poison ivy and poison oak.

Therapy. Treatment for contact dermatitis and other DTH reactions involves avoidance of the allergen or, in the case of infectious diseases, ridding the tissues of the pathogen. Corticosteroid ointments usually are sufficient treatment for contact dermatitis, but parenteral administration of the steroids may be necessary in severe cases. Infectious diseases with DTH involvement usually are not treated with corticosteroids because of the potential suppressive effects on protective immunity.

Oral Aspects. DTH reactions have been implicated in chronic infections in the oral cavity, including periodontal diseases and pulp and periapical infections. Contact dermatitis is an occupational hypersensitivity of dentists and their patients. Some of the more frequently encountered sensitizing agents in dentistry are listed in Table 8–10. These compounds can cause contact dermatitis in the clinician and the patient.

Cytotoxic T-Cells. Cytotoxic T lymphocytes mediate the second type IV hypersensitivity reaction. These CTLs kill other cells that possess membrane anti-

TABLE 8–10. SOME COMPOUNDS OF DENTAL INTEREST IMPLICATED IN CONTACT DERMATITIS

Agents	Sensitizers
Topical medicaments	Antibiotics in troches and ointments, benzocaine, formaldehyde
Metallic instruments and restorations	Nickel, gold, mercury, stainless steel
Mouthwashes and dentifrices	Antiseptics, astringents, flavoring agents
Dental materials	Acrylic monomer, latex, eugenol, rosins

Adapted from Eversole LR. J Oral Med. *1979;34:96.*

gens against which the lymphocytes have been sensitized. The CTL contacts the target cell briefly, initiates a cytolytic process, and leaves the target cell, which lyses shortly thereafter. CTLs can then go on to kill several other target cells. Cytotoxic cells are involved in autoimmune diseases and tumor immunity, but graft rejection is the most extensively studied CTL-mediated lesion and serves as the model for the reaction.

Transplantation Immunology

If a tissue is transplanted from one animal to a genetically different recipient, the graft will appear to succeed or take but then will die. This rejection of the graft can be demonstrated to be an immunologic process by observing the responses to successive grafts in the same animal. For example, if skin is transplanted to an animal, the graft initially becomes vacularized and flourishes. After about 10 to 14 days, however, the graft becomes inflamed, necroses, and sloughs off. This is called the first set rejection. If a second skin graft is made from the same donor, the second graft is rejected much more rapidly. This second set reaction occurs within 5 or 6 days. Finally, if skin from a third, genetically different animal is transplanted to the same recipient, this third graft will be rejected slowly, as a first set reaction. The rapidity and the specificity of the second set rejection indicates that it is a secondary immune response.

Several observations indicate that skin graft rejection is a CMI response. The second set sensitization can be transferred from a sensitive animal to a normal one with peripheral lymphocytes but not with serum. In addition, rejection can be prevented by previous removal of the thymus, which controls T lymphocyte maturation. Finally, histologic studies support the role of CMI in rejection. Allografts are infiltrated with mononuclear cells, and polymorphonuclear neutrophils are lacking. Unlike the lymphokine-mediated type-IV reaction, however, the majority of the mononuclear cells are lymphocytes, more specifically, CTLs that are attacking MHC antigen-bearing cells of the grafted tissues.

Although graft rejection under natural conditions is primarily a CMI response, human rejections, as a result of manipulations by physicians, also may be antibody mediated. Three types of reactions have been described in human graft rejections.

Hyperacute rejections, mediated by preformed antibody, are type II reactions that occur within minutes or hours after the graft has been placed.

Acute rejections usually occur within days after placement of the graft but also may occur several weeks after apparent acceptance of the transplant. These are mediated by CTLs.

Chronic rejections develop slowly after apparent acceptance of the graft. These are antibody-mediated type II reactions that are characterized by slow deterioration and eventual rejection of the transplanted tissues.

Types of Grafts. The success or failure of a graft is determined by the genetic relatedness of the graft donor and the recipient. Four types of grafts have been defined based on their source.

Autografts are grafts from one site to another on the same individual. These grafts, which are immunologically compatible and usually survive, include skin grafts in burn patients and blood vessel grafts.

Isografts are grafts from one individual to a genetically identical individual, that is, identical twins. These grafts usually are successful. The most common isografts are kidney transplants.

Allografts are grafts from one individual to another who is of the same species but not genetically identical. Most human grafts, such as kidney and heart transplants, are allografts. They will be rejected unless the immune response is suppressed.

Xenografts are grafts between individuals of different species. These are rejected rapidly.

Histocompatibility Antigens. Humans possess two major groups of antigens, histocompatibility antigens, which determine the success or failure of a graft. The first group consists of the blood typing antigens. These are found on other tissues as well and may be targets for the immune rejection of grafts. If the donor and recipient are not matched in terms of these antigens, the same antibodies that mediate transfusion reactions will reject the graft within minutes, that is, a hyperacute rejection. Therefore, donor and recipient absolutely must be compatible in terms of the red blood cell A and B antigens.

The second group of histocompatibility antigens are the HLA (human leukocyte antigens) antigens. The HLA antigens are found on all nucleated cells of the body and are divided into five groups designated HLA-A, HLA-B, HLA-C, HLA-D, and HLA-DR. Each individual carries the genes for these five groups, and since the HLA loci are codominant, as many as 10 HLA antigens may be expressed on an individual's cells. These antigens pose the greatest problem in transplantation medicine. Nearly all allograft rejections are the result of immune reactions against HLA antigens.

The degree of similarity in HLA antigens usually determines the success or failure of a graft. Ideally, donor and recipient should share all HLA antigens. However, a complete match of all antigens is a probability only with some siblings, since there are more than 100 different HLA antigens. Thus, the number of possible HLA antigen combinations is so great that the probability that any two randomly selected individuals might carry identical HLA antigens is one in tens of thousands.

HLA genes are codominant, and, therefore, the alleles on both chromosomes are expressed. Fortunately, the HLA loci are closely linked, and HLA antigens coded on a single chromosome usually are inherited as a unit or a haplotype. This enhances the possibility of finding a sibling match. As illustrated in Fig 8–1, a child receives one haplotype from each parent. Thus, there is a 25% chance that two siblings will share both haplotypes and be histocompatible and a 50% chance that they will share at least one haplotype.

Prevention of Graft Rejection. Since they are antigenically identical, autografts and isografts require only proper surgical management. Allografts require tissue matching and immunosuppressive treatment of the recipient in order to survive. Tissue matching involves (1) determining that the red blood cell antigens are compatible, (2) ascertaining the absence of cytotoxic antibody that may have been produced as a result of exposure to the HLA antigens through prior blood transfusions, pregnancy, or previous transplants, and (3) HLA antigen matching. If the blood group antigens are identical, if there are no cytotoxic antibodies in the recipient, and if there is sufficient similarity between the donor and recipient HLA antigens, the organ is transplanted. The transplant is accompanied by immunosuppressive therapy and constant monitoring of the status of the graft. Survival of human grafts depends on the organ transplanted. The success rate for kidney grafts approaches 90%, but it is much lower with other organs, such as the heart, liver, and lungs.

Graft-Versus-Host Disease. If lymphoid cells are transplanted to an immunocompetent recipient, the recipient's immune system overwhelms and destroys the transplanted cells. If, however, viable lymphoid cells are transplanted into an immunodeficient recipient, a graft-versus-host (GVH) reaction will occur. The donor's immunocytes recognize the recipient's antigens and mount an immune response against them; that is, the donor's lymphocytes attempt to reject the host. GVH disease was demonstrated initially in laboratory animals, but it is of clinical significance because of the difficulties it places on the treatment of immunodeficient individuals. Since many immunodeficiencies result from the absence of functional lymphoid tissues, transplantation of the necessary tissues would appear to be the treatment of choice. When this is done, however, a GVH reaction, which may be fatal, occurs. Thus, GVH disease prevents the use of what would appear to be the most obvious treatment for immunodeficiencies.

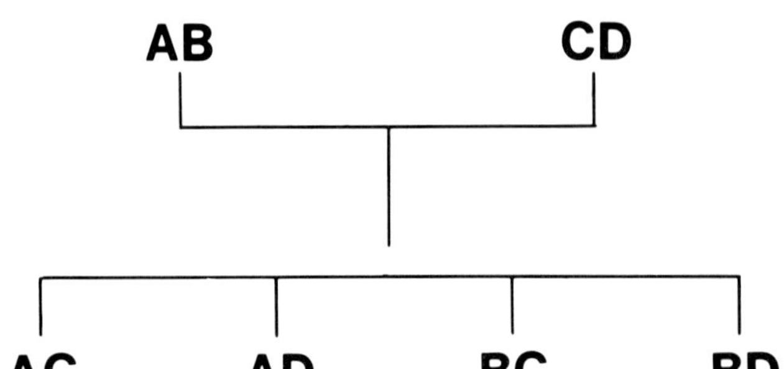

Figure 8–1. Inheritance of HLA antigens. Each child will receive a single haplotype (a or b and c or d) from each parent. Since there are only four possible combinations, there is a 1 in 4 chance that one's sibling will share the same HLA antigens.

Oral Aspects. Of all the organs and tissues available for transplantation, teeth are the most abundant and, numerically, the most needed. Tooth autografts and isografts are not rejected, but surgical management is still a problem. Unfortunately, tooth allografts are subject to the same immunologic mechanisms that affect other tissues. Transplanted teeth are rejected.

Tooth allografts, however, are retained longer than most other grafts in the absence of immunosuppression. This extended survival is assumed to occur because the antigens in teeth are less immunogenic. In addition, even when teeth are rejected and the supporting soft tissues are destroyed, the nonvital hard tissues may be retained for several years as a result of ankylosis. It is probable that rejection of teeth from a closely matched donor could be prevented with immunosuppression. However, the possible adverse reactions (ie, infections) that accompany immunsuppression far exceed any benefits that might be derived from transplanted teeth.

Like tooth transplants, allogeneic bone grafts used to correct defects caused by periodontal diseases or trauma are subject to the same immunologic problems as other tissues. Soft tissue extraction, freezing and drying, and other treatments have been used to attempt to render bone grafts less immunogenic. Although clinical investigators have reported successes with some of these treated materials, grafts using viable allogenic bone still are not possible.

Autoimmunity

The recognition of self antigens is an essential function of the immune system and critical to the well-being of the host. If this function is somehow disturbed and an immune response is mounted against self antigens, autoimmunity ensues. If the autoimmune response causes tissue injury or some functional disorder, the resulting disease is called an autoimmune disease. Autoimmunity is associated with a number of diseases, but except for some reactions involving drugs or responses to several infectious diseases, the etiology of autoimmunity is not well understood. It is often difficult, if not impossible, to determine if autoimmunity is the cause or the result of a disease process.

The reasons that the normal regulatory mechanisms that control self recognition are circumvented and autoimmunity occurs are unclear. Several theories have been proposed to explain autoimmunity, and there is scientific evidence for all of them. Indeed, there are probably multiple immunologic abnormalities that may result in autoimmunity.

One theory involves a group of antigens that are much more prone to be targets of autoimmunity than are other self antigens. These antigens include thyroglobulin and antigens in the lens of the eye, spermatozoa, and neural tissues. Since a common property of these antigens is that they are either not in contact with the circulatory system or are present only in very low concentrations, they have been called sequestered antigens. As a result of their unique anatomic location, they also are sequestered from the lymphoid system, and this appears to affect the ability of the immune system to recognize them as self antigens. The sequestered antigen theory proposes that as long as the antigens are isolated from the immune system or exposed to it only in very low concentrations, there will be no problems. However, autoimmunity can occur if, as a result of mechanical or infectious trauma, the immune system is exposed to these antigens in large concentrations. Hashimoto's thyroiditis, uveitis, and aspermatogenesis are examples of these autoimmune diseases.

Autoimmunity may result from alteration of cell membranes. Membrane antigens may be altered by haptens, such as drugs, by microbial actions and possibly by the host's own lysosomal enzymes. If the alterations are sufficient to make the antigen appear foreign to the immune system, autoimmunity occurs. Drug-induced hemolytic anemias and thrombocytopenias may be induced by haptens, such as antibiotics and analgesics. In addition, during viral infections, viral antigens may become incorporated into the membranes of infected cells, making the cells targets of an autoimmune reaction.

Autoimmunity also can be induced by heterophile or cross-reacting antigens. Antibodies directed against an antigenic determinant on a nonself antigen may react with a similar determinant on a self antigen. This occurs in rheumatic fever, in which antibody directed against *Streptococcus pyogenes* injures cardiac tissue, which shares a heterophile antigen with the streptococci. A similar mechanism has been suggested for recurrent aphthous ulcerations in which a heterophile antigenic determinant shared by *Streptococcus sanguis* and oral mucosa has been implicated.

Finally, autoimmunity may occur as a result of a defect in the regulatory mechanisms of the lymphoid system. Any malfunction of the self recognition process might release autoreactive lymphocytes from their normal controls. If, as has been proposed, T suppressor cells prevent autoimmunity, a defect in or deficiency of these cells could allow production of autoantibodies. Evidence for this possibility is supported by studies in strains of laboratory mice that develop autoimmunity as they age. This autoimmunity is considered to be a T cell defect or deficiency because the disease can be prevented or reversed by transfusion of T cells from younger mice.

Autoimmune injury may be mediated by several mechanisms. Hemolytic anemias, thrombocytopenias, and Goodpasture's syndrome, which involves the basement membranes of the glomeruli and alveoli, are mediated by type II, cytotoxic reactions. Immune complexes consisting of self antigens and autoantibodies may be deposited in the vascular walls and elicit type III reactions. Since the immune complexes often localize in the kidneys, glomerulonephritis is a frequent symptom in these diseases. Systemic lupus erythematosus and rheumatoid arthritis are autoimmune diseases characterized by immune complex reactions. Although injury mediated by sensitized T lymphocytes is not common among autoimmune diseases, it has been associated with autoimmune encephalitis.

Oral Aspects. Drug-induced autoimmune diseases are of obvious concern to dentists. Some of these drugs were mentioned previously in the description of type II reactions. In addition, oral diseases, such as recurrent aphthous ulcerations, Behcet's syndrome, and Sjögren's syndrome, are thought to be autoimmune diseases. Finally, several systemic autoimmune diseases, such as systemic lupus erythematosus, rheumatoid arthritis, and pemphigus vulgaris, are characterized by oral manifestations.

Tumor Immunology

There is a large body of evidence linking the immune response and cancer. It is, however, somewhat contradictory because the immune response may result in both protection of the host and protection of the tumor. Despite this paradox, protection does occur, and much of the new and experimental therapies for cancer are immunologically based.

Several theories have been proposed to attempt to explain why tumors occur despite immunologic surveillance. Basically, tumors occur when there is a malfunction of the immune response against these mutant cells. In the case of immunodeficient or immunosuppressed patients, immunologic surveillance is absent, and tumors succeed as a result of this absence. Tumors also might become established during a period of transient immunodeficiency. Drugs, viral infections, and malnutrition can cause such transient deficiencies, and if the deficiency were to occur coincidentally with the appearance of cancerous cells, it is possible that a tumor could establish itself.

Tumor-specific antigens have been identified in several but not all tumors, and in many cases, the antigens are only weakly immunogenic. Establishment of tumors could occur because the immune surveillance system either does not detect these antigens or fails to mount an effective immune response against the weak immunogens. Another possibility that has been proposed is antigenic overload. This could occur if a tumor is already established or if the tumor cells are reproducing too rapidly. The antigenic challenge may be so great that the immune system cannot respond rapidly enough to overcome the tumor. Finally, tumor-protective immunologic factors may be involved.

Immunologic involvement in the disease is readily apparent. For example, histologic studies reveal the presence of lymphocytic infiltrates in and adjacent to tumors. In addition, the lymph nodes draining the tumor tissues are in a reactive state indicative of an immune response. CMI and antibodies directed against tumors have been demonstrated in some humans and other animals that carry tumors. This indicates that tumors carry antigens that the immune system recognizes. There also is an increased incidence of certain types of tumors in individuals who are immunodeficient (eg, AIDS). Finally, there is an increased incidence of certain types of tumors in immunosuppressed transplant patients. Often, these tumors regress when immunosuppressive treatments are terminated.

These observations led to the formulation of a concept called immunologic surveillance. This theory proposes that mutant, potentially cancerous cells are constantly arising in the body and that it is the function of the immune system to recognize and destroy these harmful mutants. CMI factors that are thought to mediate the enforcement of immunologic surveillance include T-c cells, activated macrophages, and natural killer (NK) cells. Humoral immune mechanisms that might be involved include ADCC and complement-mediated cell lysis.

Specific T-s cells that suppress immunity against tumor antigens have been reported to be present in some patients. In addition, in vitro studies with sera from cancer patients revealed that there were substances in the sera that interfered with the CTLs and other cells thought to be involved in protection against tumors. Subsequently, several serum blocking factors, which enhance tumor formation, were discovered. One of these was antitumor antibody. Immunoglobulins (IgA and IgG, subclass 4) that do not fix complement can react with the tumor cell antigens and prevent the attachment of cytotoxic antibodies or cells. These antibodies could protect the tumor against destruction by other immune fctors.

Free tumor antigen is another blocking factor. If a tumor sheds large amounts of antigen, this soluble antigen can react with receptors on cytotoxic cells and and block attachment of these cells to the tumor cells. Free antigen also can bind to antibody, and this immune complex can react with Fc receptors of the cells that mediate ADCC and effectively neutralize their antitumor activity.

Immunotherapy of Tumors. Immunotherapy has been directed toward activating or augmenting the immune response to tumor antigens. Several forms of immunotherapy appear to be promising, but none are used routinely.

Vaccines, including live or killed tumor cells and extracts of tumor cells, have been tested in humans and laboratory animals. Some of these vaccines can prevent tumor implantation, but they are only marginally effective against established tumors.

Adjuvants have been used to augment the immune response in cancer patients. The tuberculosis vaccine, BCG, has been one of the more successful adjuvants. In addition to its antitubercle effects, the vaccine is a nonspecific stimulator of CMI. When used in association with chemotherapy, BCG has been at least partially effective in treating several human cancers, including malignant melanoma, acute lymphocytic leukemia, and acute myelogenous leukemia.

Various immune factors, such as monoclonal antibodies, interferon, IL-2, thymosin, and transfer factor, have been tested in cancer patients, but most have met with only limited success. Interferon is effective against several leukemias and lymphomas and has been accepted for routine therapy of patients with these cancers. In summary, although scientists have met with only limited success, there is still hope of developing effective methods of immunotherapy for tumors.

SUGGESTED READINGS

Altman LC. Basic immune mechanisms in immediate hypersensitivity. *Med Clin North Am.* 1981;65:941.

Genco RJ, Slots J. Host responses in periodontal diseases. *J Dent Res.* 1984;63:441.

Ivanyi L, ed. *Immunological Aspects of Oral Diseases.* Lancaster, UK, Boston: MTP Press; 1986.

Roitt IM, Lehner T. *Immunology of Oral Diseases,* 2nd ed. London: Blackwell; 1983.

Russell RRB, Johnson NW. The prospects for vaccination against dental caries. *Br Dent J.* 1987;162:29.

Sell S. *Immunology, Immunopathology, and Immunity.* New York: Elsevier; 1987.

Stites DP, Stobo JD, Wells JV, eds. *Basic and Clinical Immunology,* 6th ed. E. Norwalk, Conn: Appleton & Lange; 1987.

Strober W, Lamm ME, McGhee JR, James SP, eds. *Mucosal Immunity and Infections at Mucosal Surfaces.* New York: Oxford University Press; 1988.

CHAPTER 9

Host–Parasite Interactions

Norman P. Willett

INTRODUCTION

KOCH'S POSTULATES

PATHOGENIC PROPERTIES OF MICROORGANISMS

Virulence

HOST RESISTANCE

Constitutive Variables

Nonspecific Factors Governing Host Defense

EPIDEMIOLOGY

ORAL ASPECTS

SUGGESTED READINGS

INTRODUCTION

The details of the multifactorial relationships between host and parasite are just beginning to be understood fully. The implications of this new knowledge will force health professions to reassess the definitions of a number of terms and concepts, such as disease, infection, pathogen, and virulence. This is underscored by the recent developments of new agents being identified as pathogens, agents previously considered benign becoming important sources of infections, and the emergence of entirely new diseases, for example Legionnaire's disease, Lyme disease, and acquired immunodeficiency syndrome (AIDS).

Examples of questions that are arising are (1) What are the ecologic conditions that give rise to a particular pathogenic property? (2) What are the mechanisms by which pathogens suppress or elude host defenses? (3) What are the mechanisms of virulence at the molecular level that actually damage the cell? (4) What are the newly discovered compounds and structural elements of both host and parasite that play a critical role in their interaction?

An extremely diverse microbial flora can attach itself to various internal surfaces of mammalian species by a variety of mechanisms that are modulated by the microecologic conditions of the body and individual cells. These organisms, which are considered parasites, can establish themselves in the living host if appropriate biochemical and biophysical conditions are present and inhibitory conditions or substances are either absent or present in low amounts. This phenomenon is known as colonization. The degree of adaptation and interaction of these organisms with the host often will determine whether the colonizing organism will be a pathogen or part of the normal flora.

Achievement of a state of stability in the equilibrium between host and parasite will lead to permanent colonization of the organisms. This is called commensalism, and it is the mechanism by which most of the normal flora are established. The normal flora, initially derived by contamination from the moment of birth, may be defined as those organisms that are permanently established on and in mucous membranes and other superficial tissues. They participate in many host beneficial functions but may assume the role of a pathogen if entrance is gained to a normally sterile area of the body or a site where the organism is not part of the established flora. This may occur as a result of a decrease in host resistance or invasive medical or dental procedures. If, on the other hand, the organism is poorly adapted, that is, a pathogen, a strong interaction occurs that will result in the organism's expressing its potential of virulence, with the end result being an infectious disease. Both pathogens and normal flora can coexist on body surfaces in a state of dynamic balance until the normal physiologic conditions of the host cell or microbe are perturbed. If this occurs, as a rule, the equilibrium will shift in favor of the microbe, with consequent damage to the host and expression of clinical disease. Isolation of an organism from a surface, regardless of whether it is an actual or potential pathogen, does not constitute evidence for an infectious process. It is important to distinguish between the clinical disease state, which may sometimes be called infectious disease, and the term colonization, which is sometimes used synonymously with infection. In the case of the former, damage to the host will occur with consequent manifestation of symptoms. In the case of the latter, colonization is only the initial step in determining whether or not the organism can grow and multiply in the host. The presence of some organisms, such as *Salmonella* or *Shigella*, which normally cause disease and are not part of the normal flora, is considered part of an abnormal state, that is, subclinical infection or carrier state.

KOCH'S POSTULATES

In the nineteenth century, Robert Koch published an article that, for the first time, established a series of steps that would prove the connection between a specific microorganism and the disease caused. These proofs, known as Koch's postulates and based on the use of pure cultures, dominated microbiology for the first 75 years of their existence.

1. The organism must be regularly associated with a given disease.
2. The organism must be grown in pure culture on an artificial medium.
3. The disease must be reproduced in a susceptible experimental animal following inoculation with a pure culture.
4. The organism must be reisolated in pure culture from the experimental animal.

Although these proofs are still used today in establishing causal relationships between an etiologic agent and an infectious disease, a number of difficulties have arisen in attempting to satisfy these postulates for oral pathogens.

In mixed infections, syndromes of varied etiology, and host carriers (absence of disease syndrome), it may be difficult to satisfy the first postulate, that is, to determine if the microorganism is associated with a disease. In satisfying the second postulate, difficulties are encountered primarily with noncultivable pathogens, for example, viruses and some periodontopaths. In addition, for certain organisms, a suitable experimental mode of oral infection has not been found. Difficulties encountered with the third postulate include diseases of multiple etiology, for example, dental caries and periodontal disease, and absence of animal hosts in which the original disease is reproducible. Finally, it is difficult to distinguish the original organism from similar organisms in the oral cavity of healthy experimental animals, since the chief difference between health and disease is primarily differences in number of organisms. This is in contrast to the proof of nonoral pathogens, which is confirmed by the presence of the organism in the disease state, compared to its absence in health.

PATHOGENIC PROPERTIES OF MICROORGANISMS

The terms pathogenicity and virulence often are used synonymously. However, important distinctions must be made between these terms. Pathogenicity usually is defined as the capacity of a particular organism to produce disease within a particular host. Virulence, on the other hand, is the degree of pathogenicity of a particular organism in a host under defined conditions. This implies a quantitative aspect, since virulence can be expressed only in comparative terms because of variations in host and parasite. This can be expressed by the LD_{50}, which is the median dose for a number of microorganisms that will kill 50% of a number of experimental animals in a stated time (Fig 9–1). An alternative to this is the ID_{50}, which is the number of microorganisms necessary to produce a given effect, that is, a sign of infection in a stated time in 50% of the experimental animals.

Virulence

The conditions necessary for virulence are multifactorial and interdependent. Initially, the organism must be resistant to such external environmental factors as temperature, pH, humidity, and ecologic competition. Second, in order to survive, the organism must possess properties that enable it to spread between hosts. Transmissibility relates to the factors that modulate the transfer of organisms either from host to host or from environment to host. This can include nonpathogens as well as pathogens. The former case will be more difficult to measure, since nonpathogens do not necessarily produce an effect. Without this transfer, the organism will not survive in nature.

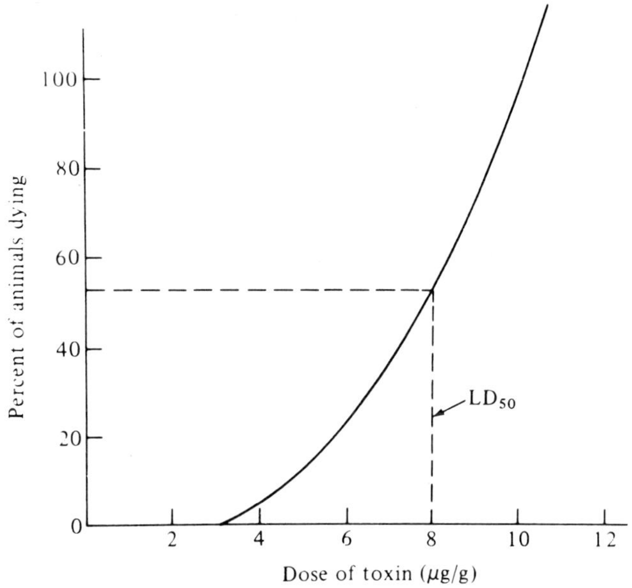

Figure 9–1. Determination of the median lethal dose (LD_{50}) for a toxin. Various doses of toxin are injected into animals. The percentage of animals that die is plotted, and the LD_{50} is extrapolated. In this figure, 8 mg of toxin per gram of animal is the LD_{50}. *(From Boyd R, Hoerl B.* Basic Medical Microbiology, *3rd ed. Boston: Little Brown & Co; 1986.)*

Once the survival and the transfer of the organism are assured, the initial prerequisite for production of infectious disease is entry into the body.

Entry. The entry of microorganisms into or onto body surfaces can occur in a number of ways.

1. The organism may be introduced into the body by a mechanical break or mediated through the bite of an infected insect or animal. Microscopic mechanical breaks may occur by means of the abrasive actions of foods on intestinal mucosa or minute fingernail and cuticle exposures in dentists.
2. A number of respiratory pathogens enter by inhalation. The dentist must be aware of the generation of dental aerosols by the high-speed drill. In order to initiate infection, organisms must avoid being caught up in mucus and removed by mechanical means through swallowing. Second, if deposited in the alveoli, they must resist phagocytosis by the macrophages or, if phagocytized, must multiply in the phagocyte.
3. The organism may be ingested directly with food or water and exert its virulence either through proliferation in the intestinal tract or by the production of toxic substances that may act on intestinal epithelium or be absorbed into the systemic circulation with other effects on host physiology.
4. Phagocytes may carry obligate intracellular parasites through mucosa. Entry of the organism into membrane-lined vacuoles in the cytoplasm of the host cell may occur by nonspecific or receptor-mediated endocytosis. These processes, which may be triggered by the adherent microorganism, are analogous to the phagocytic process and are responsible for internalizing microbes from the external environment. However, the processes differ in that in the case of the receptor-mediated endocytosis, the nature of the surface receptors does not involve immunologic components—complement or immunoglobulins. Receptor-mediated endocytosis involves specific binding of a protein ligand to the cell surface and is subject to competitive inhibition and is reversible. Examples of ligands internalized via this mechanism include polypeptide hormones, serum proteins, some viruses and bacteria, and protein exotoxins.
5. Entry can occur by direct passage through epithelial cells. The organism must be able to tolerate local biochemical and biophysical conditions, and resist various nonspecific host defenses. Organisms, both normal and pathogenic, may enter into parts of the body where they would not normally be present because of abnormalities of various body systems that may occur as a result of general impairment of host defense systems by either drugs or radiation. This may potentiate any of the previously discussed pathways of entry.

Adherence. Microorganisms may attach or adhere to and multiply on body surfaces, usually a mucous membrane. These processes, which are mediated by selective and specific binding of bacterial cell components or surface structures to host cell receptors, are critical properties that govern colonization by pathogens and nonpathogens alike. If the pathogen is not bound, its potential for virulence cannot be expressed. Therefore, the adherence of a pathogen must be considered as the next vital step in the process that may result in clinical infection. The selectivity of the binding enables both normal and pathogenic flora to attach to specific host cell surfaces. Examples of these are shown in Table 9–1. Normal flora may prevent adherence by pathogens by preempting receptor sites on the epithelium. The binding process is relatively stable and irreversible.

The structures responsible for these activities are collectively called adhesins. These include fimbriae and pili, which mediate the virulence of both gram-negative and gram-positive bacteria and are proteinaceous filamentous appendages containing man-

TABLE 9–1. EXAMPLES OF SPECIFIC ATTACHMENTS OF MICROORGANISMS TO HOST CELL OR BODY SURFACE

Microorganism	Disease	Attachment Site	Mechanism
Influenza virus	Influenza	Respiratory epithelial cell	Viral hemagglutin reacts with neuraminic acid receptor on cell
Chlamydia	Conjunctivitis Urethritis	Conjunctival or urethral epithelium	Unknown (sialic acid-containing receptors on epithelial cell?)
Mycoplasma pneumoniae	Atypical pneumonia	Respiratory epithelial cell	Foot on *Mycoplasma* surface attaches to neuraminic acid receptor on cell
Neisseria meningitidis	Carrier state	Nasopharyngeal epithelium	Pili
Vibrio cholerae	Cholera	Intestinal epithelium	Receptors are fucose and mannose
Salmonella typhi	Enteric fever	Intestinal epithelium	Bacterial adhesin attaches to mannoselike receptor on epithelial cell
Streptococcus mutans	Caries	Tooth	Bacterial production of glucosyltransferase, catalyzes glucan formation from sucrose, important in cell–cell and cell–surface adherence
Streptococcus salivarius		Buccal and pharyngeal epithelium	Bacteria bind via lipoteichoic acid on fimbriae
Treponema pallidum	Syphilis	Mucopolysaccharide on cell surface or in tissue	Bacterial mucopolysaccharide associated with virulence
Plasmodium vivax	Malaria	Erythrocyte of susceptible human	Malarial merozoite attaches to Duffy antigen on erythrocyte surface, complement not necessary

Modified from Mims C. The Pathogenesis of Infectious Diseases, *2nd ed. New York: Academic Press; 1982:22.*

nose or mannoselike compounds that bind cellular receptors. The pili mediate the initial attachment of organisms, for example, the *Neisseria,* to epithelial cells. The bacterial glycocalyx, as described in Chapter 1, which is polysaccharide in nature, also may play a key role in pathogenesis. This structure reacts with the glycocalyx of host cells and mediates the adhesion of both normal flora and pathogens. In addition to playing a vital role in the initiation of infection, adhesins are involved directly or indirectly in host injury, since the inflammatory process depends on the ability of the host to recognize bacterial surface components. Surface components involved in adherence include the glucans and mutans, which assist the adherence of *Streptococcus mutans* to tooth surfaces or to the salivary pellicle or to other bacteria, and lipoteichoic acid, which mediates the attachment of *Streptococcus pyogenes* to epithelial surfaces. Figure 9–2 depicts some of the general mechanisms by which bacterial surface components may influence host response and the initiation of infection.

Mechanisms for Damaging the Host. The mechanisms for damaging the host can be grouped into two broad categories, invasiveness and toxigenicity. Invasion leads to demonstrable damage to the host cell in the immediate vicinity of the organism. It is a complex series of phenomena involving growth and multiplication, impairment of host defenses, and consequent spread of the organisms. Toxigenicity is the ability of organisms to produce toxic substances that cause cytotoxic effects or interfere with the host's metabolic activity at sites either adjacent to the invading organism or remote from the lesion. However, toxigenicity is difficult to separate from invasiveness. Invasiveness may require factors of short-range toxicity, whereas toxicity requires at least some degree of bacterial proliferation. Together, they are two of the most important attributes of virulence.

Invasiveness

GROWTH AND MULTIPLICATION. The multiplication of organisms either on the epithelial surface or within the tissue depends on the ability to satisfy their biochemical and biophysical needs and to evade, resist, or suppress host defenses. Microorganisms require nutrients in order to multiply and carry out metabolic function. Often, these nutrients are identical to those required by the host cell. Therefore, as a result of continued growth, the organism often will compete with the cell for needed nutrients. For example, *Chlamydia psittaci,* the causative organism of psittacosis, will compete with the host cell for isoleucine and will not grow where this amino acid is limiting. Some pathogens exhibit a nutritional specificity; that is, they will only grow and multiply in tissue that supplies the specific ingredient to support growth. *Brucella abortus* requires the sugar alcohol erythritol found in the placenta of cows. As a result, the placenta becomes a target for the organism, leading to abortion in infected cows. Many organisms require iron in order to express their virulence. Iron in host tissues is not free but complexed by iron-binding host proteins called siderophores. Pathogens possess their own siderophores, which enable them to sequester iron from iron-binding proteins.

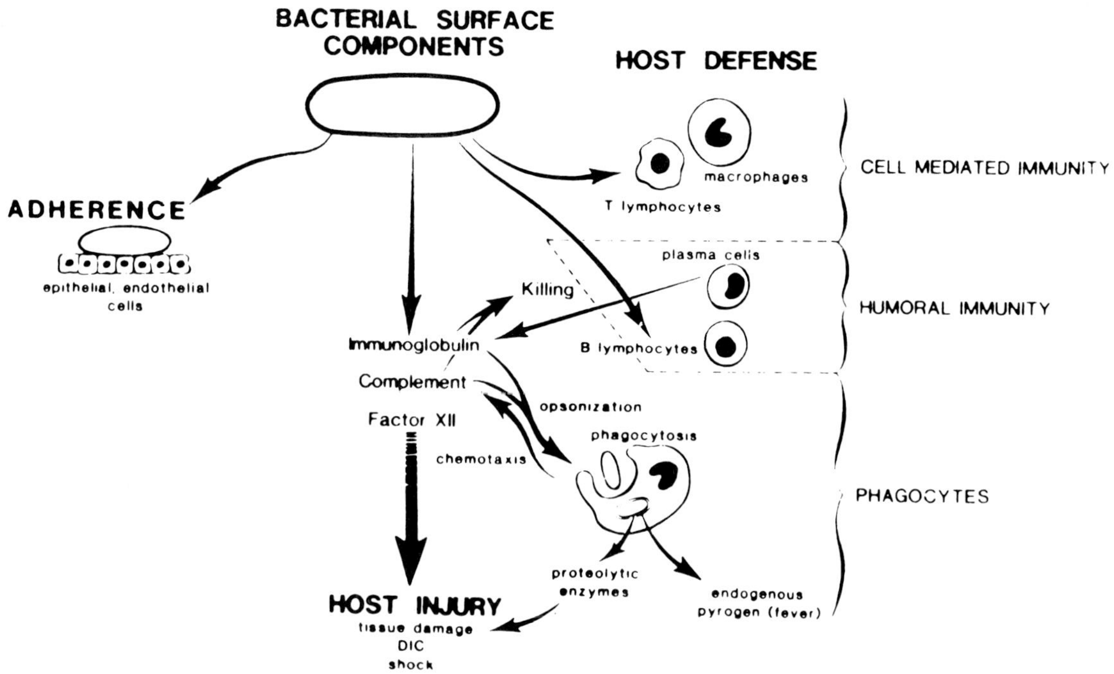

Figure 9–2. Influence of bacterial surface components on host response and the initiation of infection. *(Modified from Peterson PK, Quie D.* Annu Rev Med. *1981;32:29.)*

Iron can enhance virulence by abolishing the bactericidal action of serum as well as by reducing the lethal dose of many organisms. The best known of the iron-sequestering systems, enterochelin or enterobactin, is found in the genera *Salmonella, Klebsiella,* and *Escherichia.* Multiplication also results in the production and release of a number of extracellular enzymes that break down physical barriers, impair host defenses, or produce conditions more conducive to assimilation of growth factors.

Surface structures containing lipopolysaccharide in certain gram-negative organisms facilitate the invasive process by inhibition of the bactericidal mechanisms of phagocytosis. It should be noted that endotoxin (lipopolysaccharide) also has a stimulatory effect on phagocytosis via complement-mediated opsonization. This will be discussed in the section on Non-Specific factors, under Complement. The outer cell membrane acts as a barrier to soluble antibacterial factors, such as complement, resulting in resistance to phagocytosis for some gram-negative organisms. Another surface structure that enhances invasiveness is the flagella of gram-negative organisms, which mediate motility.

SPREAD. Another factor related to invasiveness is the pattern of spread through the body. Spread of the organism may occur on the surface before invasion of the epithelial tissue, or it may penetrate the membrane barriers by a variety of schemes before establishing systemic infection. The microorganisms may spread directly, but extension of the infection is usually localized in nature. Direct spread of the organism can be facilitated by surfaces that are covered with fluid, such as epithelial surfaces or in the intestine because of continuous flow of the intestinal contents. Direct spread also may occur as a result of enzymatic action of microorganisms. An example of this is the streptococcal hyaluronidases that hydrolyze the hyaluronic acid component of connective tissue and collagenases produced by *Bacteroides,* which are important in the destructive action of periodontal disease. Additional patterns of spread may occur via the lymphatic system or the blood. Many microorganisms are filtered out and inactivated in lymph nodes, but some viruses and rickettsia that can survive this defense can multiply in the lymph nodes, with consequent dissemination throughout the body.

The most efficient method of spreading microbes throughout the body is the blood. Many microorganisms invade the bloodstream in small numbers but are of little importance, usually being removed by the reticuloendothelial system. However, if susceptible tissue is colonized by these microorganisms, serious consequences can occur. A prime example of this may occur following rheumatic fever, in which heart tissue is injured. The scarified tissue is very susceptible to infection by blood-borne organisms. Transient bacteremias caused by dental extractions or prophylaxis can serve as the source of these infections. A more thorough discussion of this phenomenon is presented in Chapter 11. Rapid multiplication and consequent spread of certain bacterial or fungal pathogens in the bloodstream may occur. This is called septicemia and may result in the release of toxic substances, with resultant severe disease. Since viruses and rickettsia do not release toxins, they may multiply in blood for some time before producing clinical manifestations. Bacteremias result from the transitory presence of a bacterium in the blood, followed by removal from the vascular system without harmful effects. Other pathways of spread include the cerebrospinal fluid, the peritoneal cavity, and the nerves. Selected examples of patterns of spread are shown in Table 9–2.

TABLE 9–2. MICROBIAL INFECTIONS AND PATTERNS OF SPREAD

Pattern of Spread	Selected Examples of Microbe or Disease	Target System
Epithelial surface	Influenza	Respiratory tract
	Shigella sp.	Intestinal tract
	Neisseria gonorrhoeae	Urogenital tract
Microbial factors	*Streptococcus pyogenes* (hyaluronidase)	Skin
Lymphatic system	Rubella	Skin
	Mumps	Respiratory tract
Blood		
Leukocytes	Leptospirosis	Liver and kidneys
	Herpes simplex	Respiratory and central nervous system
Erythrocytes	Malaria	Liver, erythrocytes
Plasma	Poliomyelitis	Central nervous system
	Streptococcus pneumoniae	Respiratory tract
	Rickettsia	Skin, liver, spleen
Reticuloendothelial system	Brucellosis	Liver, spleen, bone marrow, placenta (cattle)
	Typhoid fever	blood, intestinal tract, lymphoid tissue
	Tuberculosis	Liver, spleen, skin, lungs
Cerebrospinal fluid	*Haemophilus influenzae*	Respiratory tract
	Cryptococcus neoformans	Respiratory tract
	Mumps	Respiratory tract
Pleural and peritoneal cavities	Abdominal bacteria and viruses	Lymphatic system
	Lung infections	Reticuloendothelial system
Peripheral nerves	Rabies	Central nervous system
	Herpes simplex	Central nervous system
	Tetanus toxin	Central nervous system

DEPRESSION OF HOST DEFENSE MECHANISMS Depression of host defense mechanisms by structural components of microbes or as a result of microbial activity can occur through a myriad of mechanisms. Perhaps the most important factors critical to survival of the organism are those that interfere with the various mechanisms leading up to and including the phagocytic process. The phagocytic process will be discussed in more detail in the section on Nonspecific Factors. The sensitive phases of the process include prevention of mobilization of phagocytes (chemotaxis), prevention of contact with the phagocytes, and interference with ingestion. The last phase of the phagocytic process can be inhibited by prevention of intracellular destruction of cells.

A number of microorganisms are capable of producing an immunosuppressive response in the host that is unrelated to the infecting organism; for example, measles virus will temporarily reduce reactivity to the tuberculin skin test. Other organisms that produce a generalized immunosuppressive effect resulting in decreased immune response include cytomegalovirus, human immunodeficiency virus (HIV), and the malarial parasite. Most of the organisms that cause generalized immunodeficiency are capable of multiplication within macrophages or lymphoid tissue. The exact mechanism of suppression is uncertain but appears to interfere with the immune functions of macrophages.

In addition to generalized immunosuppression, a number of microorganisms, primarily viruses, are capable of antigen-specific suppression in response to the infecting organism itself. Thus, the organism is able to promote its own virulence properties or factors by suppressing host defense systems. *Actinobacillus actinomycetemcomitans*, an organism associated with juvenile periodontitis, has been shown to inhibit the immune function of human lymphocytes. The immunosuppressive factors produced by this organism may play a role in suppressing immune responses not only to itself but also to other organisms involved in the pathogenesis of periodontal disease. Interference with humoral defenses is a characteristic of virulent strains of many species, including *Bacillus anthracis*, *Staphylococcus aureus*, and the Enterobacteriaceae. Siderophores are an example of this mechanism, which enables the organism to withstand the antimicrobial effect of serum. Other examples of this type include the poly-D-glutamic acid of *B. anthracis*, which interferes with the lytic action of antibody and complement.

Direct effect on host defense systems is still another mechanism by which such systems are affected. Examples of these include IgA protease, which inactivates immunoglobulin A and staphylococcal leukocidin, and toxins of *A. actinomycetem-*

comitans, which will kill PMNs directly. Some compounds, for example, staphylococcal peptidoglycan, can reduce the effectiveness of chemotaxis. Another immunologically mediated reaction that may be affected is the release of mediators as the result of inflammation. There may be pressure damage as a result of production of clots and swelling. Physical damage can occur by nonimmunologic means also because of multiplication of microorganisms to extremely high numbers, with resultant blockage of vessels.

ALTERATION OF THE BIOCHEMICAL BEHAVIOR OF THE CELL. The final mechanism that involves properties relating to invasiveness is best exemplified by viruses. In the case of a typical viral infection, the organism can enter the cell and alter the biochemical behavior of the cell to make replicas of itself. Damage to the cell may occur by interference with macromolecular synthesis or cell membrane function. More complete discussions of these phenomena are found in Chapters 24 through 31.

Production of Toxins. The second broad mechanism for damaging the host may occur when the microorganism produces a substance or conditions that directly interfere with the physiology of host cells. These toxic compounds are produced as a result of bacterial multiplication, yet do not appear to possess any function in bacterial metabolism. Toxins may be divided into two broad categories with distinct properties—exotoxins and endotoxins.

EXOTOXINS. Exotoxins are extracellular proteins synthesized and secreted by actively growing bacteria, for example, *Vibrio cholerae, Corynebacterium diphtheriae,* and *Clostridium botulinum.* These toxic substances may produce cytotoxic effects at sites remote from the site of bacterial invasion. For example, in diphtheria, the primary lesion may be in the oropharynx, but the toxin exerts its lethal effects when it spreads to other tissues, such as the heart.

The molecular action of these toxins is still being elucidated. A number of these toxins, elaborated by different organisms, enzymatically catalyze the transfer of the ADP ribosly moiety from NAD to linkage with elongation factor 2 (EF-2). This interaction inactivates EF-2 and prevents ribosomal translocation along mRNA, thus inhibiting the elongation step in polypeptide synthesis. Other ADP ribosylating toxins produced by the etiologic agents of cholera and whooping cough stimulate or activate the adenylcyclase or guanylcyclase arm, resulting in alteration of ion transport at the mucosal surface. A summary of the mechanism of some of the best understood toxins are shown in Table 9–3.

The protein nature of these substances renders them easily denatured by heat or proteolytic enzymes. Exotoxins are excellent antigens that induce the formation of toxin-neutralizing antibodies. Early microbiologists noted that formaldehyde would inactivate the toxic portion of the molecule without affecting its antigenicity. Formaldehyde-treated toxins (toxoids) are used as vaccines against diseases, such as diphtheria and tetanus, in which toxins are the primary virulence factor. Bacterial exotoxins are among the most potent poisons known, and they exhibit specific pharmacologic manifestations on certain organ sites.

In some cases, for example, enterotoxins and neurotoxins, the compounds are clearly responsible for the main pathogenic features of a disease. The toxin of *V. cholerae* is an example of the former. Some toxins formed outside the body and ingested with various foods cause thousands of cases of food poisoning annually. These intoxications most commonly are caused by *Bacillus cereus,* and *Clostridium perfringens.* Although less common, the deadliest intoxication by far is caused by the neurotoxin of *C. botulinum.* It has been calculated that a few ounces of crystalline botulinum toxin would kill the entire population of the world.

Cytolytic toxins, for example, the streptolysins produced by streptococci and some of the staphylococcal hemolysins, can be divided into two groups depending on whether or not they are activated by thiol compounds. Some of the nonthiol-activated toxins, such as staphylococcal α-toxin and *Pseudomonas* leukocidins, are capable of damaging susceptible cell membranes without causing cell death. This suggests a role of these toxins in the multiplication and dissemination of the pathogens as a result of initial permeability changes and production of lesions in the cell membrane. The thiol-activated toxins are produced by many gram-positive organisms, and it has been suggested that the toxin in the reduced state interacts with cholesterol in the cell membrane, leading to cell disruption and lysis. Other properties common to this group of toxins include cardiotoxicity, antigenic relatedness giving rise to precipitating and neutralizing antibodies. The biologic effect of these toxins can be lost by oxidation with sulfhydryl reagents and regained by reduction with thiols or other reducing agents.

ENDOTOXINS. Endotoxins are complex lipopolysaccharide molecules residing in the outer membrane of gram-negative bacteria, for example, *Neisseria, Salmonella,* and *Shigella.* They differ from exotoxins in that they remain a part of the cell structure until death and disintegration of the bacterium. An exception to this is the release of endotoxin from outer membrane vesi-

TABLE 9–3. MODE OF ACTION AND BIOLOGIC EFFECTS OF SELECTED BACTERIAL EXOTOXINS

Toxin	Organism	Mode of Action	Biologic Effect
Diphtheria toxin	*Corynebacterium*	ADP ribosylation of EF-2[a]	Damage to heart (cardiac arrest), lungs, liver, kidneys
Exotoxin A	*Pseudomonas aeruginosa*	ADP ribosylation of EF-2 Antigenically distinct toxin from diphtheria toxin	Dermatonecrosis, ocular damage, interference with cellular immune function
Enterotoxin	*Clostridium difficile*	ADP ribosylation of cellular protein	Pseudomembranous colitis following antimicrobial therapy
Pertussis toxin	*Bordetella pertussis*	ADP ribosylation of guanyl nucleotide-binding protein blocks hormonal inhibition of adenylcyclase	Hypoglycemia, regulates adenylcyclase
Cholera enterotoxin	*Vibrio cholerae*	Subunit A stimulation of adenylate cyclase, which alters ion transport at mucosal surface	Acute diarrhea
Heat-stable enterotoxin	*Escherichia coli*	Activates guanylate cyclase	Acute diarrhea
α-Toxin	*Clostridium perfringens*	Ca^{2+}-dependent phospholipase C damages cell membrane	Gas gangrene, intravascular hemolysis, food poisoning (diarrhea)
Streptolysin O	*Streptococcus*	Thiol-activated membrane damage, binds to cholesterol, leading to permeability changes	Cardiotoxin inhibits chemotaxis of neutrophils degranulation of leukocytes
Leukocidin	*Staphylococcus*	Interaction with triphosphoinositate(?), changes in cation permeability, ie, K^+ efflux, influx of Ca^{2+}, nucleotides, etc	Cytotoxin for PMNs and macrophages
Leukotoxin	*Actinobacillus actinomycetecomitans*	Unknown	Leukotoxic
Legionaella proteolytic toxin	*Legionella pneumophila*	Unknown	Cytotoxic, proteolytic, dermonecrotic
Botulinum toxin	*Clostridium botulinum*	Blockage of acetylcholine release	Flaccid paralysis, breathing and swallowing difficulty

[a]EF-2, elongation factor 2.

cles of *A. actinomycetemcomitans* and *Bacteroides gingivalis* during growth.

In addition, the lipopolysaccharide component is heat stable and cannot be converted to toxoid. The lipopolysaccharide of gram-negative bacteria consists of three components, a core polysaccharide present in most gram-negative organisms, an O-specific polysaccharide, which is responsible for serologic activity and specificity, and lipid A, which is responsible for the toxic manifestations of the compound. A schematic diagram of a lipopolysaccharide is shown in Figure 9–3.

In contrast to the specific effects of exotoxins, endotoxin affects almost every organ in the body. The most important of these are the liver and the immunologic systems. The effects may be beneficial or adverse. Included among the metabolic activities of liver that are adversely affected are depletion of carbohydrate reserves, selective inhibition of enzyme induction, and inhibition of gluconeogenesis. Beneficial effects include the immunologic responses in experimental animals, such as nonspecific polyclonal activation of lymphocytes, mitogenicity, and adjuvant activity.

Endotoxins act initially on a number of primary target cells, including the macrophages, granulocytes, B lymphocytes, and fibroblasts. Frequently, the primary cells release soluble mediators or effectors

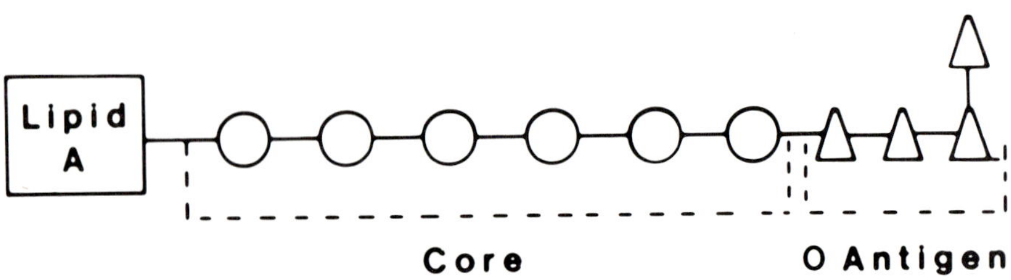

Figure 9–3. Structure of gram-negative cell wall lipopolysaccharide.

TABLE 9–4. SOME BIOLOGIC EFFECTS OF ENDOTOXINS

Adverse Effects	Beneficial Effects
Hypotension	Induction of tumor necrosis
Shock	Adjuvant
Lethality	Radiation protection
Pyrogenicity	
Generalized or local Shwartzman reaction	
Leukopenia	
Leukocytosis	
Disseminated intravascular coagulation	
Activation of complement via alternative pathway	

that activate secondary systems. Included among these factors are lymphocyte-activating factors, prostaglandins, and endogenous pyrogens. Mouse peritoneal macrophages activated in vitro by lipopolysaccharide have the capability of destroying tumorigenic cells by a cytotoxic mechanism. The combinations of effects on the primary and secondary targets extend and diversify the numerous biologic effects of endotoxins. Some of the chief effects are shown in Table 9–4. Two of the most important effects are pyrogenicity and shock. In the case of pyrogenicity, the endotoxin is phagocytized, causing the phagocyte to produce fever-producing substances termed pyrogens. Endotoxemia perturbs capillary permeability, with consequent circulatory changes and rapidly decreasing blood pressure, resulting in endotoxin shock. These changes are mediated by the release of vasoactive substances, for example, histamine and serotonin from platelets, as well as other interactions between lipopolysaccharides and platelets. Endotoxins are also involved in a type of host reaction known as the Shwartzman reaction, which results in increased sensitivity to microbial products. Endotoxins from gram-negative bacteria may initially prime and later trigger a generalized reaction, which results in intravascular clotting, that is, glomerular capillary thrombosis.

Biologic effects of endotoxin related to periodontal disease include a direct effect, by amplification of the inflammatory process, or indirectly by periodontopathogens, that is, *Bacteroides gingivalis, B. melaninogenicus,* whose endotoxins stimulate the alternative pathway of complement.

HOST RESISTANCE

The first part of this chapter concentrated on the properties and functions of the microbial portion of the dynamic host–parasite relationship. This part considers the various mechanisms of host defenses. Host defenses can be subdivided into specific and nonspecific types. Specific mechanisms of host defense involve induction of an immune response and the efficiency of the antibodies to effect protection against the invading microorganisms or bacterial toxins. These factors react only with the specific antigens of the organism that caused their production. An individual is not born with these factors. They are acquired throughout life as a result of exposure to microorganisms. Specific resistance also may be called acquired resistance. Nonspecific resistance acts against a broad spectrum of microorganisms and, in most cases, is present at birth, that is, innate resistance. Blood, secretions, for example, saliva, colostrum in milk, and gastrointestinal fluids, and phagocytic cells contain antibacterial substances, such as lysozyme, lactoferrin, and peroxidase-thiocyanate-H_2O_2 systems, that are examples of nonspecific host defense factors.

Constitutive Variables

In addition to the various nonspecific host factors, host defense is governed by a number of constitutive variables that occur in the normal individual. The mechanisms of these variables are starting to be defined only now. Included among these constitutive factors are the genetic constitution, age, and sex of the host, as well as the general physiologic state of the body. The genetic constitution of the host plays a prominent role and, many times, the critical role in determining susceptibility to infectious disease. An example of the influence of genetics at the molecular level can be demonstrated in those individuals with sickle cell trait who show an increased resistance to falciparum malaria. A simple gene in these individuals results in modification of the hemoglobin molecule by substituting one amino acid for another, thus resulting in a distortion of the cell into a sickle form when oxygen tension decreases.

Genetic susceptibility to infectious disease operates at the species, race, familial, and individual levels. Recent evidence has demonstrated the genetic control of the immune response as a factor in innate resistance. A strong genetic influence in the etiology of dental caries has been shown in human and animal experiments. Age is another important factor influencing innate host resistance. Susceptibility to specific disease may vary as a function of age, with the very young and the very old showing the least resistance. Immunologic immaturity plays a central role in the very young, whereas gradual decline in immunologic function occurs in adults over 40. Dental caries is primarily a disease of children, indicating that the tooth is more resistant in older individuals. Sex-related susceptibility to infectious diseases occurs, but little is known about the mechanisms involved. Steroid hormones elaborated during pregnancy appear to play a role in significantly increasing gingivitis as a result of changes in subgingival microflora. Physiologic factors, for example, the nutritional state, fatigue, metabolic diseases such as diabetes, and the role of hormones in maintaining homeostasis, also have effects on host susceptibility. Malnutrition inevitably predisposes to many microbial diseases, usually by interfering with various barrier mechanisms and both humoral and cell-mediated immunologic responses. The hormones most influential in regulating susceptibility are the corticosteroid hormones, which inhibit the inflammatory response. Still another physiologic response that may modulate host defense is fever. Fever usually is associated with increased resistance to infection in both bacterial and viral diseases. Among the fever-generating reactions or compounds are cell-mediated immune and humoral responses to infection, as well as specific bacterial products, for example, endotoxin. The specific mechanisms relating to the modulation of host defense systems by fever are unknown at this time.

Nonspecific Factors Governing Host Defense

Anatomic Barriers. A number of physical barriers of the host constitute the first line of defense against invading microorganisms. Included among these are the unbroken surface of the epithelium, as well as mucous membranes, enamel, and dentin (or cementum). The mucus present in nasal passages, sinuses, and the oropharyngeal region serves the dual function of a physical barrier as well as participating in the hydrodynamic action resulting from the ciliary activity. The normal flora of the various body surfaces serves a dual role as a barrier to the colonization of pathogens as well as depriving the pathogens of essential nutrients. Enamel and dentin, although effective as barriers, can be compromised by dental caries and dental instrumentation.

Antimicrobial Factors. A number of nonspecific host defense factors in body fluids possess antimicrobial properties that regulate the virulence of pathogens in concert with the various humoral and cell-mediated immune systems. Unsaturated fatty acids, for example, oleic acid, that are present in sebaceous secretions are bactericidal to many organisms. Lactic acid from sweat glands lowers the pH, providing an additional defense system.

Mucosal secretions and body fluids produce a variety of nonspecific inhibitory substances, lysozyme, lactoferrin, and peroxidase. Lysozyme is found in such fluids as tears and saliva. The antimicrobial factors present in saliva not only play a critical role in host defenses but also play a role in regulating the microbial ecology of the oral cavity. Lysozyme (present in high concentrations in saliva) is a low molecular weight protein that acts as a muramidase and attacks the peptidoglycan backbone of gram-positive bacteria. Lysozyme is also present in gingival crevice fluid and polymorphonuclear leukocytes. Lysozyme participates in a number of other host defense systems, including the lysing of gram-negative bacteria in the presence of IgA and complement, the disruption of cell membrane, and stimulation of phagocytosis.

Lactoferrin is an antimicrobial compound present in a number of body fluids, including plasma, mammalian milk, and whole parotid and submandibular saliva. Whole salivary lactoferrin originates from polymorphonuclear leukocytes in crevicular fluid. Concentrations of lactoferrin in saliva increase sharply during inflammation of the oral mucosa. Lactoferrin also functions in cellular defense mechanisms through its iron-binding properties. It is a major component of polymorphonuclear leukocytes, where it is involved in H_2O_2-dependent and independent antimicrobial action. It also promotes adherence and aggregation of PMNs on endothelial surfaces, thus amplifying the inflammatory response.

The salivary peroxidase system has multiple functions, including protecting the host from toxic accumulation of H_2O_2, generating antimicrobial products that regulate oral ecology by inhibition of growth, respiration, and metabolism, and inactivating carcinogenic and mutagenic compounds. The enzyme is part of a complex system involving thiocyanate, hypothiocyanate ions, halides, and H_2O_2. This system catalyzes the oxidation of thiocyanate ion (derived from diet) by H_2O_2 to hypothiocyanate and water. Thus, the system involves the generation of antimicrobial thiocyanate derivatives, as well as the protection of the host from toxic accumulations of H_2O_2. A diagram of the reactions is shown in Fig 9–4. Any microbial effect takes place by a number of modes of action, including halogenation of microbial protein and oxidation of sulfhydryl groups present in bacterial enzymes. Salivary peroxidase is derived from salivary gland secretions plus a contribution from leukocytes.

Additional salivary host defense factors include cationic proteins, which have both antibacterial and antifungal effects. Investigators have shown that these histidine-rich polypeptides can be either growth-inhibitory or cidal. Another cationic protein, which is found primarily in serum but also in saliva, is β-lysin, which is bactericidal against gram-positive bacteria and functions by disrupting cytoplasmic membrane function. These antimicrobial compounds are heat-stable components of serum derived primarily from platelets.

Complement. The heat-labile bactericidal activity of serum toward gram-negative bacteria has been

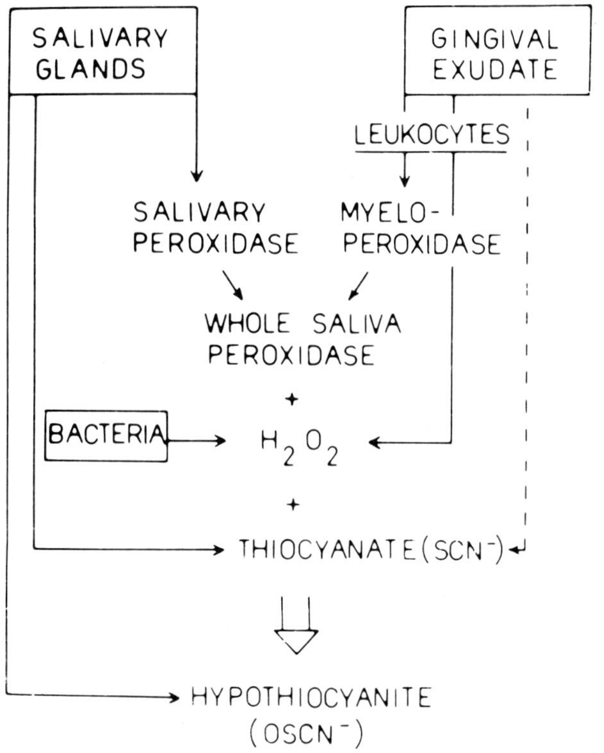

Figure 9–4. Components of the human salivary peroxidase system and their origins. *(From Tenouvo J, Pruitt KY.* J Oral Pathol. *1984;13:573.*

known for almost a century. This complex system of at least nine proteins functions by mediating and amplifying immune reactions. The initial enzymatic component is activated by binding to an antigen–antibody complex. This complex, in turn, acts on others in sequence to form large amounts of the next component. This series of reactions continues, producing a cascade reaction with a generation of high numbers of the later components of the complement system. The result of these series of reactions is amplification of the various biologic activities. This series of reactions, known as the classic pathway, attacks gram-negative bacteria and envelope viruses by causing membrane damage by action of a phospholipase. The binding of complement to immune complexes on the surface of red blood cells with resultant lysis is also the basis of complement-fixation tests discussed in Chapter 6. An alternative pathway for mediation of complement action takes place when complement reacts directly with endotoxin or bacterial capsular polysaccharide in the absence of antibody, resulting in the activation of the C3 component. The result of these steps is to promote phagocytosis via opsonization because phagocytes have receptors for complement component C3b. Complement-mediated opsonization via the alternative pathway is not as efficient as antibody-mediated complement opsonization via the classic route. In the latter case, the complement reacts with antibody attached to microorganisms, providing additional receptor sites for phagocytes. The net result is increased opsonization due to the increased number of C3 molecules produced by the cascade reaction acting in concert with the antibody. Other antimicrobial activities of complement include inhibition of attachment of virus to susceptible cells and generation of inflammatory and chemotactic factors that attract antimicrobial serum components and phagocytize at the site of infection.

Inflammation. The prime purpose of the inflammatory response is to concentrate all the circulating antimicrobial factors at the site of infection, thus playing a critical role in the outcome of the infection. Included among these are the polymorphonuclear leukocytes, macrophages and lymphocytes, as well as other components, including nonspecific factors, antibody, and complement. Increased blood supply and temperature also promote leukocyte activity. Inflammatory responses can be initiated by microorganisms in several ways. The response may have a protective effect as a result of the mobilization of leukocytes. On the other hand, if excess leukocytes migrate into the area and become activated by microorganisms, damage of surrounding tissue will occur.

A second method of initiating an inflammatory response is by production of proteases, which have the property of cleaving various complement components. Finally, bacterial products can trigger mediation systems, which may result in changes in vasopermeability and coagulation.

Immune Response to Infection. The outcome of an invasive infection will be determined in part by the ability of the host to elicit an immune response to surface virulence components of the bacterium. The antibody formed stimulates opsonization by complement component C3b and by macrophages and polymorphonuclear leukocytes. This is the usual course for successful outcome of an acute infection. In the case of chronic bacterial infection, for example, tuberculosis and periodontal disease, the outcome is more closely aligned toward cell-mediated immunity. In the case of intoxication, unless existing endotoxin is circulating, the normal course of disease will occur because the small amount of endotoxin required to produce a disease does not represent enough antigen for the host to elicit an effective immune response. A more detailed explanation of these phenomena is given in Chapters 6, 7, and 8.

Phagocytosis. The role of phagocytic cells in the protection of the host against infectious agents is perhaps the most critical component of the nonspecific host defense system. The prime functions of phagocytes are to ingest, kill, and digest invading microorganisms. The degree to which they carry out this role will determine the outcome of the course of the infection. In addition to microorganisms, phagocytes destroy damaged and foreign cells and connective tissues and eosinophils.

Phagocytes include neutrophils, eosinophils, and monocyte-macrophages. The polymorphonuclear neutrophil is smaller than the macrophage and is a nondividing, short-lived cell with granules called lysosomes, which contain a wide range of bactericidal factors and hydrolytic enzymes. It is the most abundant phagocyte in the bloodstream. Macrophages are derived from bone marrow as promonocytes, which differentiate to monocytes and then become mature macrophages. Lysosomal enzymes contained in macrophages are synthesized continuously, resulting in higher concentrations of hydrolytic enzymes in mature macrophages than at the initiation of the differentiation process of the monocyte into a macrophage. Macrophages also are present in connective tissue and are concentrated particularly in the lung, liver, and lining of the sinuses of the spleen, as well as the lymph nodes. Wandering macrophages are present in the peritoneal cavity. They are long-lived with rough-surfaced endoplasmic reticulum and mitochondria. The neutrophils act primarily against pyogenic organisms, whereas the macrophages are especially significant in the protection against intracellular bacteria, protozoa, and viruses. Eosinophils limit the extent of the immune reactions and phagocytize immune complexes. Eosinophilic granules contain blockers of inflammatory mediators, for example, histamine, in addition to hydrolytic enzymes.

The phagocytic process is preceded by direct migration of the phagocytic cell toward the focus of infection by a process called chemotaxis. This migration involves a unidirectional movement toward the highest concentration (ie, source) of various agents known as chemotactic factors. Some chemotactic agents exert their effect on cells directly, whereas others induce formation of chemotactic factors in plasma or other tissue fluids. Those that exert a direct effect are water-soluble, diffusible substances that are either protein or polypeptide in nature. Agents that induce formation of chemotactic agents indirectly often are particulate and may include proteins, polysaccharides, lipids, or small molecules, for example, guanosine. The chief mechanism by which microorganisms generate chemotactic factors is the result of the activation of serum complement. This may occur by the classic or alternate pathway. Chemotactic factors may be released during the phagocytic process, resulting in the attraction of additional cells.

After the phagocyte reaches the microorganism, a series of steps occurs. These include the adherence of the microorganism to the phagocyte plasma membrane, ingestion into a vacuole in the cytoplasm of the phagocyte, fusion of the lysosomes to form a phagosome, degranulation, and destruction of the organism by a variety of bactericidal mechanisms.

Phagocytes exercise a high degree of selectivity in recognition of the type cells that they will attack. They ingest damaged and aged host and bacterial cells but not healthy ones. Similarly, unencapsulated cells will be engulfed, but closely related encapsulated organisms will be avoided. The process of recognition has been demonstrated many times to involve surface phenomena. Recognition and subsequent ingestion are mediated by a process called opsonization, which enhances the phagocytosis. Opsonins, such as immunoglobulins (IgG) and complement, may coat an organism and facilitate ingestion by several mechanisms. Antibody may act as an opsonin by itself, or antigen–antibody reactions may mediate activation via the classic pathway of complement. Immunoglobulins may activate complement via the alternative pathway in the opsonic process. Evidence has shown that receptor molecules on the phagocyte recognize and interact with specific molecular configurations on the Fc portion of immunoglobulins and the part of the C3 component of complement that binds to the cell. This facilitates attachment of the coated bacteria. Receptor-mediated phagocytosis appears to have at least two major functions. First, the macrophages have the property of tightly sealing off a closed compartment between them and their opsonized targets. The enclosed area is useful in concentrating and protecting antimicrobial substances secreted by the phagocyte. Second, macrophages can regulate the phagocytosis-promoting capacity of their C3 receptors. This provides a mechanism of activating C3 receptors at the site of infection. Binding of the receptor on the phagocyte to the ligand on the bacterial cell cannot occur if the C3 component is in an inactive state, and, consequently, phagocytosis will not be promoted.

Adherence usually is followed by the process of ingestion. The microorganisms initially are enclosed in membrane-lined cytoplasmic vacuoles that invaginate to form a phagosome. As a result of the ingestion process, the phagosome containing the ingested microorganism fuses with lysosomal granules, which results in release of the lysosomal contents via a process called degranulation. The net result of these actions is the basis of both the oxygen-dependent microbicidal reactions called the respiratory burst and the oxygen-independent microbicidal reactions that result from the release of cationic proteins and a series of hydrolytic enzymes from the lysosomal particle.

Oxygen-Dependent Reactions. In the oxygen-dependent series of reactions, membrane-bound oxidase catalyzes the reactions, which initially accounts for oxygen consumption and production of superoxide anion. Superoxide dismutase then catalyzes the breakdown of the superoxide anion to form H_2O_2 and O_2, as shown.

$$\text{Reaction 1.}\quad 2\,O_2 + 2\,\text{NADPH} \xrightarrow{\text{NADPH oxidase}} 2\,H^+\ 2\,\text{NADP} + 2\,O^{-2}\ \text{(superoxide ion)}$$

$$\text{Reaction 2.}\quad 2\,O^{2-} + 2\,H^+ \xrightarrow{\text{superoxide dismutase}} H_2O_2 + O_2$$

The net result of these reactions results in increased glycolysis via the hexose monophosphate shunt and increases in molecular oxygen and H_2O_2. The increase in hexose monophosphate activity results from increasing availability of NADP derived from reaction 1 (above) and the formation of the reduced form of glutathione by a peroxidase. The reduced form of glutathione also functions as a detoxification mechanism by breaking down H_2O_2.

Another oxygen-dependent system is the myeloperoxidase system of the polymorphonuclear neutrophils (PMN). Myeloperoxidase (MPO) is released from the vacuole when the phagosome fuses with lysosomes or granules. The halogenation of bacterial proteins by H_2O_2 by myeloperoxidase-catalyzed reactions in the presence of halide (derived from the PMN) produces an antimicrobial effect.

$$\text{Bacteria} + 2\,H_2O_2 + \text{halide} \xrightarrow{\text{Myeloperoxidase}} \text{Bacteria–halide} + 2\,H_2O + O_2$$

This provides another pathway for detoxification of hydrogen peroxide in addition to the oxidation of glutathione. Thus, two of the most important oxygen-dependent microbicidal systems can be either myeloperoxidase-dependent or myeloperoxidase-independent. Other oxygen-dependent systems involve generation of singlet oxygen, a reactive electronically excited form of O_2 and hydroxyl radical (OH). In summary, the three reactive forms of oxygen with antimicrobial properties generated during the respiratory burst are superoxide, singlet oxygen and hydroxyl radical (OH). These are supplemented by H_2O_2, whose antimicrobial activity can function directly, independent of the myeloperoxidase system or with the myeloperoxidase system in combination with protein halogenation. The production of these metabolites of oxygen by the phagocytes results in the death of the majority of the phagocytized organisms. A summary of these reactions is shown in Fig 9–5.

Oxygen-Independent Reactions. The process of degranulation results in an oxygen-independent series of events that release hydrolytic and digestive enzymes and compounds, such as lysozyme, lactoferrin, and cationic proteins, that have antimicrobial effects. Polymorphonuclear phagocytes possess two types of granules, primary and secondary, both of which possess compounds with digestive or microbicidal properties. Included among the substances released from the primary granule are hydrolytic enzymes, for example, RNAses, lipases, and esterases, as well as lysozyme, cationic proteins, and myeloperoxidase. The secondary or specific granules (unique to the specific cell) contain hydrolytic enzymes, such as acid and alkaline phosphatases and collagenases, as well as antimicrobial compounds, such as lactoferrin and lysozyme.

Although the macrophage has a number of mechanisms for disposing of extracellular parasites, a different set of circumstances arises when the macrophage encounters either facultative or obligate intracellular parasites. Facultative intracellular organisms, for example, *Mycobacterium tuberculosis* or various *Listeria* species, survive and proliferate in the phagocytes as well as in the extracellular environment. The obligate intracellular organisms, for example, *Chlamydia,* rickettsia, viruses, and certain protozoans, will survive and proliferate only within the intracellular environment. Survival of these organisms must take place through a variety of perturbation of intraphagocytic mechanisms.

Intracellular resistance is expressed only when the intracellular environment is modified, with resultant inhibition of survival and proliferation mechanisms. Examples of these, as well as extracellular mechanisms, are shown in Table 9–5. These changes are expressed through a number of mechanisms that result in nonspecific effects that not only control intracellular pathogens but also play a role in modulation of immunity and host resistance to other physiologic and pathologic stimuli.

Many examples of nonspecific cross-resistance between antigenically related and unrelated organisms exist. Nonspecific resistance to facultative intracellular bacteria, viruses, and fungi can be shown experimentally after infection with intracellular microbes. Infections with BCG (*bacille Calmette Guerin*), a strain of the tubercule bacillus used for vaccine purposes, can stimulate nonspecific resistance against a number of bacterial, viral, and fungal pathogens. The macrophage is the effector cell in the expression of this nonspecific resistance. Details regarding the activation of these macrophages and their relation to acquired cellular immunity are discussed in Chapters 7 and 8.

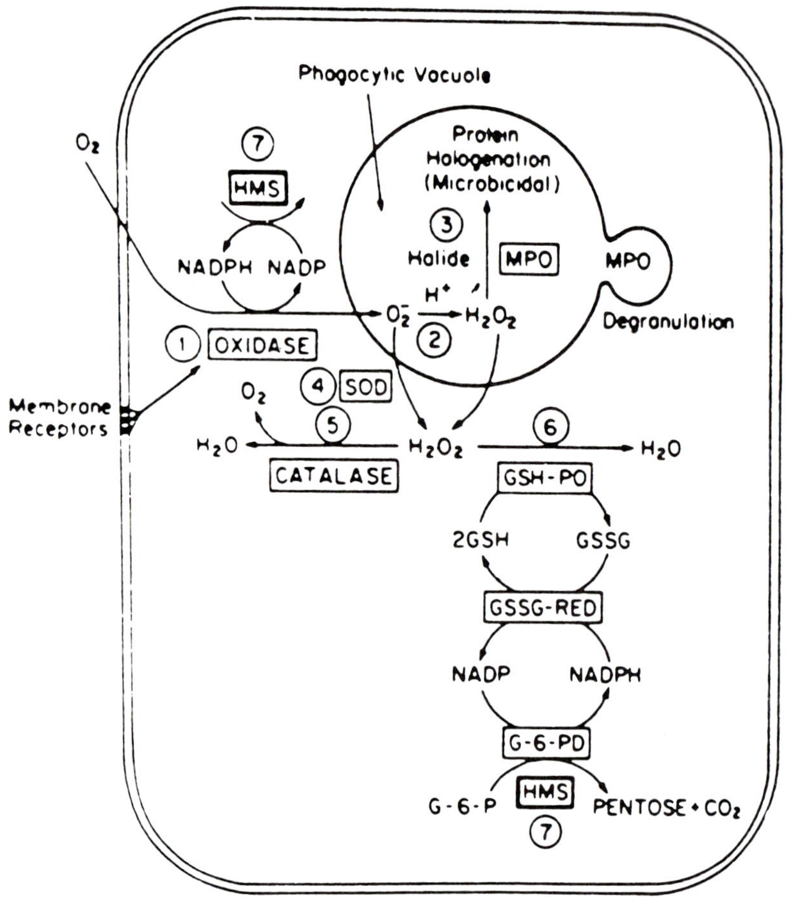

Figure 9–5. Events that occur during oxidative killing. HMS, hexose monophosphate shunt; MPO, myeloperoxidase; SOD, superoxide dismutase; GSO-PO, glutathione peroxidase; GSH, reduced glutathione; GSSG, oxidized glutathione; G-6PD, glucose 6-phosphate dehydrogenase; GG-P, glucose 6-phosphate. *(From Root RK. Antibacterial properties of polymorphonuclear leukocytes and their interactions with antibiotics. In Schlessinger D, ed.* Microbiology. *Washington, DC: American Society for Microbiology; 1981:177.)*

Phagocytic Defects. Although a number of phagocytic function defects occur, the one that has been studied most is chronic granulomatous disease (CGD). This disease is characterized biochemically by the absence of the events characterized by the respiratory burst and failure to generate peroxide. As a result, frequent recurrent infections occur despite high levels of specific circulating antibodies. CGD patients suffer from infections of lungs, spleen, liver, skin, and soft tissues with catalase-positive organisms, including staphylococci, aerobic gram-negative organisms, and opportunistic fungi. The significance of this is underscored in light of the fact that most microbes produce H_2O_2 but only some produce catalase to destroy H_2O_2. If a microbe does not make catalase, the cells of the CGD patient will use the microbial produced H_2O_2, via MPO to kill the organism. Deficiencies in MPO also occur but do not result in recurrent infections as frequently as CGD.

TABLE 9–5. SELECTED EXAMPLES OF PETURBATION OF PHAGOCYTIC DEFENSES BY MICROORGANISMS

Defense System Perturbed	Organism	Interfering Structure, Component, or Mechanism
Chemotaxis	*Pseudomonas aeruginosa*	Protease
Attachment	*Neisseria gonorrhoeae*	Antigenic heterogeneity of pili
Ingestion	*Streptococcus pneumoniae*	Polysaccharide capsule
	Streptococcus pyogenes	M protein
Microbiocidal Mechanisms		
Phagocytic oxidative response	*Legionella pneumophila*	Toxin
Lysosome–phagosome fusion	Influenza A	Depressed granulocyte function
Digestion	*Salmonella typhi murium*	Resistance to lysosomal enzymes

Effect of Antibiotics on the Host–Parasite Relationship. Recent evidence has demonstrated that antibiotics may mediate the host–parasite relationship. Studies have shown that penicillin, streptomycin, and ampicillin can alter the activity of both gram-positive and gram-negative bacteria to adhere to human epithelial cells. In addition, a number of antibiotics have been shown to increase T and B lymphocyte response. Others may alter the surface of serum-resistance gram-negative bacteria so that they may become more susceptible to lysis. Many investigations have been carried out on the interactions of antibiotics and phagocytes. The effect on chemotaxis can be either stimulatory or inhibitory, depending on the antibiotic used. Amphotericin B appears to inhibit both phagocytic and bactericidal functions, but none of the other antifungal agents have an effect. Penicillin, cephalosporins, erythromycin, and clindamycin enhance killing of antibiotic-altered bacteria by PMNs. On the other hand, aminoglycosides and tetracyclines have a depressant effect on the uptake of bacteria and fungi, but only at extremely high levels. Sulfa drugs appear to inhibit microbicidal activity. In general, studies demonstrate that most antibiotics improve killing activity of human PMNs against antibiotic-altered bacteria, but the clinical significance remains to be determined.

EPIDEMIOLOGY

Any discussion of the factors that govern host–parasite relationships and the variables that modulate their expression would be incomplete without at least a brief discussion of epidemiology. Epidemiology is the study of the factors that affect the distribution and determinants of diseases in populations. At one time, the study of epidemiology was directed primarily to understanding the factors that influence the transmission and distribution of infectious diseases in humans. The scope of epidemiology has expanded to include heart disease, cancer, and other metabolic or chronic diseases or nondisease states in humans using the same methods previously applied to infectious disease.

Because epidemiology is the study of the distribution of diseases in populations, a number of terms that deal with distribution must be differentiated. The morbidity rate is the number of cases per unit population during a given period of time (this is usually expressed per 100,000 population). This must be differentiated from the mortality rate, which is the number of deaths per unit population in a given period of time. The incidence is the measure of the rate in which new cases develop during a given period of time. It measures the probability that healthy people would develop disease during a specified period. On the other hand, prevalence is a measure of the probability of people having a disease at a given point in time and includes both new and old cases. Both incidence and prevalence rates are fundamental measures of morbidity.

The pattern of diseases in a population occurs with a particular frequency and may be referred to as endemic or epidemic. An endemic disease is one that is indigenous to a population; that is, it occurs in a given population at a fairly constant rate for a long period of time. In contrast, an epidemic occurs when a disease arises rapidly, proliferates, and infects a large number of people over a short period of time. Examples of this include the outbreak of Legionnaire's disease or the sudden occurrence of a large number of measles patients in a nursery. A pandemic is considered to be a worldwide epidemic.

The factors that control the rate of spread of the epidemic are those that are a function of the transmissibility of the organisms as well as the immunity of the population. The immunity of a group or community, known as herd immunity, is based on the relative number of immune and susceptible individuals in a population. It has been defined as the resistance of a group to invasion and spread of an infectious agent based on a high proportion of individual immune members of a group. Immune individuals act as a barrier to the spread of microorganisms from infected animals to susceptible animals. Herd immunity is an important factor governing the dynamics of epidemics and the periodicity of diseases.

Two of the most important variables in the spread of infectious disease in a population are the reservoirs of infection and the mechanisms of transmission. Reservoirs are the living organisms or inanimate matter that is the normal habitat of the infectious agent. The reservoir is the critical component of the cycle by which the microorganism perpetuates itself in nature. Examples of animate reservoirs include humans, other animals, and insects. Humans may be a reservoir of disease for other humans in the case of respiratory diseases, for example, influenza or diphtheria. Examples of animal diseases transmitted to humans include rabies, trichinosis, and brucellosis. Two of the best known of the insect-borne diseases transmitted to humans are malaria and yellow fever, in which the mosquito serves as a reservoir of infection. Inanimate reservoirs may be soil, water, or food.

The actual mechanisms of transmission of infectious agents may be direct or indirect. Direct transmission involves immediate transfer of a microorganism from an infected host or reservoir to another host. This can involve not only direct physical contact, as exemplified by sexually transmitted diseases, but also respiratory diseases, which can be transmitted by droplets through sneezing or coughing. Indirect transmission may be vehicle-borne, vector-borne, or airborne. Vehicle-born transmission involves indirect contact with inanimate objects known as fomites, which are contaminated with infectious agents. Vector-borne transmission is mediated by arthropods that may transmit the etiologic agent mechanically. In mechanical transmission, the arthropod is contaminated when feeding on blood and then contaminates the next host on which it feeds. A variation of this may occur if the infectious agent multiplies or undergos part of its cycle in the arthropod host before transmission. Transmission may be also airborne, involving either dust particles or droplet nuclei. Droplet nuclei are small particles that may be formed from the evaporation of droplets that have been projected in the air by coughing, sneezing, or talking. Droplet nuclei also may be formed by aerosolization of infective or other body fluids. The increased use of the high-speed drill generates both drops of salivary material and small aerosolized particles. Transmission of fungal spores in soil is another example of an airborne transmission by dust particles.

ORAL ASPECTS

The human oral cavity contains one of the most complex ecosystems in all of nature. This enormous concentration of microorganisms with their biochemical activities represent the major contributing factors to two of the world's most prevalent infectious diseases, dental caries and periodontal disease, as well as causing numerous systemic infections outside the oral cavity. Investigation of the dynamic host–parasite relationships that operate in regulating oral microbial ecology and their role in modulating oral and systemic disease has made much progress over the past 5 years. The best studied of the virulence factors are those produced by *A. actinomycetemcomitans.* This organism, which has been associated with juvenile periodontitis, produces a heat-labile leukotoxin that destroys human polymorphonuclear leukocytes and monocytes. It also produces a heat-labile lymphocyte suppression factor that inhibits lymphoid proliferation and antibody production. These factors have been postulated to affect local antibacterial defense mechanisms in the in vivo environment. Additional virulence factors produced by *A. actinomycetemcomitans* include large amounts of fatty acids and an endotoxin that is cytotoxic for murine peritoneal macrophages. Vibrios, fusiforms, *Veillonella,* and other gram-negative organisms also form potent endotoxins with high destructive potential for gingival tissue. The mechanisms of endotoxin damage to the periodontium may occur by activation of the complement system via the alternative pathway, which results in production of biologically active effector molecules. Direct action by macrophage can stimulate production and release of bacterial collagenase, as well as stimulation of calcium and proline release from bone. Collagenase of the black-pigmented *Bacteroides* may play a role in tissue destruction in mixed oral infections of the mucosa, periodontitis, and endodontic infections. Other hydrolytic enzymes produced by the *Bacteroides* that may be involved in tissue destruction are phospholipases, DNases, phosphatases, and hyaluronidase. Hyaluronidase has been shown to be produced by peptostreptococci associated with periodontal diseases. Other workers have shown that a number of microorganisms produce fibrinogenolytic and fibrinolytic enzymes that may be significant virulence factors in periodontal disease. Other virulence attributes of the *Bacteroides* include their ability to adhere to buccal and crevicular epithelial cells. Volatile sulfur compounds, such as hydrogen sulfide, may play a role in cytotoxicity.

The virulence factors of *S. mutans* in the etiology of dental caries have been described by many investigators. This includes the ability to adhere to hard surfaces mediated by the high molecular weight glucose polymers produced from sucrose and their ability to produce and withstand copious amounts of lactic acid. Lipoteichoic acid may be considered a virulence factor. It is involved in adherence of streptococci to buccal epithelial cells.

The host defense factors operating in the oral cavity were discussed earlier in this chapter. Recent evidence has demonstrated that lysozyme, lactoferrin, salivary peroxidase, and secretory IgA may interact in a common antimicrobial system. However, additional evidence is needed to elucidate the details. In general, the effect of any oral defense mechanism depends on the activity over the time required for development of that disease. This, of course, can be affected by such variables as microbial metabolism, salivary flow rate, and diet.

SUGGESTED READINGS

Beaman L, Beaman B. The role of oxygen and its derivatives in microbial pathogenesis and host defense. *Annu Rev Microbiol.* 1984;38:27–48.

Brubaker RR. Mechanisms of bacterial virulence. *Annu Rev Microbiol.* 1985;39:21–50.

Clark R, Leidal K, Taichman N. Oxidative inactivation of *Actinobacillus actinomycetemcomitans* leukotoxin by the neutrophil myeloperoxidase system. *Infect Immun.* 1986; 53:252–256.

Eickinberg HU, Hahn H, Opferkuch W, eds. *The Influence of Antibiotics on Host–Parasite Relationships.* New York: Springer-Verlag, 1982.

Finelay B, Falkow S. Common themes in microbial pathogenicity. *Microbiol Rev.* 1989;53:210–230.

Finkelstein R, Sciartino CV, McIntosh M. Role of iron in microbe host interactions. *Rev Infect Dis.* 1983;5:S759–S777.

Foster JW, Kinney DM. ADP ribosylating microbial toxins. *Crit Rev Microbiol.* 1985;11:273–298.

Genco RJ, Slots J. Host response in periodontal disease. *J Dent Res.* 1984;63:441–451.

Hahn H. Antibacterial defence mechanisms. *Infection.* 1983; 11:S112–S118.

Jones G, Issacson R. Proteinaceous bacterial adhesins and their receptors. *Crit Rev Microbiol.* 1983;10:229–260.

Mims C. *The Pathogenesis of Infectious Diseases*, 3rd ed. New York: Academic Press, 1987.

Mirelman D. *Microbial Lectins and Agglutinins.* New York: John Wiley & Sons; 1986.

Slots J, Genco RJ. Black pigmented *Bacteroides* species, *Capnocytophaga* species and *Actinobacillus actinomycetemcomitans* in human periodontal disease: Virulence factors in colonization, survival and tissue destruction. *J Dent Res.* 1984;84:412–421.

Tenouvo J, Pruitt K. Relationship of the human salivary peroxidase system to oral health. *J Oral Pathol.* 1984; 13:573–584.

Tsai CC, Shenker B, DiRienzo J, Malamud D, Taichman N. Extraction and isolation of a leukotoxin from *Actinobacillus actinomycetemcomitans* with polymyxin B. *Infect Immun.* 1984;43:700–705.

CHAPTER 10

Staphylococci

Robert R. White

INTRODUCTION
CLASSIFICATION
MORPHOLOGY
CULTIVATION
VIRULENCE FACTORS
PATHOGENESIS
DIAGNOSIS
IMMUNITY
TREATMENT AND CONTROL
ORAL ASPECTS
SUGGESTED READINGS

INTRODUCTION

Staphylococci are common members of the normal flora of the skin and mucous membranes of humans. There are two species of major medical significance. *Staphylococcus aureus* is the pathogenic species and is the agent for numerous human infections. The second major species, *Staphylococcus epidermidis,* is a saprophyte that is becoming increasingly important as as a nosocomial pathogen. Even *S. aureus* is not highly virulent and usually requires some predisposing factor to establish an infection. This is made apparent by the absence of disease in a carrier population that may comprise 50% or more of the normal population. If a person's resistance is compromised, however, these microorganisms may cause many infections, ranging from minor skin abscesses to life-threatening systemic diseases. As such, they are among the most important human pathogens. Staphylococci have been implicated in oral lesions, and they may pose additional problems as a result of their resistance to penicillin, an antibiotic that in the absence of sensitivity testing, is often the drug of choice of many dentists.

CLASSIFICATION

The staphylococci have been differentiated into numerous species, but only three are of medical significance. *Staphylococcus aureus* is considered to be the primary pathogenic species. *Staphylococcus epidermidis,* a saprophyte, causes disease in medically compromised individuals, and a third species, *Staphylococcus saprophyticus,* is an agent of urinary tract infections in young women. *Staphylococcus aureus* strains are classified further on the basis of their susceptibility to infection and lysis by specific bacteriophages. Four groups, I, II, III, and IV, have been identified by phage typing.

MORPHOLOGY

Staphylococci are gram-positive spherical microorganisms that usually appear in large irregular grapelike clusters when viewed microscopically (Figure 10–1). They also may occur in pairs and short chains. Staphylococci range from 0.8 to 1.0 μm in diameter. They are nonmotile and do not form spores. Some strains are encapsulated.

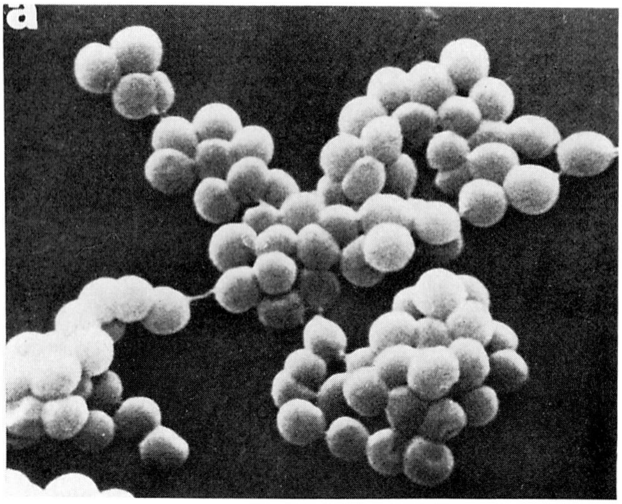

Figure 10-1. Scanning electron micrograph of *S. aureus*. *(From Watanakunakorn C, et al:* Infect Immun. *1971;4:73.*

CULTIVATION

Staphylococci are facultative anaerobes that grow readily on most laboratory media. Colonies of *S. aureus* produce a golden yellow pigment, whereas *S. epidermidis* colonies are white. The yellow pigment is not an absolute property, and some *S. aureus* colonies may be white. Staphylococci produce a catalase that can be useful in differentiating them from streptococci. Differential and selective media are available to grow and identify staphylococci. These bacteria are resistant to relatively high (7.5%) concentrations of NaCl. *Staphylococcus aureus* and *S. epidermidis* can be differentiated on the basis of mannitol fermentation—*S. aureus* ferments mannitol, and *S. epidermidis* does not. These properties are the bases for mannitol salt agar, a selective and differential medium for staphylococci. It contains 7.5% NaCl, mannitol as the sole fermentable carbohydrate, and an acid-base indicator. The salt inhibits most other bacteria, and the fermentation of mannitol (or lack thereof), as shown by the acid-base indicator, allows differentiation of the staphylococcal species. Yet another differential property is that *S. aureus* produces hemolytic toxins. These produce a zone of clear hemolysis surrounding colonies on blood agar. *Staphylococcus epidermidis* usually is not hemolytic. Hemolysis, however, also is not an absolute property of *S. aureus;* some strains do not produce hemolysis, whereas some *S. epidermidis* strains are hemolytic.

VIRULENCE FACTORS

Staphylococcus aureus produces a number of cytolytic toxins. Several of these (hemolysins) lyse red blood cells. Four hemolysins, α, β, δ, and γ, have been described. α-Toxin is lethal to laboratory animals and dermonecrotic if injected into the skin. It may contribute to the tissue necrosis that occurs in staphylococcal infections. Leukocidin is a cytolytic toxin that kills polymorphonuclear leukocytes and macrophages. The pathogenic role of these toxins is uncertain.

Exfoliative toxin (exfoliatin) causes scalded skin syndrome, a form of impetigo. This toxin lyses the attachments between cells of the granular layer of the epidermis, causing the outer epidermal layers to peel off and give an appearance resembling severely scalded skin.

Many strains of *S. aureus* produce enterotoxins (designated A through F) that cause vomiting and diarrhea. The toxins, the most common cause of food poisoning, usually are produced in contaminated foods, such as cooked meats, pastries, custards, and milk products, that are not adequately refrigerated. The toxins are not destroyed by intestinal enzymes and can survive boiling for 30 minutes.

The toxin that causes toxic shock syndrome has been demonstrated to be identical to the type F enterotoxin and exotoxin C, a pyrogenic toxin. This toxin has been designated as toxic shock syndrome toxin 1 (TSST-1) because there is evidence that additional TSSTs are produced by staphylococci. Its mechanism of action is unknown.

Protein A is a cell wall component that binds to the Fc portion of human IgG. It is possible that protein A could inhibit phagocytosis by blocking the reaction between polymorphonuclear neutrophils and the Fc part of the IgG molecule that functions as an opsonin. Peptidoglycan and lipoteichoic acid are other wall components that may be involved in staphylococcus-induced inflammation.

Staphylococci also produce many enzymes that might be be associated with disease. Coagulase is an enzyme that catalyzes the coagulation of plasma. Although coagulase-positive strains are considered pathogenic, the role that the enzyme might play in the disease process has not been determined. The enzyme causes the deposition of fibrin on the staphylococcal cell, and it has been proposed that the fibrin inhibits phagocytosis or intracellular killing. The presence of the enzyme is the key differentiating property between *S. aureus* and the less pathogenic species of staphylococci.

Other enzymes produced by staphylococci include a fibrolysin (staphylokinase) that dissolves fibrin clots, DNAse, lipase, and hyaluronidase. Some of these enzymes may aid in staphylococcal invasion of tissues, but again their actual role in pathogenicity is uncertain.

PATHOGENESIS

Staphylococcus aureus is carried by many individuals who are asymptomatic. As many as 50% of the population may carry the organism in the nose, the primary reservoir, and these numbers range much higher in hospital personnel. Most adults have high levels of circulating antistaphylococcal antibodies that appear to be effective in protecting normal individuals against infection. The mechanisms of specific immune protection are uncertain, but an intact complement system and competent polymorphonuclear neutrophils are essential. Infection usually is the result of a medically compromising factor. This may be as simple as an occluded sebaceous gland pore that allows the development of a localized abscess, or it may be a systemic factor, such as a leukocyte defect, diabetes, severe burn, or extensive surgery, that predisposes to life-threatening diseases. Staphylococcal infections include lesions within and adjacent to the oral cavity.

Staphylococci are a major cause of skin infections, such as boils, furuncles, and carbuncles, that often originate in hair follicles or sebaceous glands. Boils and furuncles are well-circumscribed, localized abscesses. Carbuncles develop in the thick skin on the nape of the neck and upper back. The impermeability of the skin promotes lateral extension of the lesion and development of a multifocal lesion that can be relieved only by incision and drainage. *Staphylococcus aureus* is also, along with *Streptococcus pyogenes,* a major cause of impetigo.

Scalded skin syndrome is an infection usually associated with newborn infants. As noted before, the toxin disassociates the epidermal cells, and the epidermis exfoliates, leaving large areas of denuded tissues. The disease usually is limited to the outer layers of skin, and although there may be extensive involvement, the disease rarely is fatal because the denuded areas dry up and the skin is rapidly replaced.

Staphylococci also affect the gastrointestinal tract. Staphylococcal food poisoning is a toxemia characterized by nausea, cramps, and diarrhea. The symptoms begin within 6 hours after ingestion of the enterotoxin and last about 24 hours. *Staphylococcus aureus* is one of several organisms that can cause an antibiotic-associated enterocolitis. This may occur if orally administered, broad-spectrum antibiotics suppress the normal intestinal flora and allow antibiotic-resistant staphylococci to establish a superinfection. The disease may range from a mild gastrointestinal discomfort to fatal systemic involvement.

Toxic shock syndrome is an acute febrile disease that may affect the renal, gastrointestinal, hepatic, central nervous, hematologic, and cardiopulmonary systems. The disease was identified originally in menstruating women who used tampons, but it is now associated also with men and nonmenstruating women with focal *S. aureus* infections. It is characterized by fever, falling blood pressure, and a desquamating skin rash. Death may occur as a result of shock, respiratory failure, and disseminated intravascular coagulation.

Staphylococcus aureus is the predominant cause of acute osteomyelitis, which occurs most frequently in young patients. Other infections include pneumonia, deep abscesses, mastitis, and meningitis. In addition, staphylococci are the most common cause of wound infections and hospital-acquired surgical infections.

Staphylococcus aureus is a major cause of nosocomial infections. This derives in part because patients in hospitals are predisposed to infections in general. In addition, hospital personnel carry pathogenic staphylococci, many of which are resistant to antibiotics, and this increases the risk of disease in an already debilitated patient.

Staphylococcus epidermidis or coagulase-negative staphylococci generally were considered to be commensals in the past but have become increasingly recognized as nosocomial pathogens that can cause serious infections in medically compromised patients. They are a major cause of infections in patients with prostheses, such as artificial heart valves, hip joints, and cerebrospinal fluid shunts. They are agents for infections associated with intravascular catheters, and they infect premature neonates, cancer patients, and immunosuppressed transplant recipients. These infections are difficult to treat because the organisms are resistant to many antibiotics.

DIAGNOSIS

Both *S. aureus* and *S. epidermidis* are members of the normal skin flora and may occur as contaminants in clinical specimens. Therefore, it may be difficult to determine if they are actually involved in a specific pathogenic process. Specimens suspected to contain pathogenic staphylococci are plated on blood agar, and the staphylococcal colonies that appear are analyzed for hemolysis, pigmentation, and production of coagulase. Production of coagulase is considered to be the definitive diagnostic property of *S. aureus* (Figure 10–2). Highly contaminated specimens may be plated on mannitol salt agar. Phage typing is not a routine diagnostic procedure, but it has been used in epidemiologic studies.

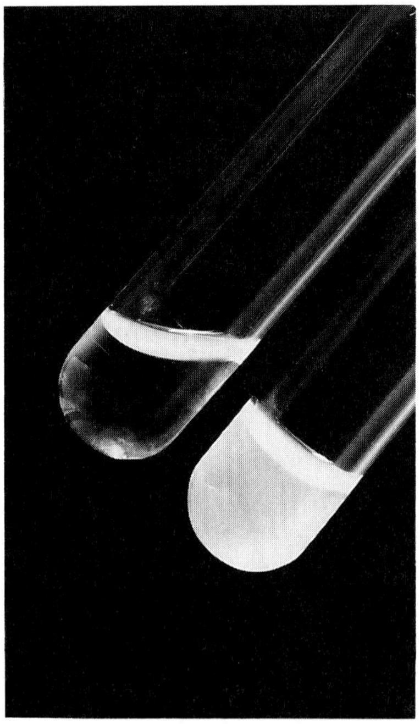

Figure 10-2. The tube coagulase test. Coagulation of plasma (lower tube) is considered definitive evidence of pathogenic *S. aureus*.

TREATMENT AND CONTROL

Staphylococcal infections are treated with antibiotics and surgical drainage. Ever since antibiotics were first introduced, staphylococci have demonstrated a remarkable ability to develop resistance, and this continues to be a serious therapeutic problem. Most clinical isolates produce β-lactamase and are resistant to penicillin G and V and ampicillin, and many are resistant to other antibiotics. Therefore, the choice of an appropriate antibotic should be based on the results of antibiotic sensitivity testing. In emergency situations, a penicillinase-resistant penicillin, such as oxacillin or methicillin, may be used before obtaining the results of antibiotic sensitivity tests. If the patient is allergic to penicillins, cephalosporin, vancomycin, or clindamycin may be used.

Control of staphylococci is difficult because they are so prevalent. Good hygiene and aseptic techniques are the most practical effective means of control. Additional precautions are required in hospital nurseries, operating rooms, and intensive care units, because patients in these areas are at high risk of contracting an infection and many hospital personnel are asymptomatic carriers of *S. aureus*. Personnel with active lesions should avoid patient contact, and carriers also may be excluded from high-risk areas. Carriers may be treated with topical antibiotics to reduce shedding of staphylococci.

ORAL ASPECTS

Dental personnel are often asymptomatic carriers of *S. aureus* and other staphylococci. In addition, the presence of these bacteria as normal inhabitants of the oropharynx, nasopharynx, and the anterior nares would seem to pose a ready source for oral infections. Despite the relatively high carrier rate and the potential for cross-infection and self-infection, oral staphylococcal infections are relatively infrequent. It appears that the resistance factors that limit staphylococcal infections in other tissues in normal subjects are effective also in the oral cavity. It has been suggested that saliva and the normal oral flora are antagonistic toward *S. aureus*. If so, they may complement the systemic resistance factors.

However, as is the case with other tissues, staphylococcal infections do occur throughout the oral cavity. They may be pure staphylococcal abscesses or polymicrobic infections. Staphylococci may infect soft tissues, salivary glands, pulp chambers, extraction sites, and bony processes ranging from the alveolar bone to the temporal mandibular joint and extending into other facial areas. These infections are especially troublesome because most staphylococci are resistant to many antibiotics, and treatment can be difficult. Since β-lactamase-producing staphylococci constitute the majority of clinical isolates, penicillin almost always is useless against staphylococcal infections.

SUGGESTED READINGS

Barnard JDW. Osteomyelitis of the jaws as a sequel to dental local anesthetic injections. *Br J Oral Surg.* 1976;13:264.

Cohen JO, ed. *The Staphylococci.* New York: Wiley-Interscience; 1972

Coke JM, McDonald P, Sanger RG. Toxic shock syndrome: Dental implications and guidelines. *J. Oral Med.* 1983; 38:62.

Easmon CSF, Adlam C, eds. *Staphylococci and Staphylococcal Infections.* London: Academic Press; 1983; vol I, II.

Kannangara DW, Thadepalli H, McQuirter JL. Bacteriology and treatment of dental infections. *Oral Surg.* 1980; 50:103.

Neihart RE, Fried JS, Hodges GR. Coagulase-negative staphylococci. *South Med J.* 1988;81:491.

Sabath LD. Mechanisms of resistance to beta-lactam antibiotics in strains of *Staphylococcus aureus. Ann Intern Med.* 1982;97:339.

Willett HP. Staphylococcus. In: Joklik WK, Willett HP, Amos DB, Wifert CM, eds. *Zinsser Microbiology,* 19th ed. Norwalk, Conn: Appleton-Century-Crofts; 1989.

CHAPTER 11

Streptococci

Robert R. White

INTRODUCTION
CLASSIFICATION OF STREPTOCOCCI
GROUP A STREPTOCOCCI
Morphology
Cultivation
Virulence Factors
Diseases
Sequelae to Acute Streptococcal Infections
Diagnosis
Treatment, Immunity, and Prevention
GROUP B STREPTOCOCCI
GROUP D STREPTOCOCCI
VIRIDANS STREPTOCOCCI
PEPTOSTREPTOCOCCUS
STREPTOCOCCUS PNEUMONIAE
Cultivation
Classification
Virulence Factors
Diseases
Diagnosis
Treatment, Immunity, and Prevention
ORAL ASPECTS
SUGGESTED READINGS

INTRODUCTION

The streptococci are a heterogeneous group of bacteria that derive their name from their spherical cellular morphology and their tendency to form chains. Streptococci are widely distributed in nature and may be saprophtyic and parasitic. They are responsible for a number of diseases in humans and other animals. In humans, these diseases include the respiratory diseases produced by *Streptococcus pyogenes* and *Streptococcus pneumoniae,* dental caries by *Streptococcus mutans,* orofacial infections, and infective endocarditis. Since the streptococci are so varied, it is not possible to describe them as a single group. Therefore, this chapter first considers *S. pyogenes,* followed by the other Lancefield groups, the viridans streptococci, and *S. pneumoniae.* The oral streptococci are described to the extent necessary to indicate their position among the streptococci and their role in disease outside of the oral cavity. Most of the information on the oral streptococci can be found in Chapters 32 and 33.

CLASSIFICATION OF STREPTOCOCCI

The streptococci are differentiated on the basis of immunologic, cultural, and biochemical properties. They can be differentiated from staphylococci on the basis of the enzyme catalase. Staphylococci are catalase-positive, and streptococci are catalase-negative. Many of the streptococci may be immunologically differentiated according to the Lancefield classification. These streptococci contain an acid-soluble carbohydrate antigen (the C carbohydrate or group carbohydrate) in their cell walls. Originally, these antigens were used to divide these streptococci into 13 groups designated aphabetically from A to O. Nineteen groups have now been identified based on these group-specific antigens. Several major groups of streptococci that do not posses Lancefield antigens are described subsequently.

Members of the Lancefield groups also possess additional distinctive cell wall antigens that allow further classification. The M protein found in group A is one of the most important. M proteins have been used to subdivide group A into over 60 serotypes. Serotyping is useful in epidemiologic studies and in predicting the potential for sequelae of acute streptococcal infections.

Many streptococci produce soluble factors that lyse red blood cells, and hemolysis of blood agar also is used to classify these microorganisms (Brown's classification). Some hemolysins cause only a partial lysis of the blood cells and produce a green or greenish brown halo around the colony. Others lyse surrounding blood cells completely and produce a clear zone around the streptococcal colony. The partial or green hemolytic reaction is called α-hemolysis, and the bacteria are called α-streptococci or viridans (green) streptococci. The clear zone of hemolysis is called β-hemolysis, and the bacteria are referred to as β-hemolytic or β-streptococci. If no hemolysis occurs, the reaction is called a γ-reaction, and the streptococci that are not hemolytic are called γ-streptococci. This use of hemolytic reactions to classify the streptococci is valid only within certain limits because some taxa are uniformly α, β, or γ reactors, whereas others are not. For example, the members of Lancefield group A, the group that contains the major human pathogens, are uniformly β-hemolytic, whereas different strains of *S. mutans* may exhibit any one of the three reactions.

In addition to serotyping and hemolysis, the effects of compounds, such as optochin, bacitracin, and sodium chloride, and various biochemical reactions are useful in characterizing streptococci. Some of these compounds are noted in Table 11–1 and are described further as they relate to the various streptococci.

GROUP A STREPTOCOCCI

Most human pathogens and the agents for the most severe infections are found in group A. Group A streptococci are all members of a single species, *S. pyogenes,* and are the agents for pharyngitis, scarlet fever, skin infections, rheumatic fever, and acute glomerulonephritis. These streptococci are uniformly β-hemolytic and often are incorrectly referred to as the β-streptococci. As noted in Table 11–1, there are several other streptococcal groups that exhibit β-hemolysis

Morphology

Group A streptococci are gram-positive, spherical organisms that usually divide in one plane and have a tendency to remain attached and to form chains. The cellular morphology ranges from spherical to ovoid or even rod shaped, and the sizes range from 0.6 to 2.0 μm in diameter (Figure 11–1). None of the streptococci are motile, and none form spores. *Streptococcus pyogenes* possesses fimbriae or pili that are involved in adherence to host cells (Fig 11–1). It also produces a hyaluronic acid capsule early in culture that is rapidly lost as the culture grows older.

Group A streptococcal L forms can be produced in vitro by treating the cells with penicillin or enzymes that lyse the cell wall. L forms occur spontaneously in patients receiving penicillin therapy, and this phenomenon has given rise to the suggestion that streptococcal L forms may be responsible for the persistence of some streptococcal infections.

TABLE 11–1. DISTINGUISHING PROPERTIES OF SELECTED STREPTOCOCCAL GROUPS

Category	Representative Species	Hemolytic Reaction	Significant Features	Diseases
Group A	*S. pyogenes*	β	Bacitracin sensitive	Pharyngitis, scarlet fever, skin infections, rheumatic fever, glomerulonephritis
Group B	*S. agalactiae*	β	CAMP test positive	Neonatal infections
Group D				
Enterococci	*S. faecalis*	α, β, γ	Growth in 6.5% NaCl and at 45°C	Infective endocarditis, urinary tract infections
Nonenterococci	*S. bovis*	α, γ	Growth at 45°C	Infective endocarditis
Viridans	*S. mitis, S. milleri, S. mutans*	α, γ, some β		Infective endocarditis, dental caries
Pneumococcus	*S. pneumoniae*	α	Optochin and bile sensitive	Pneumonia, meningitis, otitis media
Peptostreptococcus	*P. magnus*	Variable	Anaerobic	Mixed anaerobic infections

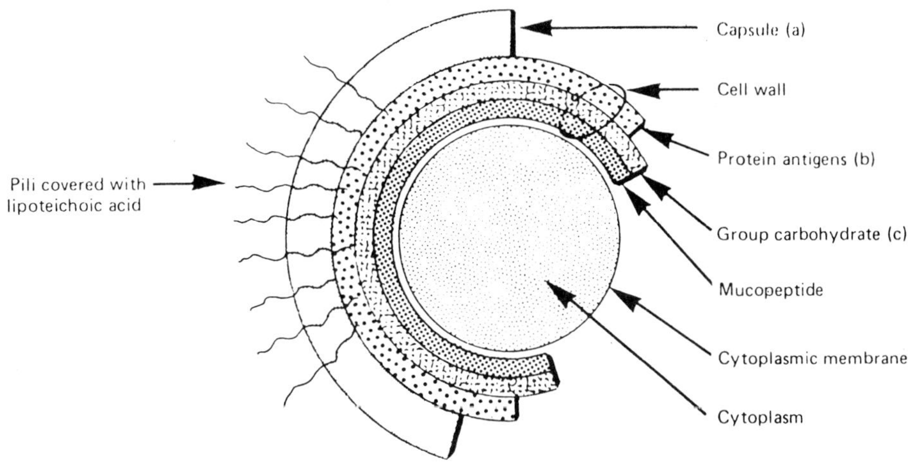

Figure 11–1. Cross-section of a group A streptococcal cell. The major protein antigen is the M protein. The pili also contain M protein. *(From Jawetz E, Melnick JL, Adelberg EA.* Review of Medical Microbiology, *16th ed. Los Altos, Calif: Lang Medical Publications; 1984.)*

Cultivation

Streptococci require complex medium that is usually enriched with blood or serum for their routine cultivation because they cannot synthesize many required nutrients. These streptococci are facultative anaerobes whose growth is optimal at 37°C.

Virulence Factors

Group A streptococci produce many possible virulence factors, but the actual roles of many of these factors in disease processes are uncertain. The M protein appears to be the most significant factor in disease. M protein is antiphagocytic and, thus, protects the organisms from the major resistance mechanism in the body. The pathogenic potential of M protein is demonstrated readily by the rapid phagocytosis of streptococci lacking M protein or those exposed to antibody specific for the M protein. M protein also has been shown to be an adherence factor in association with lipoteichoic acid.

Lipoteichoic acid is found on the fimbriae and is believed to be involved in adherence to epithelial cells. Lipoteichoic acid and the peptidoglycan or mucopeptide found in the cell wall are inflammatory and suspected of mediating injury.

A capsule composed of hyaluronic acid is produced by streptococci during the early stages of growth, but the capsule is lost because the organism also produces hyaluronidase. The capsule impedes phagocytosis, but its significance in disease is uncertain.

Streptococcal hyaluronidase also hydrolyzes the hyaluronic acid that comprises the host's connective tissue ground substance. This is thought to enhance the invasiveness of the microorganisms, and, thus, the enzyme is commonly called spreading factor. Other streptococcal enzymes include a deoxyribonuclease (streptodornase) and a fibrinolysin (streptokinase). The roles in disease of these two enzymes are uncertain. Mixtures of these two enzymes have been used in medicine to digest purulent exudates to clean lesions and facilitate healing, especially in patients with severe skin burns.

Erythrogenic or pyrogenic toxin is responsible for the diffuse skin rash that gives scarlet fever its name. The mechanism of action resulting in pyrogenicity and the skin rash is uncertain. An immune hypersensitivity reaction may be involved. The toxin is produced as a result of infection by a lysogenic bacteriophage that carries the genetic information coding for toxin production. Only those streptococci carrying this temperate phage produce the toxin. There are at least three toxin serotypes, A, B, and C.

Group A streptococci produce two hemolysins, streptolysin S and streptolysin O. Streptolysin S, which is responsible for the β-hemolytic reaction on blood plates, is a nonantigenic polypeptide. The significance of the hemolytic activity to streptococcal diseases is unknown, but it is known that streptolysin S kills neutrophils and macrophages, and the lysin may be of pathogenic significance as a result of this antileukocytic activity. Streptolysin O is a protein that is susceptible to oxidation. It also lyses erythrocytes and leukocytes and inhibits leukocyte chemotaxis. Streptolysin O is antigenic, and this antigenicity is the basis for a diagnostic test, the antistreptolysin O antibody (ASO) test. A high serum ASO titer is indicative of recent infection with group A streptococci and is useful in the diagnosis of rheumatic fever and acute glomerulonephritis.

Diseases

The most common reservoir of group A streptococci is human carriers. Five to fifteen percent of normal individuals carry these streptococci as members of their pharyngeal flora. They are transmitted by contact, either direct or by aerosol droplets. Acute streptococcal pharyngitis, the most common group A infection, is characterized by inflammation of the pharynx, tonsils, and soft palate, with a grayish yellow purulent exudate in the tonsillar areas. The disease is usually of rapid onset and is accompanied by fever, chills, malaise, nausea, and varying degreees of lymphadenopathy. The acute infection is self-limiting and resolves in about a week. In infants, streptococcal pharyngitis differs in that the onset is slower, and the illness may last for several weeks. The disease in infants often spreads to paranasal sinuses and the middle ear to cause otitis media.

Scarlet fever is caused by toxigenic strains of *S. pyogenes.* The symptoms of acute streptococcal pharyngitis are present, and they are accompanied by a diffuse erythematous rash, which first appears on the chest and spreads to other areas of the body. A white coating forms on the tongue. The inflamed fungiform papillae swell and project from the surface of the tongue, giving it a characteristic strawberry tongue appearance. The rash disappears in about a week, after which desquamation of the skin and the tongue may occur.

Group A streptococci are responsible for several skin infections, including impetigo and erysipleas. Impetigo, which most commonly occurs in children, is a superficial vesicular infection that results from streptococcal contamination of a break in the skin. The vesicles, which are highly infectious, break down and become encrusted. The disease is self-limiting. Erysipelas is a deeper infection of the skin that may result from contamination of wounds or may occur spontaneously. It is characterized by an erythematous spreading lesion with a sharply demarcated, raised margin. Erysipelas commonly occurs on the face and legs.

Sequelae to Acute Streptococcal Infections

Group A streptococcal infections are unique because of the sequelae that may follow the acute infections. Rheumatic fever occurs in 1% to 3% of individuals experiencing streptococcal pharyngitis, and acute streptococcal glomerulonephritis occurs in about 0.5% of individuals who have had acute pharyngeal or skin infections. Rheumatic fever is a cardiovascular disease that appears 2 to 3 weeks after pharyngeal infections. It is characterized by inflammation of the joints, heart, brain, and skin. Arthritis, carditis, and chorea occur, but the cardiac involvement is considered the most serious because of the injury to heart muscle and valves. The inflammation is thought to be of immunologic origin. Several of the streptococcal antigens and the host organs share antigenic determinants, and anticardiac tissue antibodies reactive with streptococci have been identified in patients. Autopsies have revealed the presence of immune complexes known as Aschoff bodies in cardiac tissues.

Acute glomerulonephritis may follow either pharyngeal or skin infections. Whereas rheumatic fever is not usually associated with any particular M protein serotypes, glomerulonephritis is most commonly caused by a limited group of serotypes, the so-called nephritogenic strains. Type 12 is the most common cause of glomerulonephritis following pharyngitis, whereas serotypes 2, 49, 55, 57, and 60 frequently are associated with glomerulonephritis following skin infections. Acute glomerulonephritis appears about 1 or 2 weeks after the initial streptococcal infection and is characterized by blood and protein in the urine, edema of the face and legs, and impairment of renal function. The disease is considered to be an immune complex disease. Immunofluorescence microscopy has revealed granular deposits of immunoglobulin and complement lining the basement membranes of the renal vasculature.

Diagnosis

It is essential that acute streptococcal infections be identified rapidly in order to initiate treatment that will prevent the development of rheumatic fever or glomerulonephritis. The organism must be isolated and identified, since the clinical features of streptococcal pharyngitis are not a reliable diagnostic aid because they are shared by several acute viral pharyngitides. In order to diagnose the disease, a throat swab should be inoculated on blood agar. If group A streptococci are present, β-hemolytic colonies will appear in 24 to 48 hours. The group A streptococci can be differentiated from other β-hemolytic streptococci by restreaking the colonies on a second plate and placing a bacitracin antibiotic disk on the inoculated area. Over 95% of the group A streptococci are inhibited by bacitracin, whereas nearly all other β-hemolytic organisms are not inhibited by bacitracin. Rapid diagnostic tests, such as latex agglutination, coagglutination, and ELISA, that are capable of detecting the streptococcal antigens picked up by a pharyngeal throat swab are now available. These diagnostic kits can identify positive group A streptococcal specimens within 5 to 10 minutes after the specimen is collected.

Serologic assays can be used to detect antibody directed against several stretococcal antigens, including streptolysin O, hyaluronidase, and streptodornase. These antibodies are of little use in diagnosis of the acute infection, since they usually appear several days after the acute infection has passed. However, they are useful in identifying the antecedent streptococcal infection responsible for rheumatic fever or glomerulonephritis.

Treatment, Immunity, and Prevention

The group A streptococci are all sensitive to penicillin G, the antibiotic of choice. Most are sensitive to erythromycin, which is used for patients allergic to penicillin. Early and extended treatment is essential to prevent subsequent development of rheumatic fever or acute glomerulonephritis. The antibiotics are administered for 10 days to ensure complete removal of the streptococci. Rheumatic fever and glomerulonephritis are not affected by antibiotics, and patients are given symptomatic therapy.

Immunity to group A streptococci is type specific. Infection by one M protein serotype will confer protective immunity against that serotype but not against others. Thus, additional infections by other group A streptococci can occur. The immune response to the infecting organisms may be abrogated as a result of rapid, effective chemotherapy, since the antigenic stimulus will be curtailed. Recovery from scarlet fever results in immunity to the erythrogenic toxin, but since there are three immunologically different toxins, an individual may contract scarlet fever more than once.

The only routine preventive measure taken against group A infections is the extended antibiotic treatment used to prevent the sequelae, rheumatic fever and acute glomerulonephritis, and reduce the numbers of carriers. Mass prophylaxis may be carried out if there are localized outbreaks of streptococcal pharyngitis in schools, institutions, or military compounds. Chemotherapy also is used in carriers in critical positions, such as hospital personnel. As a result of the large number of serotypes, an antistreptococcal vaccine currently is not practical.

GROUP B STREPTOCOCCI

Group B streptococci, represented by *Streptococcus agalactiae*, are members of the normal flora in the pharynx, gastrointestinal tract, and vagina. In the past, these organisms were not common causes of serious disease, but group B infections have been increasing in recent years. They rarely affect normal adults except pregnant women and the elderly but can cause problems in medically compromised individuals, and they are the agents of serious neonatal infections, such as septicemia, pneumonia, and meningitis. Group B streptococcal infections occur in about 0.1% of neonates. These streptococci give a positive response to a diagnostic test called the CAMP test. *Streptococcus agalactiae* is susceptible to penicillin, but it is extremely difficult to eradicate the infant infections, and the mortality rate is 50% or greater.

GROUP D STREPTOCOCCI

Group D streptococci are members of the normal flora of the gastrointestinal, respiratory, and genitourinary tracts and skin. They differ from other streptococci because they can grow at 45°C, they grow in the presence of 40% bile, and they hydrolyze esculin. Group D streptococci are divided into two groups, enterococci and nonenterococci, based on the ability of the enterococci to grow in the presence of 6.5% sodium chloride. Enterococci, of which *Enterococcus faecalis* is the major pathogen, frequently are involved in infective endocarditis, urinary tract infections, and orofacial infections. *E. faecalis* also has been shown to produce dental caries in laboratory animals. Enterococci are resistant to penicillin alone but susceptible to a combination of penicillin and aminoglycosides. Nonenterococci (eg, *Streptococcus bovis*) are infrequent pathogens of humans but have been isolated from infective endocarditis lesions. Most are sensitive to penicillin.

VIRIDANS STREPTOCOCCI

A large number of streptococci that do not fit readily into any of the established classification schemes have been relegated to a large heterogeneous group called the viridans or α-streptococci. Despite these names, many are nonhemolytic, and some are β-hemolytic. Although they often are referred to incorrectly as *Streptococcus viridans,* there is no such species. The viridans streptococci are members of the normal flora of the mucous membranes of the body, including the oral cavity, the nasopharynx, and the genitourinary tract. This group includes *S. mutans, Streptococcus milleri,* and *Streptococcus mitis,* all of which are found in the oral cavity. In addition, bacteria that carry Lancefield antigens often are included in the viridans group. For example, *Streptococcus sanguis,* which carries Lancefield group antigen H, and *Streptococcus salivarius,* (group K), are two such species.

The viridans streptococci are of major significance for two reasons. One is that they comprise a major portion of the oral flora of humans and are involved in several oral diseases, including dental caries. Their role in oral ecology and dental diseases is discussed in Chapters 32 and 33. α-Streptococci account for 50% to 70% of the cases of subacute infective endocarditis, formerly called subacute bacterial endocarditis. Infective endocarditis occurs in individuals who have a predisposing heart valve injury or defect that may have resulted from rheumatic fever, mitral valve prolapse, congenital defects, or implanted prosthetic valves. Bacteria in the blood colonize these tissues, and vegetations consisting of bacteria, fibrin, platelets, and blood cells form on the valves and cause further injury to the cardiac tissues. As the vegetations grow, fragments that break off can produce thrombi in other organs throughout the body. Symptoms include chronic fever, anemia, weakness, cardiac murmurs, and splenomegaly. The disease is usually fatal if untreated. The viridans streptococci may enter the blood from several areas of the body through natural methods or as a result of surgical procedures or instrumentation involving mucosal surfaces or infected tissues. A major source of the bacteremias is the oral cavity. Streptococci entering the bloodstream as a result of oral lesions and dental manipulations, such as extractions and cleaning and scaling of teeth, often cause infective endocarditis. Because α-streptococci are not universally susceptible to any particular chemotherapeutic agent, antibiotic sensitivity tests must be used to determine what agent will be effective against individual isolates.

PEPTOSTREPTOCOCCUS

Peptostreptococcus is a genus of anaerobic streptococci that is found in mixed anaerobic infections in the pelvis, abdomen, lungs, and oral cavity. They have been isolated from polymicrobic anaerobic lesions in the periodontium, the pulp, and other orofacial infections. Additional details concerning these anaerobic infections are given in Chapter 21.

STREPTOCOCCUS PNEUMONIAE

Streptococcus pneumoniae is a gram-positive, lancet-shaped coccus that usually occurs in pairs (diplococci) but can be found in chains. It once was designated *Diplococcus pneumoniae* and is referred to commonly as the pneumococcus. Virulent strains of *S. pneumoniae* are encapsulated. The capsule is of pathogenic and diagnostic importance. The capsule also is of historical significance, since the discovery that avirulent nonencapsulated strains could be transformed into encapsulated virulent strains with DNA from virulent *S. pneumoniae* was the first proof of the role of DNA in genetic expression.

Cultivation

The pneumococci require a complex medium, such as brain-heart infusion enriched with blood. These organisms are facultative anaerobes and produce an α-hemolytic reaction on blood agar. *Streptococcus pneumoniae* tends to lyse spontaneously as the cultures age. This autolysis is mediated by an autolytic enzyme, L-alanine-muramyl amidase, which acts on the peptidoglycan in the cell wall of the organism. This characteristic autolysis is useful diagnostically, since the enzyme's action can be accelerated by surface active agents, such as bile.

Classification

The pneumococcal capsule is a polysaccharide called specific soluble substance (SSS). There are over 80 antigenically different capsular polysaccharides, and these are used to classify the pneumococci into serotypes designated by Arabic numerals. *Streptococcus pneumoniae* does not possess Lancefield antigens, but all penumococci share a common cell wall polysaccharide antigen, the C substance, which will precipitate when mixed with serum as a result of its interaction with a β-globulin, C-reactive protein (CRP). CRP occurs in only very small amounts in normal serum, but it rises markedly during acute inflammation. Therefore, the appearance of an increased CRP–C substance precipitate in serum is used as a diagnostic aid in inflammatory diseases.

Virulence Factors

The capsule, which inhibits phagocytosis, is the only factor that has been associated definitely with virulence. Encapsulated pneumococci are virulent; nonencapsulated cells are not. Antibody directed against the capsule will protect against pneumococcal pneumonia. The mechanisms leading to the injury that occurs in pneumococcal pneumonia is unknown. The capsule is relatively nontoxic, and other potential virulence factors, such as peptidoglycan, a hemolysin (pneumolysin O), and neuraminidase, have not been proven to be of significance to the disease process.

Diseases

Streptococcus pneumoniae is spread by aerosol droplets and direct contact of diseased patients and carriers. Thirty to seventy-five percent of healthy humans carry virulent pneumococci. Despite this high carrier rate, the disease is not widespread because normal subjects are highly resistant to the disease. When the disease occurs, there is usually a predisposing factor present. It often occurs secondary to viral infection, and it is common among alcoholics whose respiratory defense mechanisms are compromised. Debilitated children and the elderly also are at higher risk of contracting pneumococcal pneumonia.

In adults, the disease is most commonly lobar pneumonia, characterized by fever, chills, and pleuritic pain. It is a disease of acute onset that lasts for 5 to 10 days and often disappears as rapidly as it appears. It is one of the most frequent types of adult pneumonias. In the elderly and young children, it frequently affects the upper respiratory regions. The pneumococcus may spread through the lymphatics and bloodstream to establish infections in other parts of the body. Mortality is about 33% in untreated patients and 5% in treated patients. It is much higher in the elderly. *Streptococcus pneumoniae* also is the most frequent cause of meningitis in adults and otitis media in children and adults.

Diagnosis

The symptoms of pneumococcal pneumonia are distinctive enough that a preliminary diagnosis can be made based on clinical signs alone. It must be verified by laboratory diagnosis, as must cases of pneumococcal meninigitis. Specimens, such as sputum or spinal fluid, should be inoculated on enriched medium containing blood, and any α-streptococcal colonies that appear must be differentiated from other α-hemolytic streptococci that are common inhabitants of the oropharynx. Presumptive differentiation can be accomplished by inoculating the suspected colonies on a blood plate and placing a filter paper disk impregnated with ethyl hydrocuprein hydrochloride (optochin) on the plate. The pneumococci will not grow in the vicinity of the optochin disk, whereas other α-streptococci, which are not sensitive to optochin, will grow. The bile solubility test may be used to differentiate presumptively pneumococci from other α-streptococci.

The pneumococci can be serologically identified using anticapsular antisera in a test called the quellung reaction. If encapsulated microroganisms are mixed with type-specific antisera and viewed with a microscope, the capsule will appear swollen. Rapid diagnostic tests, including latex agglutination and coagglutination assays, also are available for *S. pneumoniae.*

Treatment, Immunity, and Prevention

For many years, pneumococci were uniformly susceptible to penicillin, and the vast majority still are. However, sporadic penicillin-resistant strains have begun to appear among clinical isolates, and antibiotic sensitivity testing should now be carried out routinely to ensure appropriate therapy. Patients are noninfectious within 24 to 48 hours after initiating chemotherapy.

Recovery from the infection results in a strong serotype-specific immunity. Therefore, prevention has centered on immunization of high-risk groups. Although there are over 80 capsular serotypes, more than 80% of penumococcal pneumonias are caused by only 14 serotypes. The capsular polysaccharides of these 14 serotypes have been purified and combined in a polyvalent pneumococcal vaccine for adults. Immunization is recommended for the elderly and for the medically compromised, since these two groups are highly susceptible to the disease, and the fatality rate is extremely high. A second polyvalent vaccine containing 23 capsular antigens has been developed for children.

ORAL ASPECTS

The streptococci are important to the dental professional because members of this group cause primary oral infections, and the oral cavity also serves as a source of streptococci that can establish endogenous infections, such as infective endocarditis, or be transmitted to others. *Streptococcus mutans* is considered to be the primary agent for dental caries, and other oral streptococci, such as *S. sanguis, S. salivarius,* and *S. faecalis,* have been shown to cause dental caries in laboratory animals. In addition, these and other oral strep-

TABLE 11–2. SUMMARY OF RECOMMENDED ANTIBIOTIC REGIMENS FOR DENTAL PROCEDURES

Standard regimen	
For dental procedures that cause gingival bleeding, and oral/respiratory tract surgery	Pencicillin V 2.0 g orally 1 hour before, then 1.0 g 6 hours later. For patients unable to take oral medications, 2 million units of aqueous penicillin G intravenously or intramuscularly 30–60 minutes before a procedure and 1 million units 6 hours later may be substituted
Special regimens	
Parenteral regimen for use when maximum protection desired (for example, for patients with prosthetic valves)	Ampicillin 1.0–2.0 g intramuscularly or intravenously, plus gentamicin 1.5 mg/kg intramuscularly or intravenously, one-half hour before procedure, followed by 1.0 g oral penicillin V 6 hours later. Alternatively, the parenteral regimen may be repeated once 8 hours later
Oral regimen for penicillin-allergic patients	Erythromycin 1.0 g orally 1 hour before, then 500 mg 6 hours later
Parenteral regimen for penicillin-allergic patients	Vancomycin 1.0 g intravenously slowly over 1 hour, starting 1 hour before. No repeat dose is necessary

Pediatric doses: Ampicillin 50 mg/kg per dose; erythromycin 20 mg/kg for first dose, then 10 mg/kg; gentamicin 2.0 mg/kg per dose; penicillin V full adult dose if greater than 60 lb (27 kg), one-half adult dose if less than 60 lb (27 kg); aqueous penicillin G 50,000 units/kg (25,000 units/kg for follow-up); vancomycin 20 mg/kg per dose. The intervals between doses are the same as for adults. Total doses should not exceed adult doses.

From Prevention of bacterial endocarditis: a committee report of the American Heart Association J Am Dent Assoc. *1985;110:98–100.*

tococci (viridans streptococci and peptostreptococci) have been isolated from many orofacial infections, such as gingivitis, pulpitis, and soft tissues abscesses.

As previously noted, oral streptococci are the predominant agents of infective endocarditis, and dental manipulations are a major cause of the bacteremias that lead to infection of the valvular tissues. The reported rate of bacteremias resulting from extractions, periodontal scaling, restorative work, and other operations ranges from 20% to 100%. It is generally accepted that dental personnel may be responsible for many cases of infective endocarditis among individuals with a congenital or acquired predisposition to this disease. As a result, dentists bear an increased responsibility to prevent the infection. This responsibility can be satisfied only by making every effort to obtain an adequate history to determine if the patient is at risk and administering the proper prophylactic measures (Table 11–2) needed to prevent infection if the patient is found to be at risk

In addition to the oral streptococci, *S. pyogenes, S. pneumoniae,* and other streptococci frequently are seeded to the saliva from carrier colonies in the upper respiratory tract. In one study, pneumococci were found in 76% of childrens' saliva, enterococci in 42% and β-hemolytic streptococci in 22%. Thus, there is a very strong potential for self-infection or cross-infection in the dental operatory.

SUGGESTED READINGS

Bisno AL. *Streptococcus pyogenes.* In Mandell GL, Douglas RG, Bennett JE, eds. *Principles and Practices of Infectious Diseases,* 2nd ed. New York: John Wiley & Sons; 1985.

Committee on Rheumatic Fever and Infective Endocarditis of the Council on Cardiovascular Diseases of the Young. Prevention of bacterial endocarditis. *Circulation.* 1985; 70:1123A.

Durack DT, Kaplan EL, Bisno AL. Apparent failures of endocarditis prophylaxis—Analysis of 52 cases submitted to a national registry. *JAMA.* 1983;250:2318–2322.

Facklam RR. Physiological differentiation of viridans streptococci. *J. Clin Microbiol.* 1977;5:184.

Gallis HA. Streptococcus. In: Joklik WK, Willett HP, Amos DB, eds. *Zinsser Microbiology,* 18th ed. Norwalk, Conn: Appleton-Century-Crofts; 1984.

Gillespie SH. Aspects of pneumococcal infection including bacterial virulence, host response and vaccination. *J Med Microbiol.* 1989;28:237.

Mufson MA. Pneumococcal infection. *JAMA.* 1981;246:1942.

Parker MT, ed. *Pathogenic Streptococci.* Surrey, England: Reedbooks; 1979.

Quie PG, Giebink GS, Winkelstein JA, eds. The pneumococcus: A symposium. *Rev Infect Dis.* 1981;3:183–371.

Read SE, Zabriskie JB. *Streptococcal Disease and the Immune Response.* New York: Academic Press; 1980.

CHAPTER 12

Neisseria

John A. Molinari and P. H. Chandrasekar

INTRODUCTION

CLASSIFICATION

MORPHOLOGY AND CULTIVATION

NEISSERIA MENINGITIDIS
- Virulence Factors
- Pathogenicity
- Diagnosis and Treatment
- Immunity

NEISSERIA GONORRHOEAE
- Virulence Factors
- Pathogenicity
- Diagnosis and Treatment
- Prevention

ORAL ASPECTS

SUGGESTED READINGS

INTRODUCTION

The genus *Neisseria* is comprised of a group of microorganisms that share a number of morphologic and metabolic properties but vary widely in their relationship to the hosts that they infect. Members of this genus range from frank pathogens that cause diseases, such as meningitis and venereal disease, to commensal nonpathogens that colonize the mucous membranes throughout the body. *Neisseria* species are found in the oral cavity and the adjacent nasopharyngeal tissues. As a result of the predilection of *Neisseria* for these tissues, the dental professional will encounter both pathogens and nonpathogens. A significant percentage of these instances occur with *Neisseria* either in orofacial infections or in asymptomatic carriage.

CLASSIFICATION

The *Neisseria* are classified in the family Neisseriaceae, along with the genera *Moraxella, Acinetobacter,* and *Branhamella. Neisseria meningitidis* and *Neisseria gonorrhoeae* are the major pathogens of this family. Since all of these bacteria colonize mucous membranes, close observation of gram-stained preparations is necessary to distinguish the small coccobacilli of *Moraxella* and *Acinetobacter* species from the diplococci of *Neisseria* and *Branhamella.* Ultimate differentiation often relies on specific biochemical characteristics.

MORPHOLOGY AND CULTIVATION

Neisseria are flattened, gram-negative, bean-shaped diplococci (Fig 12–1). They are nonmotile and do not form spores. Some strains possess polysaccharide capsules and pili, both of which have been associated with pathogenicity. *Neisseria* are obligately aerobic, delicate microorganisms. They are killed after short periods of exposure to drying, heat, cold, sunlight, and many disinfectants, such as iodophors, phenols, and alcohols. They are extracellular parasitic bacteria that cause clinical infection only in susceptible humans.

Neisseria meningitidis and *Neisseria gonorrhoeae* are the major pathogens of this relatively fastidious ge-

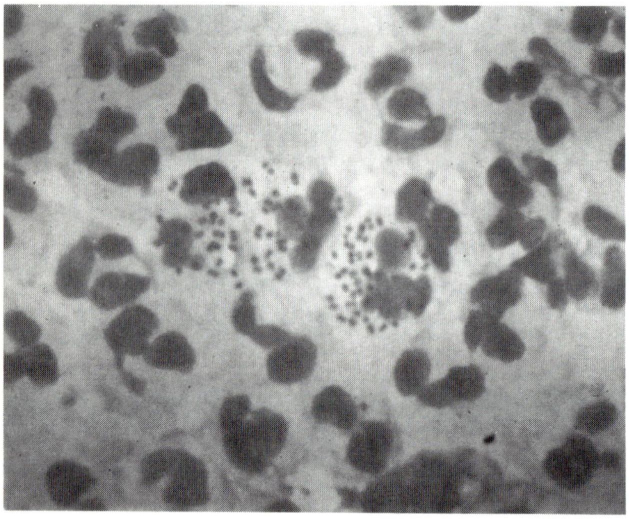

Figure 12–1. Phagocytized *Neisseria gonorrhoeae* in urethral exudate. *(Courtesy of Centers for Disease Control, Atlanta, GA.)*

nus. These are distinguished from the more saprophytic *Neisseria* by isolation on enriched selective media, such as Thayer-Martin medium or chocolate agar, and a series of fermentation reactions. Like *N. meningitidis* and *N. gonorrhoeae*, nonpathogenic commensal *Neisseria* species also have a predilection for mucous membranes, and their presence can confuse a diagnosis made strictly on the basis of a gram stain. A highly humid growth environment supplemented with 5 to 10% CO_2 is required for growth of most *Neisseria* species. Pigmentation of colonial growth is most often associated with the nonpathogenic *Neisseria*.

NEISSERIA MENINGITIDIS

Neisseria meningitidis, commonly called meningococcus, is a major cause of meningitis. The disease also is called epidemic cerebrospinal meningitis, meningococcal meningitis, spotted fever, and cerebrospinal fever.

Virulence Factors

The meningococcus possesses a polysaccharide capsule that inhibits phagocytosis. Antibody directed against the capsule can prevent disease. Nine immunologically distinct capsular antigens that are designated alphabetically have been described. In addition to their role as virulence factors, the capsules also are useful in serotyping the members of the genus. Meningococci possess an endotoxin that is thought to be responsible for the vascular injury associated with the disease. *Neisseria meningitidis* produces a proteolytic enzyme that cleaves human IgA1. The role that this protease plays in disease is not known, but the enzyme may serve to protect against secretory IgA (SIgA) on the mucosal surfaces that meningococci colonize (Table 12–1).

Pathogenicity

The disease is transmitted by inhalation of respiratory aerosols from individuals carrying the disease. Five to thirty percent of the population carry *N. meningitidis* in their nasopharyngeal flora. Just before and during epidemics, the carrier rate may exceed 80%. The microorganism colonizes the nasopharynx and passes through the mucous membranes into the bloodstream, from where it disseminates throughout the body, especially the central nervous system.

The incubation period for the disease is usually less than 1 week. Meningitis is the most common manifestation, but the disease can range from a relatively mild febrile infection accompanied by pharyngitis to a fulminating meningococcemia that can rapidly progress to shock (Waterhouse-Friderichsen syndrome) and death within hours. Diagnostic hemorrhagic skin lesions usually are observed within 12 to 36 hours after disease onset. Meningococcal endotoxin is responsible for these hemorrhagic lesions, shock, disseminated intravascular coagulation, and myocarditis. The disease occurs primarily as single, isolated cases, but localized outbreaks may occur among military personnel, in day care centers, and in schools.

Diagnosis and Treatment

The microscopic demonstration of gram-negative diplococci in acute inflammatory exudates from cer-

TABLE 12–1. PATHOGENICITY OF MENINGOCOCCI

Factor	Function
Serogroup-specific capsular polysaccharides	Major virulence factor; promotes presence of bacteria by resisting phagocytosis
Lipopolysaccharide-endotoxin complex	Resides in outer portion of plasma membrane; responsible for toxicity and skin lesions of meningococcal disease, most responsible factor for life-threatening meningococcal infection
P substance	Nucleoproteins that have some toxic effect; does not appear to be specific for meningococci
Pili	Attachment of piliated *Neisseria meningitidis* strains to nasopharyngeal cells
IgA1 protease	Excreted into extracellular environment; production limited to pathogenic *Neisseria* (ie, meningococci and gonococci); role in meningococcal pathogenesis unclear

ebrospinal fluid, snyovial fluid, and other tissues provides rapid presumptive evidence of infection. The diagnosis is confirmed if *N. meningitidis* is isolated from these specimens.

The rapid onset of life-threatening symptoms requires that antibiotic therapy be initiated while waiting for confirmation of the presumptive diagnosis. Penicillin is the drug of choice for meningococcal meningitidis. Prophylactic antibiotic therapy is recommended for even casual contacts of the patients. Since meningococcal disease is spread primarily from carriers, these individuals may be treated with sulfadiazine or rifampin to eliminate the organisms from their pharyngeal tissues.

Immunity

Protective immunity that is specific for the polysaccharide capsules develops after clinical or subclinical infections. An individual immune to one serotype may be susceptible to another. The antibody does not eliminate meningococci that have colonized the nasopharynx. Two capsular polysaccharide vaccines are available, but they are administered only to special high-risk populations, such as exposed military personnel. Bivalent and quadrivalent vaccines are both administered as single dose injections.

NEISSERIA GONORRHOEAE

Neisseria gonorrhoeae, the etiologic agent of gonorrhea, is commonly referred to as the gonococcus. Gonorrhea has reached epidemic proportions in the United States, as two to three million new cases of the disease now occur each year. *Neisseria gonorrhoeae* is second only to *Chlamydia trachomatis* (the agent for nongonococcal urethritis) as a predominant cause of sexually transmitted disease. Sexual transmission accounts for almost all adult infections. Most infections are genital, but the incidence of anorectal and pharyngeal gonorrhea has been rising steadily.

Virulence Factors

Neisseria gonorrhoeae cells possess pili through which the cells attach to mucosal epithelial cells. The pili appear to be necessary for colonization and infection because nonpiliated cells are avirulent. Antibody directed against the pili can prevent infection, and a vaccine composed of antigens derived from pili is being studied. Like *N. meningitidis,* the gonococcus also produces a proteolytic enzyme that cleaves IgA1. The actual role of this IgA protease in the disease process is unknown. These bacteria also possess a cytotoxic endotoxin that is thought to be involved in the disease process.

Pathogenicity

Transmission of the disease is by contact with infectious exudates. Genital infection in men is characterized by painful urination and a purulent urethral discharge. If left untreated, the patient may develop a chronic exudate (ie, gleet). The endocervix is the primary site of infection in women. Symptoms include a purulent exudate and an erythematous, edematous cervix. The disease frequently spreads to the endometrium, fallopian tubes, and peritoneum. These manifestations are collectively called acute pelvic inflammatory disease (PID). This systemic syndrome may be caused by other microorganisms, but *N. gonorrhoeae* is the causative agent in about 40% of PID cases. Further progression of the disease may result in disseminated gonococcal infection. About 5% of male and 50% of female patients are relatively asymptomatic, and these constitute a serious source for transmission of the disease. Protective immunity does not occur after gonococcal diseases, and subjects may be reinfected repeatedly.

Pharyngeal gonorrhea can occur either as a primary infection or as a secondary manifestation of infection at a different site in the body. Oral lesions usually are primary infections resulting from orogenital contact. Symptoms are nondescript and may include sore throat, gingivitis, foul breath, and cervical lymphadenopathy. Throat cultures are necessary to diagnose oral infections.

Anorectal gonorrhea is increasing in prevalence. Common symptoms of anorectal pain, bleeding, and discharge are seen mostly in male homosexuals. Symptomatic proctitis, however, occurs in only about 10% of patients with positive rectal cultures.

Ophthalmia neonatorum is a conjunctival disease of infants acquired from infected mothers during passage through the birth canal or in the postpartum period. In the United States, routine instillation of 1% silver nitrate into the eyes of newborns has been a very successful prophylactic measure, but opthalmia neonatorum is still an important cause of blindness among children in developing countries.

Diagnosis and Treatment

The clinical features of gonococcal and chlamydial infections in neonates and adults are remarkably similar, and gonorrhea cannot be diagnosed on symptomatology alone. Diagnosis is additionally complicated because both infections often coexist in the same site. The presence of intracellular gram-negative diplococci in urethral exudate smears is diagnostic of *N. gonorrhoeae* in males. In females, however, stained smears of cervical exudate may be as little as 50% accurate. If the organisms are found extracellularly, they must be cultivated for diagnosis. Since commensal *Neisseria* are members of the normal flora of the pharyngeal tissues, stained smears of pharyngeal exudates cannot be used for definitive diagnosis of gonorrhea. Confirmation rests on culturing the gonococcus from clinical specimens.

Aqueous procaine pencillin, ampicillin, or amoxicillin with probenicid is used to treat uncomplicated genital gonorrhea. Spectinomycin or tetracycline is used in patients allergic to penicillin. Until relatively recently, gonococci were considered to be universally susceptible to penicillin. Strains that produce β-lactamase (penicillinase-producing *N. gonorrhoeae,* or PPNG) have appeared throughout the world, however, and this has developed into a serious chemotherapeutic problem. The incidence of PPNG infections in the United States is low but increasing. PPNG are treated with spectinomycin.

Prevention

Prevention and control of gonorrhea are based on the tracing and treatment of sexual contacts of infected patients. Physicians are legally required to report gonorrheal cases to local health authorities in many states and countries. Contacts usually are treated without waiting for laboratory confirmation of gonococcal infection. Because the most common cause of treatment failure is reinfection, patient education, accurate reporting, and follow-up of patients and their contacts constitute the best means of prevention.

Although immunity to reinfection is not established as a result of prior infection, studies in human volunteers indicate that a vaccine composed of gonococcal pili may be effective. Since there is a great deal of antigenic heterogeneity among gonococcal pili, a clinically useful vaccine will have to include several different antigens.

ORAL ASPECTS

The *Neisseria* may present problems to clinicians for several reasons. Gonorrhea and the meningococcal carrier state both may involve asymptomatic or relatively asymptomatic colonization of the nasopharynx. Therefore, dental personnel obviously are at a higher risk of infection. This is probably of low concern with *N. meningitidis,* except during epidemics or where isolated cases have been reported among a clinician's potential patient population. Oral gonorrhea poses special problems for dental personnel because (1) the incidence of oral infections has increased with changing sexual practices, (2) the asymptomatic state can mask a potential infectious hazard, (3) the chances for gonococcal dissemination increase in the absence of appropriate treatment, and (4) transfer of gonococcal infection to adjacent tissues can occur via dental procedures. For example, extraction of teeth from patients with oral gonorrhea may lead to a severe gonococcal osteitis. If oral gonorrhea is suspected, precautions should be exercised until the specific infection is diagnosed. Such precautions include the provision for only emergency care initially and a heightened awareness of aseptic techniques.

SUGGESTED READINGS

Band JD, Chamberland ME, Platt T, et al. Trend in meningococcal disease in the United States, 1975–1980. *J Infect Dis.* 1983;148:754–758.

Black JR, Sparling PF. *Neisseria gonorrhoeae.* In: Mandell GL, Douglas RG, Bennett JE, eds. *Principles and Practice of Infectious Diseases.* New York: John Wiley & Sons; 1985:1195.

Centers for Disease Control. Bacterial meningitis and meningococcemia—United States 1978. *MMWR.* 1979;28:277–279.

Centers for Disease Control. Sexually transmitted diseases treatment guidelines. *MMWR.* 1985;34:75S–100S.

Chue PWY. Gonorrhea—Its natural history, oral manifestations, diagnosis, treatment and prevention. *J Am Dent Assoc.* 1975;90:1297–1301.

Dalabetta G, Hook EW III. Gonococcal infections. In: Handsfield HH, ed. *Sexually Transmitted Diseases. Infectious Disease Clinics of North America.* Philadelphia: WB Saunders; 1987:25.

DeVoe IW. The meningococcus and mechanisms of pathogenicity. *Microbiol Rev.* 1982;46:162–190.

Holmes K, Buchanan TM, Adam JL, Eschenbach DL. Is serology useful in gonorrhea? A critical analysis of factors influencing serodiagnosis. In: Brooks GF, Gotschlich E, Homes K, Sawyer W, Young F, eds. *Immunobiology of Neisseria gonorrhoeae.* Washington, DC: American Society for Microbiology; 1978;61–76.

Holmes KK, Mardh PA, Sparling PF, Wiesner PJ. *Sexually Transmitted Diseases.* New York: McGraw-Hill Book Company; 1984.

Hook EW, Holmes KK. Gonococcal infections. *Ann Intern Med.* 1985;102:229–243.

Hutt DM, Judson FN. Epidemiology and treatment of oropharnygeal gonorrhea. *Ann Intern Med.* 1986;104:655–658.

Laga M, Plummer FA, Piot P, Datta P, et al. Prophylaxis of gonococcal and chlamydial opthalmia neonatorum. *N Engl J Med.* 1988;318:653–657.

Treatment of sexually transmitted diseases. *Med Lett.* 1986; 28:23–28.

Wiesner PJ, Tronca E, Bonin P, Pedersen AHB, Holmes KK. Clinical spectrum of pharyngeal gonococcal infection. *N Engl J Med.* 1973;288:181–185.

CHAPTER 13

Corynebacteria

Robert R. White

INTRODUCTION

CORYNEBACTERIUM DIPHTHERIAE
- Morphology
- Virulence Factors
- Disease Process
- Diagnosis
- Treatment
- Epidemiology
- Prevention

DIPHTHEROIDS

ORAL ASPECTS

SUGGESTED READINGS

INTRODUCTION

The corynebacteria are a large group of bacteria consisting of saprophytes found throughout nature and pathogens of humans and other animals. *Corynebacterium diphtheriae,* the major human pathogen, is the agent for diphtheria, a disease in which infection of the pharynx and larynx serves as the source of a potent exotoxin that can cause a fatal toxemia. Diphtheria can be controlled readily by immunization, but as a result of public apathy concerning the disease, sporadic cases and epidemics still occur. This, coupled with its occurrence in an area adjacent to the oral cavity, makes it of continuing significance to dental personnel.

CORYNEBACTERIUM DIPHTHERIAE

Morphology

Corynebacteria are gram-positive, nonsporeforming rods that appear to be arranged in palisade or Chinese letter formations when viewed microscopically. The bacteria are pleomorphic, and club-shaped cells are characteristic. Intracytoplasmic granules (metachromatic granules, Babes-Ernst bodies) are visible when the cells are stained with methylene blue or toluidine blue. The granules, which contain polymerized polyphosphate, give the cells a beaded appearance. *Corynebacterium diphtheriae* is aerobic or facultatively anaerobic and grows on most laboratory media.

Virulence Factors

Diphtheria is a toxemia. The organism is only slightly invasive, but it produces a potent exotoxin that diffuses from the superficial site of infection and causes severe, sometimes fatal, systemic effects. The toxin is a heat-labile protein consisting of a single polypeptide chain with a molecular weight of 62,000. The toxin blocks protein synthesis by inhibiting polypeptide synthesis. It catalyzes a reaction that inactivates elongation factor 2 (EF-2), which is required for translocating polypeptide-transfer RNA on the ribosome. Ultimately, this results in degeneration of the cells of heart, kidney, and other tissues and demyelinization of nerve tissue.

The toxin is produced as a result of the presence of a bacteriophage within the bacterium. The phase genome carries the genetic information (the *tox+* gene) responsible for toxigenicity. Lysogenic bacteria produce the toxin, and nonlysogenic bacteria do not. The latter can be converted to the virulent, toxigenic state by infection with the phage. When this was discovered, it was the first known example of the role of lysogeny as a determinant of virulence.

Disease Process

Diphtheria is usually a localized infection, but the exotoxin produced by the bacteria causes injury in areas distant from the tissue colonized by the organism. The bacteria initially establish a superficial infection of the tonsils or pharynx (pharyngeal diphtheria). The infection may spread into the nasopharynx or down into the the larynx and trachea. Exotoxin secreted by the bacteria kills the epithelial cells, and this injury stimulates an intense localized inflammatory response. The inflammatory exudate, infiltrating leukocytes, dying epithelial cells, and bacteria form a firmly adherent grayish pseudomembrane. Rarely, it may spread into the oral cavity. The pseudomembrane may obstruct the upper respiratory tract, and intubation or tracheotomy may be required to prevent suffocation. In severe infections, enlargement of the regional lymph nodes and edema in the surrounding tissues cause a bullneck appearance.

The exotoxin diffuses into the tissues and spreads throughout the body to injure organs and tissues remote from the site of infection. Various organs and tissues may be affected, but the most serious injury occurs in the heart and peripheral nerves. Toxic myocarditis may occur, and congestive heart failure is the major cause of death from diphtheria. Diphtheria causes demyelinization of the nerves, which may be accompanied by neurologic complications ranging from mild weakness to complete paralysis.

Corynebacterium diphtheriae also can infect other areas of the body. Diphtheritic infections of skin wounds are common in tropical climates and are increasing in the southern part of the United States. The infections are superficial, and the amount of exotoxin absorbed through the skin and the subsequent systemic effects are considered insignificant.

Diagnosis

Diagnosis of diphtheria is dependent on isolation and identification of a toxigenic strain of *C. diphtheriae*. Specimens, preferably from the pseudomembrane, are inoculated on Loeffler's medium, tellurite agar, and blood agar. Loeffler's medium is selective for the diphtheria bacillus, and the blood agar is used to detect group A streptococci, which cause an infection that can be mistaken for diphtheria and also can coinfect the same site. The presence of gray or black colonies on tellurite agar is indicative of diphtheria, but this must be confirmed because colonies of other bacteria such as staphylococci may resemble *C. diphtheriae* colonies. Microscopic examination of a simple stained smear should reveal the characteristic pleomorphic cells in palisade or Chinese letter formations.

Toxin production by the isolated organisms must be confirmed by an in vitro gel diffusion test or an in vivo virulence test. In the in vitro Elek test, a strip of sterile filter paper containing diphtheria antitoxin is embedded in culture medium, and suspected strains of *C. diphtheriae* are streaked on the surface of the medium in single lines perpendicular to the filter strip. Toxin produced by virulent strains will diffuse from the line of growth and form an immune precipitate as it complexes with antitoxin diffusing from the filter strip (Fig. 13–1). The presence of the immune precipitate is confirmatory evidence of virulent, toxigenic *C. diphtheriae*. An in vivo virulence test may be carried out by injecting suspected cultures intraperitoneally into two guinea pigs, one of which previously has received antitoxin and one that is untreated. If the culture is toxigenic, the untreated guinea pig will die within 3 to 5 days. The antitoxin-treated animal will survive.

Treatment

The exotoxin is the predominant factor involved in diphtheria, and neutralization of the toxin with specific antitoxin is the only effective therapy. Antitoxin must be administered as soon as diphtheria is suspected because the toxin cannot be neutralized after it reacts with the host's tissues. In isolated cases, the antitoxin is administered immediately after confirming the presence of the organism on tellurite medium. During epidemics, antitoxin therapy is commenced as soon as a patient exhibits the pharyngeal symptoms

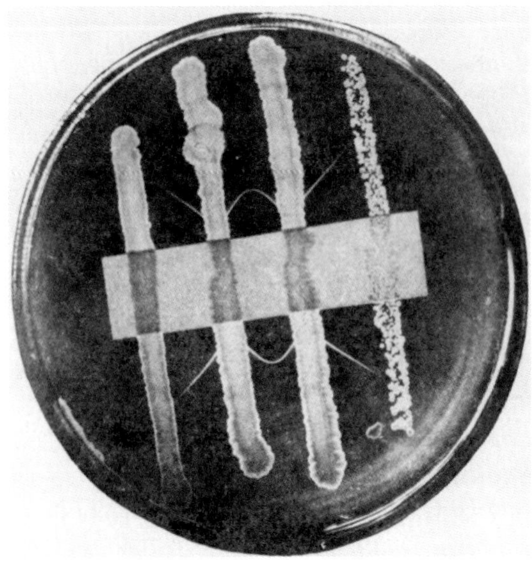

Figure 13–1. Elek test for detection of toxigenic *C. diphtheriae*. The precipitate bands confirm that the two strains in the center are toxigenic. *(From* Am J Pub Health. *1949; 39:1316.)*

characteristic of diphtheria. Before administration of the antitoxin, patients are skin tested to determine if they are allergic to the antisera, which are produced in horses and other animals.

Erythromycin and penicillin are useless against the toxemia but can affect the bacteria at the site of infection and reduce or terminate the production of toxin. Erythromycin is especially useful in reducing or eliminating the carrier state.

Epidemiology

The incidence of diphtheria declined rapidly following the introduction of the toxoid vaccine (Fig 13–2). Except when rare epidemics occur, there are usually less than 200 cases per year in the United States. The decreased incidence, although welcome, has caused problems. The decline led to a decreased awareness of the disease, with a subsequent failure of parents, especially those in lower socioeconomic groups, to have their children immunized. Therefore, despite the efficacy of the vaccine, sporadic cases and epidemics still occur. In addition, since there are fewer cases and carriers, the natural exposure to the toxin that was common before the use of the vaccine and that served as booster immunization has lessened considerably. Today, many more adults are susceptible to the disease. Whereas diphtheria was once a disease of childhood, it now occurs much more often in the postadolescent years.

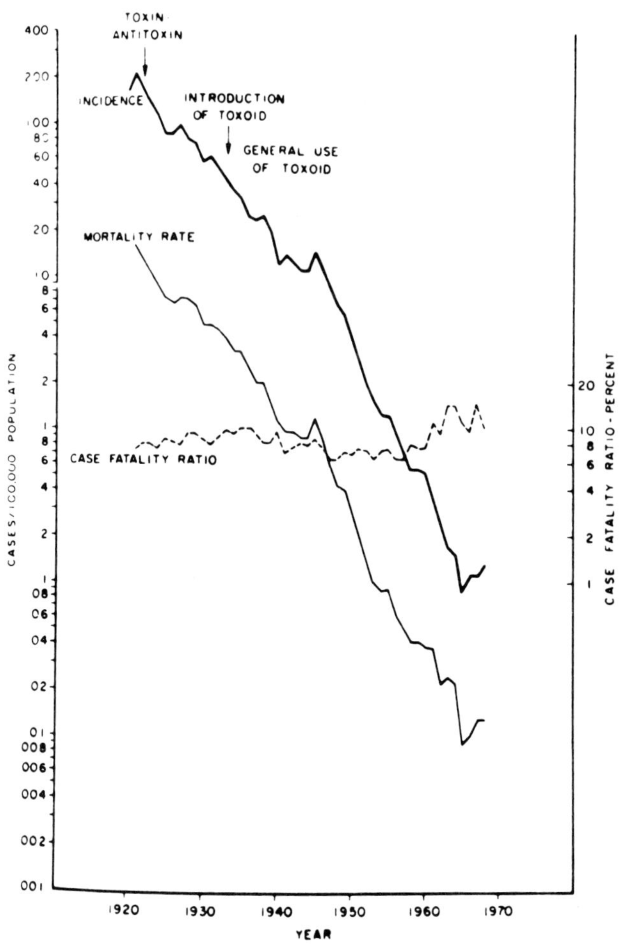

Figure 13–2. Incidence of diphtheria in the United States from time of introduction of toxoid to 1970. *(From* Morb Mort Wk Rep. *1970; 19:55.)*

Humans are the only natural host of *C. diphtheriae*, and transmission is usually by droplets from the upper respiratory tract of active cases and healthy or convalescent carriers. Cutaneous lesions also may serve as a source of infection.

Prevention

Prevention of diphtheria is accomplished by immunization against the toxin, which is of one antigenic type. A harmless toxoid that retains its antigenicity is produced by treating culture supernatants of *C. diphtheriae* with formalin. The toxoid is adsorbed to alum or aluminum phosphate, which act as adjuvants. This preparation usually is administered to children in the DPT vaccine, a mixture containing diphtheria and tetanus toxoids and killed *Bordetella pertussis* (the agent for whooping cough) cells. The recommended immunization regimen is noted in Table 8–1. Since allergy to *C. diphtheriae* antigens is common among adults, they usually are not immunized until their immune status has been evaluated with a Schick test. This skin test can determine if an individual possesses antitoxic immunity or allergy to diphtheria antigens. Adults who are found to be nonimmune may be immunized with the toxoid.

DIPHTHEROIDS

Diphtheroids is a designation referring to a variety of bacteria that are related to or morphologically similar to *C. diphtheriae*. Many reports in the literature that were derived from microscopic analyses of bacterial specimens refer to all pleomorphic gram-positive bacilli as diphtheroids. Subsequent investigations revealed that many of these diphtheroids were probably members of other genera. In addition, several species that were once classified in the genus *Corynebacterium* have been reclassified. For example, the anaerobic diphtheroid associated with acne, *Propionibacterium acnes* once was classified as *Corynebacterium acnes*.

Several corynebacteria other than *C. diphtheriae* commonly are isolated from humans. *Corynebacterium pseudodiphtheriticum* is found in the oropharynx, and *Corynebacterium xerosis* is found in the conjunctiva and on the skin. Both species grow on tellurite medium, but neither is toxigenic. *Corynebacterium ulcerans* is toxigenic, and there are several reports of diphtheria caused by this *Corynebacterium* species. One of the most frequent infections associated with these and other corynebacteria such as group JK is endocarditis in medically compromised individuals.

ORAL ASPECTS

Oral infections with *C. diphtheriae* are not common. In severe cases of pharyngeal diphtheria, the pseudomembrane may extend into the oral cavity, and instances in which the whole oral cavity was covered have been described. Palatal paralysis is one of the initial and most common neurologic complications. The tongue and muscles of mastication are involved less frequently. Recovery from paralysis is the rule. Local diphtheritic lesions of the lips, tongue, mucosa, and commissures of the mouth and in association with erupting teeth have been reported to occur in rare cases.

Carriers may be of some dental significance. *Corynebacterium diphtheriae* colonies in the nasopharynx serve as a source of bacteria that are continually disseminated into saliva. Under normal conditions, the carrier rate is so low as to not pose a problem. This potential danger, however, is accentuated during epidemics, in which carrier rates as high as 30% have been reported.

SUGGESTED READINGS

Bainton D, Freeman J, Magrath DI, Sheffield F, Smith JWG. Immunity of children to diphtheria, tetanus, and poliomyelitis. *Br Med J.* 1979;1:854.

Lipsky BA, Goldberger AC, Tompkins LS, Plorde JJ. Infections caused by nondiphtheria corynebacteria. *Rev Infect Dis.* 1982;4:1220.

McGowan JE. JK coryneforms: A continuing problem for hospital infection control. *J Hosp Infect.* 1988;11:A3581

Pappenheimer AM. Diphtheria toxin. *Annu Rev Biochem.* 1977;46:69.

Willett HP. Corynebacterium. In: Joklik WK, Willett HP, Amos DB, Wifert CM, eds. *Zinsser Microbiology,* 18th ed. E. Norwalk, Conn: Appleton & Lange; 1989.

Youmans GP. Diphtheria. In: Youmans GP. Paterson PY, Sommers HM, eds. *The Biologic and Clinical Basis of Infectious Diseases,* 3rd ed. Philadelphia: WB Saunders; 1985.

Zalma VM, Older JJ, Brooks GF. The Austin, Texas, diphtheria outbreak: Clinical and epidemiological aspets. *JAMA.* 1970;211:2125.

CHAPTER 14

Clostridium

Mary Ann Gerencser and Vincent F. Gerencser

INTRODUCTION
MORPHOLOGY, CLASSIFICATION, AND IDENTIFICATION
CULTIVATION
CLOSTRIDIUM BOTULINUM
- Virulence Factors
- Disease
- Diagnosis
- Treatment
- Epidemiology

CLOSTRIDIUM TETANI
- Virulence Factors
- Disease
- Diagnosis
- Treatment
- Epidemiology

CLOSTRIDIUM PERFRINGENS AND OTHER HISTOTOXIC CLOSTRIDIA
- Virulence Factors
- Diseases
- Diagnosis
- Treatment
- Epidemiology

CLOSTRIDIUM DIFFICILE
- Virulence Factors
- Disease
- Diagnosis
- Treatment

ORAL ASPECTS
SUGGESTED READINGS

INTRODUCTION

The genus *Clostridium* contains over 80 recognized species, many of which are soil saprophytes. Frankly pathogenic species include the agents of botulism, tetanus, clostridial myonecrosis, and antibiotic-associated pseudomembranous colitis. Pathogenic species may be found in the soil, in fresh water and marine sediments, and on the skin and in the intestinal tracts of humans and animals. *Clostridium* species are found occasionally in the human mouth, probably as transients rather than as resident inhabitants. Clostridia are the only medically important anaerobes that are found regularly in nature and cause diseases of exogenous origin. However, like other anaerobic infections, clostridial infections may be of endogenous origin. Because of their ubiquitous nature, clostridia isolated from clinical specimens are often contaminants and are not involved in the disease process. Therefore, the significance of these bacteria in clinical specimens must be assessed carefully in relationship to the patient's clinical condition and history.

MORPHOLOGY, CLASSIFICATION, AND IDENTIFICATION

Clostridia are gram-positive, sporeforming rods (Fig. 14–1). Some species lose the stain readily and appear as large gram-negative rods. Spores may be round or oval and located in a terminal or subterminal position in the cell.

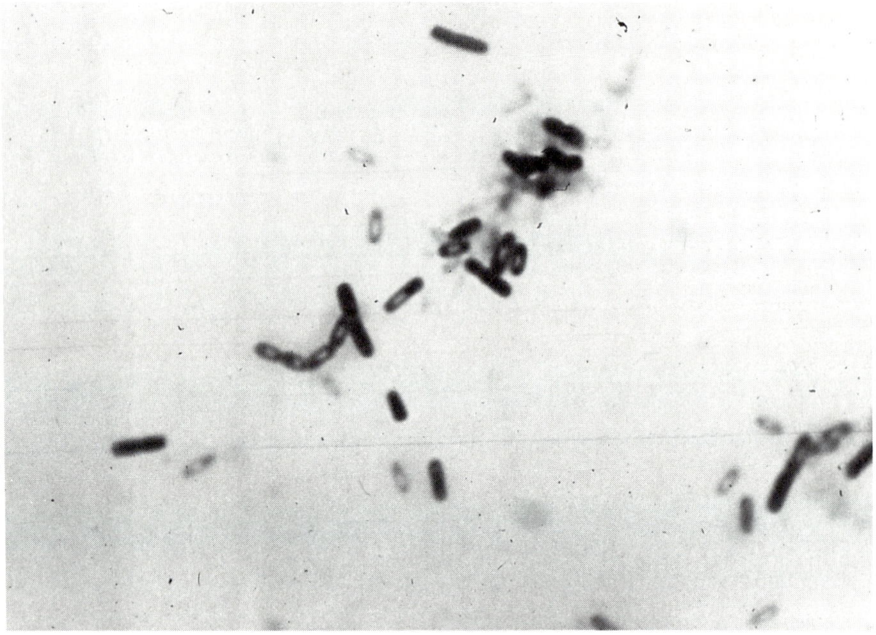

Figure 14–1. *Clostridium bifermentans* with oval, subterminal spores. *(Courtesy of Dr. V.R. Dowell, Jr., Centers for Disease Control, Atlanta, GA.)*

Clostridium species are identified on the basis of shape and position of spore, biochemical reactions, metabolic end products determined by gas-liquid chromatography, and the production of specific toxins. Some characteristics of the major pathogenic species are given in Table 14–1.

TABLE 14–1. SOME CHARACTERISTICS OF FOUR *CLOSTRIDIUM* SPECIES

Species	Important Characteristics	Disease(s)
C. botulinum	4 cultural groups; oval, subterminal spores; produces lipase; toxin test necessary for identification; toxin divided into 7 serologic types	Botulinum food poisoning (adult); infant botulism; wound botulism
C. tetani	Round, terminal spores; swarms on blood agar; asaccharolytic; 3 toxins; tetanospasmin produces disease symptoms	Tetanus
C. perfringens	Nonmotile; spores rarely found; double zone hemolysis; produces lecithinase; 12 toxins including 4 major lethal toxins	Myonecrosis (gas gangrene) and other wound infections (can be due to other histotoxic clostridia); food poisoning; enteritis necroticans
C. difficile	Oval, subterminal spores; characteristic colonies; distinctive p-creosol-like odor; produce a major peak of isocaproic acid in GLC; ferments mannitol; 2 toxins	Antibiotic-associated pseudomembranous colitis (PMC)

CULTIVATION

The clostridia are anaerobic but vary from strict anaerobes (*Clostridium haemolyticum*) to aerotolerant (*Clostridium tertium*) species. They also vary widely in nutritional and temperature requirements. Clinically important species are generally moderate anaerobes that are mesophilic and grow on routine laboratory media. Freshly poured blood agar plates are suitable for the growth and isolation of clostridia. Egg yolk medium and chopped meat glucose medium are also useful in cultivating clostridia.

CLOSTRIDIUM BOTULINUM

Clostridium botulinum, the etiologic agent of botulism, is a heterogeneous group of organisms that are given a common species name because they produce toxins with identical pharmacologic activity. The toxins are divided into seven serologic types A,B,C_1,D,E,F, and G. Recent information suggests that the toxin formerly designated C_2 is different from other botulinum toxins and is not a cause of botulism. Toxin types A, B, E, and F are the major causes of botulism in humans, whereas types C_1 and D are found mainly in birds and mammals. *Clostridium botulinum* type G has been isolated at autopsy from cases of sudden death but has not been definitely implicated in disease production.

Virulence Factors

Botulinum toxin is the most potent toxin known. One gram of toxin contains 10^8 to 10^9 mouse lethal doses, and it is estimated that 10^{-8} g is fatal to humans. The toxin is produced during the growth of vegetative cells of *C. botulinum* and is released when the cells lyse. All antigenic types of the toxin are protein with a molecular weight of about 150,000. The toxin is acid resistant and can pass through the stomach, but it is inactivated by alkali and is heat labile, being destroyed by heating at 80°C for 10 minutes. The toxins act presynaptically on peripheral nerves to prevent the passage of nerve impulses from motor nerves to the muscle by inhibiting the release of acetylcholine at the myoneural junction.

Disease

Botulism occurs in three forms: classic food poisoning, infant botulism, and wound botulism. Food poisoning is an intoxication that results from the ingestion of preformed toxin in food. Symptoms usually begin 18 to 36 hours after ingestion of the toxin but may be delayed up to 8 days. The first symptoms are gastrointestinal, including nausea and vomiting and occasionally diarrhea. These are followed by neurologic symptoms that affect the head and neck. Diplopia (double vision), dysphasia (difficulty in speaking), and dysphagia (difficulty in swallowing) are among the common symptoms. Increasing weakness of the muscles leads to flaccid paralysis. Death is most often due to respiratory paralysis. The mortality rate has declined from over 60% between the years 1899 and 1950 to 15.7% in the years 1970 to 1977. Improvement in diagnosis, the availability of antitoxin therapy, and modern respiratory support measures account for the reduced case fatality rate.

Infant botulism occurs in infants less than 6 months of age and results from the production of toxin by vegetative cells growing in the intestinal tract. The symptoms include weakness of the head, face, and throat muscles, with a depression of the suck and gag reflexes, and is called the floppy baby syndrome. Infant botulism may cause cases of sudden death that resemble sudden infant death syndrome (SIDS), or crib death.

Wound botulism, the rarest form of the disease, occurs when a wound is contaminated by *C. botulinum* from the soil. It has been associated with drug abuse in recent years. Toxin is produced in the wound, causing the symptoms of botulism.

Diagnosis

Confirmation of a clinical diagnosis of botulism requires demonstration of the toxin in patient's serum or feces or in the suspected food. Isolation of the organism from the patient's feces is helpful but is less direct confirmation of disease etiology. In infant cases, the diagnosis depends on the demonstration of toxin in the feces, since toxin has only been demonstrated rarely in the sera of infants.

Treatment

Treatment of botulism is aimed at providing general supportive care and eliminating or neutralizing any unbound toxin. Intensive respiratory support is essential. Unbound toxin in the gastrointestinal tract may be eliminated by high colonic enemas and cathartics. Trivalent A, B, E antitoxin is administered to neutralize unbound toxin in tissue and blood. Penicillin is used to eliminate the organisms growing in the intestinal tracts of children with infant botulism.

Epidemiology

Spores of *C. botulinum* are found in soil and in marine sediments throughout the world. In the United States, type A spores dominate in western soil samples, whereas type B spores dominate in the east. Type E botulinum spores are found frequently in the Great Lakes region and in Alaska.

Botulism food poisoning originally was associated with meat and meat products. The name itself is derived from the latin *botulus,* meaning sausage. In the United States, most outbreaks are associated with vegetables, such as green beans, peppers, mushrooms, or onions. Other sources may be involved, including fish, fruits, and condiments that have been home-canned. Alaskan outbreaks have been highly associated with fish or other marine foods prepared by traditional methods of the Eskimo and Indian populations. These Alaskan outbreaks are often due to toxin type E, whereas most of the foodborne botulism in the continental United States is due to toxin type A or B. No single food has been implicated in infant botulism. The only food currently considered a risk factor in infants is honey, but only a relatively few cases have been associated with it.

The use of adequate methods of food preparation and preservation is essential in preventing botulism. Any home-canned food should be heated to boiling for at least 1 minute or to 80°C for 10 minutes before being eaten to destroy any toxin that might be present.

CLOSTRIDIUM TETANI

Clostridium tetani, the etiologic agent of tetanus, is a slender bacillus with round, terminal spores that give the organisms a characteristic drumstick appearance. This species does not ferment any carbohydrates. It is actively motile and swarms on the surface of blood agar plates, producing a thin, translucent film of growth.

Virulence Factors

Clostridium tetani produces three toxins: the spasmogenic toxin (tetanospasmin), a nonspasmogenic toxin, and a hemolysin. Tetanospasmin is responsible for the typical symptoms of the disease. There is only one antigenic type. Tetanospasmin binds to gangliosides and inhibits the release of inhibitory transmitters at interneurons. Instead of causing a flaccid paralysis, as does botulinum toxin, tetanus toxin causes increasing muscle spasticity.

The nonspasmogenic toxin acts peripherally and may have some paralytic effects, but its role in human disease has not been clearly defined. The hemolysin is probably not important in human disease.

Disease

Tetanus follows the contamination of a wound with *C. tetani*. The incubation period may be from a few days to a few weeks. In generalized (descending) tetanus, the toxin is carried by the lymphatics and the bloodstream to the central nervous system. The earliest symptoms involve the head and neck, especially the masseter muscles. Spasm of the jaw muscles leads to trismus or lockjaw, which progresses to a grimace known as riscus sardonicus. The disease progresses to involve the arms, trunk, and legs, including an arching of the back called opisthotonos. Muscle spasms are frequent, intense, painful, and exhausting. Death is due to pulmonary complications or to cardiac arrest. The mortality rate for tetanus is 55 to 65%.

Occasionally, a localized form of tetanus known as ascending tetanus occurs. This form may be seen in patients with low levels of immunity. In this form, the toxin is taken up by local motor nerves and travels along the tissue spaces of the peripheral nerves to the central nervous system. Muscles near the wound are involved first, and the disease usually is confined to the extremities.

Diagnosis

The diagnosis of tetanus is based on clinical symptoms. Tetanus must be differentiated from strychnine poisoning, encephalitis, and phenothiazine reactions. Attempts should be made to isolate *C. tetani*, but it has been isolated in only about one third of the cases.

Treatment

Treatment of diagnosed tetanus is aimed at removing the source of the toxin and at neutralizing any unbound toxin. Removal of the offending organisms can be accomplished by debridement of the wound and large doses of pencillin or other suitable antibiotics. Human tetanus antitoxin is given to neutralize toxin that is not already bound to nerve tissue. Barbiturates, diazepam, or in severe cases, a curarelike drug are used to control the muscle spasms.

Prophylactic treatment of wounds should include removal of devitalized tissue and foreign bodies and administration of tetanus toxoid depending on the immunization history of the patient. In the case of clean, minor wounds, toxoid is given if the patient has not had a booster injection within 5 years. For serious wounds, both tetanus toxoid and a prophylactic dose of human tetanus immune globulin are given.

Tetanus is preventable by active immunization with a series of three doses of the toxoid (formalin-inactivated toxin), using diphtheria-pertussis-tetanus vaccine (DPT). Booster doses of the toxoid should be given every 10 years.

Epidemiology

Clostridium tetani occurs worldwide in soil and is found more frequently in cultivated soil. Sometimes, it is found in the gastrointestinal tract of humans and animals. *Clostridium tetani* can be found wherever there is dust contamination because the spores withstand both drying and light. The disease occurs sporadically. It occurs following deep, penetrating wounds, is found in heroin addicts, and occurs as tetanus neonatorum when there is improper cutting and care of the umbilical cord. Tetanus has been reported after tooth extraction, dental caries, and dental abscesses, but such cases are rare.

CLOSTRIDIUM PERFRINGENS AND OTHER HISTOTOXIC CLOSTRIDIA

Histotoxic clostridia cause a variety of wound infections, the most serious of which is clostridial myonecrosis, or gas gangrene. The most important and frequently isolated of the histotoxic clostridia is *Clostridum perfringens*, a short, plump, nonmotile rod that rarely forms spores on ordinary culture media. Typically, it produces a double-zone hemolysis on blood agar plates consisting of a narrow zone of complete hemolysis surrounded by a wider zone of incomplete hemolysis.

Virulence Factors

Clostridium perfringens produces 12 toxins, 4 of which are major lethal toxins. The species is divided into five bacterial types (A, B, C, D, E) on the basis of these 4 toxins. Most human disease is caused by strains of type A. The α-toxin (lecithinase C or phospholipase C) is the most important of the lethal toxins and is produced by all types. This toxin acts on lipoprotein complexes in cell membranes and probably on mitochondria.

Diseases

Clostridial wound infections are generally polymicrobial, containing one or more species of *Clostridium* and a variety of facultative bacteria. *Clostridium perfringens* (80%) is the most frequently isolated primary pathogen, followed by *Clostridium novyi* (40%) and *Clostridium septicum* (20%). *Clostridium sordellii, Clostridium histolyticum,* and *Clostridium fallax* are found less frequently. Clinically, wound infections may be categorized as (1) simple contamination, (2) anaerobic cellulitis, or (3) clostridial myonecrosis (gas gangrene). All these infections occur where there is a reduced blood supply producing anaerobic conditions in the tissues (trauma, surgery, or malignancies).

In simple contamination, necrotic tissue is superficially contaminated with a clostridium and a variety of facultative bacteria. Despite the isolation of clostridia, the wound usually heals normally with little or no signs of infection.

In anaerobic cellulitis, clostridia infect dead muscle tissue but do not invade healthy muscle. The disease may spread along fascial planes between muscles. Gas is produced, so that the disease may resemble true gas gangrene.

The most serious of the wound infections is clostridial myonecrosis in which the clostridia not only infect necrotic tissue but invade and destroy healthy muscle tissue. The exotoxins are released into surrounding tissue, producing additional necrosis and permitting the infection to expand. Gas is produced in the tissue, and there is a systemic toxemia not seen in anaerobic cellulitis.

Clostridium perfringens is an important cause of food poisoning in addition to its role in serious wound infections. Food poisoning due to *C. perfringens* is usually a mild disease that is very common in the United States and is caused by type A. Eight to twelve hours after the ingestion of a large number of vegetative cells, the patient experiences abdominal cramps and diarrhea. The symptoms are due to an enterotoxin that is produced when the vegetative cells sporulate in the intestine. Meat dishes, gravies, thick sauces, and casseroles are the types of food most often associated with *C. perfringens* food poisoning. A more serious gastrointestinal illness, enteritis necroticans, is also caused by *C. perfringens.* This disease is associated with type C organisms.

Diagnosis

The diagnosis of clostridial myonecrosis is based on clinical symptoms. Laboratory confirmation is based on finding large numbers of big gram-positive rods in direct smears of material from the wound and in cultures. Spores are not seen in clinical material or in cultures from *C. perfringens* infections but may be seen in material from infections with other histotoxic clostridia. Cultures are identified by gas chromatography and by biochemical reactions. It should be remembered that the mere presence of clostridia in a wound does not establish a diagnosis of gas gangrene.

Treatment

The less serious wound infections are treated by cleaning and debridement of the wound and the use of antibiotics. Penicillin is the antibiotic of choice. Clostridial myonecrosis requires immediate removal of all necrotic tissue, which may include such radical surgery as amputation. Antibiotic therapy is used to rid the wound of viable organisms. Antitoxin therapy also is used in gas gangrene, although there is some question as to its value. Another treatment that is somewhat controversial is the use of hyperbaric oxygen therapy.

Epidemiology

Clostridium perfringens, type A, is found worldwide in soil and in the intestinal tract of humans and animals. The other types are found mainly in the intestinal tract of animals and only occasionally in the soil. Infections may be from either exogenous or endogenous sources.

CLOSTRIDIUM DIFFICILE

Pseudomembranous colitis (PMC) develops in some patients following the use of a variety of antibiotics. Ampicillin, clindamycin, and cephalosporins are the antibiotics most commonly implicated, but almost all agents, with the exception of vancomycin, have been implicated in PMC. The etiologic agent of this disease is *Clostridium difficile.* It is also the agent of about one fourth of the cases of antibiotic-associated diarrhea and has been implicated in some cases of colitis following cancer chemotherapy.

Clostridium difficile is both proteolytic and saccharolytic and, like other clostridia, can be identified by cultural and biochemical reactions. A highly selective medium (closerine-cefoxitin-fructose agar) has been designed on which *C. difficile* forms large colonies that fluoresce chartreuse green. Various typing schemes, including biotying, antibiograms, detection of extracellular antigens and toxins, polyacrylamide gel electrophoresis of proteins, and bacteriophage, are being used experimentally for epidemiologic studies. In addition, there are a number of tests for the detection of the cytopathic toxin or the enterotoxin.

Virulence Factors

Clostridium difficile produces two toxins, both of which seem to be necessary for disease production. Toxin A is an enterotoxin that causes the secretion of hemorrhagic fluid into ligated intestinal loops in laboratory animals, but its mode of action is unknown. Toxin B is a cytotoxin, and its mode of action also is unknown. Diagnosis of disease due to *C. difficile* usually is based on detection of the cytotoxin in feces.

Disease

PMC usually occurs with abdominal pain and a watery diarrhea within a week of antibiotic administration, although symptoms may be delayed up to 4 weeks after treatment stops. About one half of the patients may have mucus or blood in their stools. Examination of the colon shows the presence of yellowish white exudative plaques that may coalesce to form pseudomembranes.

Disease results when some alteration of the normal intestinal flora following antibiotic usage permits colonization and overgrowth by *C. difficile*. Exactly what this alteration is is not clear, but it is probably not simply the result of the selection of an organism resistant to the antibiotic, since many strains of *C. difficile* are sensitive to the antibiotics commonly associated with PMC.

The epidemiology of disease caused by *C. difficile* is complex and not completely understood. It is not clear whether the *C. difficile* infections are of endogenous or exogenous origin or whether both sources are important. Although the organism and cytotoxin can be found frequently in healthy neonates, *C. difficile* is uncommon in the feces of healthy adults. Some evidence suggests that it may be carried in the genitourinary tract. *Clostridium difficile* also can be isolated from environmental sources. Hospital outbreaks of colitis due to *C. difficile* suggest nosocomial spread of the organism in some instances.

Diagnosis

Definitive diagnosis of the disease is made by colonoscopy or protoscopy to demonstrate the characteristic yellow plaques. As mentioned, there are tests available for the demonstration of toxins A and B and special media for isolation of the organism. However, such tests are only suggestive, since the organism often is present in asymptomatic patients on antibiotic therapy and the toxins may be present in the absence of disease.

Treatment

For pseudomembranous colitis, it may be sufficient to stop administration of the inducing antibiotic. If this does not cure the disease, oral vancomycin, metronidazole, and bacitracin are the antibiotics of choice.

ORAL ASPECTS

Clostridium species frequently are part of the flora of mixed anaerobic orofacial infections following trauma. Clostridia have been isolated from dental plaque, carious dentin, and periodontal pocket debris. Overall, these bacteria probably are present in low numbers and are transients. The presence of *Clostridium* species in relatively large numbers has been reported in a few adult subjects with periodontitis. The role, if any, of these isolates in the disease process is not clear. *Clostridium* species were found to represent about 8.0% of the cultivable flora of a group of institutionalized, retarded children. The high numbers of clostridia in these subjects is probably a reflection of their poor hygienic practices. Again, the role of the clostridia in the periodontal disease seen in such children is unknown.

The dentist may become involved in the major clostridial diseases in two ways. First and most frequently, when choosing an antibiotic for treating dental infections, the dentist should keep in mind the dangers of antibiotic-associated pseudomenbranous colitis. In particular, clindamycin, which has been recommended for oral soft tissue infections, often has been associated with PMC. Second, on very rare occasions, the dentist may see a case of tetanus before the physician. Early cases of tetanus may have only head and neck symptoms. Therefore, tetanus should be considered in the differential diagnosis, since the trismus of tetanus may be wrongly attributed to alveolar abscess, temperomandibular joint disease, or peritonsillar abscess.

SUGGESTED READINGS

Allen SD. *Clostridium*. In: Lennette EH, Balows A, Hausler WJ Jr, Shadomy HJ, eds. *Manual of Clinical Microbiology*, 4th ed. Washington, DC: American Society for Microbiology; 1985.

Brown LW. Infant botulism. *Adv Pediatr.* 1981; 28:141.

Cato EP, George WL, Finegold SM. Genus *Clostridium*. In: Sneath PHA, Mair NS, Sharpe ME, Holt SG, eds. *Bergey's Manual of Systematic Bacteriology.* Baltimore: Williams & Wilkins; 1986; vol. 2.

Centers for Disease Control. *Botulism in the United States, 1899–1974. Handbook for Epidemiologists, Clinicians, and Laboratory Workers.* Atlanta: Centers for Disease Control; 1974.

Dowell VR Jr. Botulism and tetanus: Selected epidemiologic and microbiologic aspects. *Rev Infec Dis.* 1984;6(Suppl 1):S202.

Finegold SM, George WL. Miscellaneous clostridial infections. In: Balows A, Hausler WJ Jr, Ohashi M, Turano A, eds. *Laboratory Diagnosis of Infectious Diseases, Principles* and *Practice*. New York: Springer-Verlag; 1988, vol 1.

Hatheway CL. Botulism. In: Balows A, Hausler WJ Jr, Ohashi M, Turano A, eds. *Laboratory Diagnosis of Infectious Diseases, Principles and Practice.* New York, Springer-Verlag; 1988, vol 1.

Hill EO. The genus *Clostridium* (medical aspects). In: Starr MP, Stolp H, Truper HG, Balows A, Schegel HG, eds. *The Procaryotes.* Berlin: Springer-Verlag; 1981.

Sellin LC. Botulism—An update. *Mil Med.* 1984; 149:12.

Silva JJ, Fekety R. Clostridia and antimicrobial enterocolitis. *Annu Rev Med.* 1981; 32:327.

Smith LDS. *Botulism: The Organism, Its Toxins, the Disease.* Springfield, Ill: Charles C Thomas; 1977.

Smith LDS. *The Pathogenic Anaerobic Bacteria,* 2nd ed. Springfield, Ill: Charles C Thomas; 1975.

Trnka YM, Lamont JT. *Clostridium difficile* colitis. *Adv Intern Med.* 1984; 29:85.

CHAPTER 15

Mycobacteria

John A. Molinari and P.H. Chandrasekar

INTRODUCTION

GENERAL CHARACTERISTICS OF MYCOBACTERIA
- Morphology
- Staining Properties
- Cultural and Growth Characteristics
- Virulence Factors

TUBERCULOSIS
- Pathogenesis and Disease Process
- Oral Manifestations
- Diagnosis
- Host Immunologic Responses
- Treatment and Prevention

ATYPICAL MYCOBACTERIA

LEPROSY
- Immunology
- Treatment

ORAL ASPECTS

SUGGESTED READINGS

INTRODUCTION

Mycobacteria include a large number of bacterial species that range from highly virulent human pathogens to innocuous saprophytic inhabitants of water, soil, and plants. Mycobacteria can cause a variety of human and animal diseases. Two of theses, tuberculosis (*Mycobacterium tuberculosis*) and leprosy (*Mycobacterium leprae*), are the most serious. A third group of mycobacteria, the atypical mycobacteria, also may cause human infections. The significance of mycobacteria in dental medicine becomes apparent when one considers that the primary mode of transmission of *M. tuberculosis* is by aerosolized droplets and that mycobacteria are resistant to many of the commonly used disinfectants. Both of these properties increase the occupational risks of dental personnel.

GENERAL CHARACTERISTICS OF MYCOBACTERIA

Morphology

The genus *Mycobacterium* represents a diverse group of obligately aerobic, slender, curved rods that demonstrate varying degrees of branching. They are nonmotile and nonsporeforming and do not develop capsules. The prefix *myco* refers to their funguslike property, which can result in the formation of mycobacterial filaments. The presence of cell wall peptidoglycolipid and the mycobacteria's size are two major features used to distinguish these microorganisms from fungi. The appearance of branched forms has served to place the mycobacteria in the order Actinomycetales. Mycobacteria contain significantly higher concentrations of wall lipid than either gram-positive

TABLE 15–1. REPRESENTATIVE *MYCOBACTERIUM* SPECIES

Organism	Pathogenesis
M. avium	TB in fowl, cattle, swine, and rarely in humans
M. intracellulare (Battey bacillus) (*M. avium-intracellulare*)	TB in humans that is virtually indistinguishable; opportunistic in AIDS patients
M. fortuitum	Cutaneous infection; less virulent than *M. tuberculosis*
M. bovis	Pulmonary TB similar to that caused by *M. tuberculosis;* tuberculosis of cattle
M. smegmatis	None
M. kansasii	Pulmonary infection in humans; no person-to-person spread
M. tuberculosis	TB
M. leprae	Leprosy

or gram-negative bacteria. Representative mycobacterial species are described briefly in Table 15–1.

Staining Properties

Mycobacterial species are difficult to stain by ordinary techniques primarily because of the high lipid content (60%) of their cell walls. Although mycobacteria are considered to be gram-positive, the difficulty exhibited in the microorganisms' absorption of the primary crystal violet stain makes the gram stain virtually useless.

The hallmark of this genus is the organisms' unique ability of being able to retain the dye carbolfuchsin after a decolorization attempt with 0.5% HCl in ethyl alcohol (acid alcohol). This property, termed acid-fastness, is due to the high lipid content of the cell wall of these bacteria. The differential cell wall staining technique, the Ziehl-Neelsen method, distinguishes *Mycobacterium* and *Nocardia* species from all other types and is used widely in arriving at a diagnosis of tuberculosis in infected individuals. The demonstration of acid-fast bacilli in sputum specimens, in combination with other patient signs and symptoms, is presumptive evidence of active tuberculosis.

Cultural and Growth Characteristics

Successful culture of mycobacterial species take up to 8 weeks from time of sample collection and requires enriched medium. Common features employed in the differentiation of mycobacteria are the rate of growth and demonstration of pigmented colonies, that is, the Runyon classification. The human and bovine species of *M. tuberculosis* grow more slowly than do most of the nonpathogenic species. *Mycobacterium tuberculosis* colonies are seen as rough, granular, and buff-colored colonies, whereas nonpathogenic mycobacterial species exhibit bright orange, red, or yellow colonies when exposed to light for a few days at room temperature.

Virulence Factors

Mycobacteria do not prossess any known virulence factors, but there are virulence-associated factors. A characteristic microscopic feature of mycobacteria cultured in vitro, particularly *M. tuberculosis,* is the tendency of the bacterial cells to form cords or bundles. These arrangements are referred to as serpentine cords, and their appearance is used as an indication of microbial virulence (Fig 15–1). The growth of virulent strains in serpentine cords on the surface of liquid or solid medium can be correlated with the presence of a lipid compound, trehalose 6,6′-dimycolate, called cord factor. Cord factor shares some of the

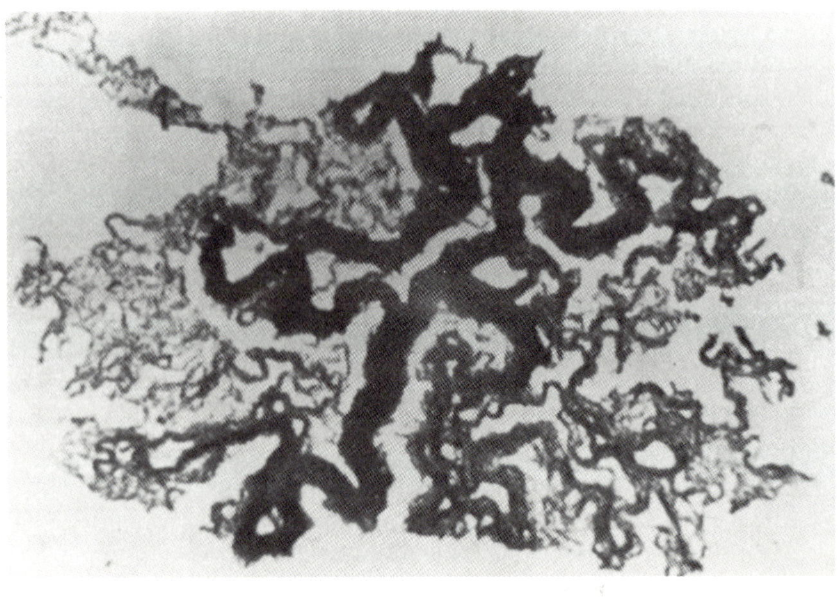

Figure 15–1. Serpentine cord formation *Mycobacterium tuberculosis*, showing in vitro parallel arrangement of acid-fast bacilli. ×70. *(From Olds RJ* Color Atlas of Microbiology. *Chicago: Year Book Medical Publishers; 1974.)*

adjuvant properties of Wax-D, which are described subsequently. Sulfolipids produced by the tubercle bacillus inhibit the intracellular killing of bacteria that have been ingested by macrophages. These substances prevent the fusion of lysosomes with the phagosomes and, thus, protect the bacteria from the hydrolytic lysosomal enzymes. This intracellular survival is of major significance in the disease because it protects the bacteria from other host resistance factors and can be overcome only by specific cell-mediated immunity.

Wax-D is a heterogeneous group of cell wall lipids that also are involved in the disease process. Their activity as immunologic adjuvants is of major importance. When Wax-D is mixed with a protein antigen, it enhances not only antibody production but also cell-mediated immunity. The cellular response is responsible for the characteristic granulomatous lesion of tuberculosis, and cell-mediated immune mechanisms are thought to be responsible for both the major part of the tissue injury in the disease and immune protection against the microorganism. This paradox has been explained as follows. The intense cellular response to the mycobacterial antigens produced by the large numbers of bacteria in an established chronic lesion injures the surrounding tissues. On the other hand, if protective immunity is present at the time of initial or recurrent infection, the same immune mechanisms mount a more moderate response that can overcome the bacteria present in lower numbers, without causing excessive tissue injury. The specific adjuvant factor in Wax-D, muramyl dipeptide, has been identified and is being studied for use with vaccines.

TUBERCULOSIS

Pathogenesis and Disease Process

Tuberculosis is primarily a chronic disease of humans. The etiologic agent, *M. tuberculosis,* is an obligate parasite that can infect both humans and primates. Other mycobacteria, in particular *Mycobacterium intracellulare* and *Mycobacterium kansasii,* are capable of producing virtually identical diseases. The incidence of tuberculosis in the United States has declined gradually in recent years (22,201 cases in 1985). The 0.2% case decrease reported for 1985, however, is significantly less than the 6.7% average annual decline observed for 1981–1984. Available evidence indicates that individuals infected with the human immunodeficiency virus (HIV), who subsequently develop AIDS, probably contribute to increased tuberculosis morbidity when they are infected with tubercle bacilli.

Tuberculosis is not a highly contagious disease. It requires prolonged or frequent contact with an infectious source for initiation of disease in a susceptible host. Casual or sporadic contact with a tuberculosis patient usually will not result in transmission. Infection in humans generally is acquired by the inhalation of respiratory microdroplets containing tubercle bacilli. The dissemination of mycobacteria via these aerosolized vehicles occurs by coughing, sneezing, or speaking. The lungs are the first tissues infected, and from that point, the organism may spread to virtually any other part of the body. The requirement of *M. tuberculosis* for oxygen predisposes to pulmonary infection.

Although the emphasis for tuberculosis transmission correctly remains with the airborne method, the disease can be spread via other routes. These include ingestion of contaminated material and direct inoculation of *M. tuberculosis* through the epithelial tissues. Gastrointestinal transmission occurs primarily from the ingestion of milk contaminated with tubercle bacilli. Infection by *M. tuberculosis* in this manner is not seen commonly because of the tuberculocidal effects of the gastric secretions. *Mycobacterium bovis* colonization and infection were noted more frequently, however, before the initiation of routine pasteurization as a public health practice. Percutaneous inoculation with mycobacteria can occur in individuals who routinely handle microbial cultures or infected tissue specimens. Individuals who work in high-risk areas, such as health personnel and laboratory technicians, are therefore at an increased risk of percutaneous exposure.

Lesions may appear anywhere in the lung parenchyma but usually are present in the periphery. Microscopically, mycobacteria can be seen within alveolar macrophages, where they are resistant to destruction following phagocytosis, even multiplying as the macrophages foster tissue dissemination of the bacteria. Onset of disease is chronic, with the gradual infiltration of polymorphonuclear leukocytes, macrophages, and T lymphocytes. The distinctive lesion is called a tubercle. The initial infection may progress to several different states depending on the extent of exposure to *M. tuberculosis* and the resistance of the patient.

Asymptomatic Primary Tuberculosis. Individuals gradually may be infected with *M. tuberculosis* without any apparent clinical manifestations. When skin-tested, these individuals display a positive tuberculin reaction, indicating that they have been infected and have developed cell-mediated immunity against the bacteria. This protective immune response prevents the continued multiplication and dissemination of the bacteria, but it does not destroy all of the bacteria present. The remaining bacteria are sequestered within tubercles in the affected tissues and may be the source of bacteria that initiate reactivation tuberculosis.

Symptomatic Primary Tuberculosis. *Mycobacterium tuberculosis* is spread via the lymphatics to cause granulomatous inflammation in both the lung periphery and hilar nodes and is accompanied by respiratory symptoms. The usual result here is one of healing and development of cell-mediated immunity. The Ghon complex, a remnant of this infection, most often occurs in infants and children and is comprised of small calcified lung nodules and lymphadenopathy of the hilar lymph nodes.

Progressive Primary Tuberculosis. A much more serious disease may develop in those individuals who are less resistant to tubercle bacilli. In these patients, microorganisms may spread throughout the body either (1) by means of the blood, resulting in miliary tuberculosis, (2) via the respiratory tissues, inducing a bronchopneumonia, or (3) through the gastrointestinal tract as a result of coughing up the organisms. In miliary tuberculosis, foci of infection occur in distant organs and tissues but develop most frequently in the meninges, lungs, liver, and renal cortex. Although cell-mediated immunity may develop in some patients, others may not react (anergy) when skin-tested with tuberculin protein preparations. Anergic patients have a poor prognosis for recovery and often die without rapid treatment.

Reactivation Tuberculosis. Reactivation tuberculosis occurs in individuals who have developed primary tuberculosis and who are asymptomatic but still carry the bacteria within tubercles. These patients exhibit positive tuberculin skin tests and, thus, demonstrate cellular immunity. Reactivation of disease is thought to be due to the activation by some alteration of host resistance of persistent bacteria in the tubercles of a previous infection. Infection is charcterized by tubercle formation, caseation, fibrosis, and further extension of the lesion. Progression may advance into a bronchus, leading to cavitation of the lung and secretion of an infectious sputum.

Oral Manifestations

Oral manifestations of tuberculosis occur in approximately 3% of patients with long-standing pulmonary or systemic infection. The bacteria infect the oral tissues and lymph nodes (scrofula) (Fig 15–2). Within the oral cavity, lesions can occur in the soft tissues and supporting bone and at tooth extraction sites. The tongue also may be affected (Fig 15–3).

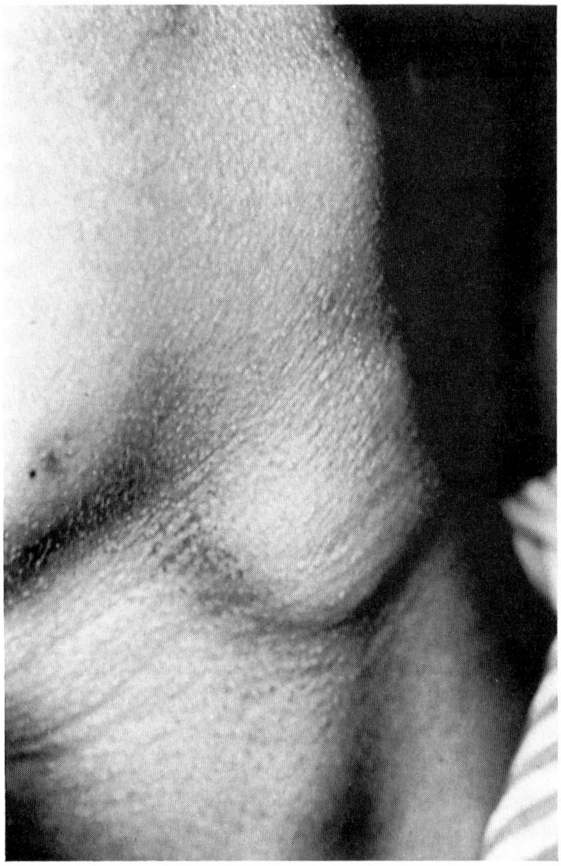

Figure 15–2. Cervical tuberculosis lymphadenitis secondary to pulmonary tuberculosis in a 16-year-old male.

Diagnosis

Presumptive diagnosis of infection relies clinically on conversion to a positive delayed hypersensitivity state, as shown by the tuberculin skin test. The antigenic preparations used for skin testing are derived from in vitro *M. tuberculosis* cultures. These extracts are a crude old tuberculin (OT) and a more purified protein derivative (PPD). PPD is used routinely in the intradermal skin test for tuberculin hypersensitivity. The antigen is administered by intracutaneous injection (Mantoux test) or by scarification or patch testing. Development after 24 to 72 hours of an erythematous, indurated swelling at the site of injection is indicative of hypersensitivity. Hemorrhage and necrosis may occur in severe reactions. A positive skin test is not necessarily proof of active disease. The patient may have an active infection or previously may have experienced tuberculosis or an immunologically related mycobacterial infection and continues to carry viable organisms. A negative skin test may occur in an infected individual in the early stages of infection or as a result (anergy) of overwhelming infection. The presence of other diseases, such as measles, also can cause a false negative reaction.

Definitive diagnosis of tuberculosis is established only by the demonstration of acid-fast mycobacteria in clinical specimens. Subsequent culture and isolation techniques can provide the means for positive identification. Sputum, gastric contents, urine, and

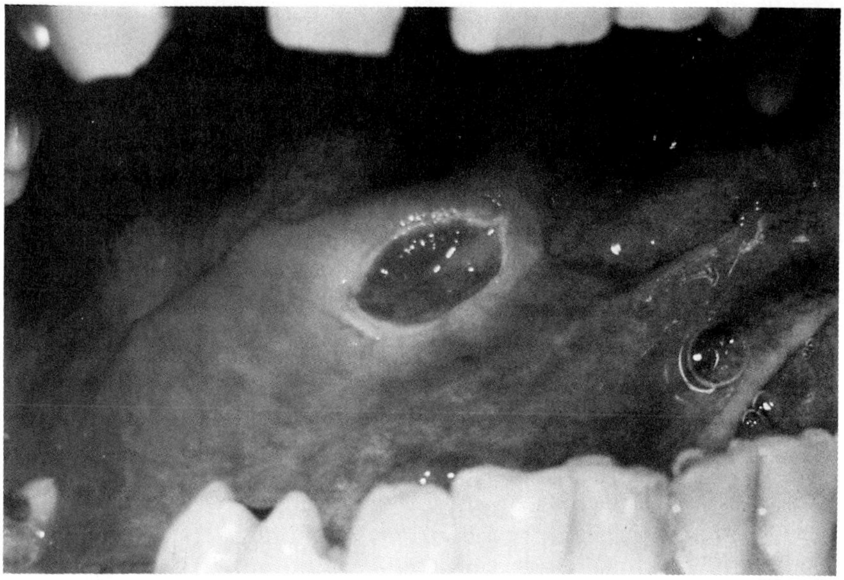

Figure 15–3. Tuberculosis ulcer of ventrolateral surface of tongue. *(Courtesy of Dr. James W. Curtis, Jr., University of Detroit, School of Dentistry.)*

other infected body fluids may be cultured on selective media.

Host Immunologic Responses

Mycobacteria are intracellular pathogens, and, therefore, antibodies are not protective. Protective immunity is a function of cellular immunity. Antigen-sensitive T lymphocytes reacting to mycobacterial antigens produce lymphokines that enhance the inflammatory response and activate macrophages. The activated macrophage possesses increased metabolic, phagocytic, and bactericidal properties that enable it to overcome intracellular pathogens. As noted, these same protective mechanisms also are the primary cause of tissue injury. However, a positive skin test, indicative of cellular immunity, usually is accompanied by an increased resistance to reinfection.

Treatment and Prevention

Multiple antibiotics are used to treat tuberculosis to ensure tissue penetration and prevent emergence of resistant organisms. Combinations of drugs are thus chosen based on the nature and site of disease. Additionally, to recover, the tuberculosis patient should have mental as well as physical rest with a buildup of nutrition (ie, patient has to gain weight).

Isoniazid (INH), rifampin, and streptomycin have cidal activity against tubercle bacilli. Tuberculostatic drugs include ethambutal and para-aminosalicylic acid. Standard therapy recommended at present is a combination of INH 300 mg daily with rifampin daily for 9 months. Hepatotoxicity is common with these drugs, and liver function usually is monitored when they are administered.

Patients who develop a positive tuberculin reaction but who do not have active disease and close contacts of patients who develop active disease are treated with INH for 1 year. BCG (*bacille Calmette-Guérin*) is a live vaccine prepared from an attentuated strain of *M. bovis.* The vaccine is only partially effective. It prevents infection in many uninfected individuals but only prevents dissemination and does not eradicate the bacteria in previously infected patients. It is used widely in Europe, but in the United States, it is recommended only for medical personnel and others who cannot avoid a high risk of exposure to the disease.

ATYPICAL MYCOBACTERIA (NONTUBERCULOUS MYCOBACTERIA)

These mycobacteria (variously known as unclassified, anonymous, or atypical mycobacteria) are found commonly as saprophytes in soil, water, and frequently in humans. In the 1950s, Runyon classified these organisms into four groups on the basis of their ability for pigment production, rate of growth, and other cultural characteristics. Clinical specimens frequently are contaminated with ubiquitous mycobacteria. At one time, these were thought to be nonpathogenic, but they are now recognized as opportunistic pathogens. Presumably, the infection is acquired by aspiration or inoculation of the organisms from a natural reservoir. Lung infections with the organisms are most common, and the clinical picture is indistinguishable from that of tuberculosis. *Mycobacterium kansasii* and *Mycobacterium avium-intracellulare* produce chronic bronchopulmonary disease in adults. Other commonly involved sites are the lymph nodes (*Mycobacterium scrofulaceum*), skin, bone, and meninges. It is noteworthy that a large number of patients with AIDS are reported to have infections due to *M. avium-intracellulare*. Atypical mycobacteria are resistant to most antituberculosis agents. Multiple drug regimens in combination with surgical resection of infected tissue is the recommended treatment.

LEPROSY

Leprosy (Hansen's disease) in the United States has been rising steadily in the last several years as a result of increased world travel and an influx of immigrants from endemic areas. Leprosy is caused by the acid-fast, slightly curved bacillus, *M. leprae*. It produces mycolic acid and shares ultrastructural properties with other mycobacteria. Humans once were believed to be the only reservoir of this organism, but naturally acquired leprosy has now been shown to occur in the nine-banded armadillo and some nonhuman primates.

Leprosy is not highly communicable. The bacilli may enter via the upper respiratory tract or through skin abrasions. The rate of multiplication of the organism within the host is extremely slow. Thus, there usually is a lag period of several years between infection and onset of clinical disease. The long incubation interval and chronic persistence of bacteria is in part due to the mechanism of *M. leprae* infection in host macrophages. After the mycobacteria enter and multiply in macrophages, there is an increased lipid production until the phagocytic cell bursts, releasing newly replicated *M. leprae*.

Clinical and Histologic Features

The spectrum of disease manifestations in leprosy is very broad. Based on clinical, histologic, and immunologic findings, the disease progresses from a limited to a more generalized form, either tuberculoid, borderline, or lepromatous. The immune status of the host, primarily a cell-mediated response, appears to decide the form of infection.

Tuberculoid Leprosy. Early lesions are large, flat, hypopigmented areas of skin, with sharply defined, circular, raised outer borders. Infiltration of dermal nerves underlying these areas causes diminished sensitivity or anesthesia. Histologically, the skin lesions are composed of granulomas with epithelioid cells, lymphocytes, and Langhans giant cells extending to the basal layer of epidermis. Bacilli are not frequently found among these lesions.

Lepromatous Leprosy. Skin involvement is extensive, characterized by erythematous macules, papules, nodules, or plaques. Diffuse dermal infiltration leads to leonine expression and thickening of ear lobes, classic signs of the disease. With progression of the disease, loss of eyebrows and eyelashes, atrophic rhinitis, destruction of nasal maxillary structures, and gynecomastic and testicular atrophy occur. Typical histologic findings of skin lesions are the foamy macrophages with numerous acid-fast bacilli. Granulomas are absent.

Borderline Leprosy. Skin lesions are multiple and mixed, seen as papules, nodules, or plaques. Histologically, the lesions contain granulomas and macrophages with acid-fast bacilli, usually within thickened nerves. These patients are clinically unstable, tending to migrate toward either end of the spectrum.

Immunology

The host's cell-mediated immune response to *M. leprae* determines the disease form. Those with the tuberculoid form display delayed-type hypersensitivity to skin tests with *M. leprae* antigens, whereas lepromatous patients are anergic. The lepromin skin test, although not diagnostic, is helpful in the classification and prognosis of patients with leprosy.

Treatment

Dapsone 4,4-diaminodiphenyl sulfone, or DDS, is the drug of choice for leprosy. The gradual emergence of both primary and secondary resistance to DDS has led to the use of multiple-drug therapy. Recent recommendations by the World Health Organization emphasize that multidrug treatment must be used for all forms of leprosy. Other drugs used to treat leprosy are clofazimine, rifampin, ethionamide, and prothiaramide. These agents must be administered for prolonged periods and, in some cases, for life.

There is no vaccine available. Prophylaxis with DDS is recommended in children who have had extended household contact with persons shedding large numbers of *M. leprae* in the nasal mucus or from open skin lesions.

ORAL ASPECTS

Dental personnel and their auxiliary staff face a constant risk of infection from oral and systemic microorganisms transmitted from their patients' mouths. A number of these, including *M. tuberculosis*, may be passed via aerosols containing saliva and sputum. Tubercle bacilli are able to survive on many surfaces for weeks and exhibit remarkable resistance to many disinfectants. These features have been recognized for their clinical importance, and as a result, bactericidal activity against *M. tuberculosis* is included as one of the major criteria employed in determining the usefulness of a disinfectant for dental practice. The lowering of host resistance also is important, as evidenced by the increased susceptibility to tuberculosis of individuals with AIDS.

SUGGESTED READINGS

Barksdale, L, Kim K. *Mycobacterium. Bacteriol Rev.* 1977; 41:217.

Centers for Disease Control. Tuberculosis—United States, 1985. *MMWR.* 1986; 35:699.

Chaisson RE, Slutkin G. Tuberculosis and human immunodeficiency virus infection. *J Infect Dis.* 1989; 159:96–100.

Enna CD, Jacobson RR, Trautman JR, et al. Leprosy in the United States (1967–1976). *Public Health Rep.* 1978; 93:468.

Jacobson MA. Mycobacterial diseases: Tuberculosis and *Mycobacterium avium* complex. In: Moellering RC, Sande MA, Volberding PA, eds. *Medical Management of AIDS. Infectious Disease Clinics of North America.* Philadelphia: WB Saunders; 1988:465.

Mani NJ. Tuberculosis initially diagnosed by asymptomatic oral lesions. Report of three cases. *J Oral Med.* 1985; 40:39.

Reichart P, Ananatasan T, Reznik G. Gingiva and periodontium in lepromatous leprosy. *J Periodontol.* 1976; 47:455.

Rosenzweig DY. Tuberculosis and other mycobacterial diseases. In: Rytel MW, Mogabgab WJ, eds. *Clinical Manual of Infectious Diseases.* Chicago: Year Book Medical Publishers; 1984:317.

Smith WH, Mason KD, Davies D, Onions JP. Intraoral and pulmonary tuberculosis following dental treatment. *Lancet.* 1982; 1:842.

Stead WW, Dutt AK. Chemotherapy for tuberculosis today. *Am Rev Respir Dis.* 1982; 125:94.

Sutton FD. TB and its fellow travelers. *Hosp Pract.* 1987

Tsukamura M. A review of the methods of identification and differentiation of mycobacteria. *Rev Infect Dis.* 1981; 3:841.

Wallace RJ, Swenson JM, Silcox VA, et al. Spectrum of disease due to rapidly growing mycobacteria. *Rev Infect Dis.* 1983; 5:657.

CHAPTER 16

Enterobacteriaceae and Related Gram-Negative Bacteria

Chris H. Miller

INTRODUCTION

MORPHOLOGY

CULTIVATION

DIAGNOSIS

VIRULENCE FACTORS
- Endotoxins
- Exotoxins
- Surface Appendages
- Capsules

DISEASES
- Salmonellosis
- Shigellosis (Bacillary Dysentery)
- Cholera
- *Escherichia coli* Diarrheal Diseases
- Coliform Diseases
- *Campylobacter* Enteritis
- Other Diseases

PREVENTION

ORAL ASPECTS

SUGGESTED READINGS

INTRODUCTION

Enteric bacteria are gram-negative bacteria capable of colonizing the intestinal tract of humans and animals. For the most part, they represent genera of the family Enterobacteriaceae (Table 16–1) and the genera *Pseudomonas, Campylobacter,* and *Vibrio* of other families. Gram-negative anaerobes, such as *Bacteroides,* also colonize the intestinal tract; these are discussed in Chapter 17.

Some enteric bacteria, such as *Salmonella, Shigella, Vibrio cholerae,* certain strains of *Escherichia coli,* and *Pseudomonas aeruginosa, Campylobacter jejuni,* and *Yersinia enterocolitica,* can cause disease when present in the intestinal tract of humans. Others, such as the coliforms (*E. coli, Klebsiella, Enterobacter, Citrobacter, Serratia,* and *Proteus*) and most *P. aeruginosa* strains, can exist in the large intestine with no harm to the host. However, if these so-called harmless bacteria are given the opportunity (frequently in a compromised host), they may cause harmful infections of the urinary tract, wounds, lung, surgical incisions, intestinal tract, tooth pulp, mouth, female genitalia, and other body sites. As direct or opportunistic pathogens, the enteric bacteria cause major health problems throughout the world. In dentistry, these bacteria may cause oral infections that often are not resolved until specific therapy based on culture and antibiotic sensitivity testing is instituted.

MORPHOLOGY

The gram-negative enteric bacilli are about 0.5 μm in diameter and vary in length from 1 to 8 μm. With the exception of *V. cholerae* and *C. jejuni,* which may appear as curved rods, they have no distinctive morphologic features except that some may possess capsules. Mo-

TABLE 16–1. EXAMPLES OF IMPORTANT SPECIES IN THE ENTEROBACTERIACEAE

Escherichia	*Enterobacter*
E. coli	*E. cloaceae*
	E. aerogenes
Edwardsiella	*E. agglomerans*
E. tarda	*Hafnia*
	H. alvei
Citrobacter	*Serratia*
C. freundii	*S. marcescens*
Salmonella	*Proteus*
S. choleraesuis	*P. vulgaris*
S. typhi	*Yersina*
S. enteritidis	*Y. enterocolitica*
Shigella	*Y. pestis*
S. dysenteriae	
S. flexneri	
S. boydii	
S. sonnei	
Klebsiella	
K. pneumoniae	

From Buchanan RE, Gibbons NE, eds. Bergey's Manual of Determinative Bacteriology, 8th ed. Baltimore: Williams & Wilkins; 1974.

tile and nonmotile species are found among the enterics, and most species possess nonflagellar surface appendages called fimbriae or pili. These structures aid in attachment of the bacteria to body cells or, as in the case of sex pili, serve as the conjugation tube important in transferring DNA from one cell to another.

CULTIVATION

The gram-negative enteric bacilli are aerobic, facultatively anaerobic, or microaerophilic bacteria that grow well on most ordinary laboratory media. Cultivation of these bacteria frequently involves their isolation from clinical specimens or environmental samples that contain other bacteria. Thus, a variety of selective and differential media is available for use. For example, detection of *Salmonella* or *Shigella* in a feces sample may involve selective enrichment. Media such as tetrathionate, selenite broth, or Hajna GN broth inhibit gram-positive bacteria and coliforms, and allow the *Salmonella* or *Shigella* to multiply to numbers much larger than were originally present in the sample. These enriched cultures can then be inoculated into various other selective or differential media.

MacConkey and eosin-methylene blue agar (EMB) are used for primary isolation of Enterobacteriaeceae species. These media contain chemicals that inhibit gram-positive bacteria and that differentiate between lactose fermenters (eg, *E. coli, Enterobacter aerogenes*) and nonlactose fermenters (eg, *Salmonella, Shigella*). The former produce colored colonies, whereas the latter produce colorless colonies. *Pseudomonas aeruginosa* also may be isolated on EMB agar as a slow or nonlactose fermenter, frequently producing a blue-green pigment and exhibiting a fruity or grapelike odor. In contrast, *V. cholerae* is inhibited on MacConkey or EMB agar but can be cultured from stool specimens on nonselective nutrient agar or bile salts agar at a slightly alkaline pH.

DIAGNOSIS

Diagnosis of all of the diseases discussed in this chapter is made, or at least is greatly aided by, isolating and identifying the causative agent. Feces, blood, or other specimens are cultured in nonselective enrichment and selective differential media, such as EMB and MacConkey agar. As mentioned under Cultivation, early determination of the ability of the isolates to ferment lactose greatly aids in the identification of gram-negative enterics. Salmonellae, shigellae, and *Proteus* do not ferment lactose, whereas *E. coli* and *Klebsiella* rapidly ferment lactose, and *Citrobactor* and some *Serratia* ferment this sugar more slowly. A key growth characteristic that aids in early classification of *Proteus* species is referred to as swarming and is observed as a rapidly spreading growth over the surface of agar, resulting from their high motility. Many strains of *Pseudomonas* produce a blue-green pigment during growth that can aid in their early detection, and some strains exhibit swarming.

Speciation or presumptive identification of the enteric isolates requires analysis of numerous biochemical properties. The laboratory diagnosis of the enterics has been greatly simplified by test systems that permit rapid analysis of as many as 20 different biochemical parameters simultaneously. The expected biochemical reactions of the enteric bacteria are described in numerous textbooks on diagnostic microbiology and are not repeated here. Frequently, biochemical testing yields only a presumptive identification, and definitive identification requires antigenic analysis of the isolate using polyvalent and specific antisera to standard strains of the organisms.

VIRULENCE FACTORS

Endotoxins

Gram-negative bacteria contain complex lipopolysaccharides, called endotoxins, in their outer membrane. In the case of enterics, they are also referred to as O, or somatic, antigens. The structure and toxic properties of these endotoxins are discussed in Chapter 9.

Endotoxin may play an important role in the clinical manifestations of human gram-negative infections. Endotoxin is pyrogenic, directly activates the C3 component of complement enhancing inflammatory reactions, depresses myocardial function, alters lymphocyte activity, and triggers platelet activity, causing occlusion of small blood vessels. Circulating endotoxin also may be responsible for many of the manifestations of toxic shock that may occur in gram-negative systemic infections.

Exotoxins

The enterics produce a variety of harmful toxins. Some strains of *E. coli* produce enterotoxins. These strains are called enterotoxigenic or enteropathogenic *E. coli* because, when present in the intestinal tract, they may cause diarrheal disease. The enterotoxigenic *E. coli* may produce a heat-stable or a heat-labile enterotoxin or both. These toxins induce hypersecretion of water and electrolytes into the bowel.

The nature and the mechanism of action of the *E. coli* heat-labile enterotoxin are similar to those of the *V. cholerae* enterotoxin. However, the cholera enterotoxin is coded for by chromosomal genes, and the *E. coli* enterotoxin is coded for by plasmid genes. It is interesting to note that these enterotoxins resemble diphtheria toxin, which exists as two subunits and causes an ADP-ribosylation reaction, but of a different substrate (elongation factor 2) (Chapter 9). Equally intriguing is the fact that most strains of *P. aeruginosa* produce an exotoxin (toxin A) that has a mode of action identical to that of the diphtheria toxin.

Shigella dysenteriae type 1 and most *Shigella sonnei* and *Shigella flexneri* produce a heat-labile exotoxin that causes paralysis and death when injected into mice. The toxin most often is referred to as a neurotoxin but apparently does not act directly on nerve cells. Its primary site of action could be the vasulature of the gray matter of the central nervous system. However, the toxin has been shown to inhibit protein synthesis in cultured human cells (HeLa cells isolated from cancerous cervical tissue) by inactivating the 60S ribosomal subunit. Apparently, the toxin binds to a glycoprotein receptor on the epithelial cell, enters the cell through endocytosis, and is activated while inside the phagolysosome. Although the pathogenisis of shigellosis suggests the action of an exotoxin, this is yet to be confirmed in human disease.

Surface Appendages

Colonization by many enteric bacteria may be promoted by fimbriae involved in binding of the bacteria to host cells (Fig 16–1). Studies on the colonization of enteropathogenic *E. coli* in bovine and porcine hosts have identified specific plasmid-mediated, fimbrial, colonization factor antigens (CFA) responsible for adherence to mucosal epithelium. In contrast, animal studies also have demonstrated the adherence of *V. cholerae* to the microvilli in the small bowel, but obvious surface pili or fimbriae are not detected.

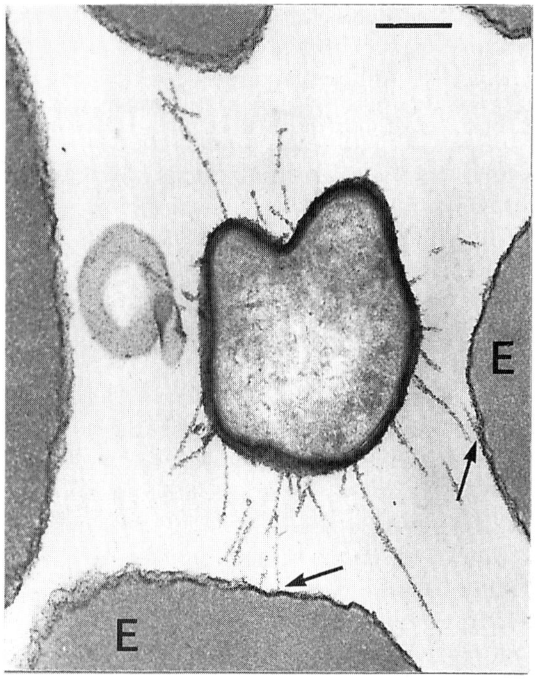

Figure 16–1. Electron micrograph showing human erythrocytes (E) agglutinated by *Escherichia coli* strain 444-3. The tips of fimbriae stained by ruthenium red can be seen to make contact with the erythrocyte membrane (arrows). Bar = 0.2 μm. *(From Knutton S, Williams PH, Lloyd DR, Candy DCA, McNeish AS.* Infect Immun. *1984;44:599.)*

Specialized surface appendages, called sex pili, are present on many gram-negative enterics. These pili serve as the conjugation tube through which DNA may be transferred to other cells. Thus, these gram-negative bacteria can transfer chromosomal genes or plasmids containing genes for virulence factors or antibiotic resistance to other members of the intestinal flora (Chapter 20).

Capsules

Many of the Enterobacteriaceae possess capsules that inhibit phagocytosis. The most noted is *Klebsiella pneumoniae,* with more than 70 capsular types that likely play an important role in the ability of this opportunistic organism to cause pneumonia and septicemia. *Pseudomonas aeruginosa* also possesses a polysaccharide capsule.

DISEASES

Salmonellosis

Harmful infections with salmonellae may manifest themselves in several ways. Enterocolitis is usually caused by *Salmonella enteritidis,* which has over 1800 serotypes. Enteric fever (typhoid fever) is usually caused by *Salmonella typhi* (one serotype), whereas

Salmonella choleraesuis (one serotype) usually produces septicemia or focal infections.

Salmonella food poisoning (enterocolitis) may be caused by ingestion of contaminated water or improperly prepared food. After colonization of the lower intestine, the organisms multiply, invade the mucosal epithelium, and cause an acute inflammatory reaction. The salmonellae that cause enterocolitis are usually of lesser virulence than other strains, and intestinal lymphatic barriers prevent their invasion of the bloodstream. However, about 4 to 5 days after ingestion of the organisms, the intestines secrete fluid and electrolytes, resulting in diarrhea. The diarrhea, which sometimes may be bloody, frequently is associated with abdominal pain, nausea, and fever. During the acute stages of the infection, the number of salmonellae commonly reaches 10^6 to 10^9 cells per gram of feces, and it may take several months for the organisms to be cleared from the intestine.

Typhoid fever also is acquired by ingesting contaminated food or water. If the *Salmonella* contaminants are of the more invasive type, such as *S. typhi,* they colonize the intestinal mucosa, penetrate epithelial cells, and invade the lamina propria, where they can enter the lymphatics. These more invasive strains resist host defenses and can survive and multiply within macrophages. Thus, these salmonellae are facultative intracellular parasites. The organims may enter the bloodstream from the lymphatics and can infect any tissue of the body, including the intestine. Infection of the gallbladder and reinfection of the intestine results in shedding of the bacteria into the intestinal tract.

Enteric fever has an incubation period of about 1 to 2 weeks, with a gradual rise in body temperature accompanied by loss of appetite, general aches and pains, and commonly a headache. During the second week, the fever may reach 104°F, with diarrhea, abdominal pain, and general weakness. Complications include intestinal perforation, abscess formation, and pneumonia, and the mortality rate varies from 2% to 10%. Chronic foci of infection may occur (frequently in the biliary tree), resulting in a chronic carrier state.

Ingestion of serotypes, such as *S. choleraeesuis,* can lead to a rapid invasion of the intestinal tract, and subsequent subclinical bacteremia or septicemia may occur with little intestinal symptomatology.

Salmonella infections usually respond to chloramphenicol, ampicillin, amoxicillin, or trimethoprim-sulfamethoxazole, with chloramphenicol being the drug of choice for enteric fevers or bacteremia. For enterocolitis, antibiotics are contraindicated unless a bacteremia also is present. Adminstration of antibiotics under these conditions tends to prolong the fecal excretion of the organisms and does not shorten the length of the illness. Management of enterocolitis must include replenishment of lost fluids and electrolytes.

Typhoid fever results in some degree of immunity to subsequent infection, but instances of additional attacks in the same person have been recorded. The immunity that does develop from natural infection or from immunization with killed vaccines is not complete. One might be protected against low doses of the bacteria but not against high doses. Also, the immune state may not protect against colonization of the intestinal tract but might modify the manifestations or the severity of the disease.

In the United States, 30,000 to 40,000 cases of *Salmonella* infections are reported to the Centers for Disease Control annually. Of these, usually less than 2% are cases of typhoid fever. The actual number of *Salmonella* cases per year is estimated to be close to 2 million in the United States alone, since many cases are never reported. The salmonellae that cause enterocolitis in humans are found in many different domestic and wild animals, including chickens, turkeys, swine, cattle, dogs, cats, and turtles. Salmonellae are somewhat hardy bacteria and can survive in meats and animal products that are not cooked thoroughly. Thus, contaminated food is the major vehicle for transmission of nontyphoidal salmonellae to humans. Transmission by contaminated water supplies or from person to person also may occur. In the case of typhoid fever, disease transmission is usually from person to person by fecally contaminated food or water, because *S. typhi* is harbored by humans and has no significant animal reservoir.

About 3% of persons infected with *S. typhi* and about 0.1% of those infected with nontyphoidal salmonellae became asymptomatic carriers. These persons serve as reservoirs for transmission of the bacteria by the fecal–oral route. Convalescent carriers may shed the bacteria for a few weeks, and the chronic carrier state may exist for years.

State health agencies restrict individuals known to be shedding salmonellae. They are excluded from food preparation, processing, or serving, patient care, or working with young children or the elderly. These exclusions apply until two or three successive fecal specimens taken at least 24 hours apart are determined by the laboratory to be negative for *Salmonella.* These restrictions apply also to providers of dental care. In 1985, students and others associated with a large U.S. medical center attended an off-campus function at which food contaminated with *Salmonella* was served. Thirty-seven dental, hygiene, and assisting students reported gastrointestinal symptoms occurring within a week after the function. When 15 of these students were found to be shedding *Salmonella* in their feces, they were restricted from patient care. Fortunately, all of the students cleared the organisms within 10 weeks after the exposure and resumed their normal dental education.

Shigellosis (Bacillary Dysentery)

Like the salmonellae, shigellae are acquired through ingestion of contaminated food and water or oral contact with contaminated hands or fomites. After ingestion, the shigellae colonize the intestinal mucosa and invade the intestinal epithelial cells. Unlike some salmonellae that invade the underlying lamina propria, the shigellae laterally invade other epithelial cells. Intestinal symptoms occur only after the bacteria have multiplied within the epithelial tissue, resulting in ulceration and shedding into the intestinal lumen up to 10 billion bacteria per gram of feces. The incubation period for shigellosis is about 36 to 72 hours. This is followed by abdominal cramps, fever, and a watery diarrhea. The disease is usually self-limiting, but young infants may die if there is a severe loss of fluids. The most serious cases usually are caused by *S. dysenteriae* type 1, also known as the Shiga bacillus. The less virulent *S. flexneri* and *S. sonnei* produce both endotoxin and exotoxin like *S. dysenteriae* but in lesser amounts.

Although many cases of shigellosis are self-limiting, antibiotic therapy can shorten the illness and more quickly eliminate the shigellae from the stools. The antibiotic of choice is ampicillin, or if the isolates are resistant, trimethoprim-sulfamethoxazole or tetracycline may be used. Replenishment of fluid loss also is important.

Some degree of protective immunity probably develops after shigellosis, but the mechanisms are not well understood. The resident population of areas where shigellosis is endemic is relatively resistant, whereas newcomers to these areas frequently develop acute disease. Parenterally administered vaccines of killed shigellae do not provide protection. However, as with other infectious diarrheas, mucosal immunity (sIgA) is probably of primary importance in protection.

Shigellae also are transmitted fecal–orally usually by hand-to-mouth contact but also by contaminated food, water, or fomites. The shigellae are restricted primarily to humans as a natural host. Shigellae are highly virulent, with as few as 200 cells capable of causing dysentery. All age groups are susceptible to harmful infection, but about 60% of the reported cases in the U.S. occur in children 1 to 10 years old. Shigellosis is prevalent in some children's institutions, hospitals for the mentally handicapped, and prisons and occurs with an above-average incidence in male homosexuals. As with salmonellosis, persons known to be infected with *Shigella* are restricted by state health agencies from food handling, patient care, or occupations involving care of young children or the elderly.

Cholera

After ingestion of *V. cholerae* in contaminated water or food, those bacteria that survive the gastric acidity colonize and multiply in the small bowel. Unlike salmonellae and shigellae, *V. cholerae* does not penetrate the intestinal epithelium but colonizes and multiplies on the epithelial surface. It secretes its enterotoxin, which causes a massive secretion of fluid from the mucosal surface. The patients first feel a slight fullness of the abdomen, with loss of appetite and sometimes vomiting. This is followed by a frequent liquid diarrhea during which the stools become almost clear, like water. About 20 L of fluid may be lost in severe cases, and death may result from loss of electrolytes, shock, metabolic acidosis, and renal failure.

Cholera is self-limiting in a few days, but death may occur in more than one half of the patients (especially children) if lost fluids and electrolytes are not replaced. The epithelial cells on the tips of the villi irreversibly bind the cholera toxin on their surface and continue to secrete fluid and electrolytes even in the presence of antibiotics. Symptoms begin to subside only when the toxin-bound cells are replaced with new epithelial cells from the mucosal crypts (2 to 4 days). Antibiotic therapy with tetracycline will reduce the number of *V. cholerae* present and will enhance its clearance from the intestine. Complete and lasting immunity probably does not occur, since reinfection with *V. cholerae* does occur in areas where the disease is endemic.

Humans are the resevoir for *V. cholerae*. This bacterium is shed in the feces from those who are obviously ill, convalescent, or transient carriers and from those with undiagnosed subclinical infections. Ingestion of fecally contaminated food or water may lead to disease. Cholera occurs worldwide but is heavily endemic in Asia (mainly in the India-Pakistan-Bangladesh area) and Africa. Occasional outbreaks occur in the U.S., usually in Louisiana and Texas.

Escherichia coli Diarrheal Diseases

Strains of *E. coli* that are pathogenic when in the intestinal tract can be grouped by serotyping as being enterotoxigenic, enteropathogenic, and enteroinvasive. The enterotoxigenic *E. coli* (ETEC) colonize the small intestine with the aid of the CFA on surface pili. As the organism multiplies on the intestinal lining, it produces one or both of the *E. coli* enterotoxins (described earlier), causing a watery type diarrhea. Disease caused by the enteropathogenic *E. coli* (EPEC) was first described as epidemic infantile diarrhea. The serotypes involved also colonize the surface of the intestine, and superficial invasion of the epithelial lining does occur. Although the EPEC produce a cytotoxin, it is apparently different from the ETEC enterotoxins.

The enteroinvasive *E. coli* first colonize and then, like shigellae, invade and destroy the intestinal epithelium, causing a bloody diarrhea with mucus. These serotypes do not produce enterotoxins.

Antibiotic therapy for *E. coli* diarrheal disease is reserved for long-term or chronic cases or for the young child in a life-threatening situation. As in other diarrheal diseases, rehydration is very important.

As with other intestinal infections, there is confusion concerning the development of subsequent immunity in *E. coli* diarrheal disease. Young children in endemic areas, as well as adult newcomers, are susceptible, whereas the incidence in older children and adults living in that area is lower. This may be due to an acquired immunity from previous or continuous exposure or to other factors.

Coliform Diseases

Coliforms and *Pseudomonas* are well noted for causing a variety of opportunistic infections involving blood, the urinary tract, surgical wounds, upper and lower respiratory tracts, the skin, and other sites. About 80% of nonobstructive urinary tract infections occurring in nonhospitalized patients are caused by *E. coli,* and other causative agents that originate from the fecal flora include *K. pneumoniae* and *Proteus. Pseudomonas* is a leading cause of septicemic death in burn patients, and a 1982 study by the Centers for Disease Control showed that coliforms and *P. aeruginosa* caused about 48% of all hospital-acquired infections.

Ampicillin, sulfanilamides, cephalosporins, tetracycline, trimethorprim-sulfamethoxazole, and nitrofurantoin have been useful in treating *E. coli* urinary tract infections. Gentamicin or tobramycin may be useful for treating infections by the gram-negative enterics, and the combination of gentamicin and carbenicillin is used frequently to treat severe *Pseudomonas* infections.

Klebsiella, Citrobacter, Enterobacter, Serratia, Proteus, and *P. aeruginosa* are found in water, soil, and to varying degrees in the intestinal tract of humans and animals. These, along with *E. coli,* frequently cause damage in people with immature or weakened body defenses as these bacteria are translocated from their normal intestinal habitat of the same person (endogenous infections) or as they contaminate the body from another person or from an environmental source (exogenous infection).

Pseudomonas is particularly important in exogenous infections because it can be free-living and can survive in water and other environments with low nutrients. Also, it is more resistant than many bacteria to chemical disinfectants. *Escherichia coli* apparently is not free-living but is an inhabitant of the intestinal tract of humans and animals. Its presence in environmental samples, water, and food is used as proof of recent fecal contamination. Thus, the occurrence of *E. coli* in water is used as an index of the suitability of the water for human consumption. As with shigellae and *V. cholerae,* there are no known important nonhuman sources of the *E. coli* strains that cause diarrheal disease. This disease occurs most commonly as a hospital-derived infection of infants in the nurseries. However, some cases occur in travelers, and there is an occasional common source outbreak involving adults.

Campylobacter Enteritis

Although *C. jejuni, Campylobacter coli,* and *Campylobacter fetus* are known to be pathogenic for humans, most interest has focused on *C. jejuni.* This organism causes as much diarrheal disease in healthy people as do *Shigella* and *Salmonella.* Ingestion and multiplication of *C. jejuni* can affect the small and large bowel, causing exudative and hemorrhagic inflammation. Those infected experience fever, diarrhea, bloody stools, abdominal pain, headache, and sometimes vomiting. The illness may last from 1 day to several weeks but is most frequently self-limiting by 7 days. As in *Salmonella* infections, *C. jejuni* may reach 10^6 to 10^9 cells per gram of feces in ill people. However, the *C. jejuni* convalescent carrier state usually lasts only 2 to 3 weeks, with a maximum of 3 months. Although infection with *C. jejuni* results in elevated serum antibody titer, it is not known if this response protects against reinfection. Some patients with *C. jejuni* colitis experience bacteremia and exhibit cellular infiltration in biopsy specimens. This suggests that the pathogenic mechanism can involve tissue invasion. In addition, *C. jejuni* produces a cytotoxin and a heat-labile exterotoxin, the latter having a mechanism of action similar to that of cholera toxin.

It is estimated that about 2 million cases of *C. jejuni* infection occur annually in the United States. *Campylobacter jejuni* is excreted in the feces of apparently healthy animals and birds, including dogs, cats, cattle, sheep, chickens, and turkeys. Human infection may result from direct contact with an infected animal or contaminated soil or ingestion of contaminated food of animal origin, water, or raw clams. Person-to-person transmission appears to be uncommon.

Although most harmful infections with *C. jejuni* resolve spontaneously, antimicrobial therapy with erythomycin or tetracycline may be indicated for more severe cases with prolonged symptoms.

Like *C. jejuni, C. coli* causes diarrheal disease in healthy persons, but the frequency is not known. *Campylobacter fetus* is considered as an opportunistic pathogen that can cause harmful infections in debilitated people, pregnant women, and newborns. *Campylobacter pylori* has been isolated frequently from gastroduodenal ulcer biopsies, but its possible role in the disorder has not been determined.

A new species of *Campylobacter, Campylobacter concisus,* was proposed in 1981 after its isolation from the human mouth. It is difficult to differentiate from other small, oral, gram-negative motile rods, such as *Wolinella recta, Bacteroides gracilis,* and *Eikenella corrodens.* Whereas the last three organisms have been implicated as possible periodontal pathogens, conflicting information on the possible role of *C. concisus* in periodontal attachment loss requires further clarification.

Other Diseases

Yersinia enterocolitica is another member of the Enterobacteriaceae that can cause infectious diarrhea. This bacterium has been isolated from domestic and wild animals and from water, raw milk, and food. Human isolates produce a heat-stable exotoxin similar to that of toxigenic strains of *E. coli.* Although the severe enterocolitis caused by this organism is more common in Scandinavia and other European countries, the causative agent is being isolated with more frequency in the United States.

PREVENTION

Infectious diarrheal diseases are best controlled by instituting or maintaining proper sanitation procedures involving sewage disposal and drinking water. It also is important to maintain proper asepsis, cooking procedures, and refrigeration during the preparation of food and food products both at home and within the food industry. Control of *Salmonella* and *Shigella* infections is enhanced by attempting to identify carriers and apply appropriate restrictions in relation to their handling of food or caring for patients, children, or the elderly.

Vaccines of killed suspensions of *S. typhi* are available for typhoid fever. Although they are seldom administered in the United States, they are used for the military and in those traveling to areas where typhoid fever is endemic. Orally administered vaccines that could control the colonization of salmonellae, shigellae, and *V. cholerae* are being investigated.

ORAL ASPECTS

Enteric bacteria, such as *P. aerugenosa, E. coli,* and species of *Klebsiella, Proteus,* and *Enterobacter,* have been isolated from orofacial infections (abscesses, postsurgical and extraction wounds, endodontic infections, sinus tracts, traumatic injuries). These bacteria usually occur in mixed infections rather than in pure cultures from these oral lesions. They occur more commonly in chronically ill and immunocompromised patients or in those receiving prophylactic antibiotic therapy that may give a selective growth advantage to gram-negative bacteria. This general pattern of occurrence of the gram-negative enterics in oral lesions reflects the opportunistic nature of these bacteria.

Another important aspect of the enteric bacteria in relation to dentistry involves survival of these bacteria in dental unit water supplies. When water is allowed to sit undisturbed in service lines or storage tanks, the antibacterial effect of chlorine in municipal-treated supplies tends to diminish. Such a decline in activity can permit the survival or growth of transient or previously colonized bacteria. These bacteria can be passed through or retained in the handpiece and air/water syringe, and in rare instances, the growth is such that a bolus of bacteria can block the waterline.

The most common isolates from dental unit water lines are *Pseudomonas* and *Klebsiella,* and because of their opportunistic nature, there is some unknown degree of risk if such contaminated water is used for irrigation procedures during surgery. In addition, use of such water during dental treatment of debilitated or immunologically compromised patients would place them at a distinct disadvantage. Elimination of this potential problem is aided by flushing the system at the beginning of each day by allowing water to flow through the handpiece, ultrasonic scaler, air/water syringe, and rinsing or drinking water dispenser for at least 2 minutes. Chlorinators also can be used, followed by flushing.

As mentioned earlier, health care professionals who are shedding salmonellae or shigellae may transmit the bacteria to their patients if personal hygiene measures, thorough handwashing, and gloving are not used. This may be particularly important in dentistry because the mouth is the normal site of entry into the body for these diseases. Although those known to be shedding these bacteria are restricted from patient care by State Board of Health Associations, prevention of transmission from unknowing carriers must rely on routine hygiene, handwashing, and gloving by all dental care providers.

SUGGESTED READINGS

Baron S, ed. *Medical Microbiology.* Menlo Park, Calif: Addison Wesley Publishing Co; 1986.

Du Pont, HL, Pickering LK. *Infections of the Gastrointestinal Tract, Microbiology, Pathophysiology and Clinical Features.* New York: Plenum Press; 1980.

Freeman BA, ed. *Burrows Textbook of Microbiology.* Philadelphia: WB Saunders Co; 1985.

Haapasalo M, Ranta H, Ranta K. Facultative gram-negative enteric rods in persistent periapical infections. *Acta Odontol Scand.* 1983;41:19–22.

Keusch GT, Donohue-Rolfe A, Jacewica M. Shigella toxin(s): Description and role in diarrhea and dysentery. *J Parmacol Ther.* 1982; 15:403–438.

Levine MM, Kaper JB, Black RE, Clements ML. New knowlege on pathogenesis of bacterial enteric infections as applied to vaccine development. *Microbiol Rev.* 1983; 47:510–550.

Rubin RH, Weinstein L. *Salmonellosis: Microbiologic, Pathologic and Clinical Features.* New York: Stratton Intercontinental Medical Book Co; 1977.

Samaranayake LP, Calman K, Ferguson M, et al. The oral carriage of yeasts and coliforms in patients on cytotoxic therapy. *J Oral Pathol.* 1984; 13:390–393.

Slots J, Rams TE, Listgarten MA. Yeasts, enteric rods and pseudomonads in the subgingival flora of severe adult periodontitis. *Oral Microbiol Immunol.* 1988; 3:47–52.

Stephenson JR. Gastrointestinal colonization and septicemia with *Pseudomonas aeruginosa* due to contaminated thymol mouthwash in immunocompromised patients. *J Hosp Infec.* 1985; 6:369–378.

CHAPTER 17

Bacteroides

Vincent F. Gerencser and Mary Ann Gerencser

INTRODUCTION
MORPHOLOGY
CLASSIFICATION
CULTIVATION
VIRULENCE FACTORS
DISEASE PROCESS
DIAGNOSIS
TREATMENT
EPIDEMIOLOGY
ORAL ASPECTS
SUGGESTED READINGS

INTRODUCTION

Members of the genus *Bacteroides* are anaerobic bacteria found in association with humans and animals. They are found in significant numbers in the oral cavity and intestinal tract. Several species cause overt disease and can be isolated from periodontal pockets and intestinal abscesses. Two groups of *Bacteroides* species, the melaninogenicus group and the fragilis group, are of major clinical significance. Species in the melaninogenicus group produce a black pigment on blood agar. Of these *Bacteroides gingivalis* and *Bacteroides intermedius* are important oral pathogens. The fragilis group is nonpigmented. In this group, *Bacteroides fragilis* is the major pathogen.

MORPHOLOGY

Bacteroides are gram-negative, non-sporeforming rods. Most species are nonmotile, although some are motile by peritrichous flagella. Sizes range from 0.4 to 1.2 μm in width and 1.5 to 7.0 μm in length. Larger cells up to 12 μm long occasionally are seen. Cultures show some pleomorphism, containing rods, spheres, and coccoid forms. Cells can occur singly, in pairs, or in short chains. Some strains have a polysaccharide capsule. Surface colonies on blood agar are small, ranging from 0.5 to 2.0 mm in size. The *Bacteroides melaninogenicus* group produces black colonies on blood agar due to the production of a hematin-containing pigment.

CLASSIFICATION

The genus *Bacteroides* is classified in the family Bacteroidaceae. This family is divided into 13 genera and contains all the anaerobic, gram-negative, straight, curved, or helical rods. Thirty-nine species are described in the genus *Bacteroides*. Before 1976, *B. fragilis* was divided into five subspecies. These subspecies are now given species rank as *B. fragilis, Bacteroides distasonis, Bacteroides thetaiotaomicron, Bacteroides ovatus,* and *Bacteroides vulgatus*. These five species constitute the fragilis group.

All black-pigmented *Bacteroides* were included in the species *B. melaninogenicus* at one time. Classification of this group has undergone a number of changes in recent years. Most of the changes result from the recognition of new species based on DNA/

TABLE 17–1. CURRENT NOMENCLATURE OF BLACK-PIGMENTED *BACTEROIDES* SPECIES

Former Name	Current Name
B. melaninogenicus subsp. *melaninogenicus*	*B. melaninogenicus* *B. loescheii* *B. denticola*
B. melaninogenicus subsp. *intermedius*	*B. intermedius* *B. corporis*
B. melaninogenicus subsp. *asaccharolyticus*	*B. asaccharolyticus* *B. gingivalis* *B. endodontalis*
B. melaninogenicus subsp. *levii*	*B. levii*
B. melaninogenicus subsp. *macacae*	*B. macacae*

Based on data from Coykendall AL, Kaczmarek FS, Slots J. Int J Syst Bacteriol. *1980; 30:559–564; Holdeman LV, Johnson JL.* Int J Syst Bacteriol. *1982; 32:399–409; Johnson JL, Holdeman LV.* Int J Syst Bacteriol. *1983; 33:15–25; van Steenberger TJM, van Winkelhoff AJ, Mayrand D, Grenier D, deGraaff J.* Int J Syst Bacteriol. *1984; 34:118–120.*

DNA homology studies. The current nomenclature of the black-pigmented *Bacteroides* is shown in Table 17–1. All of these species are found in the oral cavity except *Bacteroides asaccharolyticus, Bacteroides macacae,* and *Bacteroides levii. Bacteroides asaccharolyticus* is of nonoral, human origin, whereas the other species have been found in animals. DNA homology studies suggest that there are additional as yet unnamed species in this group. For example, a new asaccharolytic species, *Bacteroides endodontalis,* has been described that has little DNA homology with the other asaccharolytic species. *Bacteroides endodontalis* was isolated from infected dental root canals in humans. It has been proposed that the three asaccharolytic, black-pigmented *Bacteroides* species be placed in a new genus *Porphyromonas,* but it is not yet clear whether or not this proposal will be accepted.

CULTIVATION

Bacteroides are strict anaerobes with fastidious growth requirements. They must be grown under anaerobic conditions and grow best on enriched, prereduced culture media. The black-pigmented strains require hemin and vitamin K for growth. They produce pigment better on laked blood agar than on a blood agar medium with intact red blood cells. For primary isolation from clinical materials, the sample is streaked on enriched blood agar. Plates should be prereduced before inoculation and should be incubated in an atmosphere of 85% N_2, 10% H_2, 5% CO_2. A selective medium containing vancomycin and kanamycin (KVA medium), which inhibits gram-positive bacteria, also may be used to isolate *Bacteroides* and other gram-negative anaerobes. Recent evidence suggests that some black-pigmented species may be inhibited by vancomycin. Therefore, a selective medium containing kanamycin only or the use of a nonselective medium is recommended for isolation of the *B. melaninogenicus* group.

VIRULENCE FACTORS

Bacteroides fragilis is the prototype of the fragilis group. The principal virulence factors of *B. fragilis* are its polysaccharide capsule and its endotoxin. The polysaccharide capsule promotes abscess formation. Encapsulated strains produce abscesses in experimental animals, whereas unencapsulated strains fail to do so. When used by itself, the capsular polysaccharide produces similar abscesses. The capsule also promotes adherence to peritoneal mesothelial surfaces and resistance to killing by neutrophils.

The role of the endotoxin in *B. fragilis* in virulence has been questioned because it exhibits little biologic activity and because injections of pure cultures into experimental animals did not result in death. This lack of classic endotoxic activity by *B. fragilis* endotoxin may be due to its chemical composition, since it is deficient in 2-keto-3-deoxyoctonate, heptose, and β-hydroxymyristic acid in the lipid A moiety. The endotoxin does, however, activate complement by the alternative pathway. It may, therefore, act as a virulence factor.

An indication of the virulence and pathogenic potential of *B. fragilis* is the fact that it is the most frequently isolated bacterium from anaerobic infections, although it is not the most numerous *Bacteroides* species isolated from feces.

Bacteroides melaninogenicus is the prototype of the melaninogenicus group. This group contains a number of newly created species, among which is the oral pathogen *B. gingivalis.* The virulence factors of the group are listed in Table 17–2. *Bacteroides gingivalis* has no singular or unique virulence factors. However, it is able to colonize and grow on gingival tissue and cause periodontal tissue destruction. This ability resides in its surface structures and cellular products. It has pili, long surface fibers, a capsule, and lipopolysaccharide. The pili and surface fibers may be involved in attachment to oral cellular surfaces and to other bacteria. Pathogenic strains that are encapsulated are resistant to phagocytosis. The lipopolysaccharide has weak endotoxic activity probably because it lacks some of the components of typical endotoxin, but it does activate complement and stimulate bone resorption in organ tissue culture. *Bacteroides gingivalis* produces collagenase, proteases, extracellular phospholipase A, acid and alkaline phosphatases, volatile

TABLE 17–2. POTENTIAL VIRULENCE FACTORS PRODUCED BY BLACK-PIGMENTED *BACTEROIDES*[a]

Tissue-destroying factors		
Enzymes	*Toxins*	*Other*
Collagenase	Endotoxin	Abscess formation
Trypsin	Epitheliotoxin	Polyclonal B cell activators
Gelatinase	Hydrogen sulfide	Hemagglutinin
Fibrinolysin	Methyl mercaptan	
Hyaluronidase	Butyric and propionic acids	
Heparinase	Indole	
Ribonuclease	Ammonia	
Deoxyribonuclease	Fibroblast inhibiting factor	
Bone-resorbing factors		
Endotoxin		
Acid phosphatases		
Alkaline phosphatases		
Phospholipase A		
Phagocytosis-inhibiting factors		
Capsule		

[a]Not all factors are produced by all species in the melaninogenicus group.
Data derived from Slots J, Genco RJ. J Dent Res. *1984; 63:412; Slots J. In: Genco RJ, Mergenhagen SE, eds.* Host Parasite Interactions in Periodontal Disease. *Washington, DC: American Society for Microbiology; 1982:27–45.*

sulfur compounds, and other toxic factors. Thus, the main virulence factors of *B. gingivalis* are thought to be its capsule, endotoxin, and collagenase and other proteolytic enzymes. The potential pathogenicity of the *B. melaninogenicus* group was demonstrated in early studies of the pathogenicity of oral bacteria. Infectious abscesses could be produced in guinea pigs only by injection of mixtures of bacteria from the gingival crevice. *Bacteroides melaninogenicus* was found to be an essential component of any mixture that could initiate a transmissible infection. These and later studies demonstrated that *Bacteroides* play an essential role in polymicrobic anaerobic infections.

DISEASE PROCESS

Bacteroides usually depend on a synergistic relationship with other bacteria to cause infection, and, therefore, they almost always are found in mixed infections. The disease process is usually of endogenous origin but may be exogenous as a result of human or other animal bites. The typical lesion is a localized necrotic abscess.

The *B. fragilis* group, especially *B. fragilis* and *B. thetaiotaomicron,* is the most commonly found anaerobe in clinical infections. They are isolated from most intraabdominal infections resulting from spillage of fecal matter into the peritoneal cavity, causing abscess formation and peritonitis. They may be seen in infections at other sites.

The *B. melaninogenicus* group is primarily involved in oral disease. *Bacteroides gingivalis* is associated with severe adult periodontitis and may play a role in generalized juvenile periodontitis. *Bacteroides intermedius* has been implicated in acute necrotizing ulcerative gingivitis and pregnancy gingivitis.

DIAGNOSIS

Clinical characteristics that suggest the presence of *Bacteroides* in an abscess are those associated with anaerobes in general (Chapter 22). A gram stain of the clinical material is useful, since *Bacteroides* and other gram-negative anaerobes usually are pale staining and may have a distinctive morphology. Fluorescent antibody reagents are commercially available for *B. fragilis* and some of the *B. melaninogenicus* group. These reagents may be used for rapid detection of *Bacteroides* in clinical material. Definitive diagnosis requires the isolation and identication of the organisms. Pure cultures are identified by a combination of morphology, gas-liquid chromatography of acid end products, and biochemical tests.

The *B. melaninogenicus* group is distinguished from other *Bacteroides* by the production of brown to black-pigmented colonies on blood agar (Fig 17–1). *Bacteroides melaninogenicus* group colonies that have not yet pigmented can be distinguished from others because these fluoresec brick red under long wave ultraviolet light. *Bacteroides gingivalis, B. asaccharolyticus,* and *B. endodontalis* do not ferment carbohydrates, whereas the other species do. The ability to produce

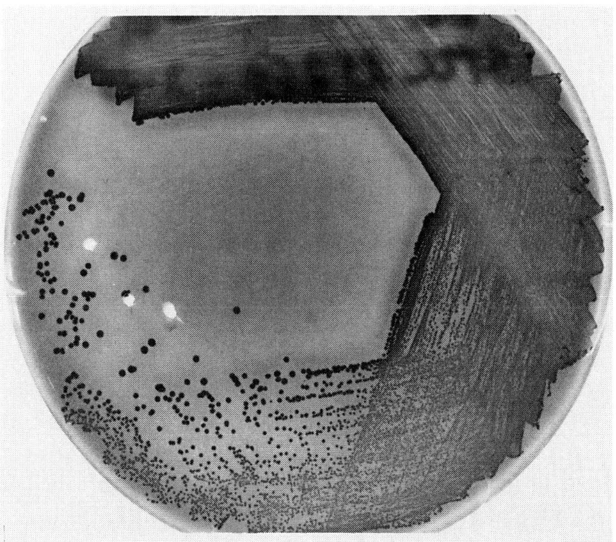

Figure 17–1. Black colonies of *Bacteroides gingivalis* (a member of the *Bacteroides melaninogenicus* group) on blood agar.

phenylacetic acid, a trypsinlike enzyme, and to agglutinate a variety of red blood cells distinguishes *B. gingivalis* from *B. asaccharolyticus* and *B. endodontalis*. Additional tests are needed to separate *B. asaccharolyticus* from *B. endodontalis*.

Identification of saccharolytic, black-pigmented species and of the members of the *B. fragilis* group is based on biochemical tests. Complete identification of these and other *Bacteroides* species may require extensive testing and a number of special media. Detailed characteristics of *Bacteroides* species can be found in *Bergey's Manual* and other standard works. Several types of test kits for the identification of anaerobic bacteria are now available commercially.

TREATMENT

Treatment of anaerobic infections involves a combination of surgery to drain abscesses and excise necrotic tissue and antimicrobial therapy. *Bacteroides* are sensitive to clindamycin, chloramphenicol, and metronidazole and are resistant to aminoglycosides. *Bacteroides fragilis*, the most common clinical isolate, is also the most antibiotic resistant of the *Bacteroides* species. The *B. fragilis* group is resistant to penicillin and the older cephalosporins because it produces a β-lactamase. The fragilis group is more susceptible to cefoxitin and moxalactam, since these antibiotics are relatively resistant to β-lactamases. About 80% of the strains are susceptible to carbenicillin. Most strains of *B. fragilis* are resistant to tetracycline, but about 70% of strains are sensitive to the tetracycline derivatives, doxycycline and minocycline. The *B. melaninogenicus* group is generally susceptible to a wide range of antibiotics. Some strains also are susceptible to penicillin and the cephalosporins, but others produce a β-lactamase and thus exhibit resistance to these antibiotics.

EPIDEMIOLOGY

Infections involving *Bacteroides* species are almost always of endogenous origin. Invasion of the tissues by members of the normal microbial flora leads to infections that are polymicrobic in nature. These infections are not transmitted from humans or from animals to humans. *Bacteroides* are found as part of the normal flora of the mouth, gastrointestinal tract, vagina, urethra, and external genitalia.

A variety of species have been isolated from the mouth, including at least 12 nonpigmented species and 6 black-pigmented species. Strains of the *B. melaninogenicus* group often are isolated from extraoral infections whose source is the oral cavity.

Bacteroides species are among the most numerous anaerobes in the intestinal tract and in feces, reaching concentrations of 10^{11} organisms per gram.

ORAL ASPECTS

A number of species of the genus *Bacteroides*, both pigmented and nonpigmented, are found as part of the normal flora of the oral cavity. The species with special significance in oral disease are *B. gingivalis* and *B. intermedius*. *Bacteroides gingivalis* is associated with severe adult periodontitis and with rapidly progressive periodontitis in young adults and may be associated with generalized juvenile periodontitis. *Bacteroides intermedius* is associated with pregnancy gingivitis and with acute necrotizing ulcerative gingivitis. The total number of these species in diseased oral sites is significantly higher than that found in normal oral sites, implying that they are playing some role in the disease process, although their exact role is not clear. Despite the current emphasis on *B. gingivalis* and *B. intermedius*, other *Bacteroides* species also may be involved in orofacial disease.

SUGGESTED READINGS

Bartlett JG. Virulence factors in anaerobic bacteria. *John Hopkins Med J*. 1982; 151:1.

Hill GB. Introduction to the anaerobic bacteria: Non-spore-forming anaerobes. In: Joklik WK, Willett HP, Amos DB, eds. *Zinsser Microbiology*. 18th ed. Norwalk, Conn: Appleton-Century-Crofts; 1984.

Holdeman LV, Cato EP, Moore WEC. *Anaerobe Laboratory Manual*. 4th ed. Blacksburg: Virginia Polytechnic Institute and State University; 1977.

Holdeman LV, Kelley RW, Moore WEC. *Bacteroides*. In: Krieg NR, Holt JG, eds. *Bergey's Manual of Systematic Bacteriology*. Vol. 1, Baltimore: Williams & Wilkins Co; 1984, vol. 1.

Lennette EH, Balows A, Hausler WJ Jr, Shadomy HJ, eds. *Manual of Clinical Microbiology*. 4th ed. Washington, DC: American Society for Microbiology; 1985:450–460.

Mayrand D, Holt B. Biology of asaccharolytic black pigmented *Bacteroides* species. *Microbiol Rev*. 1988; 52:134.

Roberts MC, Moncla B, Kenny GE. Chromosomal DNA probes for the identification of *Bacteroides* species. *J Gen Microbiol*. 1987; 133:1423.

Slots J. Importance of black-pigmented *Bacteroides* in human periodontal disease. In: Genco RJ, Mergenhagen SE, eds. *Host Parasite Interactions in Periodontal Disease*. Washington, DC: American Society for Microbiology; 1982:27–45.

Slots J, Genco RJ. Black-pigmented *Bacteroides* species, *Capnoyctophaga* species and *Actinobacillus actinomycetemcomitans* in human periodontal disease: Virulence factors in colonization, survival, and tissue destruction. *J Dent Res*. 1984; 63:412.

CHAPTER 18

Spirochetes

John A. Molinari and Virginia A. Merchant

INTRODUCTION
MORPHOLOGY
MOTILITY
CULTIVATION AND METABOLISM
TREPONEMA PALLIDUM
Clinical Features
Diagnosis
Treatment
Immunity
Prevention
Oral Aspects
LEPTOSPIROSIS
Clinical Features
Diagnosis and Treatment
RELAPSING FEVER
Clinical Features
Diagnosis and Treatment
LYME DISEASE
ORAL ASPECTS
SUGGESTED READINGS

INTRODUCTION

The order Spirochaetales consists of helically shaped, motile, gram-negative bacteria. There are five genera belonging to two families (Spirochaetaceae and Leptospiraceae) that include both free-living and parasitic species, several of which are pathogenic to humans. Major characteristics of the genera are listed in Table 18–1. In addition to being causative agents of syphilis, yaws, pinta, and relapsing fever, a number of species of spirochetes are members of the normal oral flora (Table 18–2). The numbers of oral spirochetes increase dramatically in the plaque of patients having gingivitis and periodontal disease, constituting a significant percentage of the microscopically detectable flora.

MORPHOLOGY

The spirochetes are distinguished from other prokaryotes by having one or more internal flagella or axial fibrils, which are also referred to as axistyles or axial filaments (Table 18–1). These periplasmic structures probably play a role in motility of the organism, but the mechanism is unknown. The outer sheath, a complex structure composed of protein, lipid, and carbohydrate, probably functions in cell permeability. The protoplasmic cylinder consists of the cell wall, the cytoplasmic membrane, and the intracellular contents. The cell wall peptidoglycan is chemically similar to that of other gram-negative bacteria. The spirochetes, however, contain a relatively large amount of lipid (18 to 36%) in comparison to other bacteria.

MOTILITY

Spirochetes are motile, exhibiting locomotion, rotation, and flexing motion in liquids. In addition, they have been observed to move by creeping or crawling over solid surfaces. The mechanism(s) of movement in spirochetes remain(s) to be elucidated.

TABLE 18–1. MAJOR CHARACTERISTICS OF THE GENERA OF MEDICALLY IMPORTANT SPIROCHETES

Characteristic	*Spirochaeta*	*Treponema*	*Borrelia*	*Leptospira*
Size (μm)				
Cell diameter	0.2–0.75	0.1–0.4	0.2–0.5	0.1
Length	5–250	5–20	3–20	6–12
Terminal hooks	−	−	−	+
Axial fibrils	1	3–5	15–20	1
Free-living species	+	−	−	+
Host-associated species	−	+	+	+
Species pathogenic to humans	−	+	+	+
Obligate aerobes	−	−	+	+
Obligate anaerobes	+	+[a]	−	−
Facultatives	+	−	−	−

[a]*Treponema pallidum* may be microaerophilic or facultative.

Adapted from Holt JG, ed. Bergey's Manual of Systematic Bacteriology. *Baltimore: Williams & Wilkins; 1984, vol. 1.*

CULTIVATION AND METABOLISM

Many spirochetes, including *Treponema pallidum* (the etiologic agent of syphilis), are not readily cultivable and are maintained in the laboratory by inoculation into living animals, that is, rabbits. Free-living spirochetes grow readily in prepared media. However, certain of the anaerobic host-associated spirochetes, including many oral spirochetes, require complex media supplemented with serum, serum components, ascitic fluid, or rumen fluid for cultivation.

The order Spirochaetales includes obligate aerobes and obligate anaerobes as well as microaerophilic and facultative organisms (Table 18–1). *Treponema pallidum*, once considered to be an obligate anaerobe, is now believed to be microaerophilic, requiring 1% to 5% oxygen. The free-living aerobic and facultative spirochetes all use carbohydrates as their sole source of energy and carbon, producing acetate, ethanol, and lactate as fermentation products.

TREPONEMA PALLIDUM

Treponema pallidum is the causal agent of syphilis. Like gonorrhea, syphilis is a highly infectious disease spread by either sexual contact with an infected person (ie, acquired syphilis) or by an infected pregnant woman to her fetus (ie, congenital syphilis). Its place

TABLE 18–2. SPECIES OF SPIROCHETES ASSOCIATED WITH HUMANS

Species	Site of Isolation	Associated Diseases	Transmission
Treponema pallidum	Genitalia, skin, oral cavity, systemic	Syphilis, yaws	Sexual, direct contact
Treponema carateum	Skin (lymph fluid)	Pinta	Direct contact
Treponema denticola	Normal oral flora	Isolated along with other bacteria, primarily fusiforms, from patients with acute necrotizing ulcerative gingivitis	
Treponema vincentii			
Treponema scoliodontum			
Treponema refringens	Normal flora of genitalia	Not pathogenic	
Treponema minutum			
Treponema phagedenis			
Treponema macrodentium	Gingival crevice (normal flora)		
Treponema orale			
Borrelia recurrentis	Blood	Relapsing fever	Body lice
Borrelia parkeri	Blood	Relapsing fever	Ticks
Borrelia duttoni plus 7 other species			
Borrelia burgdorferi	Blood	Lyme disease	Ticks
Leptospira interrogans	Proximal convoluted tubule of kidney/blood/CSF	Leptospirosis	Shed in urine

as a historically important disease is well established, going back to the earliest of biblical writings.

In recent years, the number of reported cases has remained constant at 25,000 to 30,000/year. Epidemiologic trends indicate that the disease most commonly occurs in lower socioeconomic groups and male homosexuals. Although the majority of infections are genital, about 20% of the patients exhibit oral or other maxillofacial manifestations.

Treponoma pallidum is a fine spirochete measuring 5.20 μm in length and 0.1 to 0.2 μm in thickness. It is difficult to observe under light microscopy, hence the derivation of its descriptive name, "pale, fine thread." Visualization of *T. pallidum* by darkfield illumination is the best form of observation. From a practical point, staining techniques for this pathogen remain unsatisfactory. Cultivation of *T. pallidum* in vitro has been unsuccessful. In nature, this microorganism is confined primarily to its human host. *Treponoma pallidum* is highly sensitive to light, air, and penicillin therapy.

Clinical Features

Syphilis is a disease characterized by a long incubation period involving a complex series of host–parasite interactions. The immune response that develops during infection appears to play a prominent role in determining the ultimate outcome of disease and residual tissue damage. *Treponema pallidum* is one of only a few microorganisms that can penetrate intact mucous membranes, but the most common passage occurs through abraded skin. It is important to note also that this spirochete is highly invasive, as evidenced by its capacity to rapidly induce a bacteremia and disseminate systemically within a short time after exposure.

Development and progression of syphilis are characterized by certain stages. These are incubation, primary, secondary, and late (tertiary) syphilis. During primary and secondary syphilis, in which there are open lesions, millions of organisms are shed, making these the most infectious stages. Patients may be infectious for months and, occasionally, for several years after most of the secondary lesions have disappeared spontaneously. The appearance of cutaneous lesions or internal tissue damage is correlated routinely with specific stages. However, the size of the treponemal inoculum and incubation period can modify the typical disease patterns.

Incubation. The incubation period is from 2 to 6 weeks after treponemal entrance into the body, with 3 to 4 weeks as the most common interval. During this time, spirochetal replication is very active at the port of entry and in many secondary sites. Clinical evidence of disease is absent.

Primary Syphilis. A characteristic lesion, called a chancre, becomes clinically recognizable at the inoculation site as the initial manifestation of syphilis (Figs 18–1, 18–2). This hard, painless lesion begins as a dull red macule that becomes papular. Erosion of the papular edges leads to ulceration of the lesion, which appears as the classic chancre. The firmness of the chancre is due to the presence of an intense cellular infiltration and mucosal and serum accumulation in the infected tissue as a response to the high concentration of spirochetes. These usually can be observed by darkfield microscopy of tissue samples. Chancres usually appear as singular lesions, although multiple chancres occasionally develop.

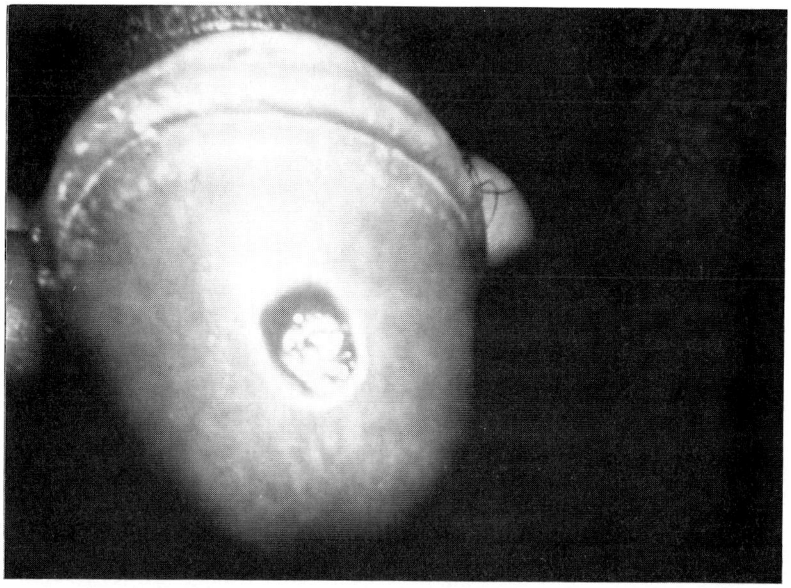

Figure 18–1. Syphilitic chancre of the penis. *(Courtesy of Centers for Disease Control, Atlanta, GA.)*

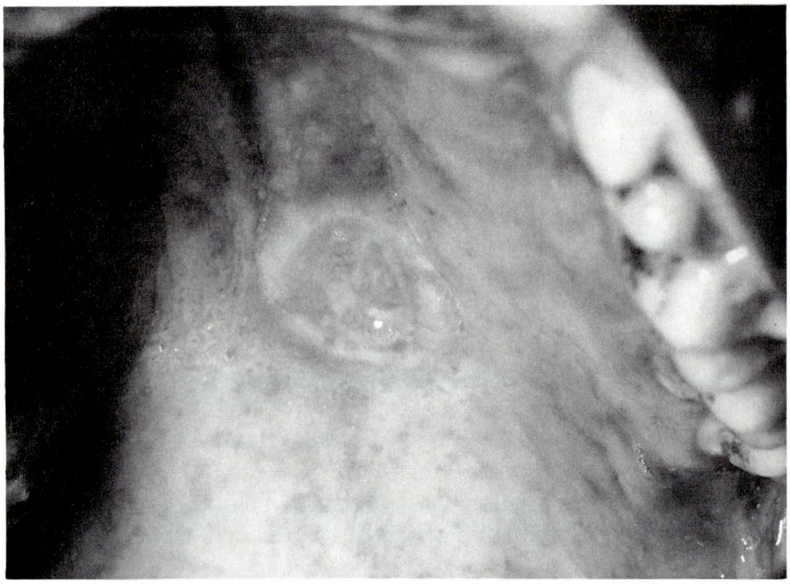

Figure 18–2. Palatal chancre in primary syphilis. *(Courtesy of Dr. James W. Curtis, Jr., University of Detroit School of Dentistry.)*

Regional lymphadenopathy, called a satellite bubo, constitutes another important diagnostic sign during the primary stage. The chancre will resolve spontaneously with little scarring in 2 to 4 weeks, even in the absence of antibiotic chemotherapy. The patient appears free of disease during the following weeks. Unfortunately, the patient may believe that the disease has eradicated itself and not seek medical assistance. This allows the dissemination of *T. pallidum* in the body to become more extensive.

Secondary Syphilis. The onset of secondary syphilis reflects a generalized spread of spirochetes. Lesions may involve mucous membranes, the eyes, bones, joints, lymph nodes, or the central nervous system. This stage signifies a period when the patient is most infectious. Mucocutaneous lesions contain the highest treponemal concentrations. Painless copper red rashes may develop on the skin (particularly the palms and soles), accompanied by fever and malaise. Oral lesions, when present, are termed mucous patches (Fig 18–3). These are painless, multiple, grayish white lesions, that arise on the tongue, gingiva, or buccal mucosa. Resolution of these syphilitic lesions also occurs spontaneously, with little scarring.

The only evidence of infection at this time is the presence of a positive serologic test for syphilis. Patients can experience relapses for up to 4 years after

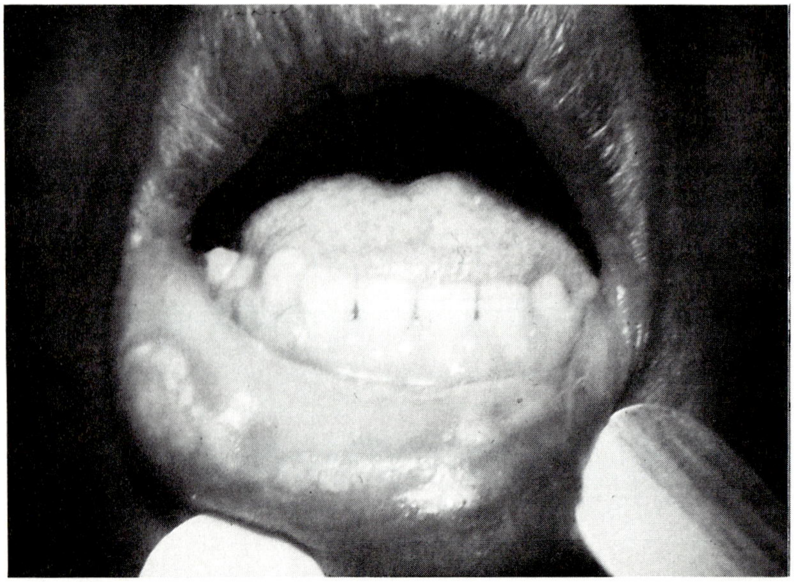

Figure 18–3. Mucous patches on lower lip. *(Courtesy of Centers for Disease Control, Atlanta, GA.)*

infections. Thus, they are still considered infectious. Lack of syphilitic manifestations within 4 years represents minimal chance for recurrence. Approximately 60 to 65% of these individuals develop immunity against *T. pallidum* and experience no further tissue damage. Over half will maintain this protection for life.

Late (Tertiary) Syphilis. The remaining one third of infected persons, whose infection does not stabilize, enter the final and most destructive stage of syphilis. Late or tertiary lesions that develop involve the deeper structures and organs of their host and interfere with their function. Chiefly affected are the central nervous and cardiovascular systems. The late lesions reflect an intense reaction that appears out of proportion to the number of spirochetes found in tissues. The presence of few, if any, *T. pallidum* detectable by either darkfield microscopy or animal inoculation techniques indicates that the patient's tissues have become highly sensitized. This is consistent with the development of an allergic response to treponemal components or metabolic products. The chief oral lesion is the gumma, a destructive, caseous lesion surrounded by fibrous tissue (Fig 18–4). Affected external sites are seen as sloughing necrotic areas. Gummas can occur in the hard palate, skin, mucous membranes, testes, liver, spleen, and bone. Cardiovascular and CNS complications also develop and often lead to death.

Congenital Syphilis. Transmission of syphilis from mother to offspring remains a common, tragic problem. *Treponema pallidum* can readily cross the placenta and infect the fetus. Sequelae range from asymptomatic to death of the baby.

Children with congenital syphilis may exhibit a wide variety of oral lesions. The Hutchinsonian triad is pathognomonic and includes hypoplasia of the incisors and molars, eighth nerve deafness, and interstitial keratitis. Not all characteristics of the triad occur simultaneously.

The enamel hypoplasia involves the maxillary and mandibular permanent incisors and the first molars. When the anterior teeth are affected they are called Hutchinson's teeth. The upper central incisor usually is notched and screwdriver shaped, with the mesial and distal surfaces of the crown tapered and converged toward the incisal edge of the tooth. The crowns of the first molars are irregular and appear to be arranged in an agglomerate mass of globules, hence, the name mulberry molars (Fig 18–5).

Not all patients with congenital syphilis will exhibit these dental manifestations, and, conversely, occasionally patients without congenital syphilis may appear to have Hutchinson's teeth. Because treponemal infection of the fetus before the fourth month is uncommon, if treatment with antibiotics is initiated before the fourth month in an infected pregnant woman, greater than 95% of the offspring of such mothers will not have the disease.

Diagnosis

Routine diagnosis of syphilis involves obtaining an accurate patient history, clinical observation, and the use of appropriate laboratory procedures. The latter include darkfield examination and serologic assays of blood or spinal fluid.

Examination of exudates, lymph node aspirates, or tissue scrapings by darkfield microscopy provides the most rapid method for direct identification of *T.*

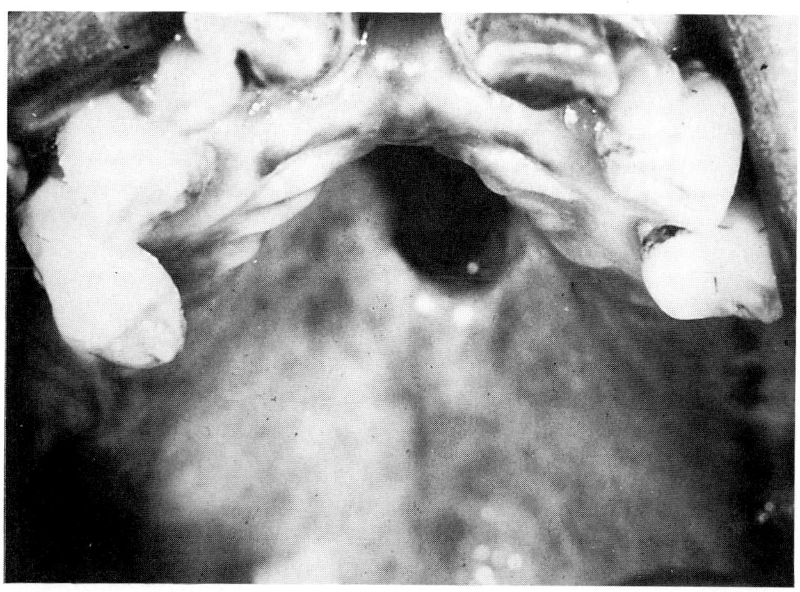

Figure 18–4. Gumma occurring on the hard palate during late syphilis.

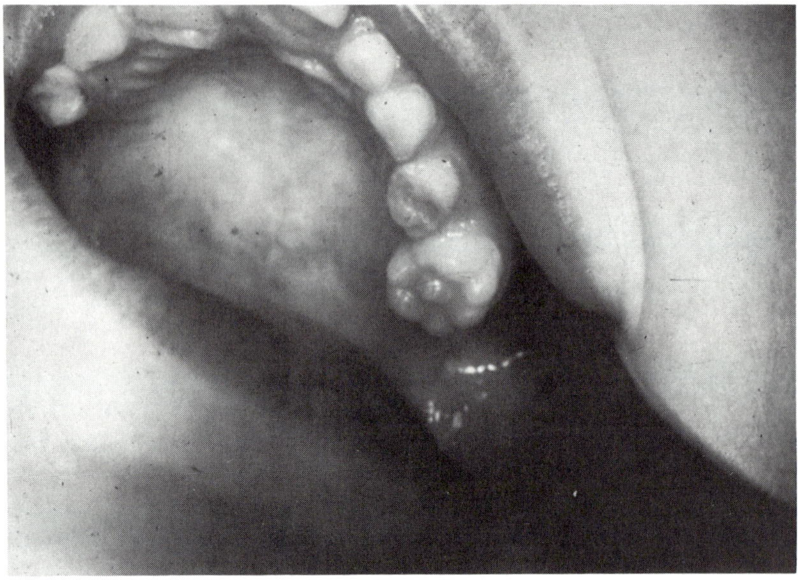

Figure 18–5. Molar hyperplasia (ie, mulberry molars) in congenital syphilis. *(Courtesy of Centers for Disease Control, Atlanta, GA.)*

pallidum in lesions during primary, secondary, and early congenital syphilis (Fig 18–6). In samples taken from oral syphilitic lesions, *T. pallidum* cannot be distinguished from the normal oral spirochetes. In these instances, aspiration of a locally involved lymph node can provide *T. pallidum* for direct observation. Unfortunately, darkfield microscopy is not always accurate, as early syphilitic chancres may not demonstrate spirochetes. Topical application of treponemicidal antibiotics, or even soap and water, also may lead to false negative darkfield results.

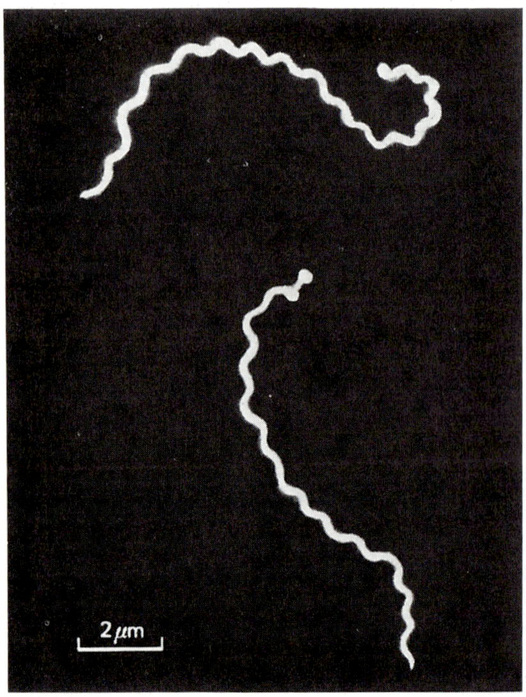

Figure 18–6. Darkfield appearance of *Treponema pallidum.*

Serologic tests constitute the most frequently employed procedures that confirm a diagnosis of syphilis. In particular, demonstration of certain immunologic markers is necessary for establishing the diagnosis during latent stages of disease. Tests are classified as nontreponemal (nonspecific) or treponemal (specific). The most frequently used nontreponemal tests at present are the rapid plasma reagin (RPR) test and the Venereal Disease Research Laboratory (VDRL) test. These detect a nonspecific antibody called reagin, which is a mixture of IgM and IgA directed against cross-reacting tissue antigens that are widely distributed in nature. Reagin appears about 4 weeks post-*T. pallidum* exposure and about 1 week after development of the chancre. Antigen for the tests is a lipid, called cardiolipin, that is extracted from bovine cardiac tissue. Although the RPR, VDRL, and other nontreponemal floculation assays provide rapid, inexpensive information, a positive test is considered to be only presumptive evidence of infection. Occasional biologic false negative results may be due to technical error or very low concentrations of syphilitic reagin in the blood specimen. More commonly, biologic false positives (BFP) may occur in the absence of syphilis. BFPs are often found when certain diseases or conditions are present. Some of the more common are malaria, leprosy, relapsing fever, atypical pneumonia, and infectious mononucleosis.

The use of highly specific treponemal assays is important in confirmation of the diagnosis for syphilis and elimination of BFPs. The primary specific antibody test employed is an indirect fluorescent antibody-absorption assay (FTA-ABS). The FTA-ABS test is expensive and, therefore, used only to confirm positive RPR or VDRL tests. Antigen for this procedure is prepared from the Nichols strain of *T. pallidum.*

Treatment

Parenteral penicillin G remains as the antibiotic of choice for treating all stages of syphillis. The recommended regimen from the United States Public Health Service for cases of primary, secondary, or latent syphilis of less than 1 year's duration is a single intramuscular injection of 2 to 4 million units. Patients with an allergy to penicillin can be treated with tetracycline hydrochloride or erythromycin. Treatment of syphilitic patients is made difficult because many infected individuals are not aware that they have the disease.

Immunity

Cell-mediated immunity provides a major portion of antisyphilitic protection. Resistance to infection may not be complete, however, and subjects may be reinfected. The host's immune system also plays a role in tissue destruction during late stages of the disease, as evidenced by gummas that are allergic reactions. As with most microbial infections, the size of the treponemal inoculation, immune status of the host, and other factors are important in determining whether syphilis develops, progresses, or is eradicated in the body.

Prevention

Because transmission of syphilis is almost entirely sexual in nature, the best preventive measure remains avoidance of an obviously infected sex partner. Syphilis is a reportable disease, requiring clinicians to notify state health departments of infected individuals. The health departments, in turn, notify the Centers for Disease Control and investigate possible spread of infection to sexual contacts of the person infected. A vaccine for syphilis is not available. Control of the disease is enhanced by early and adequate treatment with antibiotics. This minimizes the length of time during which the patient remains infectious, reducing the number of persons to whom the disease can be transmitted.

Oral Aspects

Oral lesions are common extragenital manifestations during the primary and secondary stages of syphilis. Many are open lesions discharging millions of spirochetes, thereby increasing the risk of transmission by direct contact. The routine use of barrier techniques such as gloves can virtually eliminate the possibility of dental practitioners contracting syphilis from patients.

LEPTOSPIROSIS

Leptospirosis is primarily a disease of wild and domestic animals and is caused by *Leptospirosis interrogans.* Transmission to humans occurs via direct contact with infected animals or more usually via contact with urine-contaminated water or soil and usually is acquired by occupational exposure. Rats are a common source of infection, but domestic animals, that is, dogs, livestock, and cats, also are important sources of the disease.

Clinical Features

Leptospires penetrate intact mucous membranes or abraded skin, enter the bloodstream, and are transmitted throughout the body, including to the cerebrospinal fluid and the eye. Subclinical infection is common. Clinical manifestations may be either mild (anicteric leptospirosis) or severe (icteric leptospirosis or Weil's disease).

Anicteric leptospirosis is characterized by a nonspecific, flu-like illness lasting 4 to 7 days. Weil's disease, seen in approximately 5 to 10% of patients with clinical disease is characterized by jaundice. Renal failure, hemorrhage, and cardiovascular collapse may occur in severely jaundiced patients. Death occurs in 5 to 10% of patients having Weil's disease.

Diagnosis and Treatment

Diagnosis usually is made on the basis of serology. Leptospires can be observed by darkfield microscopy, but the low numbers that occur in natural infections make direct observation difficult. The most reliable method of detection is culturing. Leptospires can be isolated from blood or CSF during the first week of illness or from urine beginning the second week.

Both penicillin G and tetracylcines have been used for treatment, but only the latter is effective in eliminating leptospires from the kidney. Vaccination of domestic animals has reduced the incidence of infection.

RELAPSING FEVER

Arthropod-borne spirochetes belonging to the genus *Borrelia* are the causative agents of relapsing fever. Epidemic relapsing fever is caused by *Borrelia recurrentis* and is transmitted from human to human by the human body louse, *Pediculus humanus.* Relapsing fever transmitted by ticks is endemic to wild small animal populations, which serve as a natural reservoir for the disease.

Clinical Features

These organisms can penetrate intact skin or mucous membranes. The tick-borne spirochetes are present in the saliva or excrement of the tick and, thus, may be released onto the skin surface during feeding.

Relapsing fever is characterized by an acute onset of high fever, severe headache, myalgia, and arthralgia. A rash is common during the end of the primary 3 to 6 day febrile attack. The disease if untreated is characterized by multiple relapses, even in the presence of specific immunity. The relapses are thought to occur as a result of antigenic variation of the spirochete. As immunity to one antigenic type develops, variants that are not affected by the immunity proliferate, and the disease recurs.

Diagnosis and Treatment

Diagnosis is based on the observation of spirochetes in blood smears taken during the febrile episode. Tetracycline, chloramphenicol, penicillin, or erythromycin can be used for treatment.

LYME DISEASE

Lyme disease, transmitted by ixodid ticks, is caused by the spirochete *Borrelia burgdorferi*. The disease, previously recognized in Europe, was first seen in Lyme, Connecticut, in 1975. It has become a serious health problem in the United States, particularly in the northeast, the upper midwest, and the Pacific states. The spirochete replicates in ticks that live in or near wooded areas, tall grass, and brush. The ticks feed on mammals, including deer, mice, domestic pets, and humans. Transmission occurs during feeding.

Like syphilis, Lyme disease occurs in three stages. Stage I occurs within several days to a few weeks after infection. Approximately 85% of patients develop an expanding erythematous rash surrounding a lighter area at the site of the tick bite. Similar but smaller additional skin lesions often develop. Many patients also exhibit flu-like symptoms, including fever, fatigue, headache, a stiff neck, myalgia, and arthralgia. If untreated, the disease progresses to stage II and early generalized disease after several weeks to months. This most commonly is manifest as an acute but transient asymmetrical arthritis. Neurologic or cardiovascular abnormalities occur less frequently. Stage III disease is the most serious and occurs months to years after infection. It consists of progressive arthritis that may be accompanied by neurologic manifestations, including intellectual deterioration or psychiatric disease.

If recognized during stage I, treatment with penicillin or tetracycline is effective in eliminating the infecsion. If the disease progresses, antibiotic treatment is less likely to prevent complications. Protection from tick bites is the best prevention.

ORAL ASPECTS

In addition to the oral manifestations of the previously discussed systemic diseases, spirochetes are prevalent in the dental plaques associated with gingivitis and periodontal disease. Five species of treponemes have been isolated from the oral cavity of humans (Table 18–2) and are considered constituents of the normal oral flora. However, the numbers of spirochetes increase significantly with the advent of gingival inflammation and periodontal disease. Metabolic byproducts of spirochetes may be responsible in part for the inflammatory reaction characteristic of gingivitis and periodontitis, but the exact role of spirochetes in these diseases remains to be elucidated.

Spirochetes, in large numbers, have been isolated from plaque in patients with gingivitis and periodontitis and appear to be directly related to the severity of disease. In addition, spirochetes have been found to penetrate intact tissue adjacent to inflamed areas in advance of other microorganisms in both acute necrotizing ulcerative gingivitis (ANUG) and periodontitis. This finding suggests that spirochetes may play an etiologic role in periodontal diseases.

SUGGESTED READINGS

Canale-Parola E. Physiology and evolution of spirochetes. *Bacteriol Rev.* 1977; 41:181–204.

Canale-Parola E. The spirochetes. In: Krieg NR, ed. *Bergey's Manual of Systematic Bacteriology.* Baltimore: Williams & Wilkins; 1984; 1:38.

Cave VG, Nikitas JA. Venereal disease—Clinical and laboratory diagnoses, *Mt Sinai J Med.* 1976; 43:795–829.

Centers for Disease Control. Continuing increase in infectious syphilis—United States. *MMWR.* 1988; 37:35–38.

Centers for Disease Control. Sexually transmitted diseases treatment guidelines. *MMWR.* 1985; 34(4S):94S–99S.

Hart G. Syphilis tests in diagnostic and therapeutic decision making. *Ann Intern Med.* 1986; 104:368–376.

Holt SC. Anatomy and chemistry of spirochetes. *Microbiol Rev.* 1978; 42:114–160.

Loesche WJ, Laughon BE. Role of spirochetes in periodontal disease. In: Genco RJ, Mergenhagen SE, eds. *Host-Parasite Interactions in Periodontal Diseases.* Washington, DC: American Society for Microbiology; 1982:62–75.

Mandell GL, Douglas RG, Bennett JE, eds. *Principles and Practice of Infectious Diseases.* New York: John Wiley & Sons; 1985:1323.

Mertz LE, Wobig GH, Duffy J, Katzmann JA: Ticks, spirochetes, and new diagnostic tests for Lyme disease. *Mayo Clin Proc.* 1985; 60:402–406.

Treatment of sexually transmitted diseases. *Med Lett.* 1986; 28:23–28.

CHAPTER 19

Actinomycetes

George H.W. Bowden

INTRODUCTION

ACTINOMYCES
- Morphology
- Classification
- Cultivation
- Clinical Features
- Epidemiology
- Diagnosis
- Treatment

NOCARDIA
- Morphology
- Classification
- Cultivation
- Clinical Features
- Diagnosis and Treatment

OTHER ACTINOMYCETES IN THE ORAL CAVITY

ORAL ASPECTS

SUGGESTED READINGS

INTRODUCTION

Actinomycetes is a collective name for members of the order Actinomycetales and related organisms and includes gram-positive bacteria that often are pleomorphic and may form branches. Several members of this group are significant pathogens in humans and animals (Table 19–1). The pathogens include the genera *Actinomyces, Nocardia, Mycobacterium,* and *Corynebacterium*. *Actinomyces* are significant among the members of the order because they are components of the normal oral flora of humans and other animals. They are uniquely oral and have not been isolated from other habitats. *Nocardia* are found free-living in soil and water and are not normal inhabitants of the mouth. The human pathogens within *Actinomyces* are *Actinomyces israelii, Actinomyces viscosus, Actinomyces naeslundii,* and, occasionally, *Actinomyces odontolyticus*. Two species, *A. viscosus* and *A. naeslundii,* have been associated with periodontal tissue destruction, and all species have been isolated from carious dentine. Recently, several new species of *Actinomyces* have been identified as components of the normal flora or pathogens in animals. These species include *Actinomyces howelii, Actinomyces denticolens, Actinomyces slackii,* and *Actinomyces hordeovulneris*. In addition to these new species, *Actinobacterium meyeri,* an organism that can be isolated from periodontal pockets has been placed into *Actinomyces* as *Actinomyces meyerii*. The most significant pathogen within the *Nocardia* is *Nocardia asteroides*.

ACTINOMYCES

Morphology

Actinomyces are gram-positive, nonacid-fast, nonsporeforming bacteria that grow as short rods or long filaments and show true branching. *Actinomyces viscosus* and *A. naeslundii* produce diffuse growth or ropy sediments in broth culture. *Actinomyces israelii* grows as masses of tangled filaments in the form of a

TABLE 19–1. DISEASES CAUSED BY ACTINOMYCETES

Organism	Infection		Notes
	Human	*Animal*	
Actinomyces israelii	Actinomycosis	Actinomycosis	
Actinomyces bovis		Actinomycosis	Lumpy jaw
Actinomyces viscosus	Mixed infections	?	Oral commensal[a]
Actinomyces naeslundii	Mixed infections	?	Oral commensal[a]
Actinomyces odontolyticus	?	?	Oral commensal[b]
Actinomyces hordeovulneris		Actinomycosis	Pathogen in dogs
Nocardia asteroides	Nocardiosis	?	
Nocardia brasiliensis	Mycetoma	?	
Actinomadura madurae	Mycetoma	?	

[a]Strains of these species can produce gingival tissue destruction in experimented oral infections in animals.
[b]Commonly isolated from carious dentine.

granule or granules with a clear supernatant. This granular growth by *A. israelii* also is evident in the lesions of actinomycosis, in which sulfur granules (small colonies) can be detected in the pus or histologic sections of the lesions (Fig 19–1).

Classification

Many of the actinomycetes resemble fungi in that they can grow as filaments, they branch, and, in some cases, they produce spores. The morphologic similarity to the fungi caused a considerable classification problem for early bacteriologists. *Actinomyces* have been shown to have a cell wall mucopeptide typical of bacteria, and they are sensitive to penicillin and other antibiotics that are ineffective against the true fungi. The *Actinomyces* cannot be differentiated easily on the basis of morphology and routine physiologic and biochemical tests. Accurate classification of the *Actinomyces* depends on demonstration of unique chemical components, for example, cell wall analysis, the acid end products of fermentation, and serology. However, routine identification in diagnosis is sometimes based on relatively simple morphologic criteria, which although useful are not necessarily accurate.

Cultivation

One broad distinction that can be drawn between *A. israelii* and *A. viscosus*, *A. naeslundii*, and *A. odontolyticus* is that *A. israelii* is usually an anaerobe, whereas the other species are facultative anaerobes. All species require an enriched medium, and growth is enhanced by carbon dioxide. Selective media employing cadmium salts or sodium fluoride have been devised for isolation of *Actinomyces* and other Actinomyce-

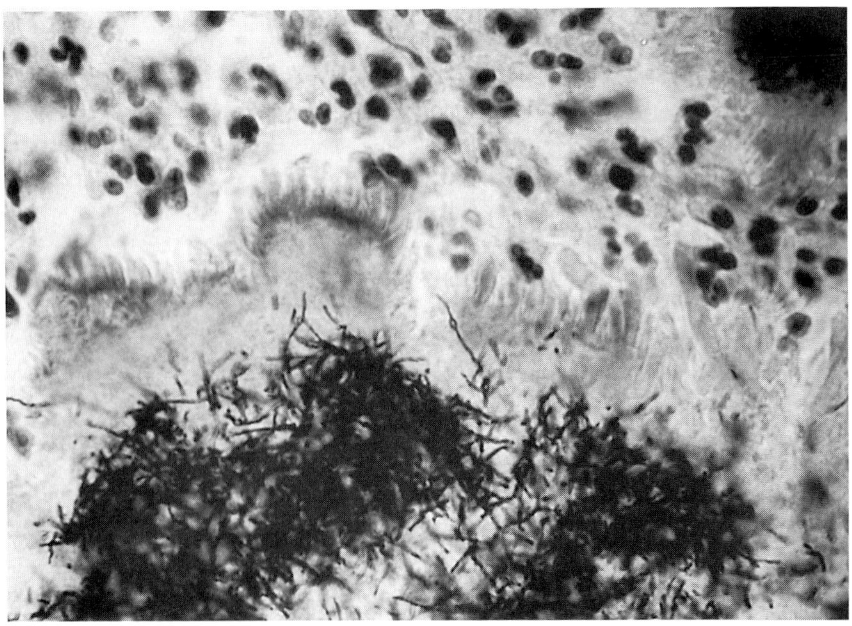

Figure 19–1. Filamentous *Actinomyces* in a sulfur granule from a human case of actinomycosis. *(From Slack JM, Gerencser MA.* Actinomyces, Filamentous Bacteria: Biology and Pathogenicity. *Minneapolis, Minn: Burgess Publishing Co; 1975.)*

taceae, since they are relatively resistant to these chemicals.

Clinical Features

The most common pathogen is *A. israelii,* and the lesions produced by infections involving this organism generally are taken as typical of the disease. The less common pathogens, *A. viscosus, A. naeslundii,* and *A. odontolyticus* do not produce lesions that include sulfur granules.

The typical lesion of actinomycosis develops as a chronic inflammatory lesion with granulation tissue and tissue necrosis. In almost all cases, the infection is mixed, with one or more organisms in the form of colonies, known as sulfur granules, within the tissue and the pus of the lesion (Fig 19–1). The lesions develop slowly and can form abscesses with draining sinuses. The disease can go unnoticed if the lesion is not obvious and associated with the surface of the body.

Cervicofacial lesions account for 60% of the cases, approximately 20% are abdominal, and 15% are thoracic. The prevalence of cervicofacial lesions might be expected, since the organism is a member of the normal oral flora. The dentist may be the first to diagnose cervicofacial lesions (Fig 19–2). The lesion is first noticeable as a swelling that may be painless and often is present on the mandible. Sinus tracts may develop with pus that may contain sulfur granules. If the infection is not treated, the lesion and sinuses will enlarge, and there is a risk of spread via the bloodstream. *Actinomyces* do not usually invade bone.

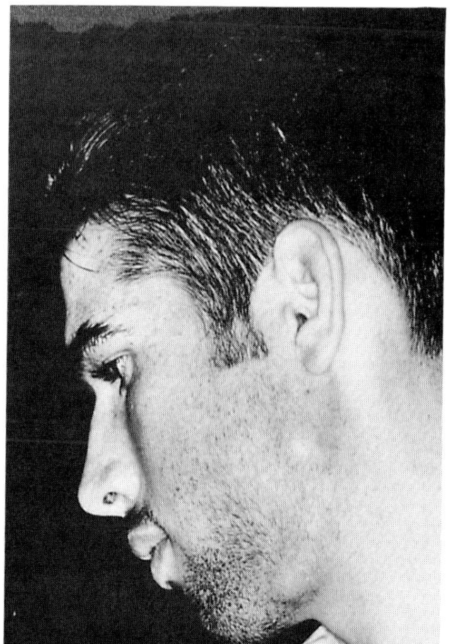

Figure 19–2. Extensive cervicofacial actinomycosis. *(From Slack JM, Gerencser MA.* Actinomyces, Filamentous Bacteria: Biology and Pathogenicity. *Minneapolis, Minn: Burgess Publishing Co; 1975.)*

Thoracic actinomycosis can develop as a direct extension from a cervicofacial lesion by inhalation or via the bloodstream. The infection will spread slowly within the lungs and may perforate the chest wall or the diaphragm. Infections of the lungs can disseminate to the brain, causing brain abscesses.

Abdominal actinomycosis may result from perforation of the diaphragm or diseases or trauma that perforate the gastrointestinal tract. Any of the abdominal tissues and organs can be involved, and as with the other forms of actinomycosis, sinuses may perforate the skin. In addition to the sites mentioned, it should be noted that actinomycotic lesions have developed from human bites. This suggests that the organisms in the oral flora can be virulent and cause disease.

Actinomyces does not produce any known toxins or factors that aid in its establishment or contribute to its virulence. The relative roles played by *Actinomyces* and the other organisms in mixed infections are not known with certainty.

Epidemiology

Actinomyces are found only in the mouth, and it is likely, therefore, that the mouth or perhaps the tonsils are the major reservoir for *Actinomyces* in humans. This means that any proposal for a route of infection must include the mouth. There is little difficulty in explaining the increased frequency of cervicofacial lesions on the basis of an initial oral infection. However, it is less easy to explain lesions in the brain or other organs. *Actinomyces* may enter the bloodstream as part of the bacteremias that occur after oral operations or even chewing. As a result of this hematogenous dissemination, the organism could establish infections at sites distant from the oral cavity. This concept of the origin of *Actinomyces* infections also would explain the presence of other oral organisms in the lesions. The risk of bacteremia increases with poor oral hygiene, and poor oral hygiene could be associated with increased risk of the occurrence of actinomycosis.

Diagnosis

The diagnosis of *Actinomyces* infection depends on demonstration of the organism by microscopy or culture. Microscopic examination can range from a simple Gram stain of the pus or granules from a lesion to the use of specific fluorescent antibody on similar specimens. In the former case, diagnosis is based on demonstration of gram-positive branching filamentous bacteria. Use of the Gram stain is a relatively inaccurate method because many actinomycetes will present this microscopic appearance. Specific fluorescent reagents are used for definite identification of *Actinomyces* species.

Treatment

Actinomyces are not more resistant to antibiotics than are other similar bacteria, but *A. israelii* cells that are sheltered within sulfur granules may survive antibiotic treatment in vitro for relatively long periods of time. Resistance to antibiotics also is a result of the granulomatous and necrotic nature of the lesion, which retards adequate penetration of the drugs. As a result of this resistance, treatment of actinomycotic lesions involves surgical drainage and removal of dead tissue coupled with long-term application of penicillin, erythromycin, or sulfonamides.

NOCARDIAE

Morphology

The nocardiae are gram-positive filamentous bacteria that form true branches and go through a unique cycle of morphologic forms. In *Nocardia,* the filaments, which are often termed hyphae, fragment into short rods or coccal forms. Thus, cultures of *Nocardia* will be found that are composed of filaments or of rods and cocci or mixtures of both. In addition to the hyphae present in the agar, *Nocardia* can produce aerial hyphae, which can divide into chains of spores. *Nocardia* strains are weakly acid-fast and nonmotile. In broth culture, *Nocardia* can form granules.

Classification

The *Nocardia* are one genus of a collection of gram-positive catalase-positive bacteria that are included in nocardioform bacteria. There are within this group several genera, including some mycobacteria, *Actinomadura, Rothia,* and *Rhodococcus,* and the true taxonomic position of some of these genera is in doubt. The taxonomy of *Nocardia* is complex, and many of the bacteria once placed in this genus have been reclassified. In the current edition of *Bergey's Manual of Systematic Bacteriology,* nine species are listed. Of these, *N. asteroides* and *Nocardia brasiliensis* are the major human pathogens. *Nocardia* are identified initially by morphologic characteristics, but accurate identification depends on sophisticated chemical analysis of the cell wall and other components.

Cultivation

In general, the *Nocardia* grow well on relatively simple media, reflecting their free-living nature. This ability to grow on such media as Sabouraud's agar (routinely used for fungi) distinguishes them from *Actinomyces.*

Clinical Features

Nocardia produce two types of disease in humans. One is nocardiosis, a pulmonary infection that can spread to other areas of the body. The second, actinomycetoma, usually affects the extremities. Both infections are usually chronic and progressive, but some mycetomas are chronic localized infections of the skin and subcutaneous tissues. The organisms probably are introduced into the body as a result of some local trauma. Mycetoma occurs most commonly in Africa, India, and South America. The lesions are often on the legs or feet and occur as chronic infections with granulomatous tissue with abscesses and sinuses. The pus from the sinuses usually will contain granules of the organisms, which may be white, red, or brown. The most common pathogen in nocardiosis is *N. asteroides,* and *N. brasiliensis* is the major causative organism in mycetoma. However, several other organisms will cause mycetoma, including *Actinomadura madurae* and some *Streptomyces.*

The normal habitat of the *Nocardia* is soil, and infections result from trauma that allows access of the organisms to the tissues or by inhalation. *Nocardia* grow slowly and do not, therefore, overwhelm the host by their rapid growth. Some strains of *Nocardia* are more virulent than others, but no toxins or other virulence factors have been identified. *Nocardia* are able to survive within phagocytes, and this property may play a role in the disease.

Diagnosis and Treatment

Diagnosis depends on the clinical symptoms, demonstration of granules, and isolation of *Nocardia* from sputum, pus, or other specimens. Sulfonamides, often used in combination with other chemotherapeutic agents, are the drugs of choice for treating *Nocardia* infection. Treatment may be extended for as long as 4 years. Nocardiosis and nocardial mycetoma are very difficult to treat.

OTHER ACTINOMYCETES IN THE ORAL CAVITY

Other members of the Actinomycetales found in the mouth include *Bacterionema* (recently reclassified into *Corynebacterium*), *Rothia,* and *Arachnia. Rothia* and *Bacterionema* generally are regarded as nonpathogenic. *Bacterionema matruchotii* has the capacity to calcify, and this has suggested a potential role for the genus in calculus formation. *Bacterionema* is one of the filamentous bacteria that grow in close association with streptococci to form the corn cobs seen in dental plaque. *Arachnia* can produce an infection indistinguishable from actinomycosis.

ORAL ASPECTS

Actinomyces are members of the normal flora of the mouth of humans and animals, and this appears to be their sole habitat. Obviously, these organisms are well adapted to survive in the mouth and are able to compete effectively with other organisms of the normal flora. Their success is reflected by the relatively high numbers of *Actinomyces* that can be found colonizing the surfaces of the teeth. This is particularly true of the interproximal area, where *Actinomyces* can comprise between 40% and 80% of the cultivable flora.

The species that predominate on the tooth surface are *A. viscosus* and *A. naeslundii. Actinomyces israelii* and *A. odontolyticus* occur in lower numbers. A second habitat in the mouth is carious dentine. Careful studies of carious lesions have revealed relatively high numbers of *A. viscosus, A. naeslundii,* and particularly *A. odontolyticus.* The last species was first isolated from carious dentine, and it is likely that this organism flourishes in this habitat. *Actinomyces* have been suspected of being involved in root caries and gingivitis. However, it is not clear whether *Actinomyces* play a specific pathogenic role in these oral diseases. Their possible roles in the oral cavity are discussed in Chapters 33 and 34.

SUGGESTED READINGS

Beaman BL. Actinomycete pathogenesis. In: Goodfellow M, Mordarski M, William ST, eds. *The Biology of the Actinomycetes.* London: Academic Press; 1984:457–478.

Bowden GH, Hardie JM. Oral pleomorphic (coryneform) gram-positive rods. In: Bousfield JJ, Calley AG, eds. *Coryneform Bacteria.* London: Academic Press; 1978:235–263.

Bowden GH. Pathogenesis of *Actinomyces israelii* infections. In: Ortiz-Ortiz L, Bojalil LF, Yakoleff V, eds. *Biological, Biochemical and Biomedical Aspects of Actinomycetes.* Orlando, Fla: Academic Press; 1984:1–12.

Bowden GH, Hardie JM. Commensal and pathogenic *Actinomyces* species in man. In: Sykes G, Skinner FA, eds. *Actinomycetales Characteristics and Practical Importance.* Society for Applied Bacteriology. Symposium Series 2. London: Academic Press; 1973:277–299.

Schaal KP. Laboratory diagnosis of Actinomycete disease. In: Goodfellow M, Mordarski M, Williams ST, eds. *The Biology of the Actinomycetes.* London: Academic Press; 1984:425–456.

Schaal KP, Beaman BL. Clinical significance of *Actinomycetes.* In: Goodfellow M, Mordarski M, Williams ST, eds. *The Biology of the Actinomycetes.* London: Academic Press; 1984:389–424.

Slack JM, Gerencser MA. *Actinomyces, Filamentous Bacteria: Biology and Pathogenicity.* Minneapolis, Minn: Burgess Publishing Co; 1975.

Sneath PHA, Mair WS, Sharpe ME, eds. *Bergey's Manual of Systematic Bacteriology.* Baltimore: Williams & Wilkins; 1986;2:1383–1418, 1459–1471.

CHAPTER 20

Rickettsiae, Chlamydiae, and Mycoplasmas

Chris H. Miller

INTRODUCTION

RICKETTSIAE
- General Characteristics
- Pathogenesis
- Weil-Felix Reaction
- Spotted Fevers
- Typhus Group
- Q Fever
- Oral Aspects

CHLAMYDIAE
- General Characteristics
- *Chlamydia trachomatis*
- *Chlamydia psittaci*
- *Chlamydia* TWAR
- Oral Aspects

MYCOPLASMAS
- General Characteristics
- Virulence Factors
- Mycoplasma Diseases
- Oral Aspects

SUGGESTED READINGS

INTRODUCTION

Rickettsiae, chlamydiae (formerly bedsoniae), and mycoplasmas are considered together because they have unique properties that differentiate them from all other bacteria. All but one of the rickettsiae and all of the chlamydiae are obligate intracellular parasites, a unique property within the bacterial world. Mycoplasmas are not obligate intracellular parasites, but they are unique among bacteria because they have no cell wall.

RICKETTSIAE

Rickettsiae are a special group of bacteria with three medically important genera: *Rickettsia,* which contains several species, and *Rochalimaea* and *Coxiella,* each containing a single species. Rickettsiae are small gram-negative bacteria that (with the exception of *Rochalimaea quintana*) can multiply only within living cells. Their natural habitat is within various arthropods (eg, ticks, lice, fleas), which may transmit these organisms to vertebrates when the arthropods obtain a blood meal. The organisms may then multiply within the new host, which then serves as another reservoir for the disease agent from which other arthropods may be infected. Thus, infected arthropods serve as vectors of rickettsial infection from animal to animal, from animal to human and from human to human.

General Characteristics

Rickettsiae are pleomorphic coccobacilli with a diameter of about 0.5 μm and a maximum length of about 2.0 μm. These gram-negative bacteria stain poorly with the usual dyes but can be visualized with special staining procedures. The composition and structure of the rickettsial cell wall are similar to those of other gram-negative bacteria. Some species possess a capsule. The uniqueness of this group of bacteria stems from their requirement of living cells for growth. Although *R. quintana* can be cultured on enriched blood agar, the other rickettsiae must be grown in tissue cultures, embryonated eggs, animals, or arthropods. In contrast to viruses, which are also obligate intracellular parasites, the rickettsiae carry out some of their own metabolism and divide by binary fission. It has been suggested that the intracellular growth requirement and the extracellular instability of rickettsiae might be explained by a defective membrane system that prevents retention of essential metabolites.

Pathogenesis

Endothelial cells lining small blood vessels are the primary target cells of rickettsial infections of humans. Rickettsiae adhere to and enter endothelial cells and multiply, causing endothelial hyperplasia, thrombosis, and a vasculitis. Rupture of the infected endothelial cells causes a rickettsemia that permits hematogenous spread of the organisms and allows for possible transmission of organisms by blood-sucking vectors.

Since experimental animals injected with large amounts of rickettsiae may die from an acute toxemia, it is possible that these bacteria possess or elaborate a toxin. There is some evidence for the presence of endotoxin-like materials in rickettsiae, but the importance of such toxins in human disease is unknown. Some rickettsiae (eg, *Rickettsia prowazekii*) are capable of lysing erythrocytes, but again, the importance of this hemolytic activity in the disease process is not known.

Weil-Felix Reaction

The Weil-Felix reaction detects antibodies produced during some rickettsial diseases and may aid in diagnosis when paired sera demonstrate a rise in these antibody titers. The antigens used to detect these antibodies are present on certain nonmotile strains of the gram-negative rod *Proteus vulgaris* and nonmotile strains, or O strains, of *Pseudomonas*. These antigens are similar to those of some rickettsiae, and the antibodies produced during the rickettsial infection cross-react and agglutinate the *Proteus* or *Pseudomonas* cells.

Spotted Fevers

Rocky Mountain Spotted Fever. Rocky Mountain spotted fever (Table 20–1) is the most frequently reported rickettsial disease in humans. It is caused by *Rickettsia rickettsii* and is acquired by contamination of a tick bite or skin abrasion with the feces or crushed body of an infected tick.

TABLE 20–1. MAJOR RICKETTSIAL DISEASES OF HUMANS

Organism	Disease	Vector
Rickettsia rickettsii	Rocky Mountain spotted fever	Rocky Mountain wood tick (*Dermacentor andersonii*) American dog tick (*Dermacentor variabilis*) Lone star tick (*Amblyomma americanum*)
Rickettsia akari	Rickettsialpox	Mouse mite (*Allodermanyssus sanguineus*)
Rickettsia prowazekii	Epidemic typhus	Human body louse (*Pediculus humanus corporis*) Human head louse (*Pediculus humanus capitis*)
Rickettsia typhi	Endemic typhus	Rat flea (*Xenopsylla cheopis*) Rat louse (*Polyplax spinulosus*)
Rickettsia tsutsugamushi	Scrub typhus	Rat mites (*Trombicula pallida* and others)
Rochalimaea quintana	Trench fever	Human body louse (*Pediculus humanus corporis*)
Coxiella burnetii	Q fever	Ticks; airborne infection

Rocky Mountain spotted fever has an incubation period of 7 days, followed by a sudden onset of fever, headache, body pains, frequent chills, and a rash after 2 to 4 days. The chance of fatality is 15% to 20% in untreated cases. Early antibiotic therapy with chloramphenicol or tetracycline is important and should be based on clinical diagnosis rather than waiting for results of diagnostic tests. The Weil-Felix reaction may be used for confirmation of infection. Prevention includes reducing exposure to ticks and careful removal of attached ticks using forceps. Recovery usually results in good immunity. Prophylactic immunization with killed organisms usually provides only partial protection.

Rickettsialpox. Rickettsialpox is caused by *Rickettsia akari*, which is transmitted to humans by the mouse mite. The disease is characterized by the development of papular skin lesions at the site of the mite bite, with associated lymphadenopathy. Within a few days, fever, headache, chills, and a generalized papulovesicular rash occur. In some cases, vesicles develop on the palate and tongue. The initial skin lesion develops into a persistent eschar. Diagnosis is based on recognizing the clinical symptoms and mainly differentiating the disease from chickenpox. Tetracycline or chloramphenicol is used for treatment.

Typhus Group

Epidemic Typhus. The epidemic nature of this form of typhus results from transmission of the causative agent (*R. prowazekii*) from human to human by the human body louse. This type of disease transmission is enhanced when environments and conditions foster crowding and poor personal hygiene. Today, epidemic typhus occurs mainly in limited areas in Africa and Central and South America. Sporadic cases occur in the United States, and recent reports have implicated the flying squirrel as possibly being involved in disease transmission.

Lice may contain *R. prowasekii* in their intestinal tract as a result of taking a blood meal from an infected human with a rickettsemia. When the louse feeds on another human and defecates, the rickettsiae often are scratched into the skin because of the irritation of the bite. Illness begins with high fever, chills, headache, and body pain. A skin rash appears frequently first on the trunk and then becomes generalized. Some outbreaks have exhibited a mortality as high as 40% in untreated cases. Chloramphenicol or tetracycline usually is effective when administered early in the course of the disease.

Recovery from epidemic typhus generally results in a long-lasting immunity to primary infection. However, mild recurrences (Brill-Zinsser disease) may occur some years later. Thus, *R. prowazekii* apparently can establish a latent infection in some patients, since Brill-Zinsser disease may occur in an individual living in an environment free of lice.

Endemic Typhus. Endemic typhus is known also as marine typhus or rat typhus. Endemic typhus is still a reportable disease in the United States and is endemic mainly in Texas and the southeastern states. In recent years, there have been less than 100 cases reported per year.

Rickettsia typhi, the cause of endemic typhus, primarily infects rats. Fleas that feed on rickettsemic rats or mice may accidently bite humans and at the same time defecate on the skin. If the feces is scratched into the skin, transmission is complete. Susceptible individuals develop an abrupt fever, headache, malaise, and chills, and a rash develops on the trunk and extends to the extremities. Clinically, endemic and epidemic typhus are very similar and often are indistinguishable except that the latter usually is more severe. Chloramphenicol and tetracycline are effective. Recovery from infection results in lasting immunity.

Q Fever

Q fever has been observed worldwide. In the United States, outbreaks have occurred in Texas, California, and Illinois. Although the causative organism, *Coxiella burnetii,* infects ticks and the ticks may transmit the organisms to animals, human infection occurs usually from contact with infected domestic animals or their products. The occurrence of nonarthropod routes of *C. burnetii* infection for humans is best explained by the high resistance of this organism to physical and chemical agents, unlike other rickettsial organisms. *Coxiella burnetii* can survive in extracellular environments for extended periods, and sources of infection include milk, soil contaminated with feces or blood of infected animals, wool, hides, and animal bedding.

Coxiella burnetii may enter the body through the skin or mucous membranes or by inhalation or ingestion. The disease is characterized by an abrupt onset of fever with chills, headache, and body aches, as in other rickettsial diseases. In contrast to other rickettsial diseases, a rash with Q fever is rare. Endocarditis, pneumonia, and hepatitis have been observed in some patients with Q fever. Tetracycline is used for treatment.

Oral Aspects

Rickettsial lesions may occur in or about the mouth. The maculopapular-vesicular rash that develops in rickettsialpox may appear on the face or be present as transient oral mucosal lesions. They may occur on the lips, tongue, buccal mucosa, hard and soft palates, and pharynx. Such lesions appear as vesicles surrounded by a zone of erythema. The rash of Rocky Mountain spotted fever may involve the mucosa of the inner cheeks and throat, and the tongue may become swollen.

CHLAMYDIAE

Chlamydiae are obligate intracellular bacteria that infect as many as 20% of all humans worldwide. There are only two species of *Chlamydia, Chlamydia trachomatis* and *Chlamydia psittaci* (Table 20–2). They are transferred to new hosts by direct or indirect contact and usually establish an inapparent infection. Harmful infections can occur in humans, and the type of disease usually relates to the site of entry into the body.

TABLE 20–2. CHLAMYDIAE

Organism	Disease
Chlamydia trachomatis	Trachoma
	Inclusion conjunctivitis, genital infection, infant pneumonitis
	Lymphogranuloma venereum
Chlamydia psittaci	Psittacosis, ornithosis, human lung infection

General Characteristics

Chlamydiae have a unique life cycle, with two developmental forms (Fig 20–1). The elementary body (EB) is adapted for survival in the extracellular environment and is the form that infects host cells. The EB is a dense spherical bacterium about 0.2 μm to 0.4 μm in diameter. It has a rigid cell wall that is similar to that of gram-negative bacteria but does not exhibit endotoxic properties. Although the EB is metabolically dormant, it contains sufficient DNA to provide for about 600 different proteins. The intracellular form is called the reticulate body (RB) and is about 0.7 μm to 1.0 μm in diameter and has a nonrigid envelope that results in pleomorphism. It is metabolically active and undergoes binary fission. It cannot survive outside the host.

The chlamydial growth cycle is initiated by adherence of an EB to a susceptible host cell through an attachment mechanism involving specific cell surface receptors. The organism enters the cell through phagocytosis and is surrounded by the invaginated host cell membrane to form the phagosome. Infectious chlamydiae prevent fusion of lysosomes with the phagosome, which prevents lysosomal digestion and permits development of the organism within the phagosome. In immune hosts, the antibody-coated EB does not prevent lysosomal fusion and is digested rapidly. In a developing inclusion, EB change into RB that mature and undergo binary fission. These daughter cells undergo conversion to EB, and by about 40 hours after initial infection, large numbers of EB are present within the host cells. The host cells begin to die, and chlamydial EB are released by lysis.

The need for intracellular parasitism of host cells by chlamydiae is thought to be related to the inability of the parasite to synthesize certain metabolic precursors or drive energy-requiring reactions. Although chlamydiae contain several genes, preformed nucleic acid polymerases, and some metabolic enzyme systems, they are unable to synthesize ATP and other high energy phosphates, and they require host purines and pyrimidines for synthesis of their own nucleic acids.

Chlamydiae possess a group-specific, cell wall antigen that may be detected by complement-fixation tests. There are also species-specific and strain-specific antigens that have been detected by indirect immunofluorescence. These tests have demonstrated at least 16 serologically distinct types of *C. trachomatis*, and typing of strains isolated from clinical disease has suggested that certain disease states may be related to certain serologic types. Further work on the antigenic composition of chlamydial isolates may aid in developing diagnostic and preventive approaches.

A B C

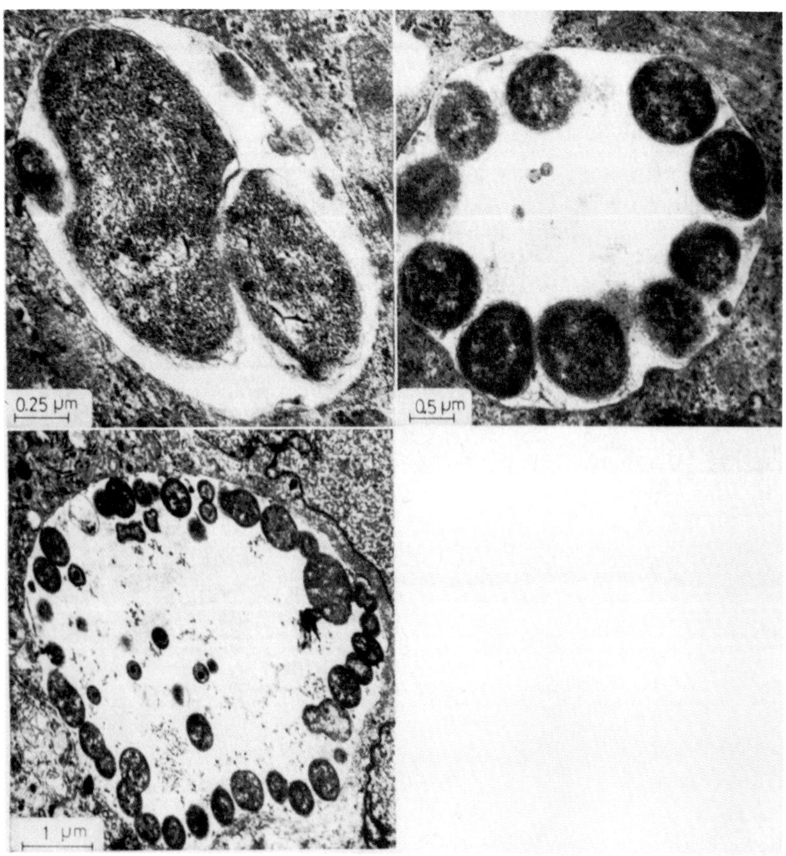

Figure 20–1. The developmental cycle of *Chlamydia trachomatis* (TE 55 strain). **A.** An initial step in the formation of the inclusion body. **B.** An inclusion body with reticulate bodies. **C.** A developed inclusion body with reticulate bodies, dividing bodies, and elementary bodies. *(From Becker Y. The agent of trachoma.* Monogr Virol. *1974;7:31.)*

Chlamydia trachomatis

Trachoma. Trachoma is a human disease of the eye that is a leading cause of blindness in many underdeveloped areas. It is usually associated with poverty and poor sanitation and personal hygiene and is endemic in Asia and Africa. *Chlamydia trachomatis* usually is transmitted by hand–eye contact or by fomites. After an initial inflammation of the conjunctivae, follicular and papillary hypertrophy occurs. Ulceration and scarring of the cornea may lead to partial or complete blindness. Little, if any, protective immunity develops as a result of infection.

Inclusion Conjunctivitis. Inclusion conjunctivitis is similar to the early stages of classic ocular trachoma and usually is self-limiting, without vision impairment. Inclusion conjunctivitis usually occurs in newborns and results from passage through a birth canal infected with *C. trachomatis*. The incidence of chlamydial newborn eye disease is related directly to cervical infection in the mothers. Ear, nose, and vaginal infection may accompany eye infections in these newborns. Outbreaks of inclusion conjunctivitis in adults have been associated with the presence of chlamydiae in unchlorinated swimming pools. Sporadic occurrences in adults possibly result from contamination of the eyes with genital exudates through autoinoculation or from sexual partners. Sulfonamides, tetracycline, and chloramphenicol are effective therapeutic agents.

Infant Pneumonia. *Chlamydia trachomatis* is a major cause of pneumonia in infants under 6 months old. The children lack systemic symptoms but do exhibit wheezing and cough. The pneumonia is preceded by chlamydial conjunctivitis in about one half of the cases.

Genital Tract Infection. Urethritis for which *Neisseria gonorrhoeae* cannot be established as the cause usually is referred to as nongonococcal urethritis (NGU). NGU may have several different etiologic agents, but *C. trachomatis* is thought to be the leading cause (as high as 50% of the cases in males). It is acquired and transmitted through sexual intercourse, and it is commonly detected in men with a history of other sexually transmitted diseases and promiscuity. The infection in women may be asymptomatic, or there may be chronic cervicitis and urethritis.

Chlamydia are associated also with some cases of postgonococcal urethritis following penicillin therapy that eliminates the gonococcus but not the chlamydiae. In such cases, it is likely that simultaneous infection by both organisms occurred.

Lymphogranuloma Venereum. Lymphogranuloma venereum (LGV) is another sexually transmitted disease caused by *C. trachomatis*. Although it most commonly occurs in tropical areas, there are about 500 cases reported per year in the United States, frequently in those who have other sexually transmitted diseases.

The disease may be contracted from symptomatic or asymptomatic carriers. A primary lesion develops at the site of entry (genital, anorectal, oral) in the form of a vesicle that ruptures, leaving a shallow ulcer that heals. This lesion commonly is painless, small, and often inconspicuous. Affected lymph nodes may abscess, and fistulous tracts may remain for years. Infections that progress to the later stages of the disease may have continued destruction of the vulva and urethra.

Diagnosis depends on recognizing clinical symptoms, recovery of *C. trachomatis* from lesions, and demonstration of an increasing complement-fixing antibody titer. Direct microscopic demonstration of the organisms in exudates using fluorescent antibody techniques is being used as a diagnostic tool. Continued development of specific DNA probes will make detection of chlamydiae more rapid and convenient. Acute cases of LGV usually are treated successfully with sulfadiazine or tetracycline. Immunity to this disease appears to be associated with the presence of low numbers of organisms remaining after disease, causing a minimal immune response.

Chlamydia psittaci

Chlamydia psittaci causes a usually fatal infection in birds. If the birds are psittacine types, such as parrots or parakeets, the disease is called psittacosis. If the birds are nonpsittacine (eg, ducks, chickens, pigeons, turkeys), the disease is called ornithosis. Humans usually contract the disease (psittacosis, ornithosis) by inhalation of organisms from infected birds or their droppings. Human to human spread also occurs. In the United States, about 100 to 150 human cases occur per year.

The disease in humans varies greatly but commonly begins with fever, body aches, and headaches, followed by pulmonary involvement with a nonproductive cough and rales and consolidation. In rare instances, central nervous system involvement results in encephalitis, coma, convulsions, and death.

Diagnosis by clinical signs is difficult, and laboratory diagnosis is based on isolation of the organism by mouse, egg, or tissue culture inoculation and identification. Direct microscopic detection with fluorescent antibody also is used. Tetracycline or erythromycin has been used with some success.

Chlamydia TWAR

A *Chlamydia* strain that is classified morphologically as *C. psittaci* has been redesignated *Chlamydia* TWAR after the laboratory designation of the first two isolates TW-183 and AR-39. Although originally isolated in 1965, it was not until the middle 1980s that TWAR strains were shown to cause outbreaks of pneumonia and to be associated with bronchitis and pharyngitis. There is serologic evidence of high rates of human exposure to TWAR strains, with up to 60% of some adult populations having antibodies. Unlike previously recognized strains of *C. psittaci,* the TWAR strains appear to be spread directly from human to human without an avian or lower mammalian host. The TWAR strains are difficult to grow in tissue culture, but microimmunofluorescence tests using TWAR antigen to detect serum antibody aid in the diagnosis.

Oral Aspects

A primary infection of the mouth and related cervical lymph nodes may result after oral sex with a partner having genital LGV. As with most sexually transmitted diseases, the mouth is the most common extragenital site of primary infection in LGV. Although the tongue is the frequently infected oral site in these primary infections, other sites may be involved. Early tongue lesions are vesicular and may be painless. With progression, the tongue enlarges, and deep grooves may form as a result of loss of superficial epithelium. These tongue lesions may become chronic and may recur after healing.

Extragenital nonvenereal infections with LGV I, II, or III may involve the fingers of dental personnel after contact with patients exhibiting oral infections.

MYCOPLASMAS

The mycoplasmas originally were called pleuropneumonia organisms (PPO) or pleuropneumonia-like organisms (PPLO) because they were first isolated from cattle with pleuropneumonia. They constitute an unusual group of microbes in that they do not have a cell wall. They are the smallest known prokaryotes that can self-replicate. The mycoplasmas belong to a special class of small prokaryotes called Mollicutes, meaning soft skins. Most of those associated with humans are placed in one of two distinct genera in the family Mycoplasmataceae (Table 20–3). Although most of these mycoplasmas are nonpathogenic and may constitute part of the normal body flora, others cause disease in humans and other animals.

TABLE 20–3. MYCOPLASMAS ASSOCIATED WITH HUMANS

Organism	Most Common Sites of Isolation	Disease
Mycoplasma		
M. pneumoniae	Oropharynx, respiratory tract	Pneumonia, tracheobronchitis
M. hominis	Genitourinary tract, oropharynx	Salpingitis, septicemia
M. orale	Oropharynx	None
M. salivarium	Oropharynx	None
M. faucium	Oropharynx	None
M. lipophilum	Oropharynx	None
M. fermentans	Genitourinary tract	None
M. primatum	Genitourinary tract	None
Ureaplasma		
U. urealyticum	Genitourinary tract	Nongonococcal urethritis

General Characteristics

Mycoplasmas range in size from 0.2 μm to 0.8 μm in diameter, and their primary mode of replication is binary fission. Because they lack a cell wall, their outer limiting structure is the cytoplasmic membrane, which contains cholesterol (a unique property among prokaryotes). Most species are spherical, but some produce branching filamentous cells. Some species also have specialized structures that may aid in motility or attachment to host cells. Mycoplasmas can be cultured on a complex cell-free medium supplemented with horse serum (for cholesterol and related sterols), nucleic acid precursors, and yeast extract. Most species are facultative anaerobes and grow slowly.

Virulence Factors

Most of the little information available on the virulence factors of mycoplasmas comes from studies with *Mycoplasma pneumoniae,* the most frequently pathogenic species for humans. Mycoplasmas attach to mucous membranes of the respiratory, genitourinary, and gastrointestinal tracts. Attachment to host cells is very important for microbial colonization of a mucous membrane body site, and at least in the case of *M. pneumoniae,* attachment to host cells apparently is required for disease production. Avirulent strains possess a specialized organelle on the tip of filamentous cells that mediates attachment to epithelial cells. *Mycoplasma pneumoniae* does not penetrate the epithelial cells but does have an as yet unexplained toxic effect on the host cell. *Mycoplasma pneumoniae* produces hydrogen peroxide, which may be cytotoxic but is not known to produce a soluble exotoxin as do some mouse strains of *Mycoplasma.* It has been suggested from tissue culture infections by *M. pneumoniae* that depletion of host cell nucleic acids (required for growth by mycoplasmas) may explain the observed cytotoxicity.

Mycoplasma Diseases

Respiratory Diseases. Up to 20% of all pneumonias in humans are caused by *M. pneumoniae.* The disease (originally called primary atypical pneumonia) is mainly endemic, with an occasional outbreak among groups of people with frequent, close contact. Spread is by droplet infection, but only a small percent of those who are infected exhibit disease. If disease occurs, it is usually an upper respiratory tract problem associated with gradual onset of fever, headache, and nonproductive cough. As the disease progresses, rales develop, but there is little physical evidence of consolidation. The pneumonia is usually mild and self-limiting and seldom lasts longer than 3 weeks.

Diagnosis of a *Mycoplasma* respiratory disease based on clinical symptoms often is difficult. Laboratory aids in diagnosis include culture and identification of the organism, but this may require up to 3 weeks because of slow growth of the isolates. Serologic diagnosis involves testing for complement-fixing antibodies. *Mycoplasma pneumoniae* is sensitive to tetracycline and erythromycin, and these agents usually reduce the clinical course of the disease but may not eliminate the organism from the respiratory tract. The development of protective immunity is questionable.

Urogenital Disease. Ureaplasmas are present in the urogenital tract of many apparently normal people, but their frequency of occurrence appears to be related to sexual activity. *Ureaplasma urealyticum* has been shown to be one of the causes (maybe as high as 30% of the cases) of NGU. This organism also is present in the mouths of a few individuals, but no relationship has been shown between its presence and the occurrence of any oral disease.

Mycoplasma hominis frequently is found in the genitourinary tract of sexually active people. Although this organism has not been shown to be related to NGU, it has been implicated in postpartum fever, pelvic inflammatory disease, and recurrent abortions.

Oral Aspects

Although several species of *Mycoplasma* may be present in the human mouth (Table 20–3), *Mycoplasma salivarium* and *M. pneumoniae* appear to be the predominant oral species. *Mycoplasma* species have been isolated from the mouths of healthy subjects and those with experimentally induced gingivitis, with chronic periodontitis, and with juvenile periodontitis. *Mycoplasma salivarium* has been shown to comprise 89% of the *Mycoplasma* species in dental plaque and gingival crevices and is present in significantly higher percentages in those with periodontal diseases than in healthy people.

Analysis of a single diseased site in a juvenile periodontitis patient has revealed the presence of *Mycoplasma* on the surface of the tooth, on the surface of pocket epithelium, and invading the gingival epithelium and adjacent connective tissue. Nevertheless, further studies are needed to determine what role, if any, *Mycoplasma* species may play in the initiation or progression of periodontitis.

Another oral aspect of *Mycoplasma* infection relates to transmission of the organisms through dental aerosols and respiratory droplets. Dental patients carrying potentially infectious *M. pneumoniae* in their oropharynx can serve as a source of infection for the dental team during procedures that generate aerosols.

SUGGESTED READINGS

Becker Y. The *Chlamydia:* Molecular biology of procaryotic obligate parasite of eucaryocytes. *Microbiol Rev.* 1978; 42:274.

Burgdorfer W, Anacker RL. *Rickettsia and Rickettsial Diseases.* New York: Academic Press; 1981.

CDC. Sexually transmitted diseases: Guidelines. *MMWR.* 1985;34 (4S):94–99.

Cox RL, Kuo C-C, Grayston JT, Campbell LA. Deoxyribonucleic acid relatedness of *Chlamydia* sp. strain TWAR to *Chlamydia trachomatis* and *Chlamydia psittaci. Int J Syst Bacteriol.* 1988;38:265–268.

Grayston JT, Kuo C-C, Wang S, Altman J. A new *Chlamydia psittaci* strain, TWAR, isolated in acute respiratory tract infections. *N Engl J Med.* 1986;315:161–168.

Handsfield HH. Sexually transmitted diseases. *Hosp Pract.* 1982; January:10.

Newman MG, Saglie R, Carranza FA, Kaufman AK. *Mycoplasma* in periodontal disease. Isolation in juvenile periodontitis. *J Periodontol.* 1984;55:574–580.

Razin S. The mycoplasmas. *Microbiol Rev.* 1978;42:414.

Schacter J, Grossman M. Chlamydial infections. *Annu Rev Med.* 1981;32:45.

Shepard MC. The recovery of pleuropneumonia-like organisms from Negro men with and without nongonococcal urethritis. *Am J Gonorrhea Vener Dis.* 1954;38:113.

Walker DH. Rickettsial diseases: An update. In: *Current Topics in Inflammation and Infection.* Baltimore: Williams & Wilkins; 1982:188.

Watanabe T, Matsuura M, Seto K. Isolation and seriological typing of *Ureaplasma* in human saliva. *Arch Oral Biol.* 1983;28:545.

CHAPTER 21

Anaerobic Infections

Robert R. White

INTRODUCTION
ESTABLISHMENT OF ANAEROBIOSIS
CHARACTERISTICS OF ANAEROBIC INFECTIONS
Polymicrobic Infections
Endogenous Pathogens
Closed Space Infections
Odors
Thrombophlebitis
VIRULENCE AND RESISTANCE FACTORS
PATHOGENESIS
DIAGNOSIS
TREATMENT
ORAL ASPECTS
SUGGESTED READINGS

INTRODUCTION

Anaerobic infections are those lesions produced by bacteria that require a tissue environment with very low concentrations of oxygen and a reduced oxidation-reduction potential (Eh). Any infection involving strict anaerobes is an anaerobic infection, but clinicians often speak of anaerobic infections when referring to a large group of polymicrobic lesions with a relatively nonspecific etiology. This group of infections is the subject of this chapter. Other anaerobic infections, including the clostridial infections, are discussed elsewhere. The anaerobic infections are of special significance to the dentist because most oral abscesses, periodontal lesions, and pulp and periapical lesions are anaerobic lesions. Some of the most commonly encountered anaerobic bacteria are listed in Table 21–1. Several of these are described further in other chapters of this book.

No absolute limits on oxygen tolerance have been designated in defining anaerobes. As noted in Chapter 2, the degree of oxygen tolerance varies from species to species and from strain to strain within species (Table 2–2). Despite their need for an anaerobic environment, it is not surprising to find anaerobic infections within the tissues. Many anaerobes inhabit the human body, and, in fact, they outnumber aerobes on some parts of the body. For example, in the colon, anaerobes outnumber aerobes 1000 to 1, on the skin, they outnumber aerobes 10 to 1, and in the oral cavity, the ratio is about 5 or 10 to 1.

ESTABLISHMENT OF ANAEROBIOSIS

Healthy tissues and surfaces of the body devoid of bacteria are well oxygenated, and the Eh is well above the requirements of anaerobes. Thus, anaerobic infections do not occur within healthy tissues. Conditions needed for an anaerobic infection can be established by several mechanisms. Interrupting the blood flow to a tissue causes oxygen deprivation that leads to a drop in the Eh and produces the environment necessary for an anaerobic infection. Any tissue injury that restricts capillary blood flow to an area of the body may cause a decrease in oxygen tension that allows

TABLE 21–1. PERCENTAGE DISTRIBUTION AND SELECTED EXAMPLES OF ANAEROBIC BACTERIA INVOLVED IN HUMAN CLINICAL INFECTIONS

Group or Species	% of Isolates
Gram-negative nonsporeforming bacilli	
Bacteroides spp	39
B. fragilis group	
B. melaninogenicus group	
B. intermedius	
B. asaccharolyticus	
B. gingivalis	
Fusobacterium spp	4
F. nucleatum	
F. necrophorum	
Gram-positive cocci	
Peptostreptococcus spp	22
P. magnus	
P. asaccharolyticus	
P. anaerobius	
Staphylococcus sp	1
S. saccharolyticus	
Streptococcus sp	1
S. intermedius	
Gram-positive nonsporeforming bacilli	
Actinomyces spp	1
A. israelii	
A. odontolyticus	
A. viscosus	
Propionibacterium sp	17
P. acnes	
Eubacterium sp	4
E. lentum	
Sporeforming bacilli	
Clostridium spp	11
C. perfringens	
C. difficile	
C. tetani	
C. botulinum	

Adapted from Lennette EH, et al. Manual of Clinical Microbiology. *4th ed. Washington, DC: American Society for Microbiology; 1985.*

colonization by anaerobic bacteria. The injury may result from surgery or accidental trauma. In addition, ischemic necrosis occurring as a result of tumor formation also may produce anaerobiosis. Having colonized these tissues, the anaerobic bacteria produce cytotoxic and other necrotizing factors that further destroy vascular tissues and thus maintain and even extend the anaerobic site.

Anaerobic conditions may be established in or on a tissue as a result of the presence of aerobic or facultative bacteria. These bacteria consume the oxygen present, and strict anaerobes can then survive and multiply. This method of establishing anaerobiosis is common on body surfaces and is the basis for the predominance of anaerobic bacteria on the skin and the mucous membranes throughout the body in both healthy and diseased states. Within the oral cavity, strict anaerobes flourish in the pits, fissures, and crevices and even on smooth surfaces covered by dental plaque and other oral debris because aerobes in the overlying materials consume the oxygen before it reaches the anaerobes.

CHARACTERISTICS OF ANAEROBIC INFECTIONS

Polymicrobic Infections

Anaerobic infections usually involve more than one species of bacteria; that is, they are polymicrobic. As many as 13 different species have been isolated from a single lesion, and they often include a mixture of aerobes and anaerobes. Several reasons have been proposed to explain the polymicrobic nature of these infections. One is that aerobes or facultative anaerobes must be present initially in order to consume any oxygen present and establish the anaerobiosis needed by strict anaerobes. Second, several of the most commonly encountered anaerobes require growth factors that they cannot synthesize. Therefore, other bacteria are needed to produce these growth factors. The black-pigmented *Bacteroides,* members of the oral flora, are a good example. These bacteria cannot synthesize vitamin K and must obtain it from other members of the polymicrobic population. This is readily demonstrated experimentally. Pure cultures of *Bacteroides* will not grow on medium devoid of vitamin K. If a vitamin K-producing organism is mixed with the *Bacteroides,* the latter will grow on the medium. This finding has been extended to in vivo studies. Experimental *Bacteroides* infections are almost impossible to initiate in laboratory animals unless other bacteria are inoculated with *Bacteroides.*

Yet another explanation for the polymicrobic nature of these infections is that they often result from contamination by or extension from the mucous membranes to submucosal areas. In fact, they often are found in close proximity to these surfaces. The mucosal surfaces are populated by a rich and varied bacterial flora containing both aerobes and anaerobes, and an infection originating from these surfaces would reflect this varied population. It is probable that all three of these mechanisms are involved to varying degrees in determining the polymicrobic nature of anaerobic infections. The multiplicity of microorganisms in these infections makes it difficult to determine what organisms have most significance. This has been a major hindrance in studying these infections.

Endogenous Pathogens

The anaerobic pathogens are usually endogenous and of low virulence; they are opportunists. Most of the bacteria listed in Table 21–1 are members of the normal flora, usually of the oral cavity and the gastrointestinal tract. Other sites in the body contribute to the populations associated with anaerobic infections, but these two sites predominate.

Closed Space Infections

The lesions usually are closed space infections into which oxygen cannot readily enter. Brain, lung, and liver abscesses commonly are anaerobic infections (Table 21–2). Pulp and periapical infections and the periodontal lesions are examples of oral closed space infections.

Odor

A foul odor often is associated with anaerobic infections. Proteolysis constitutes a major metabolic activity of anaerobes, and the amines (eg, putrescine, cadavarine) and other fermentation products are very foul smelling. The presence of these strong odors often is considered to be presumptive diagnosis of an anaerobic infection.

Thrombophlebitis

Anaerobic infections often are accompanied by thrombophlebitis. The reason for the predisposition to thrombophlebitis is unknown, but it has been proposed that it may result from the *Bacteroides* enzyme, heparinase, which breaks down the heparin that usually inhibits clot formation. In addition, endotoxins produced by gram-negative anaerobes may activate the clotting cascade through Hageman factor.

TABLE 21–2. RELATIVE INCIDENCE OF ANAEROBIC BACTERIA IN VARIOUS INFECTIONS

Type of Infection	Incidence (%)
Bacteremia	10–20
Central nervous system	
Brain abscess	89
Head and neck	
Chronic sinusitis	50
Periodontal abscess	100
Pleuropulmonary	
Aspiration pneumonia	85–90
Lung abscess	93
Intraabdominal	
Peritonitis and abscess	90–95
Liver abscess	>50
Female genital tract	
Tubo-ovarian abscess	92
Vulvovaginal abscess	74
Septic abortion and endometritis	73

Adapted from Lennette EH, et al. Manual of Clinical Microbiology. *4th ed. Washington, DC: American Society for Microbiology; 1985.*

VIRULENCE AND RESISTANCE FACTORS

The bacteria associated with anaerobic infections produce a large number of factors that may be involved in the diseases they cause. Except for the exotoxins produced by *Clostridium,* none are highly toxic substances, and none have been proven to be the specific disease-producing factors.

Endotoxins are common among the gram-negative anaerobes. The various endotoxin properties described in Chapter 9 are shared by the endotoxins found in anaerobic infections. There is a strong correlation between endotoxins and the degree of injury in pulp and periodontal lesions. In addition, many toxic metabolites, such as hydrogen sulfide and ammonia, are produced by these bacteria.

Anaerobic bacteria produce many potentially injurious enzymes. These include proteases, collagenase, heparinase, and fibrinolysins. As noted in Chapter 14, the clostridia alone produce many different enzymes. In addition, *Bacteroides fragilis* and other *Bacteroides* species produce β-lactamase, an enzyme that inactivates antibiotics such as penicillin. This enzyme probably protects not only the *Bacteroides* but also other bacteria present in the polymicrobic infection.

Polymorphonuclear neutrophils (PMNs) constitute a major resistance factor within the body, and anaerobic bacteria produce antiphagocytic factors that interfere with several PMN functions. Some anaerobic species secrete substances that inhibit phagocytosis, not only of themselves but of other bacteria in the area. In addition, some species produce inhibitors of chemotaxis and thus prevent or hinder movement of PMNs toward the bacteria. The actions of PMNs are further compromised because of the anaerobic environment. The PMNs bactericidal activity is for the most part dependent on an oxygen-dependent metabolic burst. In the absence of oxygen, this important protective factor is missing, and this enhances the virulence of anaerobic bacteria.

PATHOGENESIS

Anaerobic infections occur throughout the body, but certain disease processes almost always involve either pure anaerobic or mixed anaerobic/aerobic infections. Some of the more common extraoral infections are listed in Table 21–2. Although the incidence of these infections is low, they are significant because of their severity, the difficulties encountered in treating them, and the fact that they often occur in debilitated people.

Anaerobic infections predominate within the oral cavity. Pulp, periapical, and periodontal infections

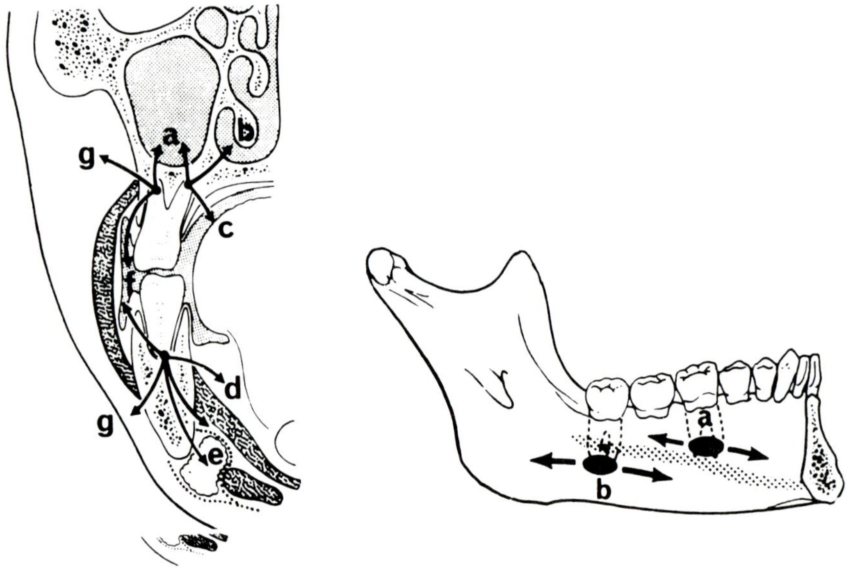

Figure 21–1. Routes of spread of orofacial infections along planes of least resistance. **Left.** Coronal section in region of first molar teeth. a, maxillary antrum; b, nasal cavity; c, palatal plate; d, sublingual space; e, submandibular space; f, intraoral presentation with infection spreading through the buccal plates inside the attachment of the buccinator muscle; g, extraoral presentation to buccal space with infection spreading through the buccal plates outside the attachment of the buccinator muscle. **Right.** Lingual aspect of the mandible. a, apices of the involved tooth above the mylohyoid muscle, with spread of infection into sublingual space; b, apices of involved tooth below the mylohyoid muscle, with spread of infection into submandibular space. *(From Chow AW, Roser SM, Brady FA.* Ann Intern Med. *1978;88:396.)*

are predominantly anaerobic infections. These are discussed in Chapters 34 and 35.

Orofacial infections, a term that generally refers to infections occurring in orofacial tissues other than the teeth and periodontium, are primarily anaerobic infections. They are polymicrobic, containing both facultative and anaerobic bacteria. These may be localized oral abscesses or may spread throughout the orofacial tissues, or even systemically. Orofacial infections are almost all of dental origin, with endodontic abscesses being the predominant source of the bacteria (Fig 21–1). They must be treated as serious infections not only because of the injury and pain they may cause in the immediate oral tissues but also because they may rapidly spread to the mediastinal, intercranial, or retropharyngeal tissues (Fig 21–2). This may result in osteomyeltitis, maxillary sinusitis, cavernous sinus thrombosis, or Ludwig's angina, all of which may be severe and possibly fatal infections.

The oral cavity is of special significance to anaerobic infections, not only because so many occur within the oral tissues but also because the mouth is a major source from which anaerobic bacteria are disseminated to the rest of the body. As noted previously, anaerobes may spread by direct extension from an oral site, such as a periapical lesion, and invade surrounding tissues. The bacteria may be spread hematogenously through bacteremias resulting from oral lesions or from tooth extractions or other dental manipulations. Both natural and iatrogenic dissemination is well documented. In addition, inspiration of anaerobes in dental plaque or calculus is considered to be a major source of the bacteria in anaerobic lung abscesses. Finally, anaerobes often are involved in the infections resulting from bites by humans and other animals. Deep, closed puncture wounds, impregnated with salivary fluids rich in anaerobes, often develop into serious, difficult to treat anaerobic infections.

DIAGNOSIS

It has become apparent that anaerobic infections play a much more important role in medicine and dentistry than was believed previously. This is not simply because there are more of these infections but rather that because of improved anaerobic culturing methods, clinical laboratories are more successful in cultivating these bacteria from clinical specimens. Success in isolation and cultivation of strict anaerobes is dependent on the application of strict anaerobic techniques during specimen collection, transport, and culture. Specimens must be taken under conditions that minimize exposure to oxygen. Oxygen-free transport media, tubes, and collecting apparatus, such as syringes and swabs, must be used to protect the anaerobes, and the specimens should be transferred to an anaerobic environment in the clinical laboratory as quickly as possible.

There are three general methods of establishing anaerobic conditions for cultivation of anerobes in the laboratory. The cultures may be sealed within a Brewer jar from which oxygen is then removed. The air within the jar is either displayed by vacuum and replaced with a nitrogen/carbon dioxide/hydrogen mixture, or the oxygen within the jar is consumed by a catalytic hydrogen-generating system that converts the oxygen to water.

A second method involves the use of oxygen-free tubed media and cannulas through which oxygen-free gas is passed into the media any time the tubes

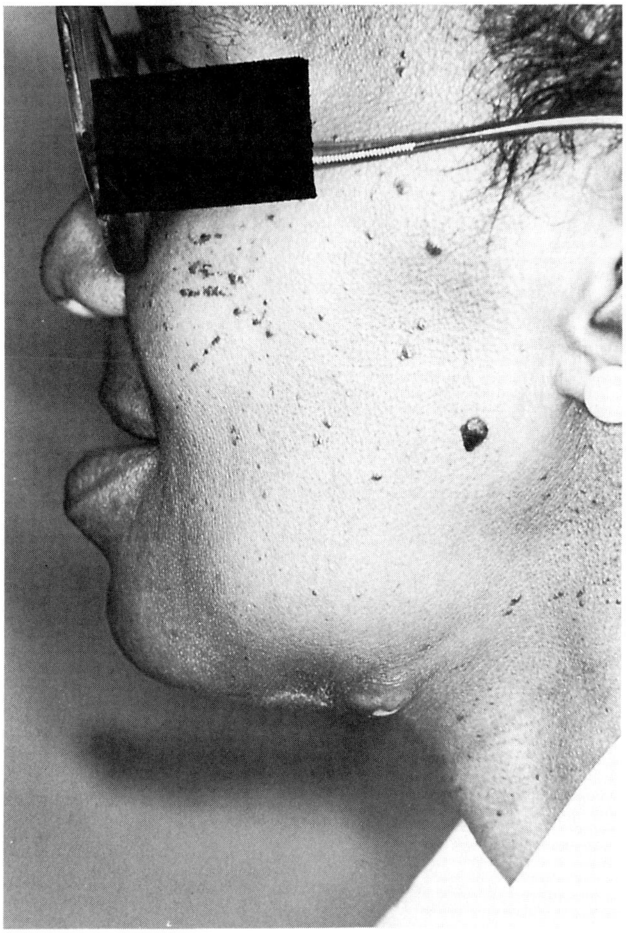

Figure 21–2. Acute cellulitis involving submandibular space. Note associated skin fistula. *(Courtesy of L. Gorzelnik, Temple University School of Dentistry.)*

are open. This constant flow of gas prevents the entry of atmospheric oxygen.

The third method is the anaerobic glove box. This is a large, transparent, airtight chamber with inverted gloves attached to its walls. The air within the chamber is replaced with oxygen-free gas mixture containing 5 to 10% H_2, 5 to 10% CO_2, and 80 to 90% N_2. Cultures can be placed in the chamber, where they may be handled with the inverted gloves without any special precautions just as one would work with aerobic cultures.

TREATMENT

Therapy almost always requires surgical drainage of the anaerobic lesion. The enclosed, anaerobic, and noxious environment retards penetration and, in some cases, the functioning of host resistance factors and antibiotics. The potential inhibition of PMN activity by oxygen deprivation was mentioned previously. The polymicrobic nature of the lesion increases the possibility that an antibiotic-degrading factor might be present. A classic example is the β-lactamase produced by *B. fragilis,* a species often found in anaerobic infections. The extracellular β-lactamase produced by *B. fragilis* can protect all of the bacteria in the lesion. Aminoglycoside antibiotics are ineffective against the bacteria present in anaerobic infections. It is believed that transport of these drugs into the bacterial cell is through an oxygen-requiring system. The oxygen levels in anaerobic lesions apparently are insufficient for the transport system to operate, and, therefore, aminoglycosides are ineffective.

For many years, penicillin has been considered to be universally effective against all clinically important anaerobes except *B. fragilis.* Recent reports, however, indicate that as many as 20% to 30% of other anaerobes isolated from clinical specimens are resistant to penicillin. This includes the black-pigmented *Bacteroides.* In general, however, penicillin still is considered to be useful against all anaerobes except *B. fragilis.* Carbenicillin, clindamycin, and β-lactamase-resistant cephalosporins also are effective against many anaerobes. Clindamycin must be used with caution because of its potential for predisposing to pseudomembranous colitis.

ORAL ASPECTS

Anaerobic bacteria are numerically dominant within the oral cavity, both as members of the normal oral flora and as agents of disease. Pulp, periapical, and periodontal lesions and orofacial abscesses are almost always polymicrobic infections containing strict anaerobes. The oral cavity serves as a reservoir from which other tissues of the body may be infected. Thus, the oral anaerobic bacteria are extremely important in dentistry and medicine.

SUGGESTED READINGS

Allen SD, ed. Anaerobic bacteria. In: *Manual of Clinical Microbiology.* 4th ed. Washington, DC: American Society for Microbiology; 1985:413–472.

Bartlett JG. Recent developments in the management of anaerobic infections. *Rev Infect Dis.* 1983;5:235–245.

Brook I. Encapsulated anaerobic bacteria in synergistic infections. *Microbiol Rev.* 1986;50:452–457.

Chow AW, Roser SM, Brady FA. Orofacial odontogenic infections. *Ann Interm Med.* 1978;88:392–402.

Finegold SM, George WL, eds. *Anaerobic Infections in Humans.* San Diego, Calif: Academic Press; 1989.

Hofstad T, Digranes A, eds. Pathogenesis and treatment of anaerobic infections. *Scand J Infect Dis.* 1985;46 (Suppl).

Schonfeld SE. Orofacial infections of odontogenic origin. *CDA J.* 1982;14:49–51.

Sutter VL. Anaerobes as normal oral flora. *Rev Infect Dis.* 1984;6:S62–S66.

Sutter VL, Citron DM, Edelstein MA, Finegold SM. *Wadsworth Anaerobic Bacteriology Manual.* 4th ed. Los Angeles, Calif: Star Publishing; 1985.

Youmans GP, Paterson PY, Sommers HM. *The Biologic and Clinical Basis of Infectious Diseases.* 3rd ed. Philadelphia: WB Saunders; 1985.

CHAPTER 22

Miscellaneous Organisms of Public Health Significance

Samuel Rosen, John A. Molinari, and Norman P. Willett

INTRODUCTION

ANIMAL PATHOGENS TRANSMISSIBLE TO HUMANS
- *Brucella*
- *Yersinia*
- *Francisella*
- *Listeria*

HUMAN RESPIRATORY PATHOGENS
- *Haemophilus*
- *Bordetella*
- *Legionella*

ORAL ASPECTS

SUGGESTED READINGS

INTRODUCTION

The etiologic agents grouped together in this chapter, although heterogeneous in morphology, pathogenesis, epidemiology, and treatment, have a common thread in that they have public health significance far beyond the total number of cases of diseases they cause (Table 22–1). They are classified into two large groups, animal pathogens transmissible to humans and human respiratory pathogens. With two exceptions, they are all notifiable diseases to local and federal health authorities. Some, such as bubonic plague, evoke fear because of their history. Others, such as Legionnaire's disease, have emerged recently as important respiratory pathogens, especially in health care facilities. Still, others, such as whooping cough, once thought to have been all but eliminated due to successful vaccination programs, have increased when these programs were dropped because of questions relating to side effects of the vaccine.

ANIMAL PATHOGENS TRANSMISSIBLE TO HUMANS

Brucella

Brucellae are obligate parasites of animals and humans. *Brucella melitensis* typically infects goats, *Brucella suis* infects swine, *Brucella abortus* infects cattle, and *Brucella canis* infects dogs. The disease in humans may be caused by any of the aforementioned species and is known as brucellosis, undulant fever, or Malta fever.

Morphology, Cultivation, and Classification. The organisms are gram-negative, nonmotile, nonspore-forming rods. Short coccobacillary forms predominate in young cultures. Brucellae are adapted to an intracellular habitat, and their nutritional requirements are complex. Fresh specimens from animal or human sources usually are inoculated onto trypticase-soy agar or into blood culture media. *Brucella abortus* requires 5

TABLE 22–1. PUBLIC HEALTH SIGNIFICANCE OF SELECTED BACTERIAL DISEASES

Disease	Organism	Average Cases/year 1980–1985
Brucellosis	*Brucella abortus*	205
Bubonic plague	*Yersinia pestis*	28
Tularemia	*Francisella tularensis*	214
Listeriosis[a]	*Listeria monocytogenes*	?
Haemophilus meningitis[a]	*Haemophilus influenzae*	8000 (est)
Haemophilus arthritis[a]		
Whooping cough	*Bordetella pertussis*	2640
Legionnaires' disease	*Legionella pneumophila*	794

[a]Not notifiable.

From Summary of Notifiable Diseases, United States. *Atlanta, Ga: Centers for Disease Control; June 5, 1987.*

to 10% CO_2 for growth, whereas the other species grow in air and are considered strict aerobes.

Virulence Factors. *Brucella* has an endotoxin to which hosts may become sensitized. The typical virulent organism forms a smooth colony. On culture, it tends to change to the rough form, which is avirulent. *Brucella* antigens stimulate a strong cell-mediated immune response and hypersensitivity reactions directed against these antigens and may play a role in the disease process.

Pathogenesis, Diagnosis, and Immunity. Brucellae are essentially animal pathogens transmitted in animal populations by contact with feces, urine, milk and infected tissues. About 15% of cattle herds are infected in the United States. Infection of humans is accidental, through contact with these same infected materials. In farmers, veterinarians, and slaughterhouse workers, most infections remain asymptomatic.

Infections occur via the skin or conjunctiva as a result of contact with infected animals. The organism spreads through the lymphatic system and localizes in regional lymph nodes. Multiplication occurs within macrophages, followed by invasion of the blood and subsequent formation of lesions in liver, kidneys, spleen, and bone marrow. *Brucella abortus* uses the sugar alcohol erythritol, which is present in significant concentration in the placenta of various domestic animals. As a result, the organism localizes in that organ, resulting in abortion.

In humans, the incubation period is 1 to 6 weeks. The onset is insidious, with malaise, fever, weakness, aches, and sweats. Lymph nodes enlarge, and the spleen becomes palpable. These symptoms of generalized *Brucella* infection generally subside in weeks or months, although localized lesions and symptoms may continue. Following the initial infection, a chronic stage may develop, characterized by weakness, aches and pains, low-grade fever, nervousness, and other nonspecific manifestations compatible with psychoneurotic symptoms.

As a rule, brucellae can be cultivated from patients only during the acute phase of the illness or during recurrence of activity. Species differentiation among four *Brucella* species is made possible by their characteristic sensitivity to dyes and production of H_2S, as shown in Table 22–2. Finding substantial IgG antibody levels indicates active infection. IgM antibodies may persist after recovery. Some resistance to subsequent attacks is produced by the initial infection.

Treatment and Control. Brucellae may be susceptible to tetracyclines or ampicillin. Symptomatic relief may occur within a few days after treatment with these drugs is begun. However, because of their intracellular location, the organisms are not readily eradicated completely from the host. For best results, treatment must be prolonged. Control rests on limitation of spread and possible eradication of infected animals, pasteurization of milk and milk products, and reduction of occupational hazards whenever possible.

Yersinia

The most significant disease, from a public health standpoint, caused by *Yersinia* is bubonic plague. This disease has caused pandemics responsible for the deaths of millions of people from the sixth century until the late nineteenth century. More recently, the disease, at least in the southwestern United States, has become established in wild rodent populations, resulting in deaths among individuals who come in contact with the rodent.

Morphology and Cultivation. The typically coccobacillary, nonmotile, gram-negative rods are predominant in cultures and in smears from infected tissues. Capsules frequently are present. On prolonged incubation or in an unfavorable environment, the rods are pleomorphic. *Yersinia* grow on ordinary bacteriologic media, but they grow more rapidly on media containing tissue fluids or blood. Gray, viscous colonies are

TABLE 22–2. DIFFERENTIATION OF *BRUCELLA* SPECIES

Species	Growth on Dye Media: Thionin	Growth on Dye Media: Basic Fuchsin	H_2S Produced	CO_2 Required
B. abortus	–	+	+	+
B. melitensis	–	+	–	–
B. suis	+	–	+	–
B. canis	+	–	–	–

Adapted from Jawetz E, Melnick JL, Adelberg EA. Review of Medical Microbiology. *17th ed. E. Norwalk, Conn: Appleton & Lange; 1987.*

formed from virulent tissue inocula, but irregular rough colonies occur frequently.

Virulence Factors. Among the virulence factors produced by these organisms are an intracellular toxin that causes irreversible shock and death in experimental animals and lipopolysaccharide–protein complexes that act to prevent phagocytosis. In addition, all virulent strains produce a capsule.

Epidemiology and Pathogenesis. *Yersinia pestis* is a parasite of various rodents, for example, rats and squirrels. It is transmitted from one rodent to another through the bites of fleas that have become infected by ingesting the blood of an infected animal. The plague bacilli proliferate in the intestinal tract of the flea and eventually block the lumen of the proventriculus completely so that no food can pass through. The hungry flea bites ferociously, and the aspirated blood is regurgitated with the plague bacilli into the bite wound. Thus, plague infection is transmitted from rodent to rodent and, occasionally, from rodent to human. It is not usually transmitted from human to human by fleas. When in the course of human infection pneumonia develops, droplets containing plague bacilli are coughed up. Such droplets are highly infectious by the airborne route and can result in primary pneumonic plague in humans. This is usually fatal without chemotherapy and is readily transmitted from person to person. Some plague strains are so highly virulent that infection with a single organism may be lethal.

Yersinia generally produce disease by rapid invasion of the host, multiplying in many tissues until overwhelming sepsis occurs. When the population of *Yersinia* reaches a high level, autolysis liberates sufficient toxin to be harmful to the host tissues. When plague bacilli enter the host through the bite of a flea, they extend via the lymphatic channels to the regional lymph nodes. Along the lymphatics and in the lymph nodes, there is a rapidly spreading hemorrhagic inflammation, and the node becomes greatly enlarged, forming a bubo. Such buboes usually are located in the groin or axilla and may undergo necrosis. In the less severe forms of plague, the infective process stops there. Often, however, organisms progress via efferent lymphatics and the thoracic duct to the bloodstream, which rapidly disseminates them to all organs, especially to the spleen, liver, lungs, and central nervous system.

Treatment and Control. Bubonic plague can be treated with streptomycin, chloramphenicol, or tetracycline. A formaldehyde-inactivated vaccine has proved effective in protecting individuals in high-risk groups. The chief control procedures are directed toward keeping rat populations at a low level and eliminating both rat and human fleas. All patients with suspected plague must be isolated, especially if pulmonary infection is involved.

Francisella

Tularemia is a significant disease of wild rodent origin caused by *Francisella tularensis*, which is transmissible to humans from rodents by biting flies, ticks, and the rabbit louse. Although it occurs on a worldwide basis, it was first noted in the United States. It also may be caused by the handling or ingestion of infected animal products.

Morphology and Cultivation. The etiologic agent is a small, gram-negative coccobacillus. Older cultures are characterized by a high degree of pleomorphism. It is an aerobe, and it requires a rich medium supplemented by blood for growth.

Epidemiology and Pathogenesis. Biting flies, ticks, rabbit lice, and others all transmit the infection among the rodent population and thus maintain the reservoir of infection. Rabbits and muskrats are the main sources of disease in humans. Handling, skinning, or eating such infected animals or drinking water contaminated by them may result in human infection. *Francisella tularensis* may enter the host via the skin or mucous membranes, through the bites of arthropods, or via the respiratory or gastrointestinal tracts. An ulcerating papule often develops at the site of penetration of the skin or mucous membranes, and the regional lymph nodes enlarge and suppurate. Transitory bacteremia establishes the organisms in various parenchymatous organs, where granulomatous nodules form that often undergo necrosis. As the disease progresses, tularemic pneumonia and septicemia develop that are fatal if untreated. Often the primary lesions are limited to the portal of entry. Thus, the clinical picture may be oculoglandular following infection via the conjunctiva, ulceroglandular following entry through the skin, or pneumonic following primary inhalation of infectious droplets. At other times, there may be no primary lesions whatever and only a febrile systemic illness.

Gram-stained smears often show pleomorphic, gram-negative organisms ranging from coccal forms to long rods. When tularemia is suspected, immunofluorescence staining can identify the organism rapidly.

Treatment and Control. Streptomycin is currently the drug of choice, although tetracycline, gentamicin, and chloramphenicol are also useful. An attenuated vaccine is available for high-risk individuals (eg, hunters).

Control of the wild animals is difficult, and hunters or anyone handling rodent carcasses should wear gloves.

Listeria

The significance of listeriosis as a disease of public health importance has increased dramatically over the past several years. The transmission of the etiologic agent *Listeria monocytogenes,* an animal pathogen, to humans has been documented in recent outbreaks. It is spread by dairy products or raw vegetables.

Morphology, Classification, and Cultivation. *Listeria monocytogenes* is a short, gram-positive, nonsporeforming rod. It is a facultative anaerobe, and its cultivation on media is greatly enhanced by addition of blood, ascitic fluid, or glucose.

Pathogenesis and Diagnosis. *Listeria monocytogenes* is an obligate intracellular parasite that may cause meningoencephalitis in adults, with immunosuppressed patients being especially susceptible.

Perinatal human listeriosis occurs as a result of intrauterine infection and may result in death of the infant before or after delivery. Infections in adults occur most often in immunosuppressed patients, resulting in meningitis. Diagnosis is based on isolation of the organism from blood or spinal fluid.

Treatment and Prevention. Antibiotics that have been used successfully clinically include ampicillin plus gentamicin and tetracycline. The ubiquitous occurrence of the organism in nature and its ability to survive without significant loss for months in both moist and dry environments, its tolerance for preserving agents, and its ability to grow at refrigeration temperatures pose a potential risk for refrigerated food. Because much is unknown regarding the degree of transmission through infected dairy and animal products, the only prevention available at this time involves strict adherence to pasteurization and sterilization protocols for those involved in the preparation of these products and appropriate surveillance carried out by agencies, such as the Center for Disease Control.

HUMAN RESPIRATORY PATHOGENS

Haemophilus

Haemophilus influenzae is a respiratory and central nervous system pathogen that cause diseases in young children but rarely in adults.

Morphology, Classification, and Cultivation. Haemophilus influenzae are short, coccoid, gram-negative bacilli, sometimes occurring in short chains. Long rods and large spherical bodies also are found. *Haemophilus* species get their name because of their affinity for blood-enriched culture media. Specimens are grown on enriched chocolate (heated blood) agar until typical colonies can be identified with a capsule swelling test.

Identification of organisms of the *Haemophilus* group depends, in part, on demonstrating the need for certain growth factors called X and V. Factor X acts physiologically as hemin, which is required for the organism's heme-containing cytochrome system as well as catalase. Factor V can be replaced by nicotinamide adenine nucleotide (NAD) or other coenzymes important in intermediate metabolism. The requirement for X and V factors of various *Haemophilus* species are listed in Table 22–3.

In addition to requirements for X and V factors, *H. influenzae* is differentiated from related gram-negative bacilli by hemolysis on blood agar and by immunologic means. Around staphylococci on blood agar, the colonies of *H. influenzae* grow much larger (satellite phenomenon) because of the release of the V factor by the staphylococci.

Isolates of *H. influenzae* may be classified or serotyped according to their capsular polysaccharide or are nontypable if no capsule exists. There are six recognized serotypes, a, b, c, d, e, f, but type b is the most important pathogen.

Pathogenesis and Virulence Factors. Probably the chief virulence factor is the capsule, which inhibits phagocytosis in the absence of specific antibody. The resistance of the organism to the bactericidal antibody of serum also may be considered a virulence factor. It is related to some undetermined antigenic sites that may be located in the capsule, outer membrane protein, or lipopolysaccharides. However, the specific role of these sites is not yet clearly understood. *Haemophilus influenzae* type b enters by way of the respiratory tract in small children and produces a nasopharyngitis, often with fever. Other types rarely produce disease. There may be local extension, with involvement of the sinuses or of the middle ear. *Haemophilus influenzae* type b and pneumococci are the two most common etiologic agents of bacterial otitis media. The organisms may reach the blood stream and be carried to the meninges or, less frequently, may establish themselves in the joints to pro-

TABLE 22–3. CHARACTERISTICS AND GROWTH REQUIREMENTS OF SOME HEMOPHILIC ORGANISMS

Organism	Hemolysis	Requires X	Requires V	Capsule
Haemophilus influenzae	−	+	+	+
Haemophilus parainfluenzae	−	−	+	+
Haemophilus haemolyticus	+	+	+	−
Bordetella pertussis	+	−	−	+

Adapted from Jawetz E, Melnick JL, Adelberg EA. Review of Medical Microbiology. *17th ed. E. Norwalk, Conn: Appleton & Lange; 1987.*

duce septic arthritis. *Haemophilus influenzae* is now the commonest cause of bacterial meningitis in children age 5 months to 5 years. Clinically, it resembles other forms of childhood meningitis, and diagnosis rests on bacteriologic demonstration of the organism. *Haemophilus* meningitis is increasing in incidence.

Occasionally, a fulminating obstructive laryngotracheitis develops in infants and requires prompt tracheostomy as a lifesaving procedure. Pneumonitis and epiglottitis due to *H. influenzae* may follow upper respiratory tract infections in small children and old or debilitated people. Prominent among late complications of influenzal meningitis is the development of a localized subdural accumulation of fluid that requires surgical drainage. In addition, some investigators have reported that *H. influenzae* can cause cellulitis in young children because of the affinity of the organism for soft orofacial tissue. This may be considered an opportunistic infection, since the organism is normally a resident of the nasopharynx.

Immunity. Infants under 3 months of age may have serum antibodies transmitted from the mother. During this time, *H. influenzae* infections are usually asymptomatic but may result in respiratory disease or meningitis. By age 3 to 5 years, many children have protective antibodies. There is a correlation between the presence of bactericidal antibodies and resistance to major *H. influenzae* type b infections. It is not known, however, whether these antibodies alone account for immunity.

Diagnosis. When organisms are present in large numbers in specimens, they may be identified by immunofluorescence or may be mixed directly with specific rabbit antiserum (type b), after which a capsule swelling test is performed. Counterimmunoelectrophoresis with spinal fluid may be done with specific antiserum to *Haemophilus*.

Treatment and Control. Many strains of *H. influenzae* type b are susceptible to ampicillin, but up to 30%, which produce β-lactamase, are resistant. Most strains are still susceptible to chloramphenicol. It is common practice to initially treat suspected *H. influenzae* meningitis with both chloramphenicol and ampicillin until definitive microbiologic diagnosis and drug susceptibility are established. Prompt diagnosis and antimicrobial therapy are essential to minimize late neurologic and intellectual impairment.

Contact with patients suffering from *H. influenzae* clinical infection poses little risk for adults but presents a definite risk for siblings and close contacts under age 4 years. Prophylaxis with rifampin for 4 days is recommended for such children.

Vaccines are available for children over 2 years of age, especially those at high risk. They are suggested also for adults without bactericidal antibody.

Haemophilus ducreyi. *Haemophilus ducreyi* is the cause of chancroid, a sexually transmitted disease that is distributed worldwide. The organism is differentiated diagnostically from other hemophilic organisms by the fact that it requires X but not V factor, whereas *H. influenzae* requires both X and V factors. The disease is characterized by genital ulcers, with swelling and tenderness. Antimicrobial therapy is complicated by the fact that two thirds of clinical isolates produce β-lactamase. However, excellent clinical results have been obtained with erythromycin and sulfamethoxazole-trimethoprim.

Bordetella

Bordetella pertussis is the etiologic agent of whooping cough, a debilitating respiratory disease of infants and children. This is an easily transmitted respiratory disease that can be spread rapidly in a dental or medical office under suitable circumstances.

Morphology, Classification, and Cultivation. *Bordetella* are short, ovoid, gram-negative bacilli resembling *H. influenzae*. Bipolar metachromatic granules can be demonstrated. A capsule is present. *Bordetella* are strict aerobes. This genus does not require X and V factors but produces hemolysis. In other respects, *Bordetella* resembles *H. influenzae*.

Primary isolation of *B. pertussis* requires enriched medium. Bordet-Gengou medium (potato-blood-glycerol agar) that contains penicillin G or blood-charcoal agar that contains cephalexin is used.

Virulence Factors. The best-documented virulence factor of *B. pertussis* is its exotoxin. It has many biologic effects that have an impact on the disease, including a histamine-sensitizing factor and a lymphocytosis-promoting factor. Pertussis is another of the many exotoxins that catalyze ADP ribosylation, as described in Chapter 9. *Bordetella pertussis* also produces an adenylcyclase that catalyzes the conversion of endogenous ATP to cyclic AMP in target cells, with resultant multiple effects on the various phases of phagocytosis. *Bordetella pertussis* also possesses an endotoxin with the usual associated biologic effects (Chapter 9).

Pathogenesis and Epidemiology. Transmission is largely by the respiratory route from early cases and possibly via carriers. *Bordetella pertussis* survives for only brief periods outside the human host. The organism adheres and multiplies rapidly on the surface of the epithelium in the trachea and bronchi and interferes with ciliary action. Systemic spread does not occur.

After an incubation period of about 2 weeks, the catarrhal stage develops, with mild coughing and sneezing. During this stage, large numbers of organisms are sprayed in droplets, and the patient is highly infectious but not very ill. During the paroxysmal stage, the cough develops its explosive character and the characteristic whoop on inhalation. This leads to rapid exhaustion and may be associated with vomiting, cyanosis, and convulsions. Convalescence is slow. Rarely, whooping cough is followed by encephalitis of unknown origin.

Whooping cough is endemic in most densely populated areas all over the world and also occurs intermittently in epidemic outbreaks. The source of infection is usually a patient in the early catarrhal stage of the disease. The communicability is high, ranging from 30% to 90%. Most cases occur in children under age 5 years, and most deaths occur in the first year of life.

Immunity. Recovery from whooping cough or adequate vaccination is followed by immunity. Second infections may occur but are mild, although reinfections occurring years later in adults may be severe. It is probable that the first defense against *B. pertussis* infection is the secretory antibody that prevents attachment of the bacteria to the cilia of the respiratory epithelium.

Diagnosis. Mucus or aerosol droplets are cultured on Bordet-Gengou or blood-charcoal agar. The antibiotics in the media tend to inhibit other respiratory flora but permit growth of *B. pertussis*. Organisms are identified by immunofluorescence staining or by slide agglutination with specific antiserum.

Treatment and Control. *Bordetella pertussis* is susceptible to several antimicrobial drugs in vitro. Administration of erythromycin during the catarrhal stage promotes the elimination of the organisms and may have prophylactic value. Treatment after the onset of the paroxysmal phase rarely alters the clinical course.

Control of whooping cough rests mainly on adequate immunization of all infants. Every infant should be immunized against *B. pertussis* during the first year of life. The vaccine, a suspension of killed bacteria, is given in combination with diphtheria and tetanus toxoids (DTP vaccine). Rarely, the *B. pertussis* component can cause neurologic reactions, but most experts do not consider this possible adverse reaction to be of sufficient magnitude to discontinue routine use of this very effective vaccine.

Legionella

An outbreak of pneumonic illness of an American Legion Convention in 1976 led to the discovery of *Legionella* species. In ensuing years, 14 *Legionella* serotypes have been discovered and classified in the Legionellaceae family. It has been demonstrated that these organisms cause a fairly common type of pneumonia in both nosocomial and communal locations. Although the organism is a facultative intracellular parasite, it is ubiquitous in soil and water environments.

Morphology, Classification, and Cultivation. *Legionella* are motile, fastidious, gram-negative bacilli, which are very difficult to stain using the Gram stain technique, and, therefore, special staining is required for visualization of bacteria in infected tissue specimens.

Since the initial isolate was obtained from the Legionnaires' disease episode, the etiologic agent was designated *Legionella pneumophila*, and the nomenclature for *Legionella* species has been formulated in part from their sources of isolation (Table 22–4).

Legionella pneumophila is difficult to culture in artificial media and has been found to require special enriched agars. Optimum growth occurs at 35°C in an atmosphere of 2.5% CO_2. Legionellae, especially *L. pneumophila*, produce unique fatty acids that are useful in differentiating them from other bacteria. Approximately 80% of these molecules are branched, chained fatty acids. These are highly unusual because the fatty acids in other living organisms are linear. This finding is so distinctive that it provides the basis for a definitive gas chromatographic marker useful in the identification of isolated unknown gram-negative bacilli as *Legionella*.

Virulence Factors. The intracellular location of the organism (Fig 22–1) and its ability to multiply in monocytes and interfere with the entire series of phagocytic events by inhibiting phagosome–liposome fusion must be considered one of its most important attributes of virulence. Resistance to the immune

TABLE 22–4. CLASSIFICATION OF *LEGIONELLA* SPECIES

	Source of Isolation	
Species	***Clinical***	***Environmental***
L. pneumophila	Yes	Yes
Serogroup 1		
2		
3		
4		
5		
6		
L. micdadei	Yes	Yes
L. bozemanni	Yes	No
L. dumoffi	Yes	Yes
L. gormanii	No	Yes
L. longbeachae	Yes	No

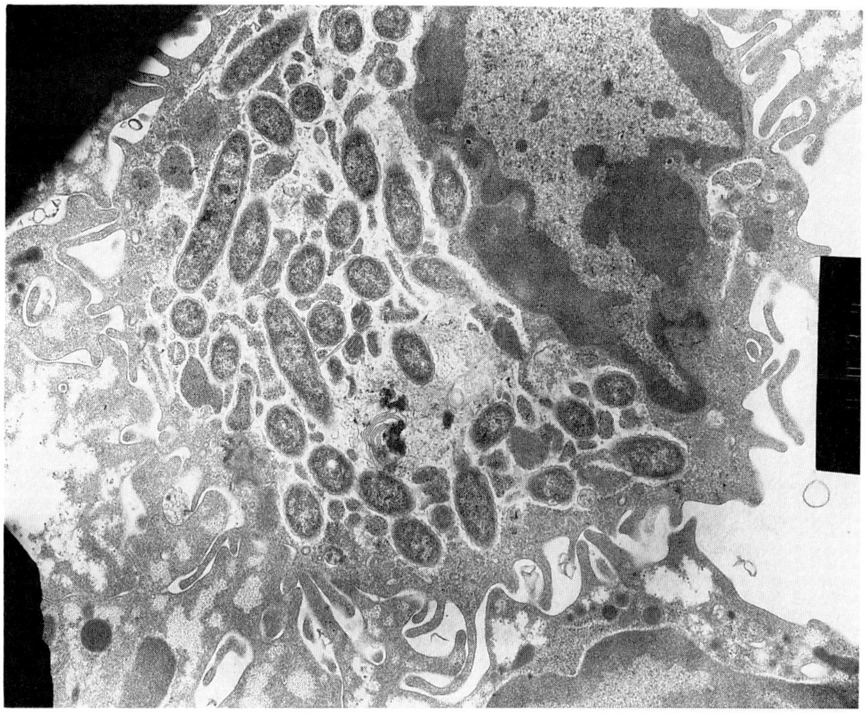

Figure 22–1. Electron micrograph of *Legionella pneumophila*, serogroup 1, in alveolar macrophage of guinea pig lung after aerosol infection. ×10,000. *(Courtesy of W. Winn, University of Vermont School of Medicine.)*

system and many antibiotics is directly related to these phenomena. The acute inflammatory infiltration and febrile nature of the disease appear consistent with the biologic manifestations of released endotoxin in tissues.

Pathologic changes resulting from the pneumonia caused by *L. pneumophila* have been reproduced in experimental animals by administration of a protease produced by the organism. In addition, a number of studies have demonstrated that some species possess cytolytic activity against tissue culture cells.

Pathogenesis. *Legionella pneumophila* causes a severe pneumonia that can result in a mortality rate of 15% to 28%. The microorganism appears to be localized in the lungs. A less severe form of *L. pneumophila* infection also has been documented, that is, the 1968 Pontiac fever syndrome in Pontiac, Michigan. In addition to a shorter incubation period (1 to 2 days), patients infected during this outbreak failed to manifest any evidence of pneumonia. Overall, *L. pneumophila* mainly appears to cause a self-limiting, treatable respiratory infection.

The other major respiratory pathogen is *Legionella micdadei,* commonly referred to as Pittsburgh pneumonia agent (PPA). This bacterium has been associated with a similar type of opportunistic pneumonia occurring in immunocompromised patients after high-dose corticosteroid therapy. The infection may become clinically manifest in 4% to 50% of exposed individuals and constitutes an important nonviral pneumonia that frequently can be fatal in compromised patients and the elderly. The outbreak associated with PPA in patients on corticosteroid therapy also identifies this group of microorganisms as an important source of nosocomial infections. Abdominal cramps, vomiting, and diarrhea are common and may be used to distinguish pneumonias caused by *Legionella* from other pneumonias.

Diagnosis. The diagnosis of legionellosis may be accomplished by cultivation from infected tissues or aspirates, direct or immunofluorescent staining of clinical specimens, and detection of *Legionella* antigens in the patient's urine.

Treatment. The antibiotic of choice for treatment of clinical infection is erythromycin. The bacteria also are susceptible to rifampin, and some cases that have not responded to erythromycin alone have been treated effectively with a combination of erythromycin and rifampin. Oxygen serves as an important supportive adjunct to chemotherapy in severe cases of illness.

Epidemiology. The infectious agent is transmitted from fomite to susceptible individual. There does not appear to be any significant evidence to suggest person-to-person spread of the disease. Environmental sources of *Legionella,* such as air conditioning systems and cooling towers, have been traced as the origins of Legionnaires' disease, Broad Street pneumonia (both in Philadelphia), and Pontiac fever epidemics. The organism also has been isolated from creek water near the site of another outbreak at the University of Indiana.

ORAL ASPECTS

The occurrence of *Bordetella, Legionella,* and *Haemophilus* as respiratory pathogens and the presence of hemophilic organisms in dental plaque make these organisms of prime significance to dental health personnel. The etiologic agent of whooping cough, *B. pertussis,* is a common inhabitant of the oropharyngeal region. The recent decrease in the use of the vaccine because of actual and potential side effects had led to observations that this highly contagious disease, once thought to be a rare occurrence, can again be a hazard to the general population, especially to those health professionals, such as pediatricians, pedodontists, and dental hygienists, who deal with children. *Legionella* has acquired a dental significance as a result of a number of reports from dental clinics in the United States and Europe of increasing antibody titers to *Legionella* directly related to number of years of clinical experience. This suggests that *Legionella* may be present in the dental clinic environment, possibly the water supply, creating an increased risk for clinical personnel and patients.

Recent studies have shown that *Haemophilus* species are ubiquitous in both supragingival and subgingival plaque of adults. However, they represent only a small percentage of the total plaque flora. The relationship of *Haemophilus aprophilus* and other hemophilic organisms to oral health is uncertain at this time, but another very closely related organism, *Actinobacillus actinomycetemcomitans,* until recently classified as *Haemophilus actinomycetemcomitans,* has been strongly associated with juvenile periodontitis bacteriologically and immunologically.

SUGGESTED READINGS

Albritton WL. Infections due to *Haemophilus* species other than *H. influenzae. Annu Rev Microbiol.* 1982;36:199–216.

Berche P, Gaillard JC, Sansonetti P, Geoffrey C, Alouf J. Towards a better understanding of the molecular mechanisms of intracelluar growth of *Listeria monocytogenes. Ann Inst Pasteur Microbiol.* 1987;138:242–246.

Boyle JM *Francisella tularensis* (tularemia). In: Mandel GL, Douglas RG, Bennett JE, *Principles and Practice of Infectious Diseases.* New York: John Wiley & Sons; 1985;1290–1294.

Broome V. Epidemiology of pertussis: Risks and benefits of the current vaccination program. *Microbiology.* 1984;158–160.

Centers for Disease Control. Update prevention of *Hemophilus influenzae* type B disease. *MMWR.* 1988;37:13–16.

Fotos PG, Westfall HN, Snyder IS, Miller RW, Mutchler BM. Prevalence of *Legionella*-specific IgG and IgM antibody in a dental clinic population. *J Dent Res.* 1985; 64:1352–1355.

Hull HF, Montes M, Mann J. Septicemic plague in New Mexico. *J Infect Dis.* 1987;155:113–118.

Keen M, Hoffman PS. Characterization of a *Legionella pneumophila* extracellular protease exhibiting hemolytic and cytotoxic properties. *Infect Immun.* 1989;57:732–738.

Kovick JA, Yu V, Fang G. *Legionella* species as a respiratory pathogen. *Semin Respir Infections.* 1987;2:34–47.

Kuenberg JE. Outbreaks of listeriosis/listeria contaminated food. *Microbiol Sci.* 1988;5:355.

Liljemark WF, Bloomquist CG, Uhl LA, Schaffer EM, Wolff, LF, Philstrom BL, Bandt CL. Distribution of oral *Haemophilus* species in dental plaque from a large adult population. *Infect Immun.* 1984;46:778.

Muder R., Yu V, Woo A. Mode of transmission of *Legionella pneumophilia. Arch Intern Med.* 1986; 146:1607–1612.

Taylor W, Carter JB. Buccal cellulitis in an infant due to ampicillin-resistant *Haemophilus influenzae. J Oral Maxillofac Surg.* 1986;44:234.

Weiss A, Hewitt E. Virulence factors of *Bordetella pertussis. Annu Rev Microbiol.* 1986;40:661–686.

Young EJ. Human brucellosis. *Rev Infect Dis.* 1983;5:821.

CHAPTER 23

Medical Mycology

Carl M. Allen

INTRODUCTION
- Morphology
- Cultivation
- Host Response
- Diagnosis
- Treatment

CANDIDIASIS
- Morphology
- Cultivation
- Virulence Factors
- Disease Process
- Diagnosis
- Treatment

HISTOPLASMOSIS
- Disease Process
- Diagnosis and Treatment
- Epidemiology and Prevention

BLASTOMYCOSIS
- Disease Process
- Diagnosis and Treatment

CRYPTOCOCCOSIS
- Disease Process
- Diagnosis and Treatment

COCCIDIOIDOMYCOSIS
- Disease Process
- Diagnosis and Treatment

OTHER FUNGAL INFECTIONS

DERMATOPHYTES
- Disease Process
- Diagnosis, Treatment, and Prevention

ORAL ASPECTS

SUGGESTED READINGS

INTRODUCTION

Modern biologic concepts place the fungi in their own separate kingdom apart from both the higher plants and the simpler bacteria and protozoans. The fungi are a diverse group of eukaryotic organisms that lack chlorophyll and reproduce by either sexual or asexual means. Examples of commonly encountered fungal organisms include mushrooms, molds, and yeasts. Between 100,000 and 200,000 species of fungi are found in a wide variety of environments, but only about 145 of these cause significant medical problems. The study of fungal organisms is termed mycology, and the branch that deals with fungi that are pathogenic for humans is known as medical mycology. Although fungal diseases are not seen as commonly as bacterial or viral diseases, they still represent an important cause of illness and death. The dentist should be aware of the oral manifestations of fungal infection, since the implications of such infections may be very significant for the patient.

MORPHOLOGY

The majority of fungi that cause human disease are classified as yeasts and molds. These organisms generally reproduce by asexual means and belong to the group known as Deuteromyces or Fungi Imperfecti. Molds typically grow by forming filamentous tubular structures known as hyphae (Fig 23–1), and a collection of a large number of hyphae is termed a myce-

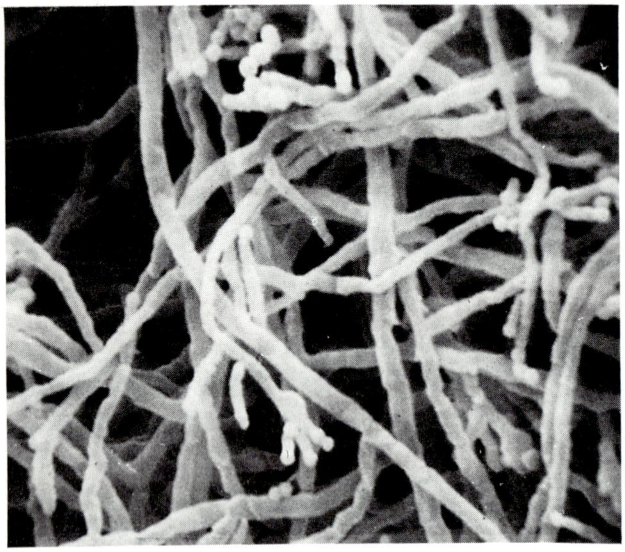

Figure 23–1. Hyphae are tubular, branching structures that make up a mycelium. Junctions between individual cells usually can be seen.

lium. Since fungal organisms lack chlorophyll, they must assimilate nutrients from their environment, whether it be a decaying log or an artificial medium prepared in a laboratory. The portion of the mycelium that grows below the surface of the substrate or medium, acting to carry nutrients, is termed the somatic (or vegetative) mycelium. The aerial mycelium, in contrast, grows above the surface of the substrate.

The mycelium produces germinative structures called spores. Spores are equivalent to the seeds of higher plants, and they may be produced by meiosis and fusion (sexual) or by mitosis (asexual). The asexual types are more common, and they are known as conidia. A wide variety of sporulating structures are produced, and they are useful in classifying the fungi. Some spores are contained within a structure called a sporangium, and they are referred to as sporangiospores. Others are produced at the sides or ends of hyphae. Other spores include the chlamydospore (chlamydoconidia), which is formed by the thickening and enlargement of the hyphal cell wall, and the arthrospore (arthroconidia), which is derived from segments of the hypha. Spores are particularly adapted to survive harsh conditions and have the ability to produce new fungal growth when they encounter the proper environment.

The growth of yeasts is characterized by a budding process whereby a daughter cell is produced mitotically by a parent cell (Fig 23–2). Some yeasts, however, can produce a mycelial phase under certain circumstances. Usually, these organisms appear as a mold when cultivated in the laboratory but grow as yeasts in the human host. (*Candida albicans,* the yeast most commonly encountered by the dentist, is a notable exception to this rule.) This biphasic quality is termed fungal dimorphism, and it frequently confused early medical mycologists, in some instances leading them to believe that they were dealing with two different organisms.

Fungi generally have thick cell walls made up of biologically resistant substances, such as polymeric carbohydrates (glucans and mannans) or glycoproteins (chitin). The cell membrane, which lies beneath the cell wall, differs from that found in mammalian cells in that the fungal cell membrane contains ergosterol rather than cholesterol. Like mammalian cells, however, the fungi maintain chromosomal material within a membrane-bound nucleus. The nucleus re-

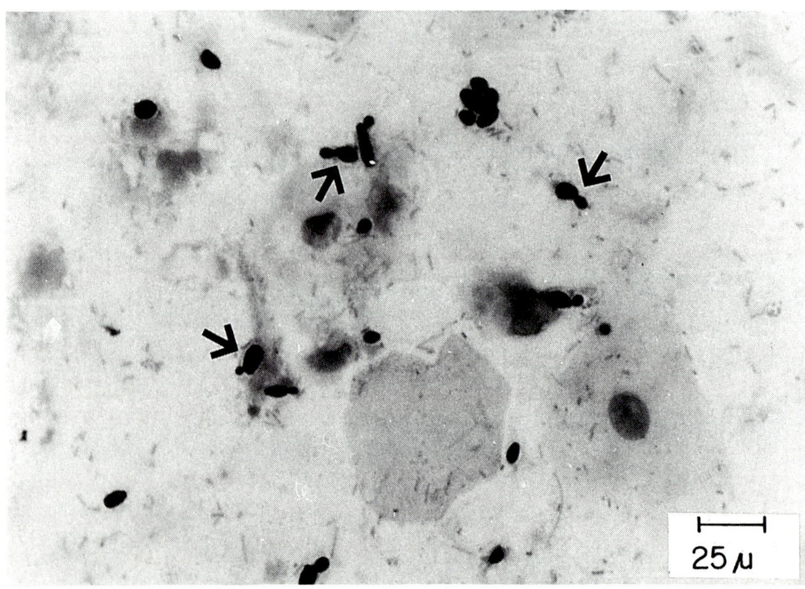

Figure 23–2. Yeasts typically reproduce by a process known as budding, in which a daughter cell grows from the parent cell, eventually breaking away to form a new yeast cell. These yeasts are in various stages of the budding process.

sides within the cytoplasm, which contains the usual organelles necessary for cellular function, such as ribosomes, mitochondria, and endoplasmic reticulum.

CULTIVATION

The cultivation of fungi for purposes of identification has been carried out traditionally using Sabouraud's medium, an agar gel that contains 4% glucose and has a pH of 5.6. The high sugar content and low pH provide conditions that greatly favor the growth of fungi and discourage the growth of bacteria. This medium was developed in the late nineteenth century, and many of the initial descriptions of fungal organisms were based on their appearance when grown on this medium. Because the appearance of a fungal colony can differ considerably depending on the substrate on which it grows, a constant type of culture medium is necessary in order to make comparisons between organisms, and Sabouraud's agar has been accepted as that standard medium.

HOST RESPONSE

Fungal infection will elicit an immune response consisting of antibody production and a cell-mediated reaction. The cell-mediated immune response is the more critical in controlling and resolving a fungal infection. A classic granulomatous inflammatory infiltrate consisting of activated macrophages and T lymphocytes occurs in most instances. The importance of an intact cell-mediated limb of the immune system in protecting against fungal disease is dramatically illustrated in patients affected by congenital thymic aplasia. These individuals have virtually no T lymphocytes and are prone to repeated severe fungal infections. These include not only the fungi described in this chapter but also some such as *Aspergillus* and *Geotrichum,* which never cause disease in normal individuals. Similarly, patients affected by acquired immunodeficiency syndrome (AIDS) have great difficulty in fighting off fungal infections because of the destruction of T helper lymphocytes by the human immunodeficiency virus (HIV).

Unfortunately, the immune response may act as a two-edged sword in that the inflammatory infiltrate causes damage to the host tissue, with resultant scarring and loss of organ function. This injury is the result of delayed hypersensitivity reactions mediated by T lymphocytes responding to fungal antigens. The lymphocytes produce lymphokines that enhance the inflammatory process. Although inflammation generally is considered to be protective, it also may injure the surrounding tissue, as described in Chapter 8. Thus, to a large degree, the damage to the immunocompetent host is not caused by toxins or enzymes produced by the fungal organism. Instead, the host response to the invading organism is responsible for much of the tissue damage.

DIAGNOSIS

The effective treatment of fungal infections depends on an accurate diagnosis, and this is best accomplished by culturing for the causative organism in order to examine such characteristics as colony morphology, microscopic morphology, and types of spores produced. Carbohydrate fermentation and nitrogen source usage are also important in identifying the yeasts. Tentative identification of a fungal organism may be made by microscopic examination of biopsy or cytology specimens, but this method of diagnosis based on microscopic morphology of the organism is not as definitive as the information obtained from culture.

Skin tests that measure delayed hypersensitivity to fungal antigens also are used in diagnosis. Antigenic extracts of suspected fungi are injected intradermally, and the response at the site of inoculation is examined 48 hours later. A positive test only indicates that an individual has been exposed to fungal antigen at some time in the past and does not necessarily mean that active infection is present. A negative skin test may either indicate that a patient has not been exposed to that particular fungus or that he or she has become anergic. Anergy is a condition in which the host cannot mount an immune response, and it is commonly seen in patients with disseminated fungal infections. Therefore, interpretation of the skin test results must be made in a clinical context.

TREATMENT

The treatment of fungal diseases relies on the use of special antifungal agents because antibiotics used to treat bacterial diseases usually have little or no effect on fungal organisms. The differences that separate the bacteria from the fungi both biochemically and structurally are responsible for the differences in response of these organisms to antibiotics. Similarities between the fungal cell structure and mammalian cell structure have caused problems. Many antifungal drugs are also quite toxic to the host. The differences between fungal and mammalian cells that are apparent have been used to develop new antifungal drugs, such as the imidazoles, which are much less toxic. The imidazole compounds seem to impair ergosterol metabolism in the fungal cell membrane, resulting in lethal injury to the fungal organism. Because mammalian cell membranes contain cholesterol instead of ergosterol, imidazole has little effect on the host. Despite such advances in therapy, fungal diseases continue to be a significant cause of illness and death, particularly in the immunocompromised patient.

CANDIDIASIS

Candidiasis is by far the most frequently encountered fungal infection in the oral cavity, and it exhibits a wide spectrum of clinical disease, ranging from a mild mucosal involvement to fatal systemic infection. The causative organism, *Candida albicans,* is a dimorphic yeast that typically exists in the mouths of up to 45% of the adult human population and can be cultured frequently from the stools of normal, healthy individuals. Usually, the transition from the asymptomatic saprobic state to the disease-producing parasitic state is accompanied by a change in either the immunologic status of the host (eg, cancer patients) or a disruption of the microbial ecology (eg, prolonged antibiotic usage). When the term candidiasis is used, it generally is assumed to refer to infection with *C. albicans.* However, other species of the *Candida* genus may be found in the mouth. *Candida tropicalis, Candida stellatoidea, Candida krusei,* and *Candida parapsilosis* occasionally are recovered from the oral mucosa, yet they rarely are the cause of clinically significant disease except in the severely immunocompromised patient.

Morphology

When cultured on an enriched medium at 25°C (room temperature), *C. albicans* grows in the yeast phase, characterized by 4 to 7 μm, round to ovoid cells that multiply by budding. At 37°C (body temperature), the pseudohyphal form of the organism predominates. Pseudohyphae are not true hyphae but superficially resemble them. Pseudohyphae are essentially elongated, tubular cells, approximately 4 μm in diameter, that branch and typically are attached to each other, forming filamentous structures of varying lengths (Fig 23–3). When cultured under adverse conditions (eg, on cornmeal agar), a characteristic sporulating body termed a chlamydospore (chlamydoconidia) is formed. Chlamydospores are relatively large (12 μm) and are essentially diagnostic for *C. albicans* (Fig 23–4). If the yeast form of the organism is inoculated into serum at 37°C, the formation of structures called germ tubes can be observed (Fig 23–5). Germ tube formation also aids in the identification of *C. albicans,* since very few yeasts display this property.

Cultivation

Sabauraud's agar is the medium most commonly used to grow *C. albicans. Candida* colonies are creamy, round, and dome-shaped, with a yeasty odor (Fig 23–6). Other media frequently used to cultivate *C. albicans* include Sabouraud's broth, BiGGY (bismuth, glycine, glucose, yeast extract) agar, mycologic agar, and Pagano-Levin agar.

Virulence Factors

Candida albicans does not possess any known virulence factors. Experimental evidence suggests that there are differences in pathogenicity among various strains of the organism. There is usually a predisposing factor present, such as pregnancy, endocrine disturbances (eg, diabetes mellitus), broad-spectrum

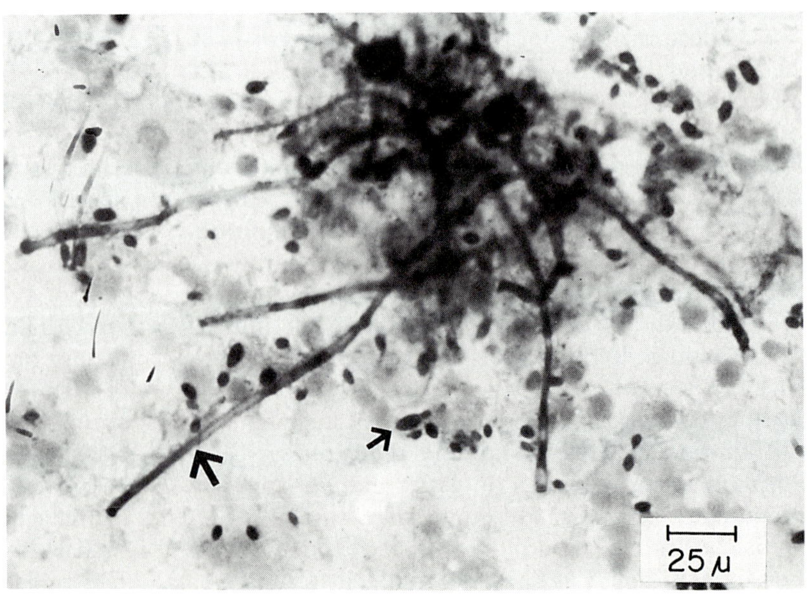

Figure 23–3. This photomicrograph shows a cytologic smear of *Candida albicans* obtained from a patient with acute pseudomembranous candidiasis. The yeast form of the organism (smaller arrow) is seen in association with numerous filamentous pseudohyphae (larger arrow).

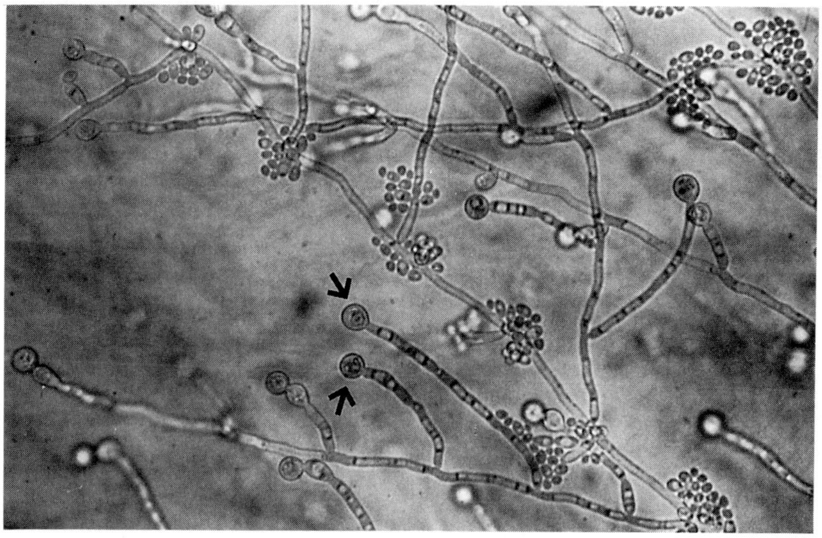

Figure 23–4. These large sporulating bodies, termed chlamydospores, are formed by *Candida albicans* when it is grown on a nutrient-poor medium, such as cornmeal agar.

antibiotic usage, corticosteroid usage, and developmental or acquired deficits of the immune system.

Disease Process

The broad spectrum of diseases produced by *C. albicans* can be related to three factors: (1) host immune status, (2) mucosal/skin environment, and (3) organism characteristics. The clinical presentation of candidiasis depends on the relative contribution of each of these factors, resulting in a wide range of disease. Systemic candidiasis is relatively uncommon and is confined to those patients whose immune systems are severely compromised, usually due to cancer chemotherapy (toxic to white blood cells) or to a malignancy (such as leukemia or lymphoma, which replaces the normal white blood cells with a malignant cell population). With an impaired immune system, the host offers little resistance to the spread of the organism to the lungs, kidneys, brain, and other organs, and death is a frequent outcome.

Similarly, very debilitating cases of chronic mucocutaneous candidiasis are seen in association with specific immunologic defects. Although these patients rarely die of their disease, severe involvement of the skin, nails, and oral and other mucosal surfaces is observed. Abnormalities of the immune system that have been identified in these patients include a lack of migration inhibition factor, failure of lymphocytes to respond to *Candida* antigen, lack of antibodies to *C. albicans,* and reversed T lymphocyte helper/suppressor cell ratio.

Candidal involvement of the skin of immunologically normal patients is seen typically in areas of the body that are continually moist, such as intertriginous areas or the inframammary region. Without

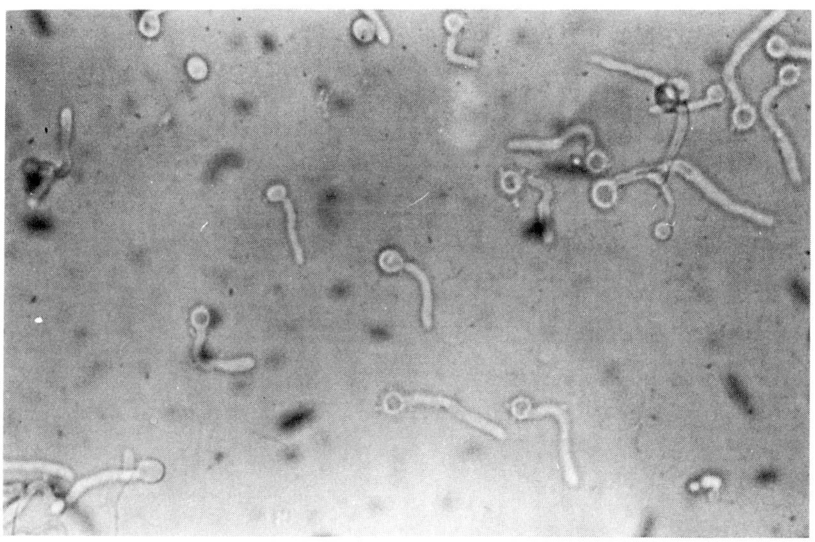

Figure 23–5. When inoculated into serum at 37°C, the yeast form of *Candida albicans* characteristically forms structures called germ tubes within 2 to 3 hours. These structures basically represent the initial transformation of the yeast form to the pseudohyphal form of the organism.

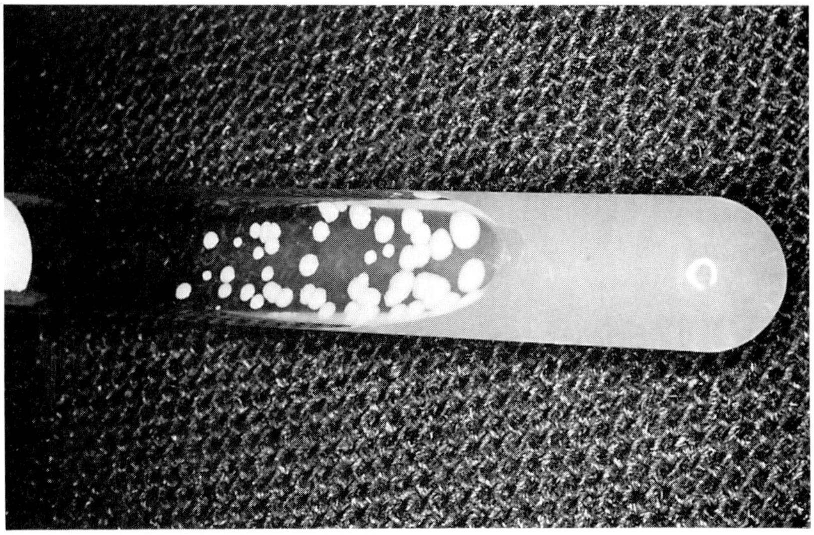

Figure 23–6. When cultured on a slant of Sabouraud's agar, colonies of *Candida albicans* appear as creamy white, round, smooth-surfaced, dome-shaped colonies that have a yeasty odor.

alteration in the skin environment, cutaneous candidiasis is quite uncommon.

Oral candidiasis may occur in one of four different forms: (1) acute pseudomembranous, (2) acute atrophic, (3) chronic atrophic, and (4) chronic hyperplastic. The acute pseudomembranous form of candidiasis is the most widely recognized form of oral candidiasis and is commonly known as oral thrush. Acute pseudomembranous candidiasis usually occurs in individuals whose immune systems are not optimally functional; for example, infants, the elderly, patients taking steroids, and AIDS patients. The lesions appear as creamy white flecks, resembling curdled milk, set on an erythematous oral mucosa (Fig 23–7). As with the other forms of oral candidiasis, the organism in this setting is a superficial parasite. The candidal pseudohyphae which characterize the disease state are very superficially invasive, limited to penetrating only the parakeratin layer of the epithelium. Consequently, these white flecks, composed of organisms and desquamated squamous epithelial cells, can be removed relatively easily, leaving an erythematous base.

Acute atrophic candidiasis usually is seen following tetracycline therapy and is probably due to the effect of decreasing the bacterial population, allowing an overgrowth of the yeast. The patient frequently complains of a burning mouth, and the mucosa appears quite erythematous, without evidence of the white flecks seen in acute pseudomembranous candidiasis.

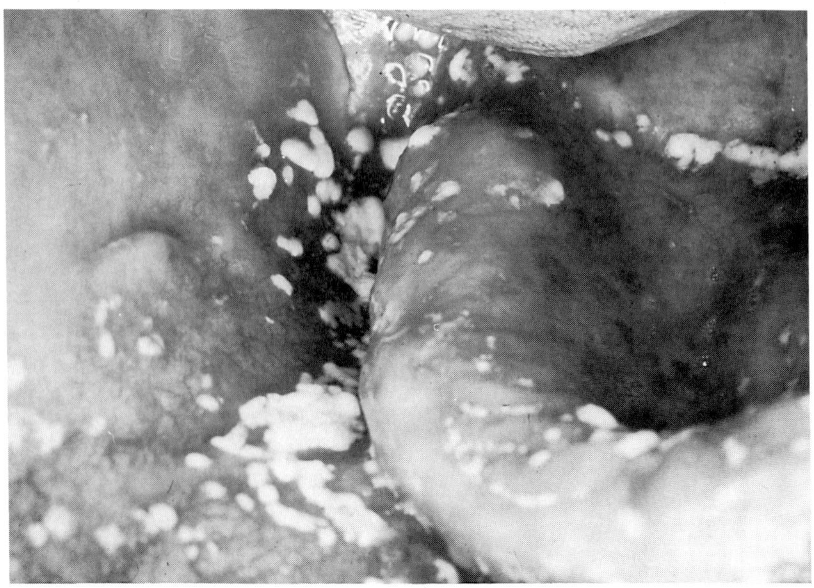

Figure 23–7. These whitish flecks set against an erythematous mucosa are seen typically in acute pseudomembranous candidiasis (thrush). Composed of yeasts, pseudohyphae, and desquamated epithelial cells, these white aggregates can be wiped off without much difficulty. This patient had a history of corticosteroid usage.

Chronic atrophic candidiasis, or so-called denture stomatitis, occurs under a maxillary denture that is removed infrequently from the patient's mouth. The mucosa appears erythematous, either in a diffuse or patchy pattern, and some degree of inflammatory papillary hyperplasia (papillomatosis) may be present. The patient usually is unaware of the lesion, which is typically asymptomatic. The role that *C. albicans* plays in the development of this lesion is somewhat controversial. Invasion of the epithelium by candidal hyphae is not frequently noted in this disease, leading some investigators to conclude that *C. albicans* may not be an etiologic agent. On the other hand, the organism frequently can be cultured from the mucosa and the tissue surface of the denture, and the condition often resolves after treatment with an antifungal agent such as nystatin.

Chronic hyperplastic candidiasis is seen infrequently and has been termed candidal leukoplakia because of its clinical appearance as a white patch that cannot be rubbed off (Fig 23–8A). These lesions are principally located on the buccal mucosa, tongue, and floor of the mouth, and microscopic examination occasionally shows changes in the host epithelial cells which suggest premalignancy. The relation between this form of candidiasis and the development of oral

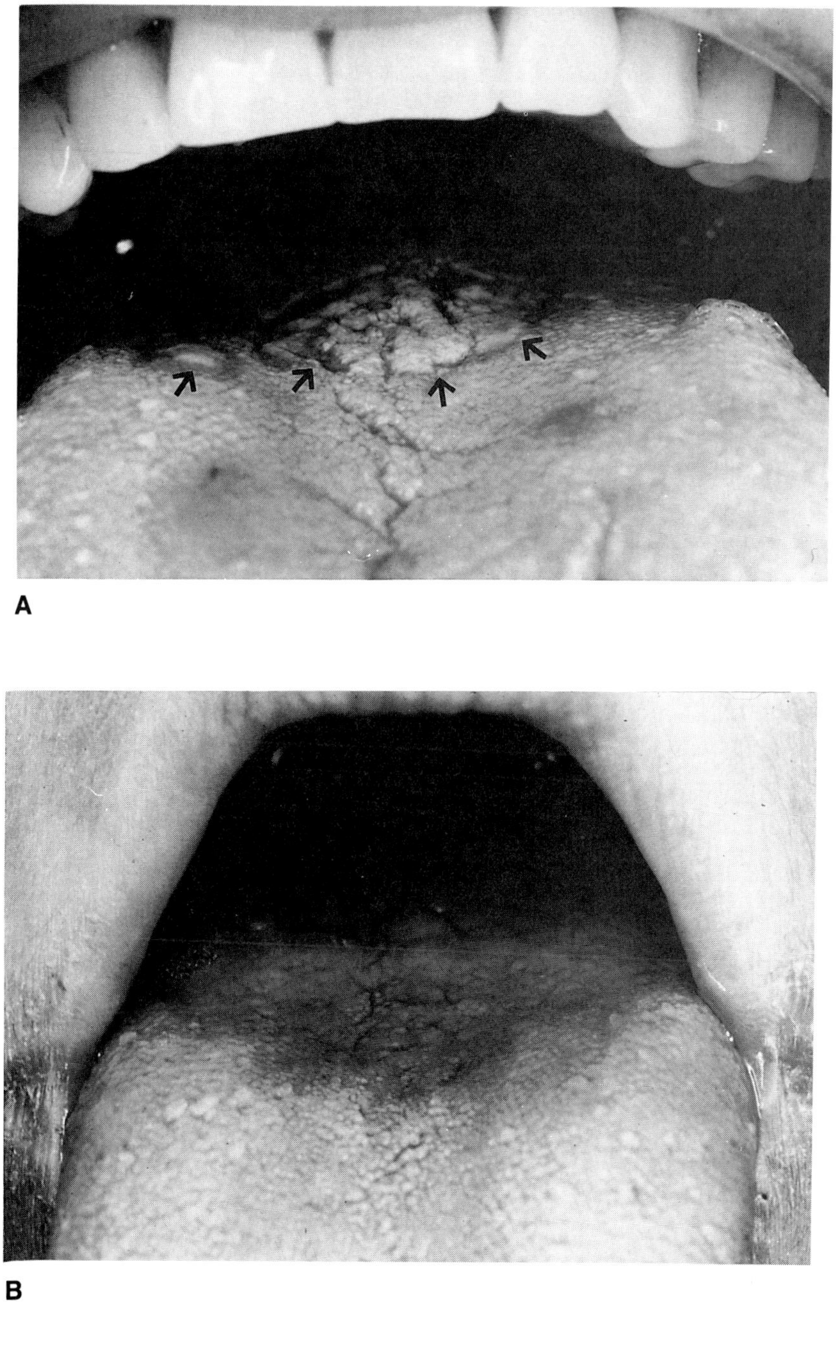

A

B

Figure 23–8.A. Chronic hyperplastic candidiasis, seen here on the midline posterior dorsal tongue (indicated by arrows), appears as a white patch that cannot be rubbed off. Immunologic survey of this patient revealed a lack of antibodies against *Candida albicans*. **B.** The same patient following treatment with the antifungal agent ketoconazole. Notice the dramatic clearing of the leukoplakic lesions of the midline posterior dorsal tongue.

cancer is unclear. Occasionally, immunodeficiencies, both congenital and acquired, have been noted in patients with oral chronic hyperplastic candidiasis.

Diagnosis

The diagnosis of oral candidiasis should be established by means of culture on Sabouraud's agar and oral cytologic preparation. Culturing the oral cavity of a patient suspected of having candidiasis would not yield an entirely reliable result if the culture was positively, simply because the yeast is found so commonly as a saprobic organism. Thus, a cytologic preparation should be stained using a technique that will identify fungal organisms (eg, periodic acid-Schiff method), and the slide should be examined for the candidal pseudohyphae that characterize the invasive or parasitic form of the organism (Fig 23–3).

Treatment

Therapy for candidiasis depends on the severity of the disease. Most oral lesions respond well to the antifungal agent nystatin, a polyene antibiotic that binds to the fungal cell membrane, causing irreversible damage. This drug is extremely effective as a topical medication. However, it is not absorbed by the gastrointestinal tract.

Systemic infections of *C. albicans* have been treated with another polyene antibiotic, amphotericin B. This drug usually is administered intravenously, and it has significant nephrotoxic properties for most patients. Therefore, its use in the United States has been restricted to patients who have systemic life-threatening candidal infections.

Similarly, the fluorinated pyrimidine known as 5-fluorocytosine (5-FC) has been used in treating systemic candidal infections. Unlike amphotericin B, 5-FC can be given orally, and it acts as an antimetabolite, resulting in impaired protein synthesis in the fungal cell. Two major problems usually preclude routine use of 5-FC in clinical settings, however. In addition to being toxic to bone marrow, approximately half of the *C. albicans* infections are resistant to the drug, and resistant strains may even emerge during treatment.

A recent development in drug therapy is the antifungal agent ketoconazole, an imidazole derivative that may be taken orally and is well absorbed across the gastrointestinal tract. It exhibits activity against a variety of pathogenic fungi, including *C. albicans* (Fig 23–8B), by damaging the cell membrane. The only drawback at this time is an apparent idiosyncratic liver toxicity that occurs in approximately 1 in 10,000 to 15,000 of the patients who take the drug. Another imidazole, clotrimazole, has been introduced and has fewer potentially life-threatening complications. Thus, it is greatly favored over ketoconazole for treating routine oral mucosal candidiasis. Because of its ubiquitous nature, prevention of candidiasis has not been considered feasible. Prophylactic nystatin administration for leukemic patients has not reduced significantly the incidence of oropharyngeal or systemic candidal infections.

HISTOPLASMOSIS

Histoplasmosis is a fungal disease that is initiated by inhalation of the spores of the organism *Histoplasma capsulatum*. A wide range of disease may result, and the signs and symptoms often mimic tuberculosis clinically. *Histoplasma capsulatum* is a dimorphic organism, growing as a 2 to 5 μm yeast at 37°C and as a white to brown mold at temperatures below 30°C. The organism is cultivated on Sabouraud's maltose agar, but growth is slow, and it may take 3 or more weeks for colonies to form.

Disease Process

Following inhalation of spores into the lungs of the host, the yeast is phagocytized by the cells of the monocyte–macrophage system, which actually may serve to protect and harbor the infecting organisms to a certain extent. The clinical presentation of histoplasmosis depends on the patient's age, the competence of the immune system, and the status of the lungs. The three typical patterns of the disease include the primary acute form, the severe disseminated form, and the chronic cavitary form. Primary histoplasmosis, which is the most common, affects only the pulmonary system. It has been estimated that 80% to 100% of the population in endemic areas have experienced primary acute histoplasmosis by 18 years of age. The disease is usually asymptomatic, but it may produce fever, muscle and joint pains, chest pains, coughing, and shortness of breath. The cells of the macrophage–monocyte system phagocytize the invading yeasts and destroy them, resulting in spontaneous recovery. Chest radiographs may show residual calcified granulomas even years later.

Severe disseminated histoplasmosis is more likely to occur in infants, the elderly, or the immunocompromised patient. Fever, anemia, weight loss, and enlarged lymph nodes are present. Pulmonary symptoms may be minimal. Granulomatous lesions with red, irregular, ulcerated surfaces occur on the oral and genital mucosa (Fig 23–9). Unlike the normal patient whose macrophages destroy the yeast, the phagocytic cells of these patients are unable to kill the organism and may disseminate the yeast throughout the body.

Chronic cavitary histoplasmosis usually affects an adult male population who exhibit chronic obstruc-

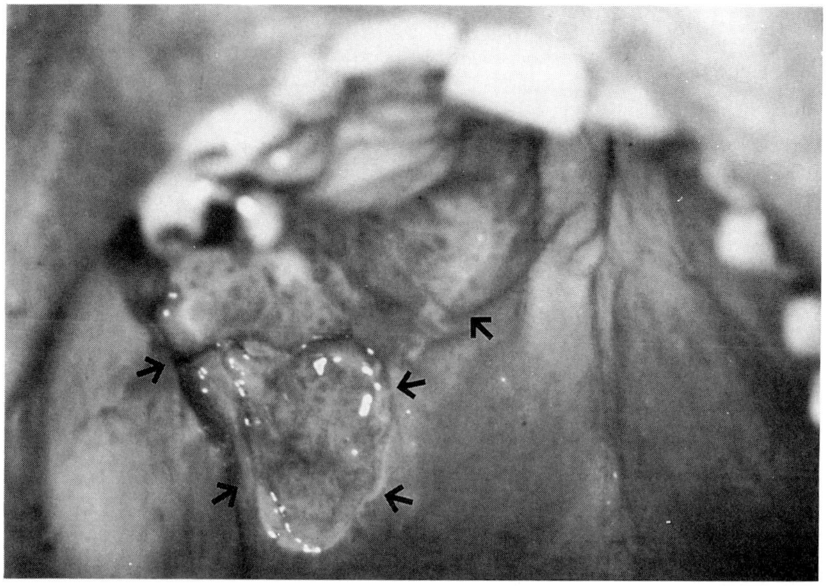

Figure 23–9. This large ulceration of the right palate and alveolar process in a 62-year-old male represents oral histoplasmosis. The patient was treated subsequently with ketoconazole, and the lesion eventually resolved. *(Courtesy of Drs. Bela Toth and Robert Frame, M.D. Anderson Hospital and Tumor Institute. Reprinted with permission from the CV Mosby Company.* Oral Surg. *1983;55:597–600.)*

tive lung disease, for example, emphysema, and have an intact immune system.

Diagnosis and Treatment

The organism may be seen within the cells in biopsy material (Fig 23–10), but definitive diagnosis requires that the yeast be cultured from the specimen. The mycelial growth phase of the organism produces diagnostic sporulating bodies called tuberculate macroconidia (Fig 23–11). The majority of cases of histoplasmosis need no treatment. Amphotericin B has been used for the more aggressive and disseminated forms of the disease. However, good therapeutic results are being obtained in noncompromised patients with ketoconazole, which has relatively minor side effects in comparison to amphotericin B.

Epidemiology and Prevention

The natural habitat of *H. capsulatum* is the soil, particularly soil enriched by bird or bat droppings. Therefore, it is not surprising that many outbreaks of the disease are associated with activities such as cave exploring or the demolition of an old chicken roost. These isolated incidents are comparatively minor when one considers that an estimated 500,000 individuals in the United States are infected yearly. Classi-

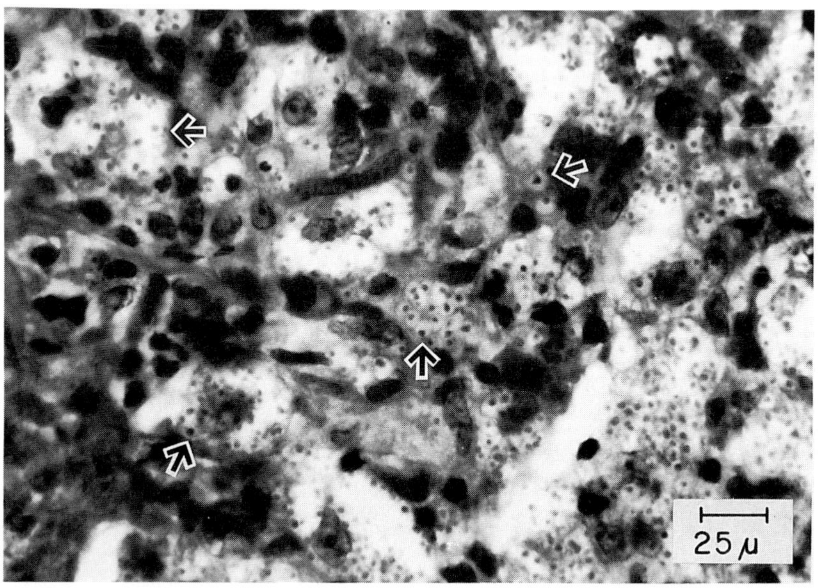

Figure 23–10. Photomicrograph of tissue sampled from an oral lesion of histoplasmosis. The macrophages frequently show the small *Histoplasma capsulatum* organisms intracellularly (arrows).

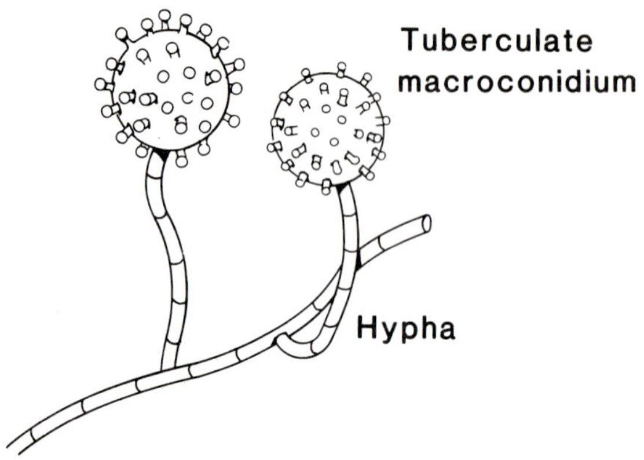

Figure 23–11. The mycelial form of *Histoplasma capsulatum* produces characteristic sporulating structures called tuberculate macroconidia.

cally, the distribution of endemic histoplasmosis has been described as the area associated with the Ohio and Mississippi River valleys. However, the disease has been shown to exhibit a worldwide distribution. In endemic areas, little can be done to prevent exposure to the spores of *H. capsulatum.*

BLASTOMYCOSIS

Blastomycosis is a fungal disease resulting from infection with the organism *Blastomyces dermatitidis,* a dimorphic organism that probably resides normally in the soil. *Blastomyces dermatitides* in tissues or in culture at 37°C is a thick-walled, spherical yeast measuring 8 to 15 μm in diameter. Below 30°C, it grows as a white to brown mold with broad, short, thick-walled hyphae. The organism may be cultured on Sabouraud's agar below 30°C or on blood agar at 37°C, allowing at least 4 weeks incubation for the slow-growing colonies to form.

Disease Process

Blastomycosis probably begins with inhalation of the fungal spores, resulting in an acute pulmonary infection that is characterized by a productive cough, fever, joint and muscle aches, and chest pains. This initial infection may resolve spontaneously, or it may disseminate to skin, bone, kidneys, and central nervous system. This latter course frequently is fatal. The skin lesions have a red, granular appearance (Fig 23–12), whereas the oral lesions appear as erythematous papillary growths.

Most cases of blastomycosis are found east of the Mississippi River, predominantly in the states of Mississippi, Kentucky, Arkansas, North Carolina, and Tennessee. Interestingly, this appears to be a disease that primarily affects males, with a 9:1 male/female ratio, although this may be due to increased exposure of males to sites that might harbor the organism.

Diagnosis and Treatment

The diagnosis of blastomycosis may be suggested through microscopic examination of scrapings from a lesion (usually with a 10% potassium hydroxide preparation) or from biopsy material, but a definitive diagnosis requires cultivation of the organism. Amphotericin B and ketoconazole are used for therapy.

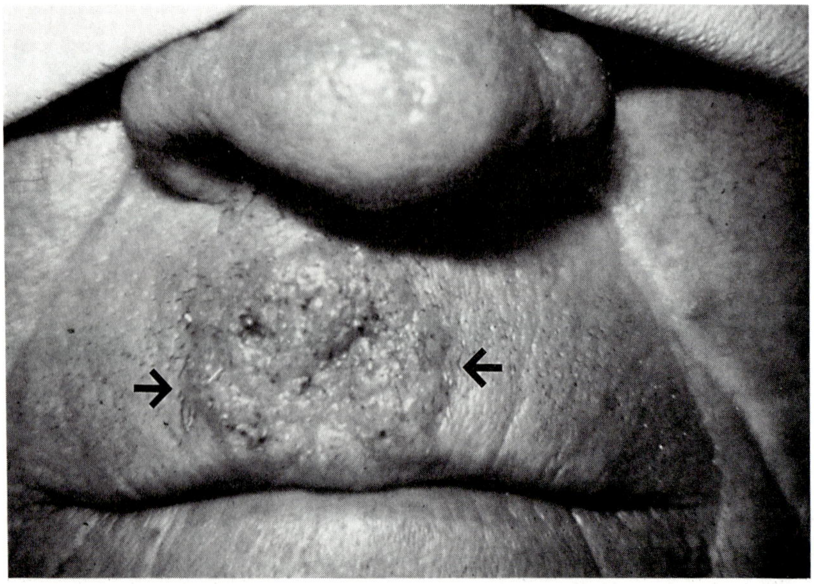

Figure 23–12. This rough-surfaced erythematous lesion of the upper lip (indicated by arrows) was noticed by this 58-year-old male for the past 4 ½ months and was slowly enlarging. Biopsy and culture established the diagnosis of blastomycosis. *(Courtesy of the Armed Forces Institute of Pathology.)*

CRYPTOCOCCOSIS

The fungal disease cryptococcosis is caused by the monomorphic yeast *Cryptococcus neoformans,* an organism with a worldwide distribution. This spherical yeast may measure from 5 to 20 μm in diameter, and it frequently exhibits a thick gelatinous capsule. Unlike most other pathogenic fungi, *C. neoformans* rarely exhibits dimorphism, growing only in a yeast form in most settings. Culture produces creamy to brownish mucoid colonies that grow well at 37°C. The gelatinous capsule probably protects the organism from destruction by the host, since both capsulated and unencapsulated forms exist, but only the encapsulated strains are capable of producing disease in humans.

Disease Process

Patients exhibiting immune deficiency are particularly prone to develop cryptococcosis. These include patients with T lymphocyte deficiency, leukemia, lymphoma, sarcoidosis, and diabetes mellitus. The disease is initiated by inhaling dust containing the organism, resulting in a pulmonary lesion. Many of these cases of pulmonary cryptococcosis are probably asymptomatic, and if symptoms do occur, they are frequently low-grade fever, weight loss, cough, malaise, and chest pain. Systemic dissemination occurs in 10% to 15% of patients, with lesions involving the skin, meninges, lymph nodes, and bone. Meningeal involvement has classically been associated with *Cryptococcus,* but the reasons for the organism favoring this site are unclear.

The fact that *C. neoformans* is so widely distributed undoubtedly relates to the association of the organism with the pigeon. The yeast lives in the bird's gut but does not produce infection, and thus pigeon droppings frequently are contaminated with this organism. *Cryptococcus neoformans* is particularly resistant to drying and will remain viable in dust for 10 to 24 months.

Diagnosis and Treatment

The diagnosis of cryptococcosis is established by culturing the organism on Sabouraud's agar or blood agar at 37°C. Scrapings of a lesion, when viewed microscopically with an India ink preparation, show the typical thick gelatinous capsule as a clear zone surrounding the yeast. Therapy consists of amphotericin B.

COCCIDIOIDOMYCOSIS

Coccidioidomycosis is a fungal infection caused by *Coccidioides immitis.* It occurs in the southwestern part of the United States. This condition occurs naturally in wild rodents and domestic animals as well as humans.

Coccidioides immitis is a dimorphic fungus that grows as a mold in its natural state. The mycelium produces barrel-shaped spores called arthrospores, which initiate infection following inhalation. In host tissue, the organism appears as a round, thick-walled structure termed a spherule, measuring 20 to 200 μm in diameter and containing numerous 2 to 5 μm endospores. *Coccidioides* is cultivated on Sabouraud's agar and must be handled carefully because highly infectious arthrospores are produced by the mycelial phase.

Disease Process

Coccidioidomycosis is a disease that occurs more commonly in males and affects nearly any age group. In the overwhelming majority of patients, inhalation of spores results in primary pulmonary coccidioidomycosis. Of these, approximately 60% will be asymptomatic, with the remaining 40% exhibiting flu-like symptoms—malaise, aches and pains, fever, night sweats, productive cough, loss of appetite, and weight loss. Only a small percentage of these patients will progress to a disseminated form of the disease, in which the skin, subcutaneous tissues, bones, joints, and viscera become involved due to hematogenous spread of the organism.

Diagnosis and Treatment

The organism may be seen in cytologic smears and biopsy material, but definitive diagnosis is established by culture. Most cases of coccidioidomycosis do not require treatment. Disseminated coccidioidomycosis is treated with amphotericin B or ketoconazole.

OTHER FUNGAL INFECTIONS

Medically compromised patients may become infected with a variety of fungal organisms that, under normal circumstances, would not be pathogenic for humans. Zygomycosis (previously known as phycomycosis or mucormycosis) is caused by genera of the Zygomyces family, usually *Mucor* or *Rhizopus.* Infection by these organisms often occurs in the head and neck region, usually starting in the paranasal sinuses of poorly controlled diabetic patients. This rhinocerebral form of zygomycosis produces marked facial swelling and extensive tissue destruction. It must be recognized early and treated aggressively with surgical debridement of infected tissue in combination with systemic amphotericin B. Even with such treatment, the prognosis is guarded.

Aspergillosis, caused by any one of several species of *Aspergillus,* also may be seen in the paranasal sinus region. This disease usually affects immunocompromised patients, particularly those with leukemia or lymphoma who are neutropenic (deficient in neutrophils) secondary to their cancer chemotherapy. As with zygomycosis, aspergillosis will occur as a diffuse swelling of the maxillary and zygomatic area, and a similar degree of necrotic tissue destruction may be seen. If the patient's hematologic status cannot be corrected, the prognosis for aspergillosis is poor despite systemic amphotericin B therapy.

DERMATOPHYTES

Dermatophytic infections are among the most common infectious diseases of the skin, commonly called athlete's foot and ringworm. The dermatophytoses are caused by a group of fungal organisms representing different species of *Trichophyton, Microsporum,* and *Epidermophyton.* They grow as molds on Sabouraud's agar.

Disease Process

The dermatophytes are usually superficial parasites, subsisting only on the keratinized structures of the host, that is, hair, skin, and nails. Infection may produce annular (thus the term ringworm) lesions composed of itchy, red, scaly papules. These lesions gradually enlarge and expand (Fig 23–13), with an advancing border and central clearing.

Dermatologists refer to these infections as tineas, and they are named basically for the area that is infected, for example, tinea capitis (scalp), tinea corporis (trunk), tinea barbae (beard), tinea pedis (athlete's foot), tinea unguium (nails), and tinea cruris (groin–jock itch).

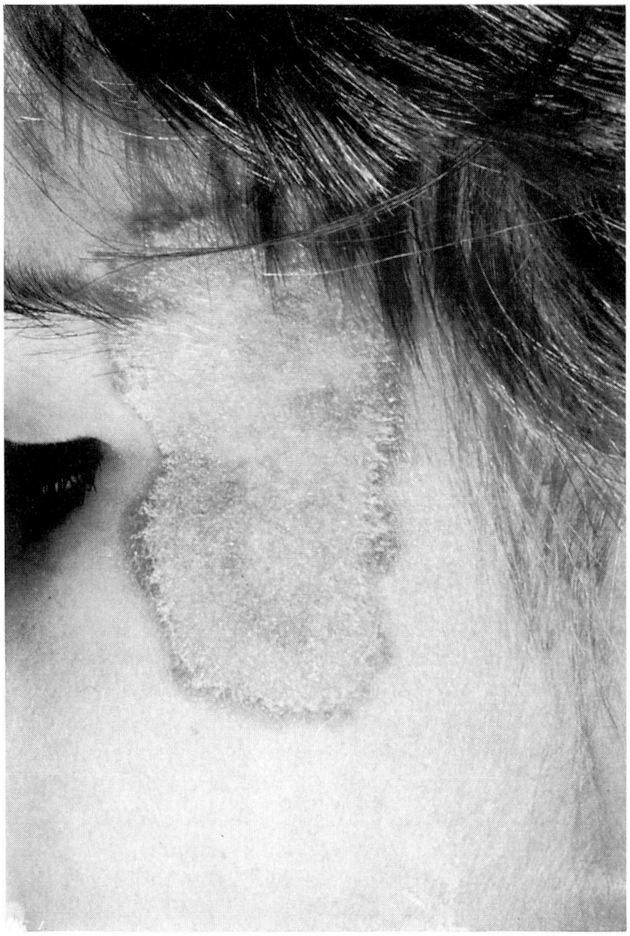

Figure 23–13. Dermatophytic infection involving the side of the face of a young girl. *(Courtesy of Charles Camisa, M.D., Cleveland Clinic, Cleveland, Ohio.)*

Diagnosis, Treatment, and Prevention

The microscopic identification of characteristic fungal hyphae and spores in a 10% potassium hydroxide preparation of lesional scrapings is evidence of the presence of a dermatophytic infection. Identification of the organism in culture is necessary for definitive diagnosis. Dermatophytic infections usually respond to the topical application of such antifungal agents as haloprogin, tolnaftate, miconazole, and clotrimazole. If these medications fail to control the infection, systemic treatment with griseofulvin, another antifungal drug, might be indicated. However, patients given this medication should be monitored carefully because griseofulvin has numerous side effects. Ketoconazole, another systemic antifungal agent, has also proven successful in the management of these stubborn infections. Prevention consists of disinfection, usually by means of a mild sodium hypochlorite solution, of areas that may come into contact with infected skin, such as floors in public showers.

ORAL ASPECTS

Candidiasis is by far the most common and usually the least morbid of mycotic infections of the oral mucosa. The clinical presentation of candidiasis is variable, and these variations have been discussed in some detail. Often the candidal infection is initiated iatrogenically through the use of broad-spectrum antibiotics or corticosteroids. The presence of oral candidiasis without an apparent predisposing condition should alert the dentist to the possibility of AIDS, particularly if the patient is in a high-risk group for that disease. Oral candidiasis is frequently an initial sign of HIV infection, and the dental practitioner may have the opportunity to first suggest the diagnosis of AIDS.

The other fungal infections that involve the oral mucosa are decidedly uncommon and typically are seen in the immunocompromised patient. These lesions are characterized by a raised, irregular, erythematous surface that frequently is ulcerated, and often the clinician believes that he or she is dealing with a malignancy because of this appearance. Biopsy will show the granulomatous tissue response to the organism, and special stains will demonstrate the characteristic morphology of the organism. Culture of the lesion generally provides the definitive diagnosis. Patients exhibiting mycotic infections of the oral mucosa should be evaluated medically for signs of involvement at other sites, and the competency of their immune system also should be examined. Oral manifestations of fungal disease, although relatively rare, may provide the first clue for the presence of systemic infection and thus result in treatment of a potentially life-threatening problem.

SUGGESTED READINGS

Allen CM, Beck FM. Differences in mucosal reaction related to *Candida albicans* isolates. *J Oral Pathol.* 1987;16:89–93.

Chandrasekar PH, Molinari JA. Oral candidiasis: Forerunner of acquired immunodeficiency syndrome (AIDS)? *Oral Surg.* 1985;60:532–534.

DeGregorio MW, Lee WMF, Ries CA. *Candida* infections in patients with acute leukemia: Ineffectiveness of nystatin prophylaxis and relationship between oropharyngeal and systemic candidiasis. *Cancer.* 1982;50:2780–2784.

Graybill JR. Potential and problems with ketoconazole. *Am J Med.* 1983;74:86–90.

Klein BS, Vergeront JM, Weeks RJ, et al. Isolation of *Blastomyces dermatitidis* in soil associated with a large outbreak of blastomycosis in Wisconsin. *N Engl J Med.* 1986;314:529–534.

Koneman EW, Allen SD, Dowell VR, et al. *Color Atlas and Textbook of Diagnostic Microbiology.* 3rd ed. Philadelphia: JB Lippincott Company; 1988.

Macher A. Histoplasmosis and blastomycosis. *Med Clin North Am.* 1980;64:447–459.

Milroy CM, Blanshard JD, Lucas S, Michaels L. Aspergillosis of the nose and paranasal sinuses. *J Clin Pathol.* 1989;42:123–127.

Rippon JW. *Medical Mycology.* 2nd ed. Philadelphia: WB Saunders Co; 1982.

Smith L. *Principles of Microbiology.* 10th ed. St. Louis: Times Mirror/Mosby College Publishing; 1985.

Wheat LJ, Slama TG, Eitzen HE, Kohler RB, French LV, Biesecker JL. A large urban outbreak of histoplasmosis: Clinical features. *Ann Intern Med.* 1981;94:331–337.

CHAPTER 24

Basic Virology

James D. Kettering

INTRODUCTION
NATURE OF A VIRUS
STRUCTURE AND COMPOSITION OF A VIRUS
REACTIONS TO PHYSICAL AND CHEMICAL AGENTS
VARIATIONS IN VIRUS STRUCTURE
ANIMAL VIRUS GROWTH
Virus Invasion and Replication
Synthesis of RNA Animal Viruses
Synthesis of DNA Animal Viruses
Virus Growth
PATHOGENESIS
VIRAL IMMUNOLOGY
CONTROL AND PREVENTION OF VIRAL INFECTIONS
Immune Protection
Antiviral Chemotherapy
Interferon
BACTERIAL VIRUSES
SUGGESTED READINGS

INTRODUCTION

Viruses are causative agents of human diseases. They are well recognized to be common causes of acute disease, and more are being identified as etiologic agents of a variety of chronic diseases, including those arising from latent viral infection. As agents that can be responsible for oral disease, the clinician must understand the role that viruses play in medicine and dentistry. An understanding of the biology and epidemiology of such viral diseases as hepatitis, herpes, and AIDS is of prime importance in order to prevent their transmission in a dental setting. The ability of viruses to survive on surfaces varies from virus to virus, with hepatitis B being highly resistant to many commonly used antiseptics and disinfectants. Dental personnel should understand the special problems that viruses present when considering which sterilization and disinfection techniques to use. It is also important to recognize that viruses differ from bacteria in many ways, and these variations may require alternate considerations by the dental clinician in the management of his or her patients.

NATURE OF A VIRUS

Viruses appear to be among the smallest agents capable of causing infection of higher organisms, with the smallest of these ranging in size from 20 to 30 nm. A virus essentially consists of two main components, a genetic element enclosed in a protein coat. A virus contains only one type of nucleic acid, either ribonucleic acid (RNA) or deoxyribonucleic acid (DNA), but never both. The nucleic acid contains all the information that a virus needs to infect a host cell, replicate its essential parts, and assemble into mature, infective virus particles, or virions. The genome of a virus is protected from the environment by means of the protein coat, often made up of only one or a few pro-

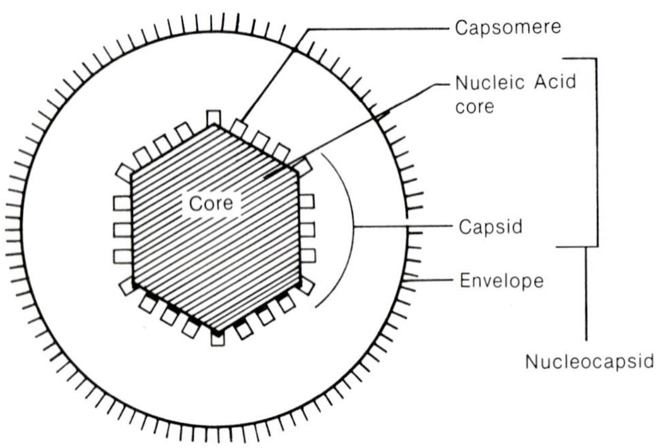

Figure 24–1. A schematic representation of the various components that comprise a typical animal virus.

teins. The nucleic acid core and protein covering together form the nucleocapsid. (Fig 24–1) Viruses are strict intracellular parasites and reproduce only in specific host cells. They depend on host cells because they do not have the requisite enzyme systems to perform the metabolic functions necessary to produce copies of the genome or essential enzymes and structural proteins. Figure 24–2 illustrates shapes and sizes of many commonly recognized viruses. Smaller, even less complex agents just starting to be recognized and studied include viroids (nucleic acid segments only) and prions (protein only).

STRUCTURE AND COMPOSITION OF A VIRUS

The symmetrical protein coat that surrounds the nucleic acid core is called a capsid. It is made up of proteins called capsomeres, which are clusters of polypeptides that are coded for by the viral genome. When completely assembled, they form the capsid. One of the most important functions of the capsid is that of protecting the viral nucleic acid from nucleases (enzymes that destroy RNA or DNA) that could destroy it. Components on the protein coat also often serve as important locations for the attachment of the virus to receptor sites on a host cell membrane. The proteins determine the antigenicity of the virus, which in turn can be useful in establishing a classification scheme. Antibodies formed against the capsid proteins often are protective of the host, either inactivating the virus particle itself or preventing attachment to the host cell.

As indicated before, the genome of a virus con-

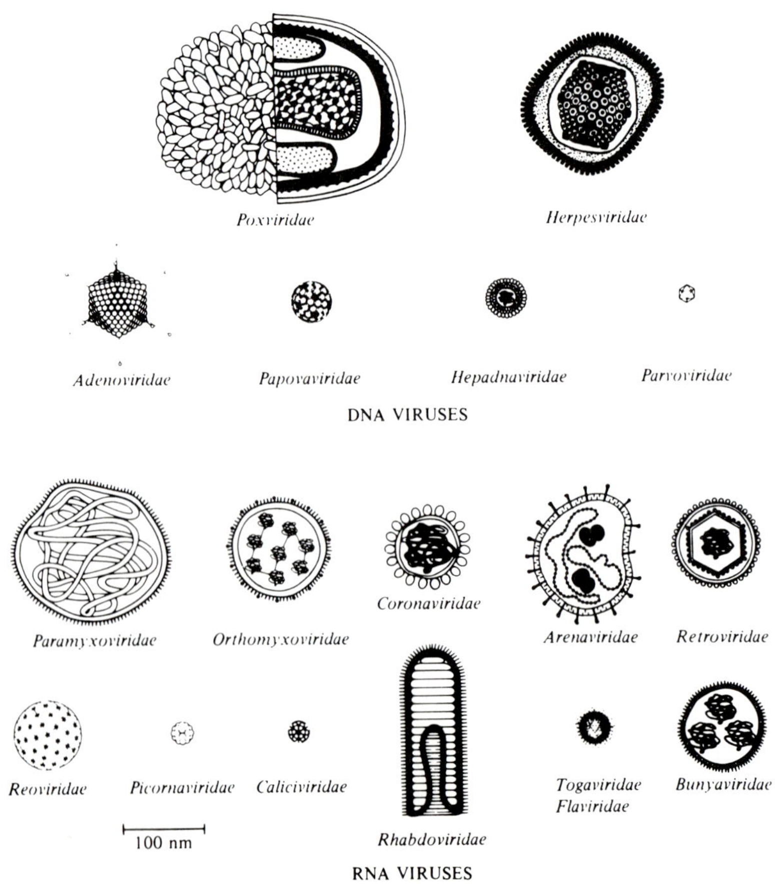

Figure 24–2. Diagram illustrating the shapes and sizes of animal viruses of families that include human pathogens. Although drawn to scale, artistic license has been used to represent virion structures. *(From White DO, Fenner FJ.* Medical Virology. *3rd ed. Orlando, Fla: Academic Press; 1986:24.)*

tains all the genetic information and is composed of nucleic acid. The genome of all higher organisms consists only of double-stranded DNA (DS-DNA). By comparison, viruses can possess a genome composed of either DNA or RNA, both of which may be either double stranded or single stranded. The nucleic acid of a virus may be linear or circular in structure. The genome of most viruses consists of an unbroken strand but is found to be segmented into a number of subunits in several groups.

Some viruses possess an additional structure, the envelope, which surrounds the capsid. The envelopes of viruses are derived, in part, from either the host cell's cytoplasmic or nuclear membrane in the final stages of viral assembly and release from the host and are composed primarily of lipids and proteins. The proteins on the outside of the envelope may possess biologic properties that can be recognized and used in the laboratory for characterizing viruses. Several viruses possess a protein spike, or peplomer, called hemagglutinin, which allows the virus to attach to erythrocytes and cause agglutination of the red blood cells. Another example is neuraminidase, an enzyme that cleaves neuraminic acid from its bond with galactose. This function appears to be used to release mature viruses from host cell membranes.

The envelope and proteins are exposed to the environment and are capable of being altered or destroyed. Organic solvents, such as ether, readily destroy lipid envelopes. Disinfectants that solubilize lipids also can inactivate viruses in the same manner. Destruction of the envelope by means of antibody and complement is another means of neutralizing viral infectivity.

The envelope assumes an important role in the initial stages of infectivity of those viruses possessing them. Fusion of the envelope with the host's cellular membrane gives the nucleocapsid access into the cytoplasm.

REACTIONS TO PHYSICAL AND CHEMICAL AGENTS

By recalling that a virus is composed of a nucleic acid core surrounded by a protein coat, it is easier to understand the effect that certain chemical and physical agents have on a virus. Most viruses are destroyed by being heated from 45°C to 60°C for 30 minutes. Hepatitis B virus can withstand this, however. Cold is ideal for storing viruses for long periods of time. Refrigeration (4°C) is least effective in maintaining viability, whereas −70°C (dry ice temperature) and −185°C (liquid nitrogen) permit survival indefinitely. Many viruses can be stabilized by molar concentration of salts, such as Mg and Mn. Virions usually are stable in the pH range of 5 to 9. Ultraviolet (UV) light will inactivate the viability of a virus by damaging the nucleic acid genome.

Chemical agents that are effective in killing a virus include detergents, oxidizing agents, and heavy metal ions. These all contribute to the actual destruction of either the capsid coat or the envelope. A 5% solution of regular household bleach is a good, all-around viral disinfectant. Chemical agents with little antiviral activity include 70% alcohol, cyanide, fluoride, and quaternary ammonium compounds. These latter are primarily compounds that appear to interfere with enzyme system functions.

VARIATIONS IN VIRAL STRUCTURE

Animal viruses can be separated into three categories on the basis of capsid symmetry (Fig. 24–3). Some RNA viruses have a helical symmetry. These possess a rodlike structure, with the nucleic acid molecule located inside a spiral arrangement of protein subunits that make up the capsid. Several RNA and most DNA virus families display a cubic or spherical symmetry. Their capsid is an icosahedral structure—a regular polyhedron with 20 faces, each one an equilateral triangle. The size of the virus is determined by the number of capsomeres that make up each triangle. A small poliovirus, for example, possesses only 32 capsomeres, whereas the larger adenovirus has 252. A final category, complex symmetry, is found in the poxvirus group. Among the enveloped viruses, the nucleocapsid is helical in some viruses and cubic in others.

Physical properties play an important role in the current classification of animal viruses as do their chemical and biological features. Table 24–1 illustrates a typical classification scheme recognized today.

ANIMAL VIRUS GROWTH

Cultivation of animal virions is essential for identification and study of viruses, assay of viruses and their products, and production of viral vaccines. Because viruses are obligate intracellular parasites and multiply only within living cells, efforts made to culture them in the laboratory have resulted in the development of three basic host systems: whole animals, embryonated eggs, and tissue culture.

Virologists initially used whole animals. Viruses, however, are host cell specific and will only grow in certain tissues. Some factors that determine the susceptibility of an animal to a virus are age, species, and route of inoculation. Certain enteroviruses, for example, will grow in 1- to 2-day-old suckling mice and not

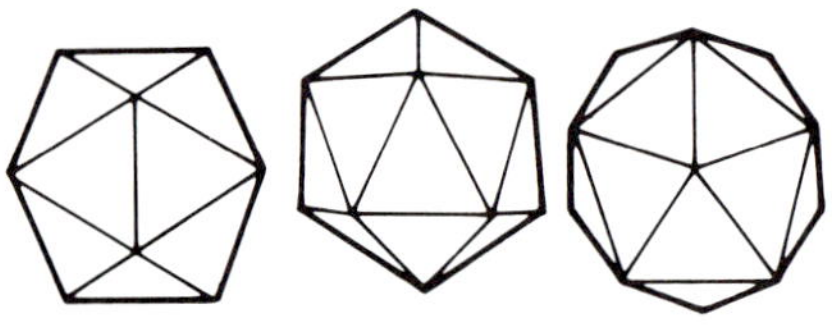

The three symmetry axes of a regular icosahedron.

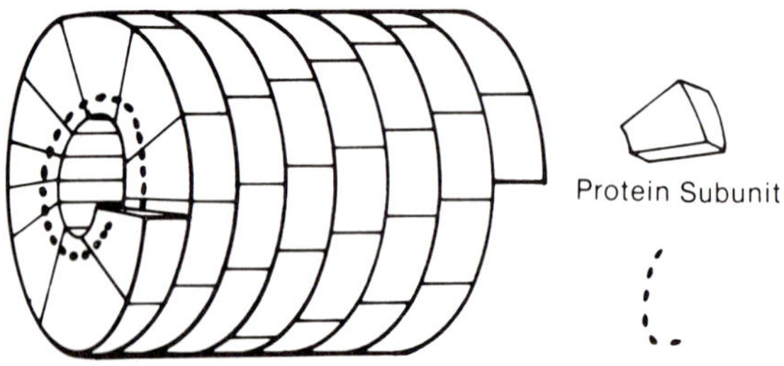

Diagram of a model helical virus.

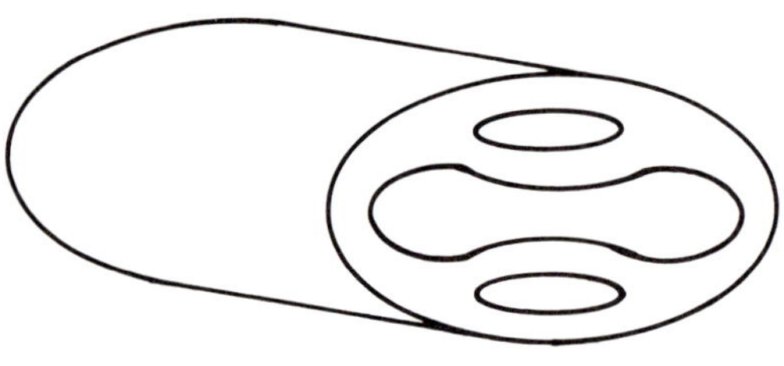

Complex viral symmetry.

Figure 24–3. Diagrams illustrate the three basic structures found for animal viruses. Cubic, or spherical, viruses appear round due to the icosahedral structure shown here, which illustrates the three axes of symmetry normally found. The nucleic acid is found within the cubic structure. The rod-shaped helical viruses are more simple in construction. The rods are flexible and bend in nature. The complex viruses contain nucleic acid in the center.

at all in adult mice. Laboratories have used mice, guinea pigs, rabbits, ferrets, monkeys, and hamsters to grow various viruses. The use of whole animals is an expensive and inefficient propagation method. Embryonated chicken eggs represent a second, more efficient and cost-effective system for a limited number of viruses. Age and route of inoculation are also important factors when considering these as a growth model. This method is used extensively today to propagate influenza viruses used in vaccine production.

The most efficient and most recent host systems are cell or tissue cultures. Three general types, primary, diploid, and established cells, may be used. Primary cell cultures represent individual cells obtained directly from a tissue source. The cells are separated by treatment with a proteolytic enzyme, such as trypsin, and then placed in a vessel along with a growth medium that supplies all nutrients. Primary cells are relatively inefficient because they can be used only one time and cannot be passed indefinitely by subculture. They do represent, however, a sensitive host system for a large number of viruses affecting humans. These are used extensively in viral diagnostic laboratories. Diploid cell strains usually are derived from fetal tissues and can be passed successfully about 50 times without loss of viral receptivity. The diploid, or 2N, chromosome number is maintained throughout the life of the cell line. Once the total limited number of passages is reached, the cells die due to a built-in senescence mechanism. Continuous or established cell lines are derived from diploid cells, grow very efficiently in vitro, and support the growth of a rather large number of viruses affecting humans. They are of limited value for vaccine development because many such cell lines represent transformation from a normal cell state to one similar to that of a cancer cell.

Viral Invasion and Replication

In order to infect a cell, a virus first attaches, or adsorbs, to a cell by means of ionic attraction between the host cell and virion. This interaction is brought about by a random collision of the two agents. Occasionally, positively charged ions (cations) may be necessary to ensure this attraction, since both cells and viruses are normally negatively charged at neutral pH. Following attachment, a second and more specific reaction takes place between the virus and the host cell. Molecular epitopes on the surface of cells act as the receptors for viruses, interacting specifically with proteins on the viral capsid or envelope. The ability of certain viruses to infect only a limited number of cell types appears to be related directly to the presence of compatible receptors.

The next step involves penetration of the cell by the adsorbed virion. Nonenveloped virions usually are phagocytized and taken directly into the cytoplasm (pinocytosis or viropexis) and remain morphologically intact. Enveloped viruses, on the other hand, enter after fusion occurs between the viral envelope and the host cell membrane. The nucleocapsid is then released into the cell cytoplasm. The virus may continue its replication within the cytoplasm, or it may enter the nucleus.

Regardless of the mechanism of entering the cell, at least partial uncoating must take place in order for transcription of the viral genome to occur. Uncoating is the separation of the protein coat from the nucleic acid and varies with the type of virus. Although the actual mechanism for most viruses has not been elucidated, it has been suggested that interaction of capsid proteins with the cellular receptors may bring about conformational changes in the capsid. These changes

TABLE 24–1. ANIMAL VIRUS GROUPS AND THEIR BASIC PROPERTIES

Group	Nucleic Acid Configuration	Capsid Symmetry	Capsomer Number	Envelope	Virus Particle Size (nm)
DNA viruses					
Parvovirus	SS	Icosahedral	32	No	18–26
Papovavirus	DS[a]	Icosahedral	72	No	45–55
Adenovirus	DS	Icosahedral	252	No	70–90
Herpesvirus	DS	Icosahedral	162	Yes	100
Poxvirus	DS	Complex		Complex	230 × 400
Hepadnavirus	DS[a]	Complex		Complex	42
RNA viruses					
Picornavirus	SS	Icosahedral	32	No	20–30
Reovirus	DS[b]	Icosahedral		No	60–80
Togavirus	SS	Icosahedral	32(?)	Yes	30–90
Arenavirus	SS[b]	Complex		Yes	50–300
Coronavirus	SS	Complex		Yes	80–130
Retrovirus	SS[b]	Complex		Yes	100
Bunyavirus	SS[b]	Helical		Yes	90–100
Orthomyxovirus	SS[b]	Helical		Yes	80–120
Paramyxovirus	SS[b]	Helical		Yes	150–300
Rhabdovirus	SS	Helical		Yes	70 × 175

[a]Circular.
[b]Segmented.

weaken the capsid structure so that the genome may be freed, or the coat is at least altered to permit enzyme access to the viral nucleic acid so that mRNA production can be initiated. Poliovirus RNA has been described as being easily liberated by means of a steric rearrangement of capsid proteins after cell entry. The uncoating of adenoviruses, on the other hand, is a multistage process. The nucleocapsid first loses its penton, the capsomer at the vertex of the particle, soon after it enters the cytoplasm. The hexon subunits are lost next, leaving a DNA–protein complex, which enters the nucleus. The uncoating of papovaviruses appears to occur entirely in the nucleus. Figures 24–4 and 24–5 illustrate the general steps involved in RNA and DNA viral replication cycles.

Once the viral nucleic acid gains access to the appropriate region of the cell, reproduction of the viral components may begin. In general, enzymes discussed here can be thought of as coming from three different sources: (1) those contained within the virion particles themselves, (2) those that are host derived and used by the virus, and (3) those that are entirely viral coded, host-produced, and present only at the time of infection. Enzymes that are needed for nucleic acid and protein synthesis are made by the host or used if they are ready present, and these processes then proceed independently. In addition to use of host enzymes for some of the steps involved in viral synthesis, there are several enzymes that play a very important role in virus replication that are found to be contained within the virion particle of certain viruses. The enzymes that have received the most study are the polymerase or replicase enzymes used in viral nucleic acid replication. Five examples are noted. (1) The first example is the positive strand RNA (positive meaning the same configuration as mRNA) viruses whose genomes act directly as mRNA to start viral replication. A virally coded RNA polymerase is produced that controls the production of additional copies of the viral nucleic acid. (2) Viruses with minus strand RNA (minus meaning an RNA that is complementary to mRNA) genomes (orthomyxoviruses, paramyxoviruses, and rhabdoviruses) have an RNA-dependent RNA polymerase that will make a positive strand RNA copy that will function as mRNA and initiate replication. (3) The complex DNA viruses (poxviruses) have a DNA-dependent RNA polymerase within their virions to produce mRNA and initiate the synthesis of mRNA. (4) Other DNA viruses (herpesviruses, adenoviruses, and papovaviruses) use DNA-dependent RNA polymerase of host origin. (5) The retroviruses have a DNA polymerase that uses single-stranded RNA as a template to make a double-stranded DNA copy, hence the name reverse transcriptase. This provides a mechanism that can allow the integration of the viral genome (called a provirus) into the host cell chromosome.

SYNTHESIS OF RNA ANIMAL VIRUSES

The RNA animal viruses can be separated into five different classes based on the nature of the RNA in the virions, using the conventional designation that mRNA is the positive or plus strand and nucleic acid complementary to the mRNA is the negative, or minus, strand (Table 24–2).

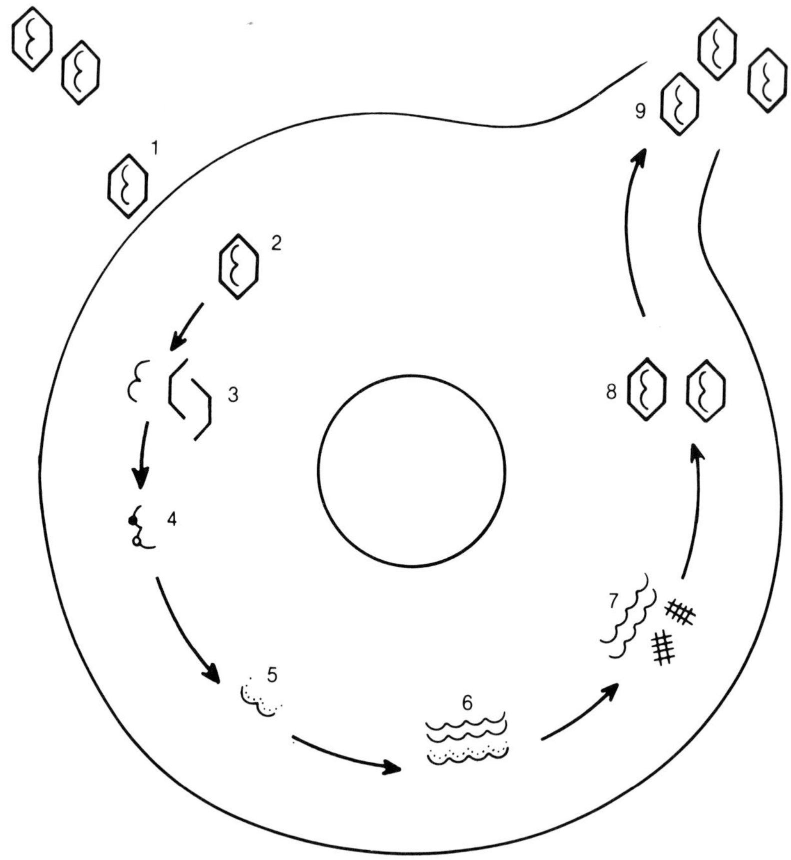

Figure 24–4. Steps in the synthesis of a representative RNA virus (poliovirus). (1) Free polioviruses attach to specific receptor sites on the host cell membrane, losing one virus polypeptide (VP4). (2) Virions are taken into the cell by viropexis (a cellular function) and (3) uncoated, releasing the RNA into the cytoplasm, where it serves as its own mRNA. Early translation occurs (4), producing RNA polymerase, nucleases, and other inhibitors, directly causing the formation of double-standard replicative intermediate RNA molecules (5). Inhibitors of cellular RNA and protein synthesis stop these host cell functions. Viral RNA minus and plus strands result in step 6, with the plus strand either serving as mRNA, a template for continued RNA synthesis, or becoming encapsulated in the protein capsid. Late translation (7) generally results in structural proteins being produced at about the same time as RNA synthesis. Step 8 completes the production cycle as RNA molecules are enclosed in the protein capsid, which is released when the cell undergoes lysis (9).

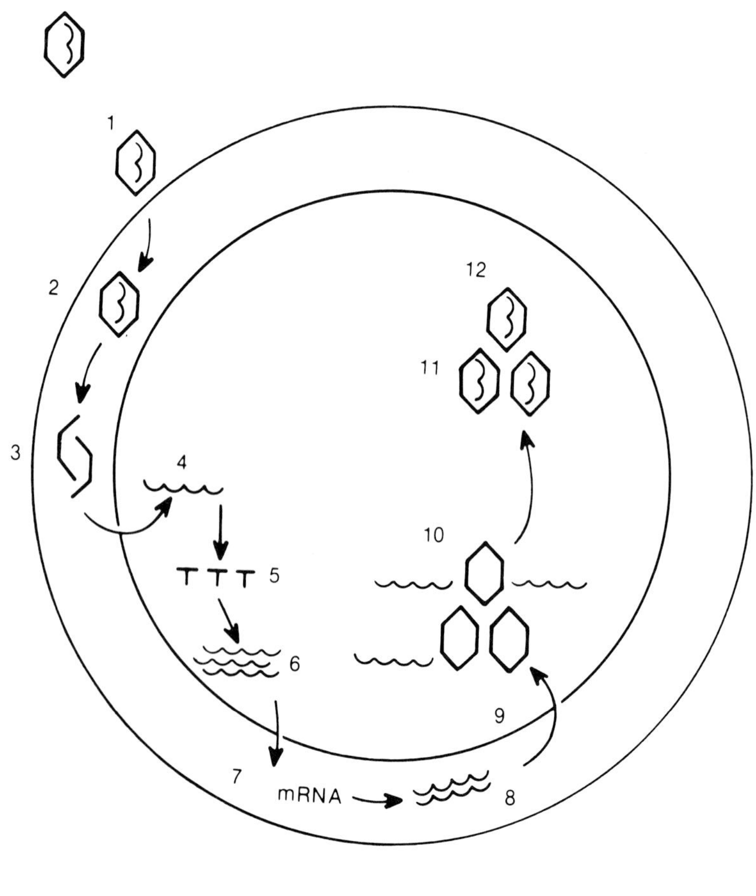

Figure 24–5. Steps in the synthesis of a representative DNA virus (adenovirus). Attachment (1) and penetration (2) steps are similar to those described for poliovirus. Uncoating (3) is thought to occur through the action of cellular proteolytic enzymes, and the viral DNA is released to migrate into the host cell nucleus (4). Specific mRNA is transcribed from viral DNA (5), where virus-specific proteins (tumor antigen and enzymes for DNA replication) are produced. Viral DNA is synthesized (6), and late mRNA is produced at about the same time. Messenger RNA (6) migrates to the cytoplasm (7) and is translated into proteins for virus capsids (8). These viral proteins now migrate to the nucleus (9), where the components are assembled into virus capsids (10). Maturation (11) occurs when the viral DNA is enclosed by the protein subunits, resulting in complete virions. Release (12) is by cell lysis.

TABLE 24–2. CLASSIFICATION OF RNA ANIMAL VIRUSES USING NUCLEIC ACID CONFIGURATION

Class	Nucleic Acid Polarity	Virion Polymerase	RNA Infective	Examples
I	+	No	Yes	Poliovirus, Togavirus
II	−	Yes	No	Paramyxovirus
III	−	Yes	No	Orthomyxovirus
IV	−	Yes	No	Reovirus
V	+	Yes	No	Retrovirus

In class I viruses, the viral single-stranded RNA (SS-RNA) molecules have the same polarity as their RNA. Proteins derived from this are necessary for viral replication. With picornaviruses, the mRNA has the same length as the genome RNA. The mRNA is polycistronic, being responsible for polyproteins produced by ribosomes. The polyproteins are then cleaved to produce enzymes that are involved in viral RNA synthesis, as well as viral structural proteins. Togaviruses and caliciviruses synthesize at least two forms of mRNA in the infected cell. One is the same size as virion RNA, whereas the other is a smaller fragment. Each is responsible for a separate polyprotein, which is cleaved into enzymes and structural proteins, as for the picornaviruses.

Class II viruses include paramyxoviruses and rhabdoviruses whose viral SS-RNA is complementary to mRNA (negative polarity). A virion-contained transcriptase functions in synthesis of messenger RNA.

Class III viruses, orthomyxoviruses, bunyaviruses, and arenaviruses, have viral SS-RNA that is segmented. The pieces (eg, eight in influenza) are of negative polarity. A virion-contained transcriptase is responsible for the synthesis of messenger RNA.

Class IV viruses, reoviruses and arbiviruses, have viral DS-RNA that is segmented. The orthoreoviruses contain 10 RNA segments, and rotaviruses contain 11 RNA segments. A virion transcriptase produces a transcript from each segment into separate monocistronic mRNAs.

Class V viruses, retroviruses, contain segments of viral SS-RNA that have messenger polarity. The virions contain reverse transcriptase, which transcribes each segment into a DNA–RNA hybrid and then into DS-DNA. The DNA is integrated into a host chromosome, and mRNA is transcribed from it.

In those classes of viruses in which the virions contain transcriptase enzymes necessary for viral RNA replication, the RNAs alone cannot be infectious, since the purified viral RNAs are unable to replicate themselves in a suitable host cell in the absence of these enzymes. Class I virions can initiate viral growth from purified RNA, however.

SYNTHESIS OF DNA ANIMAL VIRUSES

The DNA animal viruses can be separated into three classes based on structural differences in their viral genomes.

The mode of replication of Class I double-stranded linear DNA viruses is generally conservative. Members of this class, however, vary with respect to the origin of the nucleic acid polymerase that each uses for DNA replication. Adenoviruses, for example, use a DNA polymerase, which is probably of host origin. Herpesviruses have a viral DNA replication that depends on immediate and delayed early proteins coded for by the viral genome and on host cell enzymes. Poxviruses have a viral DNA-dependent RNA polymerase, present in the core, that is necessary for viral DNA replication.

Class II double-stranded circular DNA viruses include papovaviruses, which have supercoiled cyclic DNAs that replicate via cyclic intermediates. The polymerase is of host origin. Hepadnavirus contains circular DNA molecules that are mostly double stranded (one strand has a constant 3182 bases; the other varies between 1700 and 2800 bases). Each virion does contain a DNA polymerase which makes fully double-stranded molecules from the one complete strand and the incomplete strand. This must be accomplished before the growth cycle can begin.

Class III single-stranded linear DNA viruses are represented by the parvoviruses. Each virus contains only a plus or minus strand of DNA. Replication and capsid assembly take place in the nucleus of the infected cell. Once inside a host cell, the strands fuse to form a regular DS-DNA molecule. The growth process can then proceed. Host enzymes are most likely used in these processes.

Viral Growth

There is a part of the viral growth cycle that is known as the eclipse phase. This represents the molecular biology stage, when nucleic acid replication and protein synthesis (enzymes and structural components) are taking place. If the infected cell was examined by electron microscopy, no evidence of whole virions would be found, nor can infectivity be demonstrated during this period. The eclipse phase ends when mature virus particles are produced by enclosure of the nucleic acid genome with the structural coat proteins. Then the virus is ready to be released.

Maturation of virions occurs as whole viruses are assembled in the host cell cytoplasm or nucleus, depending on the type of virus. Liberation depends on the type of virus and cell. It may take place gradually as viruses are formed (eg, budding) or more suddenly if the host cell is lysed. Whereas lysis of the host results in total destruction of the cell, budding occurs as a gradual, ongoing process that takes place as viruses mature. As the virions become enclosed in a lipid envelope, they are released from the cell without harming the host. The actual mechanism of release has been best studied with the myxoviruses.

Inclusion bodies are a type of cytopathic effect (CPE) resulting from virus growth within host cells. Not all viruses cause the formation of these, and the exact role that inclusions play in the growth cycle is mostly unknown. Characterization of these may help to identify certain viruses. Cells containing viral inclusion usually are stained with hematoxylineosin, a standard histologic staining preparation. Inclusions will stain either red (eosinophilic) or blue (basophilic). Adenoviruses have a typical intranuclear inclusion that stains basophilic. There is some dissimilarity within the group, however. Type 2 adenovirus produces a multiple, well-defined eosinophilic inclusion early in the growth cycle, which later becomes basophilic and granular throughout the nucleus. Type 3 adenovirus, on the other hand, produces a large, basophilic inclusion that covers the entire nucleus. Rabies virus produces a cytoplasmic inclusion, the Negri body, in infected nerve cells. These inclusions are eosinophilic and spherical, measuring 2 to 10 μm across. They may be found in the brain and the spinal cord. Once the Negri bodies themselves were used as a diagnostic aid, but the specific viral antigens are now demonstrated by immunofluorescence. The herpesviruses typically produce large intranuclear inclusion bodies. Herpes simplex growth typically produces basophilic inclusions early in the growth cycle, and as viruses move into the cytoplasm, the inclusions are converted into an eosinophilic mass. Interpretation of the types of viruses involved based on inclusion bodies requires a person well skilled in pathology.

PATHOGENESIS

In order to produce disease, viruses must enter a host, grow within susceptible cells, and produce cell injury. Not a great deal is known about these processes in many viral infections. Studies are in progress to help understand what is happening at the molecular level so that effective antiviral strategies may be designed. These studies are mostly being done using various virus–animal models.

Most human viruses enter their hosts through the mucosa of the respiratory or gastrointestinal tract or the eye. Some may be introduced into the body by needle sticks (AIDS, hepatitis B) or insects (arboviruses, arthropod-borne viruses), bypassing the skin, which provides a tough and impermeable barrier to virus entry. It is important to realize that most viral infections are probably inapparent or subclinical. Whether or not virus infection will produce disease appears to depend on the nature of the virus, the degree of the host's immunity, and ability of the virus to reach target organs.

Many viruses reproduce at the primary site of entry, where they may or may not produce evidence of disease. Respiratory viruses (influenza, respiratory syncytial virus) and gastrointestinal viruses (rotaviruses) produce their main symptoms at the portal of entry sites. These are mostly self-limited in severity and duration.

Other viruses, though, produce disease at sites distant from the portal of entry. Disseminated infections are caused by primary multiplication at the site of entry and regional lymph nodes. A primary viremia spreads progeny virus through the bloodstream and lymphatics to additional organs for further viral replication. A second viremia often then sends the viruses to target organs, causing cell damage, pathologic lesions, and clinical disease.

Several viruses are capable of crossing the placenta and causing teratogenic effects in the developing fetus. Rubella and cytomegalovirus are most often associated with congenital defects. Herpes simplex, varicella-zoster, and Coxsackie B viruses also have been implicated.

Persistent infections, using several mechanisms, also are recognized. Latent infections represent a situation where the viral genome (called a provirus) becomes incorporated into some segment of a human chromosome. No human disease is manifested unless the provirus is dislodged by some mechanism, and the virus may then produce a clinical lesion. Herpes simplex types 1 and 2, for example, produce virus only during intermittent episodes. These usually follow a trauma of some kind, such as exposure to ultraviolet irradiation in sunlight, which may result in the production of cold sores. During chronic infections (hepatitis B and Epstein-Barr viruses), the virus is present in small amounts, and disease may be either absent or associated with pathologic symptoms. Slow virus infections, with incubation periods of several years, result in a slowly progressive disease that is usually fatal. Subacute sclerosing panencephalitis (SSPE), for example, is now known to be caused by a defective measles virus infection experienced 20 or more years earlier.

Oncogenic viruses have long been suspected as factors in human malignancies, but this has been extremely difficult to prove by direct experimentation. Many animal tumors have been shown definitely to be caused by members of five of the six DNA virus families and several RNA viruses. Herpes simplex 2 virus is implicated in cervical carcinoma, and Epstein-Barr (another herpesvirus) may cause Burkitt's lymphoma. Hepatitis B virus is strongly associated with liver cancer. The recent reports of human T lymphocytotrophic viruses (HTLV) show that some forms of human lymphomas can be caused by viruses.

VIRAL IMMUNOLOGY

Viruses contain antigens that usually stimulate strong immune responses in their host. These antigens are found in the envelope and capsid and within the virions. The immune response, which includes both humoral and cellular immunity, is useful in protection against and diagnosis of viral infections. Antiviral antibodies usually are detected by enzyme-linked immunoassays, complement fixation, hemagglutination inhibition, and neutralization assays. Skin tests can be used to evaluate cellular immunity.

Humoral immunity appears to be the main protection against primary viral infections in areas of the body that are accessible to blood and other body fluids. Neutralization of virus infectivity by antibodies appears to be interference with initial stages of virus infection of the host cell. Neutralization has been calculated to be a one-hit reaction. One antibody molecule per virion theoretically is capable of accomplishing the task. This could occur by (1) steric hindrance caused by antibody molecules that bind to antigenic determinants on or near the host cell receptors on the envelope or capsid, (2) agglutinating virus particles into large aggregates that cannot penetrate the host cell's membrane, and (3) destruction by a complement-mediated reaction of an essential component of the virus. At least one virus, the poliovirus, can enter a host with antibody attached to its capsid. The poliovirus still is neutralized because uncoating is inhibited and viral growth is prevented. All of these mechanisms may be involved to some degree among the different viral infections.

Infected cells often express nonself antigens on their membranes, and these antigens can serve as targets of the immune response to a viral infection. Immune lysis of the infected cell can reduce the numbers of viral particles. Lysis may be mediated by antibody and complement or by antibody-dependent cell-mediated cytotoxity (ADCC). In the latter, specific antibody reacting with the nonself membrane antigens serves as the bridge between the infected host cell and the killer cells that lyse the infected cell. Both types of antibody-mediated cytolysis have been demonstrated in vitro and may occur in vivo.

Cytotoxic T lymphocytes (CTL) also are important in localization of and, ultimately, recovery from viral infections. Their significance in immune protection apparently is based on experiences with immunodeficient and immunosuppressed subjects who often contract severe viral infections. The CTLs can react directly with virus-induced host cell membrane antigens and kill the infected cell. The CTL and infected cell must share class I MHC antigens. Natural killer cells also may play a role in protection against viral infections, but this has not yet been demonstrated in humans.

Several viruses can directly suppress the immune system. The primary example is HIV, the agent for AIDS. This virus invades and kills helper T cells and other immunocytes. Other retroviruses, herpesvirus, measles, and mumps virus are among a large group of viruses that display immunosuppressive properties.

CONTROL AND PREVENTION OF VIRAL INFECTIONS

The simplest concept that can be envisioned in controlling a viral disease is to break a link in the cycle of infection. Interruption of a single link may control a disease even if the biology or etiology is not completely understood. Even though a great deal is known about the epidemiology of many viral diseases, very little has been accomplished in control by environmental changes, except for arthropod vector control for the arboviruses.

Improved water supplies, proper sewage disposal, and improved personal hygiene potentially could decrease the incidence of virus infections transmitted by the fecal–oral route, but generally the results are disappointing because alternative pathways of infection exist. In addition, such measures may delay the age of exposure to later life, when infections possibly are more severe.

Immune Protection

Pooled gamma-globulin has been used in the prophylaxis of several viral infections. Standard immune serum globulin (ISG) randomly collected from adult volunteers has been used to treat individuals exposed to infectious hepatitis (hepatitis A) and measles (rubeola). More potent globulin preparations also are used prophylactically. Hepatitis B immune globulin (HBIG) is prepared from patients who have recently recovered from serum hepatitis, and antirabies globulin (RIG) is prepared from the blood of hyperimmunized volunteers. The efficacy of these immune globulins varies with the patient, the time of administration, the degree of exposure, and other factors.

Vaccines have reduced dramatically the morbidity and mortality associated with viral diseases, such as poliomyelitis, measles, rabies, and hepatitis B. Smallpox was eradicated primarily through use of a vaccine. Immunization was, and in some cases still is, the most effective means of dealing with viral infections. These vaccines are composed of live attenuated viruses, inactivated viruses, or subunits of the virion. As noted in Chapters 7 and 8, there are risks associated with vaccine administration, but the greater problem is the absence of effective vaccines for the majority of viral diseases. However, through the use of modern molecular biologic techniques, it may soon be possible to develop safe and effective vaccines against almost all viral pathogens.

Antiviral Chemotherapy

An antiviral compound may be a natural, synthetic, or semisynthetic material that prevents viral infection or alters the host–virus interaction in a way or manner that is beneficial to the host. Random screening has been successful in identifying several effective antiviral agents, but more specific methods are used now. The increase in our knowledge of the basic biochemistry of viral replication and of virus–host interrelationships has revealed not only an understanding of the targets on which existing antiviral agents exert their inhibitory effect but also new potential targets.

Various targets for which antiviral agents have been demonstrated to exert an inhibitory effect or which are potential targets for future drug development include all steps in the growth cycle of a virus, ranging from interference with specific viral-specified enzymes to prevention of viral release from the host cell. Ideally, knowledge is needed concerning what the three-dimensional structural requirements are for a compound to interact with a specific target site. Data from molecular virology studies can be subjected to computer analysis, which now assists in the design for the synthesis of drugs.

Since a number of appropriate targets are known, this knowledge can be exploited for the development of selective antiviral drugs or to use the available drugs more effectively. With the exception of amantadine, the clinically approved drugs are targeted against only certain herpesvirus infections. Need exists to find targets for development of new and better drugs to attack infections due, in part, to the following viruses: Epstein-Barr (infectious mononucleosis), cytomegalovirus, rhinovirus (common cold), respiratory syncytial virus, rotavirus (diarrhea), human papilloma virus, and HIV (AIDS).

Some specific examples of antiviral drugs include the nucleoside analogs. Acyclovir (acycloguanosine) strongly inhibits herpes simplex virus but has little effect on other DNA viruses or on host cells. The specific target is the virus-coded thymidine kinase enzyme. Cytomegaloviruses and Epstein-Barr viruses are not as susceptible because they rely on the host cell enzyme. Vidarabine (adenine arabinoside) is a purine analog that probably works by inhibiting virus-specified enzymes, such as DNA polymerase. This has been especially useful against herpes simplex and varicella-zoster infections. Idoxuridine (IDU), a halogenated pyrimidine, also inhibits thymidine kinase but is not as useful as acyclovir or vidarabine because of the emergence of drug-resistant mutants.

Ribavirin (Virazole) is a synthetic nucleoside related to guanosine and is effective to varying degrees against many RNA- and DNA-containing viruses in vitro. Its mechanism of action appears to be interference with the function of viral mRNA molecules. It is effective against influenza and respiratory syncytial virus infections when administered as a small-particle aerosol.

Azidothymidine (AZT) is a promising drug to combat HIV infection. This virus uses the unusual enzyme, reverse transcriptase, to make a DNA copy of its RNA genome. AZT inhibits the reverse transcriptase enzyme and has proven its clinical efficacy. Its mechanism of action centers on terminating the growth of the DNA chain, effectively stopping viral growth. It, however, does not affect the intracellular virus and only reduces the total virus load.

Amantadine, a synthetic amine, is specific for influenza A infections. It blocks viral penetration into the host cell or virus uncoating. It must be administered prophylactically to be effective. A newer derivative, Rimantadine, has the same spectrum of activity with less toxicity.

At this stage of antiviral chemotherapy development, we must recognize that a benefit-versus-risk situation exists. The short-term and long-term toxicity of the available antiviral agents is the most important reason to use a careful approach in clinical practice. Toxic effects may be accurately recognized only with increased time and drug usage. The main problem is that since viruses are obligate intracellular parasites, using human cells as hosts, the target selectivity is much more crucial than that of antibiotics and bacteria. Because very specific targets that are used in virus growth are so close to normal cell metabolism, the range of selective toxicity (harms the virus but not the host) is rather narrow. Vidarabine appeared relatively nontoxic in short-term controlled trials but later was recognized to be neurotoxic in various circumstances. Even greater concern has been expressed about the potential long-term adverse effects of antiviral drugs that interfere with DNA or protein synthesis. There is even some evidence that some drugs may have teratogenic or carcinogenic potential. Cases have been reported where viruses become resistant to various drugs. With all this in mind, obviously antiviral chemotherapy has to be used with caution and close patient monitoring. The positive effects of this type of therapy are overwhelmingly evident, however, in terms of lives saved (eg, herpes simplex encephalitis) and reduction of morbidity. A great deal of work is being conducted currently to seek new agents and refine the use of drugs now being utilized.

Interferon

Interferons (IFN) are a group of glycoproteins that interfere with the multiplication of both DNA and RNA viruses (Fig 24–6). IFNs are produced by many animal cells and are species specific. That is, they are most effective in the animal species that produces them or in a closely related species. IFNs are not virus specific. An IFN produced in response to one virus will inhibit many other virus species. Humans produce three main groups of IFNs ranging from 20,000 to 40,000 daltons. Type I consists of IFN-α, which is produced by leukocytes, and IFN-β produced by fibroblasts. Type II, or IFN-γ, is produced by lymphocytes undergoing an immune response.

Once IFN is released from the virus-infected cell, it binds to the surface of another cell via specific cell receptors and sends a signal to the nucleus of that cell. This signal activates a gene coding for antiviral protein (AVP). AVP acts primarily to inhibit the translation of mRNA into proteins. If both viral and cellular mRNAs are blocked, the cell may die. However, the spread of the virus is prevented. At least three enzymatic mechanisms appear to be involved in the prevention of translation. (1) AVP can act as an enzyme to synthesize an adenine trinucleotide with an unusual phosphodiester linkage. (2) This linkage plus a minute amount of DS-DNA activates an endonuclease, which destroys mRNA. (3) Small amounts of DS-RNA can initiate phosphorylation of a preexisting inactive protein of cell origin and thus produce an active protein kinase. This last enzyme inactivates the factor needed for initiation of translation. Interferons are produced within hours of virus infection, and virus production decreases. Since antibodies against viruses take several days to appear, the temporal relationship suggests that interferons play a primary role in the defense of the host against these infections (Fig 24–7).

It is now known that interferons exhibit a wide variety of cell regulatory activities, including cell growth and differentiation. Of greatest significance in our discussion is the ability of these products to modulate an immune response. For example, NK cells can have enhanced activity when exposed to IFNs. Interferons play significant regulatory roles involving macrophages as well as T and B lymphocytes when the immune system responds to a viral infection. Interferons also have been shown to have potential as anticancer reagents based on their ability to regulate cell functions and to modulate the immune system. Clinical trials testing antiviral and anticancer potentials are being conducted.

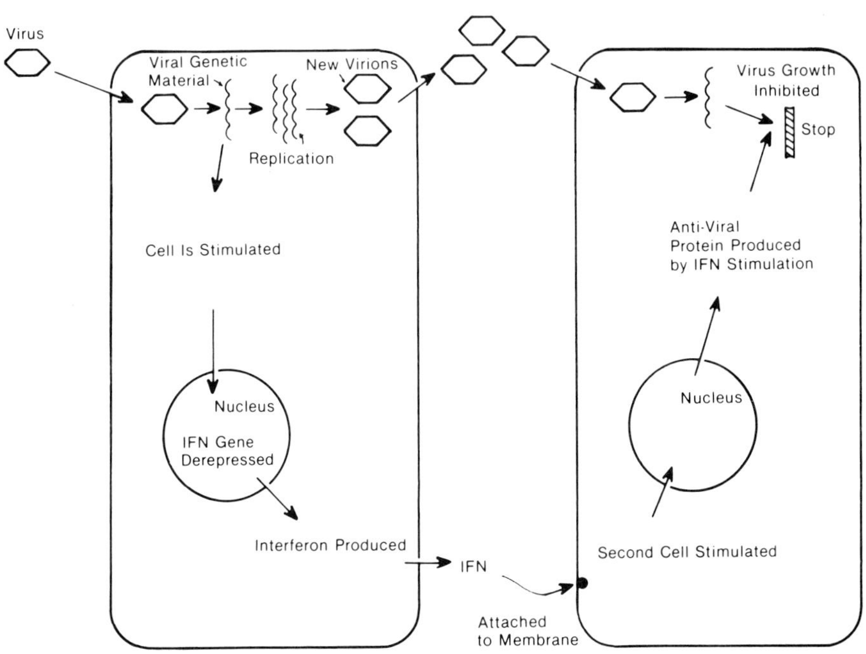

Figure 24–6. Mechanism of interferon inhibition of virus growth.

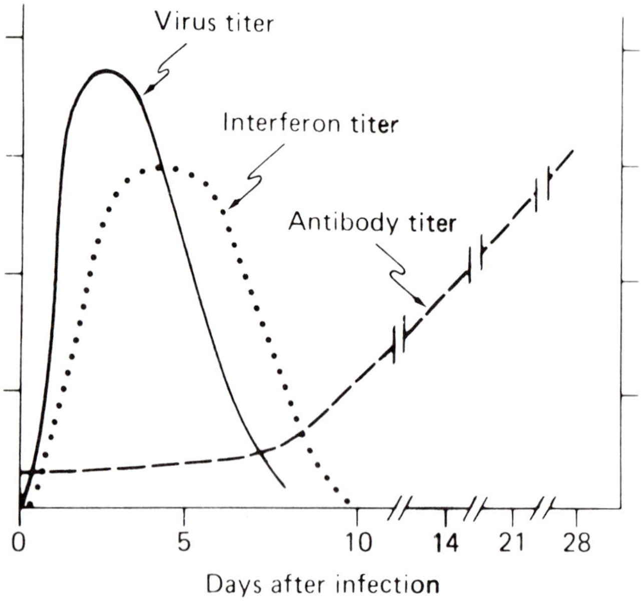

Figure 24–7. Illustration of kinetics of interferon and antibody synthesis after respiratory virus infection. The temporal relationships suggest that interferons are involved in the recovery process. *(From Jawetz E, Melnick JL, Adelberg EA.* Review of Medical Microbiology. *17th ed. E. Norwalk, Conn: Appleton & Lange; 1987:391.)*

BACTERIAL VIRUSES

Bacteria are host to a group of viruses called bacteriophage, or phage. Phages are important, since they provide ideal materials for studying host–parasite relationships, virus multiplication, and molecular genetics. The best known groups of phages are those that infect *Escherichia coli.* Virulent phages (eg, T series of *E. coli* B) always destroy their host, whereas temperate phages (such as λ) may exist as a latent form and not always destroy the host.

The steps in the process are well known. Tail fibers (eg, T series phage) adsorb to specific receptor sites on the bacterial host cell surface. The base plate then attaches to the surface, and the tail sheath contracts, pushing the core through the cell wall to the outer surface of the cytoplasmic membrane. The DNA molecule is injected as a single thread into the periplasmic space and then spontaneously crosses the cell membrane into the cytoplasm. This starts the eclipse phase of phage reproduction, during which there is no evidence of whole viral particles inside the host cell if examined with an electron microscope.

The proteins made at this time are responsible for stopping cellular DNA, RNA, and protein synthesis by degrading the host's DNA chromosome, and the virally induced enzymes required for replication of viral nucleic acid are made. Structural proteins are produced later. Maturation occurs once infectious virions have been assembled. This stage marks the end of the eclipse period. Release of the phage follows as a result of host cell lysis. Each bacteriophage infection results in a genetically determined number (burst size) of viruses.

The temperate phage cycle includes initial steps (attachment, genome insertion, early protein production) similar to those described in the lytic phage infection. The genome (prophage) of a temperate phage has the ability to be physically incorporated into the host's chromosome, becoming part of the genetic information possessed by the host cell. A few viruses have a prophage that exists as a free plasmid in the host's cytoplasm. The phenomenon is called lysogeny, and the bacteria are said to be lysogenic. The prophage produces a repression molecule that will prevent the growth of identical or closely related phages that may contact and invade the bacterium.

A lytic reproductive cycle can be induced in the prophage using such agents as ultraviolet light or carcinogenic chemicals. The phages lyse the bacterial cell and invade others in which they can reestablish the lysogenic state.

Lysogenic conversion refers to the addition of new physiologic properties to the bacterial cell as a result of the incorporation of the prophage into the host's chromosome. New genetic expression capabilities are added, some of which are recognized as harmful to a human. Examples include the diphtheria toxin from *Corynebacterium diphtheriae,* the erythrogenic toxins of scarlet fever in *Streptococcus pyogenes,* and the addition of various antigens on *Salmonella* species. If the prophage is lost, the host cell loses the ability to produce the toxin or antigen.

Temperate bacteriophages have been found to be associated with a wide variety of oral microorganisms. Realizing the consequences of lysogenic conversion has led to the speculation that lysogeny may be involved in caries or periodontal disease. No clinical studies have shown this at this time, however.

When bacteriophages were discovered in the early 1900s by Twort and d'Herelle, it was recognized that the phages actually destroyed human pathogenic bacteria in a test tube. Because this was decades before sulfa drugs and antibiotics were available, it was hoped that phages could be used as a medical treatment to destroy these organisms within the human body and lead to recovery from disease. Except for minor successes with *Shigella* dystentery, these hopes have not been realized.

SUGGESTED READINGS

Bart KJ, Hinman AR, Jordan WS Jr, eds. International Symposium on vaccine development and utilization. *Rev Infect Dis.* 1989;11:S491–S667.

Basler K, Oesch B, Scott M, et al. Scrapie and cellular PrP isoforms are encoded by the same chromosomal gene. *Cell.* 1986;46:417–428.

Diener TO. The viroid—A subviral pathogen. *Am Scientist.* 1983;71:481–488.

Evans AS, ed. *Viral Infection of Humans.* 3rd ed. New York: Plenum; 1986.

Fields BN, ed. *Fundamental Virology.* New York: Raven Press; 1986.

Galasso GT, Merigan TC, Buchanan RA, eds. *Antiviral Agents and Viral Agents of Man.* 2nd ed. New York: Raven Press; 1985.

Hooks JJ, Jordan GW, eds. *Viral Infections in Oral Medicine.* New York: Elsevier/North Holland; 1982.

Ljungman Fridell E, Lonnquist B, et al. Efficacy and safety of vaccination of marrow transplant recipients with a live attenuated measles, mumps and rubella vaccine. *J Infect Dis.* 1989;159:610–615.

Mathews REF, ed. Third Report of the International Committee of Taxonomy of Viruses: Classification and nomenclature of viruses. *Intervirology.* 1979;12:129.

Notkins AL, Oldstone MBA, eds. *Concepts in Viral Pathogenesis.* New York: Springer-Verlag; 1986, vol II.

Specter S, Lancz GJ. *Clinical Virology Manual.* New York: Elsevier; 1986.

Stringfellow DA. *Interferon and Interferon Inducers.* New York: Marcel Dekker; 1980.

White DO, Fenner FJ. *Medical Virology.* 3rd ed. Orlando, Fla: Academic Press; 1986.

CHAPTER 25

The Herpesviruses

Paul A. Farber

INTRODUCTION
MORPHOLOGY AND CLASSIFICATION
HERPES SIMPLEX VIRUS
Pathogenesis
Primary HSV-1 Infection
Latency of HSV
Skin Infections
Herpetic Whitlow
Herpetic Keratitis
Genital Infection
Neonatal Infection
Recurrent Perioral Herpetic Infections
Diagnosis, Treatment, and Prevention
HSV Vaccine
HSV and Cancer
VARICELLA-ZOSTER VIRUS
Chickenpox and Shingles
Treatment and Prevention
CYTOMEGALOVIRUS
Congenital and Perinatal Infection
Infections in Adults
CMV and Cancer
Diagnosis, Treatment, and Prevention
EPSTEIN-BARR VIRUS
Infectious mononucleosis
The Chronic Mononucleosis Syndromes
ORAL SIGNIFICANCE
SUGGESTED READINGS

INTRODUCTION

The herpesvirus group (family name: Herpesviridae) includes five human viruses that share some common properties. This group has assumed increasing importance as the cause of widely occurring infections, such as cold sores and genital herpes. The propensity of herpesviruses for latency and a lifelong association with the host present special problems in disease control. The dentist should be knowledgeable about herpes because this group of viruses is responsible for the majority of the virally induced oral lesions that might be encountered in clinical practice (Table 25–1).

MORPHOLOGY AND CLASSIFICATION

The major criterion for categorizing DNA viruses into this group is their architecture. The double-stranded DNA core is relatively large, having a molecular weight of approximately 100×10^6 daltons. The virus capsid is composed of 162 icosahedral capsomeres and is surrounded by a glycoprotein and lipid-containing envelope that is derived from host cell membrane and renders the virus sensitive to ether. The five human herpesviruses, herpes simplex virus 1 (HSV-1), herpes simplex virus 2 (HSV-2), varicella-zoster virus (VZV), cytomegalovirus (CMV), and Epstein-Barr virus (EBV), differ in their DNA and pro-

TABLE 25–1. HERPES SIMPLEX (HSV) INFECTIONS IN THE UNITED STATES

Disease Syndrome	HSV Type	Estimated Cases per Year
Primary oral—herpes gingivostomatitis	99% type 1	500,000
Recurrent oral—herpes labialis	99% type 1	100 million
Primary or first episode genital herpes	50 to 92% type 2	60,000–500,000
Recurrent genital herpes	Mostly type 2	2–20 million
Herpes keratoconjunctivitis	97% type 1	400,000
Herpes encephalitis	98% type 1	1,000
Neonatal herpes	67% type 2	399–500

From Overall JC. In: Rapp F, ed. Herpes virus. *New York: Alan Liss; 1984:17.*

tein components. Only HSV-1 and HSV-2 share significant DNA sequence homologies. Infection with these viruses is fairly common, and most adults have antibodies against several types. Although the herpesviruses are morphologically similar, they can be classified into subfamilies based on differences in their biologic properties. Alphaherpes (HSV and VZV) are rapidly growing and cytolytic and have a wide host range. Betaherpes (CMV) have a narrower host range, are slow growing, and frequently produce enlargement (cytomegaly) of infected cells. Gammaherpes (EBV) have the narrowest host range and replicate only in lymphoblastoid cells (B lymphocytes) and tumor cells of nasopharyngeal carcinoma.

The interaction of herpesviruses with susceptible cells may result in more than one outcome, including cytocidal infection, latent infection, and oncogenic transformation. Most members of this family have a special affinity for cells of ectodermal origin, with a tendency for focal cytopathogenicity resulting in the production of vesicles or pocks on the skin. Primary infections occur in nonimmune hosts, and secondary or reactivation infection results from induction of latent virus. Several herpesviruses have been linked to cancer in humans.

HERPES SIMPLEX VIRUS

Pathogenesis

Herpes simplex virus, types 1 and 2, primarily infect epithelial cells, and the subsequent viral proliferation leads to cell death. HSV infection is detected histologically by the presence of multinucleated cells and intranuclear inclusions (Figs 25–1, 25–2). Following a primary infection, which occurs in a nonimmune host, HSV becomes latent by moving along sensory nerves to the corresponding ganglion, where the virus remains quiescent in a noninfectious form. Reactivation of the virus and subsequent replication can be induced by a number of stimuli, such as fever induced by another virus, immunosuppression, local trauma to the ganglion or the epithelium it innervates, hormonal changes, and psychogenic factors.

The two serotypes of herpes simplex, types 1 and 2, share many similar properties and can be differentiated in the laboratory only by restriction endonuclease analysis of DNA or by serologic typing using monoclonal antibodies. Differentiation can more easily be made on clinical and epidemiologic grounds, by the body sites that each type infects and by their method of transmission. HSV-1 is associated with lesions above the waist, particularly the oral region,

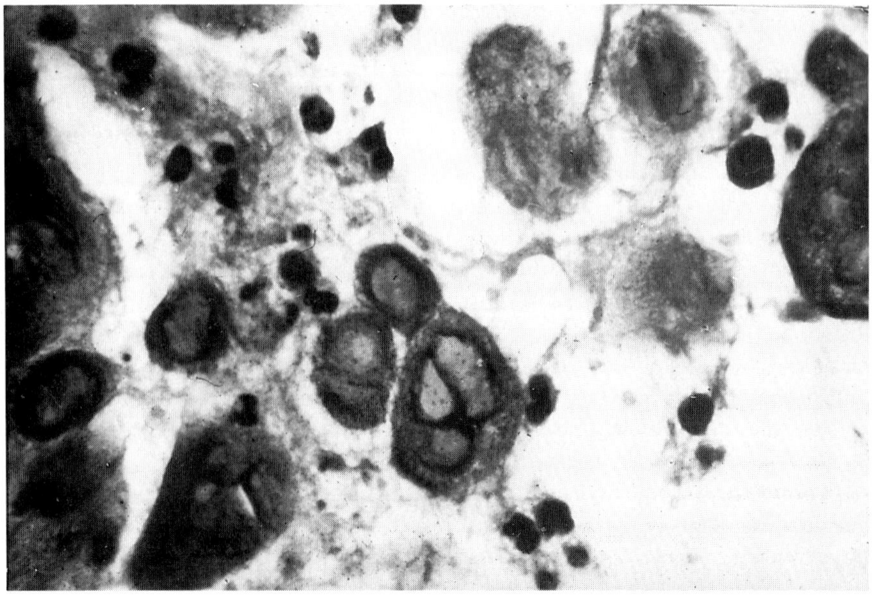

Figure 25–1. Cytologic smear (Tzanck smear) of an oral herpetic vesicle, showing infected epithelial cells with multiple nuclei with marginal condensation of chromatin. Some lymphocytes are seen.

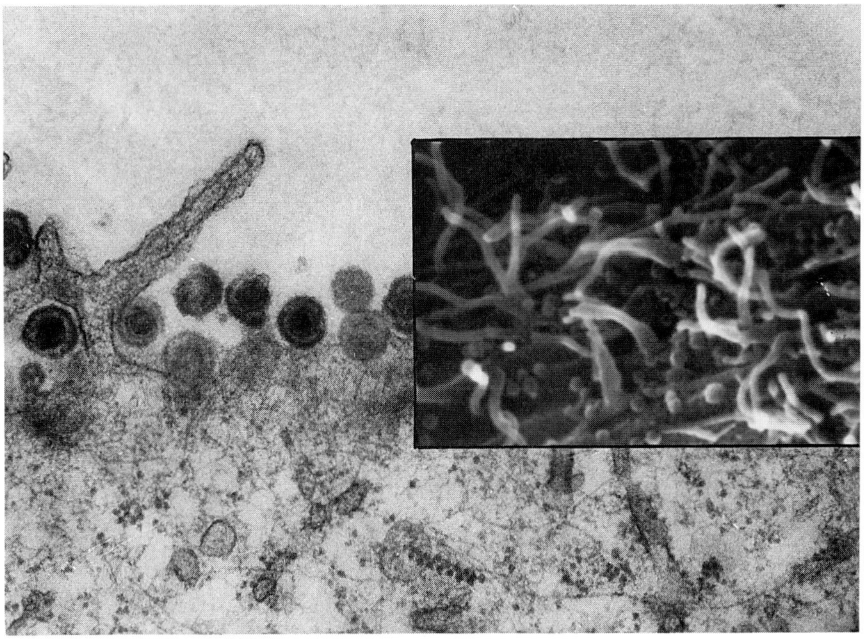

Figure 25–2. Transmission electron micrograph of herpes simplex virus, type 1, infecting Hep-2 cells in tissue culture. ×30,000. Inset. Scanning electron micrograph of budding virus particles among villus processes of Hep-2 cells infected with HSV. ×20,000.

and is spread by oral secretions or contact with oral tissue. Primary infection usually occurs in children aged 6 months to 6 years and presents clinically as gingivostomatitis. The site of viral latency is the trigeminal ganglion, and reactivation causes herpes labialis. HSV-2 produces primary infection in adolescents and older individuals and is spread through venereal contact, with lesions usually confined to areas below the waist, primarily the genital region. The virus assumes a latent form in the sacral ganglion, and recurrences occur on the genitalia. These clinical distinctions can be modified by factors such as high socioeconomic status which ensure that some individuals are exposed to HSV later in life, after the onset of sexual activity. In such cases, oral lesions might be caused by type 2 and genital lesions by type 1.

Primary HSV-1 Infection

Most primary HSV-1 infections are asymptomatic, and it has been estimated that only 10% of patients with serologic evidence of infection (ie, presence of HSV-1 antibodies) actually experience clinical disease. The virus is ubiquitous and can be demonstrated not only from lesions of infected individuals but also in about 1% of healthy subjects. The peak incidence is between 6 months and 4 years of age, and the major clinical finding is a generalized gingivostomatitis. This begins as erythema and edema and rapidly progresses to vesiculation, followed by ulceration. In younger individuals, the painful lesions are found on the buccal mucosa, tongue, soft palate, lips, and gingiva (Fig 25–3). Lymphadenopathy in cervical and submandibular nodes and fever and malaise are also frequently present. In adolescent and adult patients, primary HSV-1 infection produces a severe pharyngotonsillitis. Complications are rare, and there is complete recovery in 2 to 3 weeks.

Latency of HSV

The pathogenic spectrum of HSV infection includes alternating cycles of virus latency and virus activity. The establishment of latent virus in ganglia occurs at an early stage of primary infection. Following local virus replication at the mucosal or skin site of inoculation, the virus migrates via nerve endings as a noninfectious nucleocapsid to the local ganglion. The latent virus remains in an inactive state within neurons of the ganglion for prolonged periods, often a lifetime. When reactivated, the noninfectious form is induced to undergo at least one cycle of vegetative replication. The mature virions migrate from the ganglion to the site it innervates. Recurrent lesions, such as herpes labialis, result when this ganglion-derived virus replicates in oral tissues. Individuals who harbor latent virus may periodically shed virus in oral or genital secretions without producing clinical lesions. The maintenance of the latent state requires active surveillance by the immune system. Factors that produce only subtle alterations in one or more immune processes are capable of allowing escape of latent virus.

Skin Infections

Herpetic infection of the skin is usually a self-limiting infection. However, in certain instances where the integumental natural defenses are damaged by intercurrent allergic reactions, superimposed herpetic infections are extremely severe and even life-

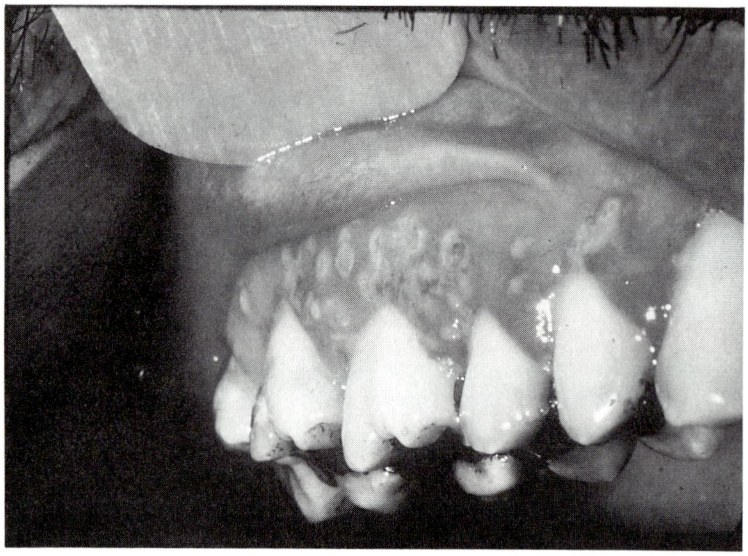

Figure 25–3. Primary herpetic gingivostomatitis in a dental student showing ulcers on attached gingiva. Patient also had severe pharyngitis and herpetic whitlow (Fig 25–4). *(Courtesy of Dr. John Fantasia, Long Island Jewish Medical Center, New Hyde Park, NY.)*

threatening. This occurs in children and young adults who suffer from skin disorders, such as eczema, contact or atopic dermatitis, or seborrheic dermatitis, and is referred to as eczema herpeticum. Extensive crops of vesicular lesions appear on face, scalp, and hands. Bacterial superinfection becomes a problem as these vesicles rupture to leave large areas of ulcerated skin. The virus may spread from the skin to involve visceral organs, resulting in pneumonia or encephalitis. Physical damage to the skin, such as superficial abrasions resulting from contact sports, also can predispose to HSV infection.

Herpetic Whitlow

Herpetic infection of the digits (herpetic whitlow) is a recognized occupational hazard of medical and dental personnel (Fig 25–4) and may be contracted through treatment of patients with oral herpetic lesions. Similar to other types of herpes infection, primary infection occurs in those individuals who have not been exposed to HSV. The dentist or hygienist, in turn, may transmit this infection to other patients. Herpetic whitlow usually occurs through a break in the skin and results from localized virus replication, which causes swelling, redness, and tenderness, with subsequent vesiculation. Healing follows in 2 weeks and, as in other HSV infections, latency and periodic reactivations are common. One report on an outbreak of HSV infections in a dental practice traced the source to a whitlow on the finger of a dental hygienist. She treated 46 patients when she was infected, and 20 of these developed clinical signs and symptoms of severe primary HSV gingivostomatitis, including fever, sore throat, and dysphagia (Fig 25–5).

Herpetic Keratitis

Herpetic keratitis of the eyes is second only to trauma as the leading cause of blindness in the United States. The most frequently encountered form is keratoconjunctivitis, which can occur alone or simultaneously with oral infection. It is almost always unilateral and begins as a conjunctivitis together with herpetic vesiculation of the eyelids. If the infection is confined to the conjunctiva alone, symptoms resolve in a few days with no residual effects. Extension to the cornea

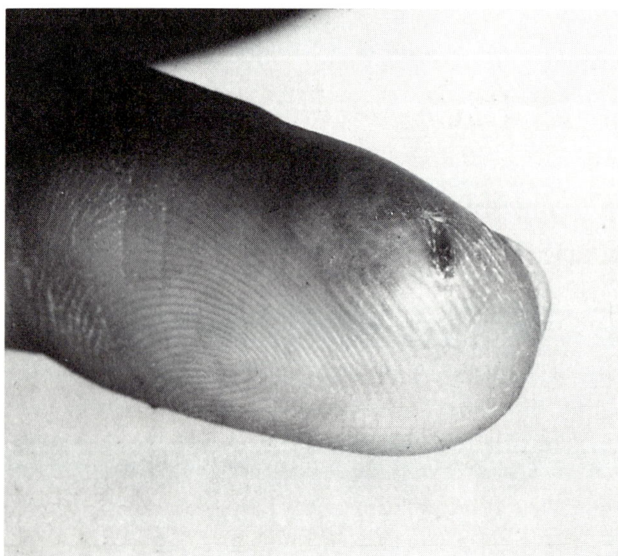

Figure 25–4. Herpetic whitlow in same patient as in Fig 25–3. The finger became infected with herpes simplex virus shed from oral lesions. *(Courtesy of Dr. John Fantasia, Long Island Jewish Medical Center, New Hyde Park, NY.)*

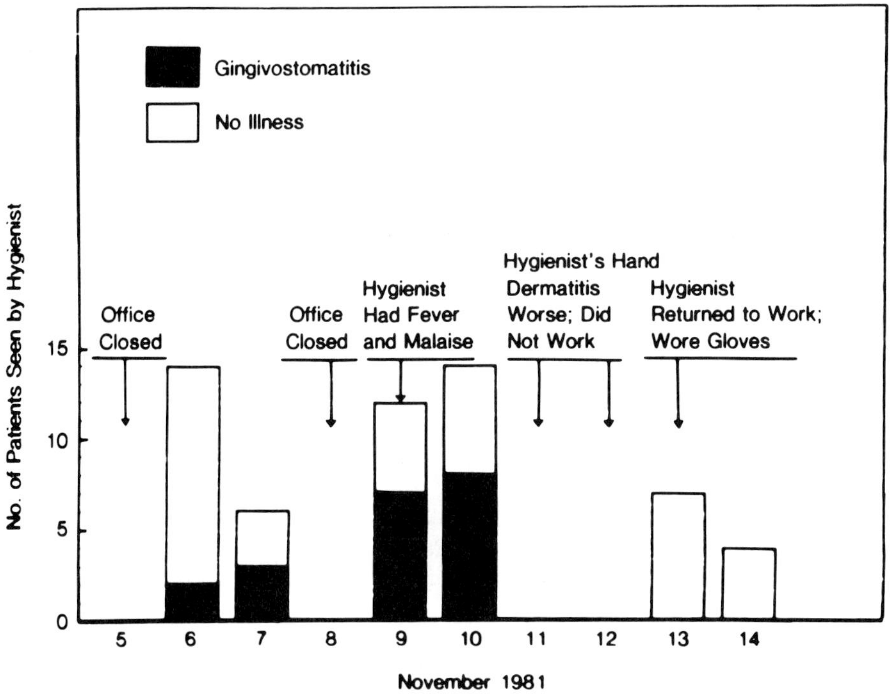

Figure 25–5. Incidence of gingivostomatitis in patients treated by a dental hygienist who contracted primary herpes and herpetic skin infection while treating one of her patients. The hygienist transmitted the virus to 20 of 46 patients in a 4-day period. *(From Mazella JP, et al. An outbreak of herpes simplex virus type 1 gingivostomatitis in a dental hygiene practice.* JAMA. *1984;252:2019–2022.)*

results in vesicle formation and subsequent ulceration, which in turn may produce vision impairment. Following primary infection, recurrent herpetic episodes occur in about one fourth of patients. These recurrences may be more extensive than the primary infection, and subsequent scarring can result in blindness.

Genital Infection

Genital infection, which is associated with HSV-2 in almost 90% of cases, is one of the most common venereal infections (Table 25–1). The virus is contracted during sexual intercourse and infects the vaginal mucosa or penile epithelium, producing vesicular eruptions after an incubation period of 2 to 7 days. In males, lesions may extend into the urethra and cause dysuria or urinary retention. Systemic signs, such as fever and malaise, often accompany the local lesions as well as regional lymphadenopathy. First episodes of genital herpes in patients with prior HSV-1 infections are less severe and heal faster than in those with no history of virus contact. It has been estimated that 50% of primary genital infections are asymptomatic, thereby complicating control. A direct correlation has been established between the incidence of genital herpes and the level of sexual activity, prostitutes having the highest rates of infection.

Neonatal Infection

Neonates become infected during birth to women with active genital herpes. More than half of these babies will have skin lesions, usually on the scalp or in the perianal area. Viral infection of the eyes also may occur. Vesicles quickly break down and become encrusted or infected with pyogenic bacteria. Constitutional symptoms, such as fever, vomiting, or failure to eat, also occur. Newborns are particularly susceptible to herpes, especially if they are inoculated during the birth process. Over 50% of infected children succumb, and the survivors suffer from permanent mental or physical deficits. Involvement of the central nervous system is a cardinal feature of herpes neonatal infection, with frequent infection of the liver and adrenals as well. It is recommended that cesarean section be performed before rupture of the membranes in any pregnancy in which HSV infection is known to have occurred in the months before delivery. HSV-1 infection may be acquired through postnatal contact of the newborn with family members who have oral herpes.

Recurrent Perioral Herpetic Infections

The reactivation of latent herpesvirus in the trigeminal ganglion results in secondary herpetic infections, colloquially known as fever blisters, cold sores, or herpes labialis. This is the most common form of herpes infection, and one third of the population may have this disease, with each individual averaging two occurrences per year. The preferred site is the lower lip, with the upper lip second. Other less frequently affected skin sites include the nose, chin, and cheek. Intraorally, vesicular lesions can occur on the gingiva and hard palate. The appearance of recurrent herpetic lesions often is preceded by prodromal symptoms at the site. These include paresthesia (numbing sensation) or a tingling sensation that occurs 12 to 24 hours before frank vesiculation. Direct trauma to the trigeminal ganglion during surgical procedures is invariably followed by the appearance of herpetic vesicles. Virus can be isolated from oral tissues during the first 3 days. The vesicles rupture within 36 to 48 hours, leaving an ulcerated surface that crusts and heals by the tenth day. In healthy subjects, these lesions produce only local discomfort. However, the severity and duration of herpes labialis are increased in older individuals and in those with depressed immunity. Recurrent oral herpetic lesions may trigger erythema multiforme, an acute dermatitis of unknown etiology in which there is extensive oral vesiculation as well.

Diagnosis, Treatment, and Prevention

Herpes simplex infections usually are diagnosed by clinical criteria. Isolation of virus or cytologic smears (Tzanck smear, Fig 25–1) of vesicles are confirmatory. Differentiation between types 1 and 2 is achieved using monoclonal antibodies, nucleic acid hybridization techniques, or the polymerase chain reaction (PCR). Serodiagnosis of primary HSV infection requires the demonstration of a significant rise in antibody titers to the virus. A rise in antibody may also be observed following recurrent infections.

Recently, several antiviral compounds have been developed that are effective against herpes simplex. The most effective of these is acyclovir (Zovirax), which inhibits viral DNA polymerase without affecting host cell DNA metabolism. Primary genital herpes infections respond well to intravenous acyclovir. This is reflected in most clinical parameters, including amelioration in symptoms, facilitated healing, and reduced virus shedding. The FDA has approved the oral form of acyclovir as effective both in treatment and as a prophylactic agent against reactivation infection in high-risk immunosuppressed patients. Topical application of 5% acyclovir speeded healing and reduced painful symptoms of primary genital herpes but had little effect on recurrent lesions. Acyclovir has not proven effective in treatment of recurrent oral lesions. A major difficulty in treatment of herpes labialis is the rapid evolution of the lesions, which mature from macule to papule in less than 12 hours. Application of topical agents to lesions when they are clinically visible may be too late to affect healing or abort viral replication significantly. Antiviral drugs must be applied during the prodromal stages to produce any demonstrable effect. At present, topical acyclovir is recommended for herpetic lesions only in immunologically compromised hosts where lesions tend to persist and spread.

The emergence of resistant virus strains argues against trivial usage for minor infections. The best success for treatment of herpetic infections has been obtained with the use of topical agents in herpes keratitis. One of the first was idoxuridine (IDU), which interferes with viral nucleic acid replication. Its effectiveness is limited as viral resistance develops rapidly. Adenine Arabinoside and trifluorothymidine (F_3T) are more effective and produce less toxic side effects. The use of topical steroids, formerly recommended to impede scarring of the cornea, has been shown to suppress antiviral immune processes and actually enhance virus replication. Their use is contraindicated in herpes infections.

To prevent the spread of HSV to either dentists or other patients, it is recommended that dental treatment for patients with oral herpetic lesions be postponed until the lesions resolve. If treatment is necessary, protective measures, such as the placement of rubber dams to prevent contact with lesions as well as the use of disposable surgical gloves, be employed.

HSV Vaccine

Although strides have been made in formulating effective antiviral drugs, none so far have been able to prevent the establishment of viral latency. The need for an effective vaccine that would prevent recurrent infections is obvious. Development of a subunit vaccine composed of HSV surface glycoproteins would eliminate the oncogenic potential of a live vaccine. These viral components induce both humoral and cell-mediated responses that protect experimental animals from lethal HSV infection and also prevent the establishment of latency.

HSV and Cancer

The oncogenic potential of HSV is discussed in Chapter 31.

VARICELLA-ZOSTER VIRUS

Varicella-zoster virus is responsible for two diseases, varicella (chickenpox) and zoster (shingles). VZV is difficult to obtain in pure form because when it is grown in tissue culture cells, such as human fibroblasts, the virus remains cell-associated and can be freed of cellular components only by sonication or enzyme treatment. Because VZV is one of the most labile of viruses, it loses infectivity rapidly during the purification procedures. It has been placed in the alphaherpes group by virtue of its biologic properties such as latency in ganglia and short reproductive cycle.

Chickenpox and Shingles

Chickenpox represents primary infection with VZV, whereas shingles results from reactivation of latent virus. Varicella is a disease of childhood, with most cases occurring in the first decade of life. Varicella is among the most contagious of diseases and, unlike HSV, primary VZV infection usually is symptomatic. It is characterized by an incubation period of 10 to 20 days, followed by the appearance of cutaneous papular-vesicular lesions that appear in crops, appearing first on the face, then on the trunk, and finally on the extremities. The virus is spread by the respiratory route, with subsequent viral replication in local lymph nodes followed by a viremic phase. Virus is captured in the liver and spleen, followed by a second viremia and the appearance of cutaneous lesions. The skin rash that appears usually on the 14th day develops rapidly and evolves from papules to vesicles in a period of hours. Vesicles can be found on the oral mucosa, particularly the palate. These rupture in a short time, leaving painful ulcers. The disease is usually self-limiting, and recovery is uneventful except in children who have immunosuppressive illnesses such as leukemia. These individuals are subject to serious complications, such as pneumonitis and encephalitis.

Zoster is essentially a disease of adults, and almost 70% of cases occur in patients 50 years or older. The skin lesions resemble those of varicella, but their distribution follows the innervation of sensory nerves supplied by the dorsal roots of thoracic, cervical, lumbar, and trigeminal ganglia (Fig 25–6). Patients have antibodies to VZV, indicating a prior encounter with the virus in the form of clinical or, occasionally, subclinical chickenpox infection. During the primary infection, VZV establishes a latent infection in the sensory ganglia. Later in life, the virus is reactivated by many of the stimuli associated with recurrent HSV. Zoster is preceded by localized pain and tenderness along the sensory distribution of the involved dorsal, spinal, or cranial nerve roots. Virus replicates in the sensory ganglion and then is transported down the nerve and released around the nerve endings in the skin. Patients who are immunosuppressed are particularly susceptible to zoster. Almost 50% of Hodgkin's disease patients experience shingles. Postherpetic neuralgia is a frequent complication, especially in patients past the age of 60, and may persist even after the skin lesions have healed.

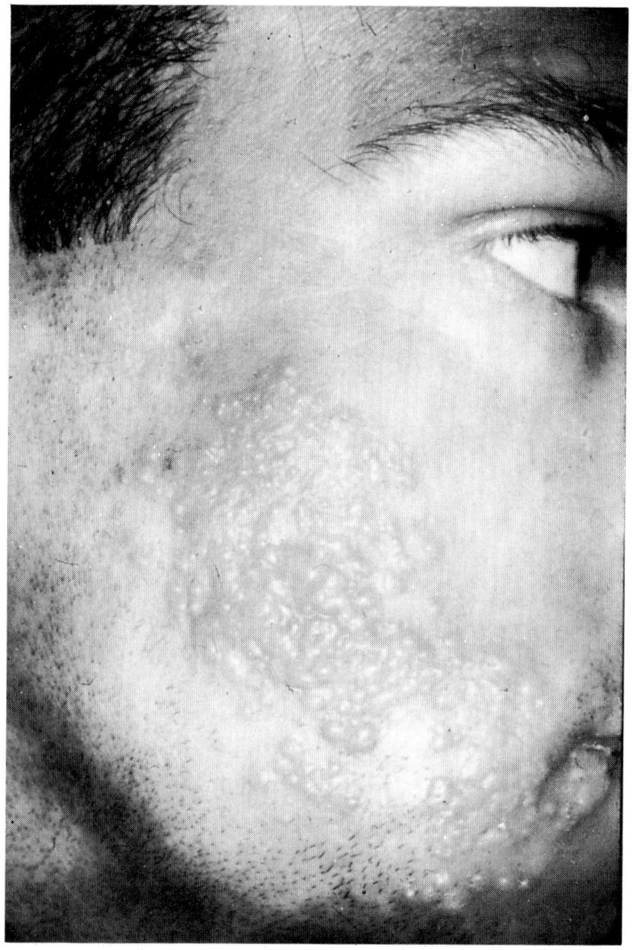

Figure 25–6. Herpes zoster infection. The vesicular lesions are distributed over the skin area supplied by the maxillary division of the trigeminal nerve.

Treatment and Prevention

The treatment of VZ with antiviral drugs has been effective in controlling infection, particularly in high-risk groups. ARA-A treatment has been shown to accelerate healing, decrease cutaneous dissemination, and reduce the duration of postherpetic neuralgia in zoster. The FDA has approved the use of ARA-A in the treatment of VZ in compromised patients. Intravenous acyclovir also is useful in preventing the development of varicella pneumonitis in exposed, susceptible, immunocompromised children and is effective against zoster in adults. Passive immunization with human immune serum globulin in susceptible patients who have been exposed to VZ also is effective in reducing the severity of lesions. An attenuated virus vaccine has been developed in Japan and has been used extensively in that country to immunize high-risk children.

CYTOMEGALOVIRUS

This member of the herpesvirus group derives its name from the large intranuclear inclusions it produces in infected cells. This inclusion measures 8 to 10 μm in diameter and appears in a cell swollen to almost four times its normal volume. Members of this group also infect nonhuman species, such as dogs, monkeys, and guinea pigs, producing the pathognomonic cell enlargement in salivary gland ductal cells. Its propensity for salivary glands initially led investigators to name the agent salivary gland virus. CMV has been established as a primary human fetal pathogen capable of inducing a variety of congenital anomalies. It also infects a majority of the adult population, resulting in a lifelong latent association in the host, with reactivation occurring during immunosuppression induced by illness or as a consequence of therapy for cancer or organ transplantation. The hallmarks of cytomegalovirus infection in humans are its asymptomatic association in a vast majority of cases and the prolonged virus shedding that occurs after primary infection.

Congenital and Perinatal Infection

CMV is ubiquitous, and neonates often contract infection through asymptomatic maternal infection. CMV also may be transmitted by close personal contact through secretions, such as urine, semen, saliva, and breast milk. The most important clinical features of acute neonatal infection include hepatosplenomegaly (Fig 25–7), jaundice, petechial rashes, microcephaly, chorioretinitis, and cerebral calcifications. Clinical disease represents only 5% of the total spectrum of CMV association with neonates, and asymptomatic infection is the rule. A variety of congenital anomalies can result, including nonspecific cardiovascular, gastrointestinal, and musculoskeletal defects. Yellow discoloration and hypocalcification of enamel have been noted in 40% of children with severe CMV infection. Hearing loss and psychomotor retardation also are associated with CMV. There is speculation that a great many schoolage children with learning disabilities, the so-called slow child, might be suffering from the effects of congenital CMV infection.

Infections in Adults

CMV in adults is an opportunistic pathogen that produces clinical disease mainly in immunosuppressed patients. This is especially true in renal transplant procedures, where hepatitis, pneumonitis, and kidney infection are frequent complications. The infection rate in patients with prior exposure to the virus is almost three times that seen in those with primary infections. This would indicate that these CMV infections result from reactivation of latent virus caused by the depressive effects of drugs on the immune system. Many hospitalized patients contract primary CMV infections through transfusion of blood containing either whole virus or leukocytes with latent virus. Fulminant infection occurs in those with AIDS, in whom the major dysfunction is a lack of helper T cells. CMV is also a causative agent of infectious mononucleosis (IM), although it produces fewer cases than does Epstein-Barr virus. CMV mononucleosis is similar in many respects to IM induced by EBV; both result in fever and lymphocytosis with large numbers of atypical lymphocytes. Unlike EBV, CMV-induced IM is not usually associated with pharyngitis or lymphadenopathy. The major differentiation is the absence of a positive heterophil test in CMV. Almost half of all cases of heterophil-negative IM are caused by CMV. This syndrome may result from transfusion of blood and occurs most commonly in children.

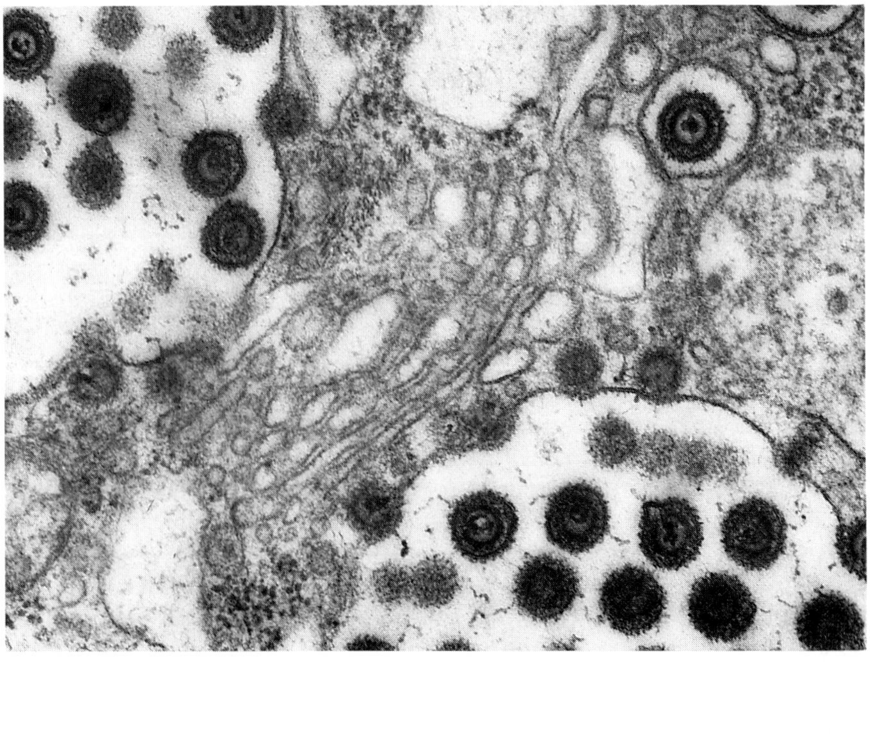

Figure 25–7. Electron micrograph of cytomegalovirus hepatitis in a 3-week-old infant. Virus is seen adjacent to the Golgi zone of the infected bile duct cells. ×40,000. *(From Balaz M. Electron microscope examination of congenital cytomegalovirus hepatitis.* Virchows Arch [Pathol Anat]. *1984;405:119–129.)*

CMV and Cancer

CMV, similar to other members of the herpesvirus group, has been associated with the establishment of the malignant state, both in vitro and in vivo. This topic is discussed in Chapter 31.

Diagnosis, Treatment, and Prevention

Diagnosis of CMV infection is accomplished by clinical criteria and isolation and serologic identification of virus. Presence of typical inclusions in sedimented urine cells may be used as a confirmatory test. Attempts to treat CMV infection with antiviral compounds that are effective against other herpes infections have met with little success. The antigenic diversity of CMV has prevented the development of an effective vaccine. The relative contributions of cellular and humoral immunity in CMV remain to be defined.

EPSTEIN-BARR VIRUS

Epstein-Barr virus (EBV), the most recently discovered of the herpesviruses, is distinguishable from the other agents in this group by its narrow host range, which is limited to lymphocytes and certain epithelioid cells. Lymphocyte infection can result in lysis without release of mature virions or, more usually, with persistence and minimum expression of the viral genome. The reproductive cycle of EBV is slow, and infection of cells often is difficult to establish. For this reason, the virus has been placed in the genus with the intriguing name of *Lymphocryptovirus*. EBV has been associated with IM and two human neoplasms, Burkitt's lymphoma and nasopharyngeal carcinoma (Fig 25–8).

Infectious Mononucleosis

Clinical cases of IM occur in developed countries and most often affect college students, white collar workers, and members of the military. Under low socioeconomic conditions, virtually all individuals acquire EBV in the first 3 years of life as an asymptomatic infection. With higher living standards, a segment of the population escapes this early infection, and clinical illness does not appear until adolescence.

Pathogenesis The disease is characterized by fever, pharyngitis, lymphadenopathy, and the presence of small petechial red spots on the uvula and the junction of the hard and soft palate. The oropharynx is the site of initial infection with EBV, where the virus infects epithelial cells, especially cells in the salivary glands. IM is known colloquially as the kissing disease because of its transmission involving exchange of infected saliva. Sixty percent of IM patients shed virus in their saliva. The virus also replicates in lymphoid tissue of the oropharynx, and infected lymphocytes migrate to other lymphoid organs to produce a generalized lymphoid infection. The interaction between EBV and B lymphocytes results in cell proliferation, or immortalization, because many of these infected lymphocytes can be maintained in culture indefinitely. B lymphocytes transformed by EBV carry multiple viral genome copies in nonintegrated episomal form, which replicates in coordination with the cell.

The only viral footprints detectable in these cells is the EBV-associated antigen, EBNA, which is important in host recognition of infected cells. Although EBV infection enhances the proliferation of B lymphocytes, the majority of the increased number of normal appearing circulating lymphocytes seen in IM are actually T lymphocytes responding to EBNA antigens. Many of these responder cells represent cytotoxic cells that specifically attach to and kill EBV-infected B cells. Another subset of T cells, the suppressor cell, also is increased in IM. These cells control the proliferation of B lymphocytes through the release of inhibi-

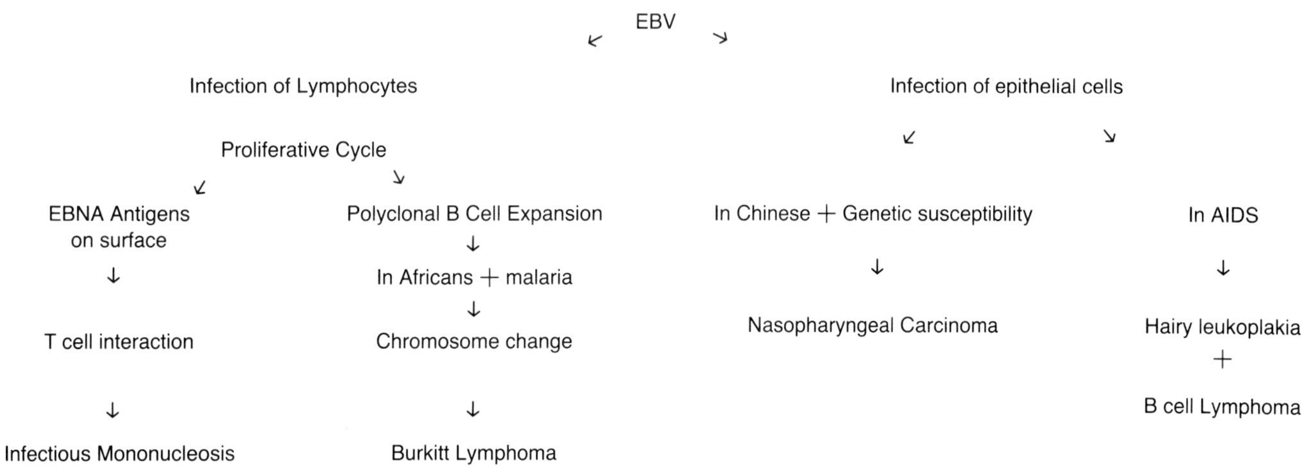

Figure 25–8. Diagram illustrating the possible outcome of EBV infection and the relationship between EBV and infectious mononucleosis, Burkitt's lymphoma, nasopharyngeal carcinoma, leukoplakia in AIDS, and B cell lymphoma.

tory substances and may be important in limiting the growth of EBV-infected cells. One side effect of this unique host response to virus infection is a generalized depression of normal lymphocyte function, resulting in immunodepression, which occurs during the acute phases of IM. These derangements in immune responsiveness are reversed in the convalescent patient.

Diagnosis and Treatment Diagnosis is confirmed by laboratory findings, which include lymphocytosis, the presence of large numbers of atypical lymphocytes in the blood, the presence of heterophil antibodies (Paul-Bunnell test), and a rise and persistence of antibodies to EBV. Heterophil antibodies are IgM antibodies that agglutinate horse and sheep red cells. The abnormal lymphocytes seen in IM are distinguishable from blast forms seen in leukemia. IM is, for the most part, a benign, self-limiting disease with complications occurring in less than 1% of cases. Complete recovery can be expected for most patients in 4 to 6 weeks. Treatment is purely symptomatic—warm saline gargles to relieve the pharyngitis and avoidance of strenuous physical activity to decrease the danger of splenic rupture. IM, because of its self-limiting nature, has not been the object of concerted attempts at antiviral therapy.

The Chronic Mononucleosis Syndromes

Although the majority of IM cases run their course in several weeks, there are instances where EBV infection becomes chronic and symptoms persist. Chronic mononucleosis encompasses several syndromes in which there is serologic evidence of EBV infection (rise in antibody titers) and certain symptoms consistent with classic IM, namely, low grade fever, recurrent sore throat, and swollen lymph nodes. Longstanding fatigue is the most common denominator, and in many cases, there is no indication that EBV is the primary cause. The involvement of other infectious agents has not been ruled out. Clinicians prefer to call this condition chronic fatigue syndrome.

Although IM for the most part represents the successful control and full recovery from EBV through a vigorous immune response, Burkitt's lymphoma and nasopharyngeal carcinoma are more serious manifestations with higher mortalities. The oncogenic properties of EBV are discussed in Chapter 31.

ORAL SIGNIFICANCE

The five human herpesviruses produce a wide range of clinical diseases involving multiple organs in a broad age group. Persistance and latency contribute to their role as opportunistic pathogens, allowing reactivation when immunosurveillance is compromised. The practicing dentist will most commonly encounter recurrent oral lesions caused by HSV-1. Oral lesions also occur in VZV and EBV infections. It is, therefore, important for the dentist to recognize these viral lesions and to keep abreast of new developments in the prevention and control of herpes infections that will facilitate proper therapy.

SUGGESTED READINGS

Amstey MS. Treatment and prevention of viral infections (HSV, CMV, HPV, HBV). *Clin Obstet Gynecol.* 1988;31: 501–509.

Corey L, Spear PG. Infections with herpes simplex viruses. *N Engl J Med.* 1986;314:686–691, 749–757.

Galasso GJ, Myers MW. The five herpesviruses: Infection, prevention and treatment. *Adv Intern Med.* 1984;29:25–58.

Greenspan JS, Greenspan D, Lennette ET, et al. Replication of Epstein-Barr virus within epithelial cells or oral "hairy" leukoplakia, an AIDS-associated lesion. *N Engl J Med.* 1985;313:1564–1571.

Hanshaw JB, Dudgeon JA, Marshall WC, eds. *Viral Diseases of the Fetus and Newborn.* 2nd ed. Philadelphia: WB Saunders; 1985.

Katz BZ, Andiman WA. Chronic fatigue syndrome. *J Pediatr.* 1989;113:944–947.

Klein RJ. Initiation and maintenance of latent herpes simplex virus infections: The paradox of perpetual immobility and continuous movement. *Rev Infect Dis.* 1985;7:21–30.

Kohl S. Herpes simplex virus immunology: Problems, progress and promises. *J Infect Dis.* 1985;152:435–440.

Schlossberg D. *Infectious Mononucleosis.* New York: Praeger; 1983.

Straus SE, Ostrove JM, Inchauspé G, et al. Varicella-zoster virus infections: Biology, natural history, treatment and prevention. *Ann Intern Med.* 1988;108:221–237.

CHAPTER 26

Adenoviruses, Papovaviruses, Parvoviruses, and Poxviruses

Paul A. Farber

ADENOVIRUSES
Structure and Morphology
Adenovirus Infections
PAPOVAVIRUSES
Structure and Morphology
Papillomaviruses
Polyoma and SV40 Viruses
JC and BK Viruses
PARVOVIRUSES
Structure, Morphology, and Classification
Human Parvoviruses
Adenosatellite Viruses (Dependoviruses)
POXVIRUSES
Structure and Morphology
Vaccinia
Molluscum Contagiosum
Treatment
Other Poxviral Infections
ORAL ASPECTS
SUGGESTED READINGS

ADENOVIRUSES

Adenoviruses were first isolated from cultured human adenoid tissues, hence, the name. They have been identified as the etiologic agent in a variety of human infections involving the respiratory, gastrointestinal, and urinary tracts as well as the conjunctiva. The dentist is most likely to encounter adenovirus infection in younger patients in whom pharyngitis is the chief sign. Adenoviruses also have been implicated in infections of immunocompromised patients, particularly in bone marrow and renal transplants. In experimental animals, certain adenovirus strains are oncogenic, but no association with human cancer has been demonstrated.

Structure and Morphology

Adenoviruses are medium sized, measuring 70 to 80 nm, and so-called naked because they lack a lipid envelope. Their DNA is double-stranded and has a molecular weight of 20×10^6 daltons. The protein coat of the virus has an interesting structure, containing a total of 252 capsomeres in icosahedral symmetry, with 240 six-sided capsomeres (hexons) and 12 five-sided capsomeres (pentons) as well as fibers with knobs projecting from each penton (Figure 26–1).

Adenovirus Infections

Pathogenesis. Over 30 different serotypes of adenovirus have been identified. Individuals become infected early in life, and approximately 5% of respiratory illnesses in children under 5 years old are caused by these agents. The symptoms are nonspecific and can be confused with those of a number of other microbial infections. In children older than 5 years, infection may result in a pharyngitis that may mimic strep throat. In fact, many cases of pediatric pharyngitis

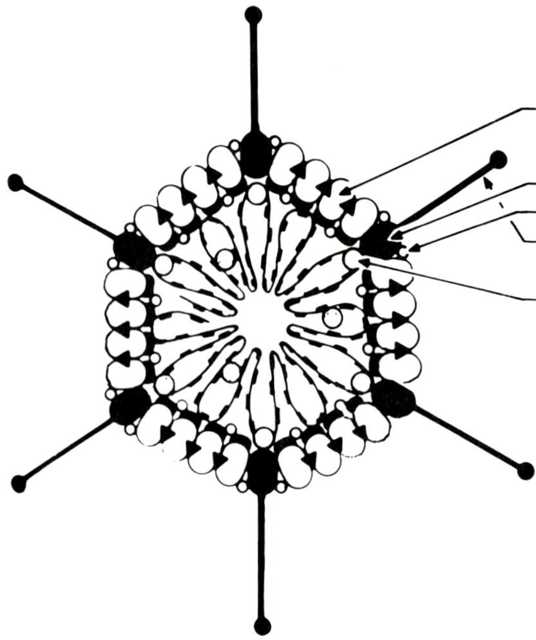

Figure 26–1. A model of adenovirus particle. The virion is composed of an icosahedral capsid containing 252 capsomeres. There are 240 hexons and 12 capsomeres at the vertices, which are referred to as pentons since they have five neighbors. Each contains a penton base and an elongated protein, the fiber projecting out from the penton base. *(From Nierhaus KH. Regulation of adenovirus gene expression.* Curr Top Microbiol Immunol. *1982;97:159.)*

from which bacteria cannot be isolated probably are caused by adenoviruses. A significant proportion of lower respiratory problems in children, such as bronchitis, croup, and pneumonia, may be associated with adenoviral infection.

The first recognized infection associated with adenovirus was an epidemic syndrome unique to military recruits called acute respiratory disease (ARD). Among the symptoms are fever, running nose, cough, pharyngitis, adenitis, and pneumonia in severe cases. This condition occurs when residents of varied geographic origin are crowded together, as occurs in military training. It lasts approximately 10 days, has a low mortality rate, and has not been reported in civilian populations. Types 4 and 7 are the adenoviral subtypes usually associated with ARD.

Pharyngoconjunctival fever is an illness characterized by pharyngitis, conjunctivitis, and fever. Eye involvement is its most distinguishing feature. Because of its association with swimming pools, it is often referred to as swimming pool conjunctivitis. This disease often occurs in sporadic epidemics that can be traced from a single source, a pool or a lake, and has been linked to inadequate chlorination.

Epidemic keratoconjunctivitis was seen first in shipbuilding facilities during the first, and subsequently the second, world wars and therefore was called shipyard eye. At present, it is more common to find outbreaks whose point source is a contaminated ophthalmologic instrument. Adenoviruses are hardy agents, relatively resistant to topical disinfection by alcohols that are used routinely on devices such as tonometers, which contact corneal tissues. These instruments serve to spread the virus among patients. The virus also may be carried by contaminated fingers or ophthalmic ointments or solutions. Unlike the conjunctivitis in pharyngeal conjunctival fever, that of epidemic keratoconjunctivitis may result in more serious and deeper involvement of the eye, which might end in visual impairment. Adenovirus types 8 and 19 have been isolated from a majority of cases.

Adenoviral infection also occurs in patients who have received bone marrow transplants. Graft-versus-host crises often accompany such procedures and may be followed by adenoviral pneumonia and renal infection. The incidence of such infections in bone marrow procedures is about 5%.

Prevention and Treatment. Prevention of some adenovirus infections has been achieved with vaccines, particularly in ARD epidemics in military populations. Initially, inactivated adenovirus vaccines were used against types 4 and 7 with mixed results. A live virus vaccine was developed that was administered orally using enteric coated gelatin capsules. The virus multiplies in the gastrointestinal tract to a limited extent without producing disease but induces serum as well as secretory antiviral antibodies that protect against natural respiratory infections. There have been no efforts to extend this procedure to control other adenovirus infections in either children or immunosuppressed adults. The oncogenic potential of certain adenoviruses in baby hamsters has dampened efforts to use a live viral vaccine.

PAPOVAVIRUSES

The papovaviruses are DNA viruses and include the human papillomavirus, which is associated with benign epithelial proliferations, such as warts, condylomas, and papillomas. These can occur in the oral cavity and represent one of the more common virus-associated lesions encountered by the dentist. Papillomaviruses have been implicated also in squamous cell carcinomas in the skin, oral cavity, and genital tract.

Structure and Morphology

The name papova was derived from three viruses that were shown to share common properties: human papillomavirus (HPV), mouse polyomavirus, and simian vacuolating virus (SV40). These viruses, whose double-stranded DNA has a molecular weight of 3 to 5×10^6 daltons, measure 40 to 50 nm. Their protein coat is composed of 72 capsomeres in icosahedral symmetry, with no lipid envelope. In 1981, the papovavirus family was divided into two new genera based on their relative sizes, *Papillomavirus* and *Miopapovavirus*. Papillomaviruses are larger (55 nm versus 45 nm) and have a larger DNA molecule (3×10^6 versus 5×10^6 molecular weights) than the polyoma and SV40 viruses, now grouped in the miopapovaviruses.

Papillomaviruses

The first virus to be isolated in this genus was the rabbit papillomavirus, which was discovered by Shope. Subsequently, similar viruses have been isolated from human warts and other hyperplastic epithelial lesions, such as papillomas and condylomas. Information on the growth cycle of these viruses is limited because, as yet, no tissue culture system has been found that allows vegetative growth. Papillomaviruses induce tumors of keratinocytes, and although keratinocytes in culture may harbor the virus as a stable replicating episome, there is no viral growth nor are the keratinocytes transformed. At least 50 types of HPV have been detected in various lesions. The typing of HPV was based initially on the absence of serologic cross-reactivity. DNA hybridization techniques have provided a more sensitive mechanism for identifying and distinguishing between various HPV types. There is a tendency for HPV types to be associated with a particular lesion (Table 26–1).

TABLE 26–1. HUMAN PAPILLOMAVIRUS TYPES

Virus	Source
HPV-1	Plantar warts and other verrucae
HPV-2	Hand warts, oral papillomas, carcinoma of tongue, oral verrucous carcinoma
HPV-3, 10	Flat warts
HPV-4	Small verrucae
HPV-5, 8, 9, 12, 14, 15, 20, 22	Papillomas in epidermodysplasia verruciformis (EV)
HPV-6, 11	Venereal warts (condyloma), laryngeal papillomas, leukoplakia (type 11)
HPV-7	Butcher's warts, HIV-associated oral warts
HPV-16, 18	Cervical carcinoma, leukoplakia (type 16), oral carcinoma (type 16), oral papilloma (type 16)

Pathogenesis and Disease Processes. The most common lesion associated with HPV infection is the papilloma. Papillomas are epithelial growths made up of numerous papillary projections that lend a roughened or cauliflower-like surface appearance (Fig 26–2). Papillomas may appear on the skin as warts (verruca vulgaris) or on urogenital skin or oral mucosa as condylomas. Papillomas also may occur as ingrowths or inverted papillomas in salivary gland ducts, larynx, or intestines. The cell tropism of HPV is restricted specifically to keratinizing cells of the epithelium. Electron microscopic examination of plantar warts (on the soles of the feet) and papillomas in rabbits (Fig 26–3) have shown virus particles in the nucleus and occasionally the keratinized cells.

Genital and Oral Papillomas. Genital infection with HPV is one of the four most common sexually transmitted diseases. The estimated annual incidence of genital warts (condylomas) in the United States is almost 1 million cases. Cervical condylomas appear on the genital skin or mucosa of either sex but are more common in women. These lesions are spread venereally, and like other venereal infections, their rate of occurrence is related to the degree of sexual activity and the number of different sexual partners. Virus particles are found in the outermost epithelial cells and are few in number. Papillomavirus DNA was shown in restriction enzyme analysis to be type 6 in two thirds of cases and type 11 in most of the remaining cases. Malignant conversion of condylomas has been reported, and HPV DNA has been detected in these carcinomas. Types 16 and 18 have been identified in over 50% of cervical dysplasias and cervical carcinomas. These two HPV types are associated with only 7% of condylomas but can be detected in most dysplasias and carcinomas-in-situ. The high frequency of HPV DNA in genital carcinomas does not establish their etiologic role conclusively. Epidemiologic and other data point to the involvement of other viruses, such as herpes. Transformation by papillomavirus may require the synergistic effect of other cofactors or carcinogens.

In the oral cavity, hyperplastic epithelial lesions such as papillomas occur frequently, and viral antigens have been demonstrated, usually by immunohistochemistry using antibodies to papillomavirus (Fig 26–4). Complete virus particles have not been seen in most cases, although viral antigens have been demon-

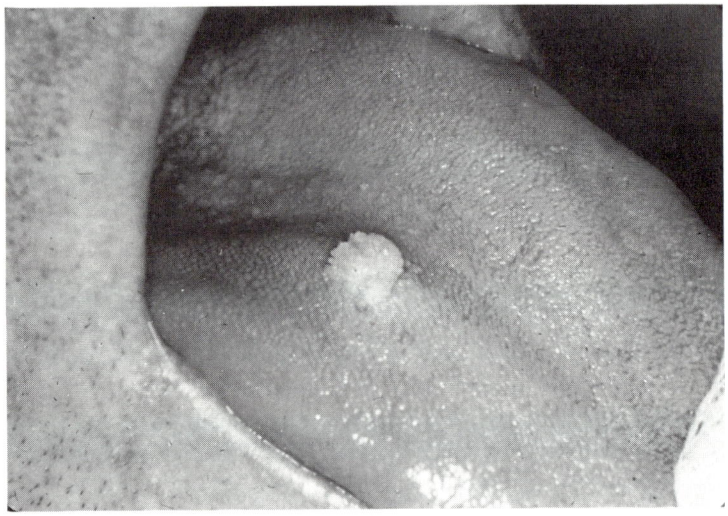

Figure 26–2. Papilloma on the tongue. *(Courtesy of Dr. C. Leifer, Temple University School of Dentistry, Philadelphia, PA.)*

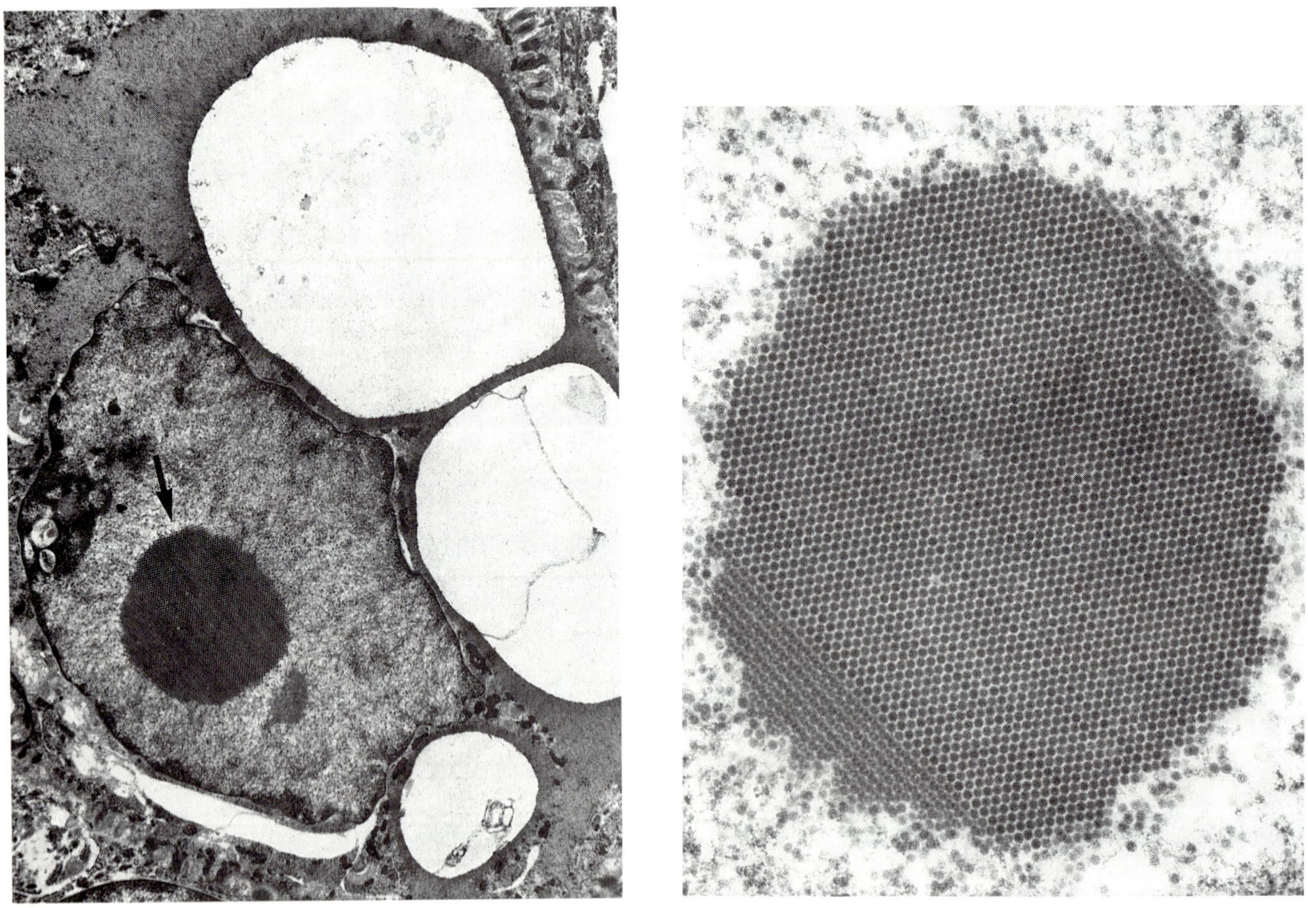

A **B**

Figure 26–3. A. Electron micrograph of papillomavirus particles in the nucleus of upper spinous cell of focal epithelial hyperplasia in the rabbit oral mucosa. ×10,700. **B.** Crystalline viral aggregates of papillomavirus in the nucleus (arrow). ×50,000 *(From Chen S-Y. Focal epithelial hyperplasia in rabbit oral mucosa.* J Oral Pathol. *1979;8:213–223.)*

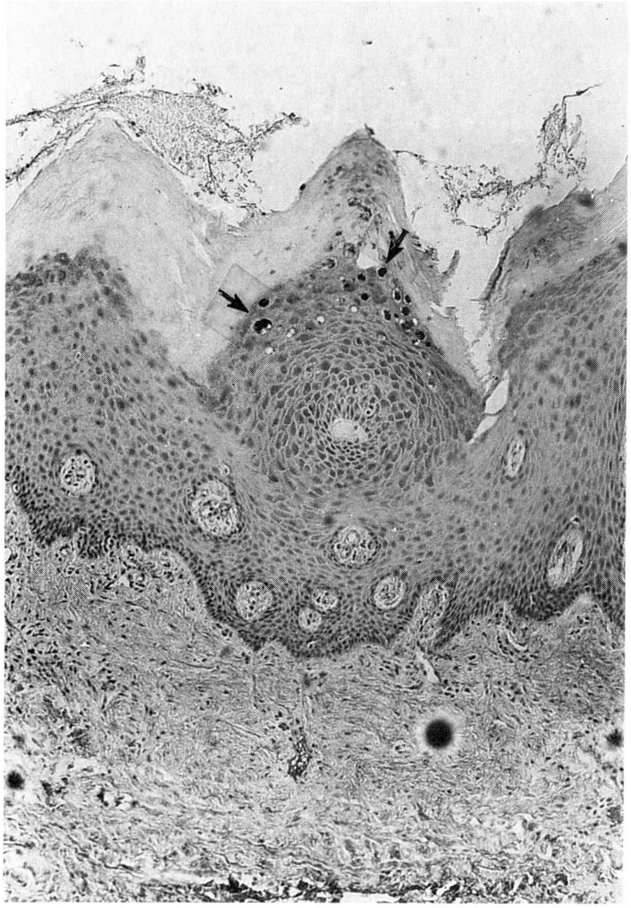

Figure 26–4. Verruca from hard palate. Papillomavirus structural antigens are identified by positive PAP (peroxidase-antiperoxidase) reactions (arrows) in outer squamous epithelial cells. ×197. *(From Jensen AB, et al. Frequency and distribution of papillomavirus structural antigens in verrucae, multiple papillomas and condylomata of the oral cavity.* Am J Pathol. *1982;107:212–218.)*

strated for a majority of condylomas (warts, verrucae) and single or multiple papillomas. More recently, evidence of HPV antigens in other oral epithelial lesions such as leukoplakia has been presented. HPV types 11 and 16 have been identified in these premalignant lesions as well as in certain well-differentiated oral carcinomas.

Respiratory Papillomatosis. The respiratory tract, particularly the larynx, is a common site for papillomas. These lesions can result in hoarseness or voice change, particularly in children under 5 years of age, who are at greatest risk of developing respiratory papillomatosis. Neonates may contract HPV during birth if the mother has genital condylomas. There is a tendency for papillomas to spread from the larynx to the trachea and even the lungs. Persistent recurrence of papillomas is an important feature, which necessitates repeated surgical intervention to maintain an open airway. In comparison to skin warts whose cells are often laden with virus particles, laryngeal papillomas do not contain many virions. Identification of HPV capsid antigens by immunostaining has been positive in about 50% of respiratory papillomas. Detection of viral DNA using more sensitive methods has shown a higher correlation between HPV and respiratory lesions. HPV types 6 and 11 have been detected most often. Malignant conversion of laryngeal papillomas is rare but is more likely to occur in cases of long duration, particularly in juvenile onset conditions.

The role of HPV in human cancer is discussed in Chapter 31.

Treatment. Papillomas and warts have a high rate of spontaneous remission, so that treatment is often not necessary. Curettage performed under local anesthesia and topical application of dessicants are the favored procedures for treatment. Lesions in the oral cavity may be treated by a light application of liquid nitrogen, and the carbon dioxide laser has been used for the removal of cervical condylomas. Multiple recurrences of respiratory papillomas may require the use of antivirals such as interferon.

Polyoma and SV40 Viruses

These viruses are discussed in Chapter 31.

JC and BK Viruses

JC virus was isolated from a case of progressive multifocal leukoencephalopathy (PML), a rare human brain disease characterized by demyelinization of the cerebral white matter. Clinically, there is an insidious loss of neurologic function, with decreased mental acuity, loss of vision, and cranial nerve dysfunction. In most cases, the disease occurs in older patients who have another disease, such as leukemia or lymphoma, or in younger patients with AIDS. Although only about 200 cases of PML have been reported, infection with JC virus is common in the general populace, with 70% of normal adults having antibodies. PML may, therefore, represent reactivation of latent virus. Although this virus induces brain tumors in monkeys, there is no evidence associating JC virus with human malignancies.

BK virus was isolated initially from a renal transplant patient who was on immunosuppressive therapy. Along with JC virus, it is encountered frequently in urinary tract infections, especially where there is stenosis of the ureters. It also is found in renal transplant patients who are given large doses of steroids. BK virus has been implicated in respiratory infections in children, where the only evidence was the detection of viral DNA in their tonsillar tissues.

PARVOVIRUSES

Most members of the parvoviruses infect animals other than humans. Human parvovirus (B19) infection is widespread, since antibodies have been detected in 50% of healthy blood donors. Two illnesses in humans, aplastic crisis and fifth disease, have been attributed to this DNA virus.

Structure, Morphology, and Classification

Parvoviruses are the smallest of the DNA viruses. Membership in this group is based on morphology and uniqueness in nucleic acid structure. Their DNA is single-stranded. The viruses measure 18 to 26 nm in diameter and contain 32 capsids in icosahedral symmetry. The virus lacks a lipid envelope and thus is resistant to ether. In susceptible cells, multiplication is limited to the nucleus. The Parvoviridae family is subdivided into three genera: *Parvovirus, Dependovirus,* and *Densovirus.* Only the *Parvovirus* and *Dependovirus* contain agents that are found in humans. *Densovirus* infects insects.

Human Parvoviruses

The B19 parvovirus, because of its small genetic capacity (only 5000 bases), replicates primarily in actively dividing cells, such as erythroid cells in the bone marrow. Infection occurs only in persons with chronic hemolytic diseases, such as sickle cell anemia or thalassemia. Transient aplastic crisis is characterized by a short-lived arrest of erythropoiesis, with rapidly worsening anemia. Although recovery usually occurs within 1 to 2 weeks, the severe anemia may require transfusion. Children are particularly prone to such episodes. B19 parvovirus has been isolated consistently from serum, and elevated anti-B19 antibodies have been detected in affected individuals.

A more common disease entity that has been associated with parvovirus is erythema infectiosum, or fifth disease. This condition occurs most commonly as epidemics in children. The most striking clinical feature is an erythematous rash that usually begins on the face and then appears on the trunk and extremities. There are few constitutional symptoms except for arthralgia, which may be experienced by adult patients. Parvovirus has been isolated from the sera of affected patients, and elevations in antibodies have been measured. Recently, parvovirus infection has been cited as an etiologic factor in rheumatoid arthritis.

Adenosatellite Viruses (Dependovirus)

These viruses are defective and cannot multiply autonomously in susceptible cells unles another (helper) virus is present. The helper virus usually is an adenovirus and occasionally herpesvirus. Dependoviruses require rapidly multiplying cells for replication and are found commonly as contaminants of viral stocks and from certain tumors. They are only of interest to laboratory researchers studying the dynamics of viral replication and have not been associated directly with any human disease.

POXVIRUSES

The best known poxvirus is variola virus, the agent of smallpox. It has been officially declared eradicated by the World Health Organization, the result of a successful vaccination program. Smallpox is of historic importance because no case of natural human infection has been reported since 1978. Smallpox was responsible for devastating epidemics, particularly in the seventeenth and eighteenth centuries. In 1776, an English country physician, Edward Jenner, introduced the first vaccine. He had observed that prior infection with the relatively mild cowpox virus conferred complete resistance to the deadly smallpox. Jenner introduced the first virus vaccine by scraping material from cowpox lesions and using it to inoculate the general populace. His procedure was successful, and the name, vaccination, coined from the latin *vacca* for cow, serves as a permanent reminder of its bovine origin. The original cowpox strain used by Jenner has mutated or been contaminated so that is no longer identical to present-day cowpox strains. The vaccine strain of poxvirus is called vaccinia virus to mark this distinction. The eradication of smallpox has largely eliminated the need for vaccination. The only people who require smallpox vaccination are laboratory workers directly involved in handling the virus or other closely related poxviruses. Molluscum contagiosum and cowpox are the major pox diseases in humans.

Structure and Morphology

The poxviruses are the largest of the DNA viruses and the most complex in structure. They measure 250 by 400 nm, are brick-shaped, and lack the symmetrical capsid morphology seen in the other DNA viruses that infect humans (Fig 26–5). In the infected cell, poxviruses multiply in the cytoplasm, where they produce alterations that are seen as inclusion bodies.

Vaccinia Virus

The present-day vaccinia virus is used in smallpox vaccines, and severe human infection may result following vaccination. The curtailment in vaccine use has resulted in a decreased incidence in vaccinia infection. Individuals who are at extreme risk include those with immunodeficiencies, pregnant women, and those who suffer from skin allergies, such as eczema. In normal vaccination, vaccinia virus undergoes limited multiplication, with minor vesiculation at the local site that scabs over and heals in a few days. In generalized vaccinia, there is extensive virus

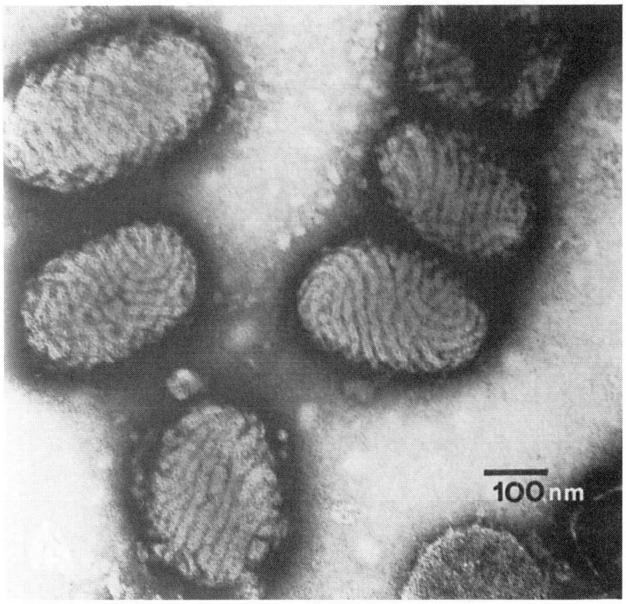

Figure 26–5. Electron micrograph of poxvirus. A. Milker's node virus stained with phosphotungstic acid. *(Courtesy of Dr. John A. Holowczak, Rutgers Medical School, Piscataway, NJ.)*

replication, the area of vesiculation is extensive, and there is widespread skin necrosis. The virus may spread to other organs and produce encephalitis or pneumonitis, with a resulting high mortality.

Molluscum Contagiosum

Molluscum contagiosum is a benign skin condition with characteristic clinical appearance. The virus of molluscum replicates in the cytoplasm of the prickle and granular cell layers and stimulates mitotic activity in the basal cell layer. This results in a raised lesion with a central crater. Histologically, there is downgrowth of hyperplastic epithelium into the dermis. Cytoplasmic inclusion bodies (molluscum bodies) are sites of the poxvirus multiplication. This virus only has been identified morphologically and has not been grown in tissue culture. The disease usually occurs in children and is characterized by the appearance of painless, wartlike papules on the skin, usually on the face, trunk, and anogenital areas. The oral cavity is only rarely involved, and lesions do not develop on the hands or soles of the feet, distinguishing them from the lesions of papillomavirus. The epithelial growths may persist for months, but spontaneous regression usually ensues without any scarring. Molluscum contagiosum has been reported in epidemic form, particularly in institutions or family groups, where the virus is easily spread by direct contact or through contaminated fomites.

Treatment. Generalized vaccinia virus infection has been treated with immune globulin or interferon with only limited success. Vaccinia is one of the favored vectors for the administration of vaccines developed from recombinant DNA, so that more widespread usage is possible. Before its eradication, smallpox was successfully treated with ARA-A.

Other Poxviral Infections

The rest of the poxviruses include agents that primarily infect animals and humans are infected accidentally. These include cowpox (milker's nodes) and contagious pustular dermatitis contracted from sheep and caused by orf virus. These infections usually are limited to the skin, where the viruses produce pocklike lesions resulting from the proliferation of basal cells and degeneration of other epidermal cells. These lesions heal spontaneously without scarring.

ORAL ASPECTS

The DNA viruses discussed in this chapter, the adenoviruses, papovaviruses, parvoviruses, and poxviruses, are associated with a variety of infections. Adenoviruses cause pharyngeal and ophthalmic infections, usually in epidemic form. Papillomaviruses produce benign epithelial neoplasms that are commonly found in the genital and respiratory tracts as well as the oral cavity. The association of papillomaviruses with malignancy is discussed in Chapter 31. Parvovirus infection may result in aplastic crises and fifth disease, and poxviruses produce the skin infections of molluscum contagiosum and cowpox. The most common virus in this group that the dentist is most likely to encounter is the human papillomavirus, which is associated with oral papillomas and condylomas.

SUGGESTED READINGS

Foy HM, Grayston JT. Adenoviruses. In: Evans AS, ed. *Viral Infections of Humans, Epidemiology and Control.* 2nd ed. New York: Plenum; 1984:67–84.

Greenspan D, de Villiers EM, Greenspan JS, et al. Unusual HPV types in oral warts in association with HIV infection. *J Oral Pathol.* 1988;17:482–487.

Katz SL. Poxviruses. In: Joklik WK, Willett HP, Amos DB, eds. *Zinsser Microbiology.* 18th ed. Norwalk, Conn.: Appleton-Century-Crofts; 1984:991–995.

Krebs H-B, ed. Genital human papillomavirus infection. *Clin Obstet Gynecol.* 1989;32:105–213.

Milde K, Loning T. Detection of papillomavirus DNA in oral papillomas and carcinomas: Application of in situ hybridization with biotinylated HPV 16 probes. *J Oral Pathol.* 1986;15:292–296.

Moss B, Flexner C. Vaccinia virus expression vectors. *Annu Rev Immunol.* 1987;5:305–324.

Mounts P, Shah KV. Respiratory papillomatosis: Etiological relation to genital tract papillomaviruses. *Prog Med Virol.* 1984;29:90–114.

Young N. Hematologic consequences of B19 Parvovirus infection. *Semin Hematol.* 1988;25:159–172.

CHAPTER 27

Orthomyxoviruses and Paramyxoviruses

Walter K. Long

MYXOVIRUSES
ORTHOMYXOVIRUSES
Viral Structure
Pathogenesis
Epidemiology
Prevention and Treatment
PARAMYXOVIRUSES
Viral Structure
Parainfluenza Virus
Respiratory Syncytial Virus
Mumps Virus
Measles Virus
ORAL ASPECTS
SUGGESTED READINGS

MYXOVIRUSES

Myxoviruses are helical enveloped viruses with single negative-stranded RNA genomes. The replicative cycle requires the generation of positive strands of RNA complementary to the virus genome. This is achieved using a virion-associated transcriptase. The resulting positive strands serve as mRNA and as a template for the synthesis of new negative-stranded viral genomes. Two families of myxoviruses have been described, the Orthomyxoviridae and the Paramyxoviridae.

ORTHOMYXOVIRUSES

Virus Structure

Members of this virus family include influenza viruses types A, B, and C. In addition to the previously described features, there are several characteristics unique to orthomyxoviruses that differentiate these agents from paramyxoviruses. The genome is composed of single-stranded RNA with a molecular weight of approximately 6×10^6 daltons. In influenza virus types A and B, this RNA exists as eight separate segments, and as seven segments in type C influenza viruses. Each genome segment is associated with its own helical capsid, which is composed of the internal viral protein NP. A complete complement of genome segments and their associated capsids are enclosed in a lipoprotein envelope, the basic matrix of which is the M protein, and the lipid component of which consists primarily of phospholipid and unesterified cholesterol (Fig 27–1). The precise lipid composition resembles that of the host cell plasma membranes from which the envelope is derived in the replication process.

The virus type, A, B, or C, is determined by the NP and M proteins. Two antigenically distinct types of glycoprotein projections, or spikes, termed hemagglutinin and neuraminidase, protrude from the surface of the envelope. These structures determine the antigenic subtype of virus. Protective antibodies are directed against these structures. Therefore, antigenic changes in these proteins can have significant consequences with respect to potential for initiating an epidemic.

Pathogenesis

Influenza virus initially infects and replicates in cells lining the upper respiratory tract, killing ciliated co-

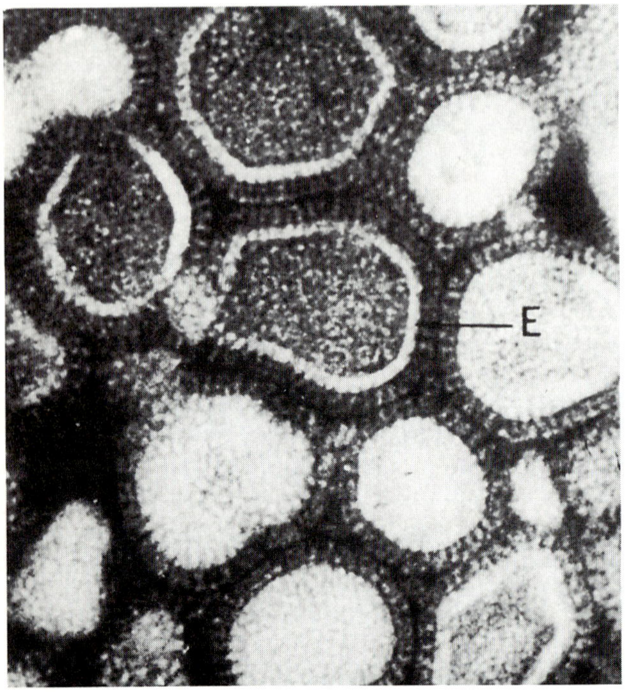

Figure 27–1. Electron micrograph of intact influenza virus particles embedded in phosphotungstate, showing the variation in size and shape. The hemagglutinin and neuraminidase spikes are visible as projections on the envelope (E) of the particles. *(From Hoyle L, Horne RW, Waterson HP.* Virology. *1961;13:4484.)*

lumnar epithelial cells. Many of the symptoms of the disease are a direct result of this cellular destruction. Nonspecific host defenses are impaired by the loss of these ciliated cells, facilitating deeper invasion of the respiratory tract by the influenza virus. This may lead to influenzal pneumonia or bacterial superinfection.

Infection generally occurs via ingestion or inhalation of droplets containing infectious virus. Clinical signs of infection appear within 1 to 3 days and include fever, chills, muscular aches, headache, malaise, and loss of appetite. Other possible symptoms include sore throat, conjunctivitis, and congestion. The course of the disease usually is uncomplicated, with resolution occurring within 1 week. However, in a minority of cases, serious complications can occur. The most serious of these are the pneumonias brought on by bacterial superinfection or the influenza virus itself. Groups at highest risk include those with severe chronic disorders of the cardiovascular or pulmonary systems and residents of nursing homes or other chronic care facilities. The majority of influenza deaths are attributable to bacterial pneumonias, and a considerably smaller number are attributable to pneumonia of an influenza virus etiology, with about 90% of the deaths occurring among individuals age 65 or older.

Epidemiology

Influenza epidemics occur periodically and usually spread rapidly around the world. The reasons for these observations can be attributed to the molecular biology of the influenza virion. Changes in the antigenic makeup of the virion's hemagglutinin (H) and neuraminidase (N) glycoproteins play a significant role in the dynamics of these epidemics. Five different subtypes of the hemagglutinin antigen have been identified in type A human influenza viruses. Two subtypes of the neuraminidase antigen have been identified in type A viruses, whereas all type B viruses thus far isolated appear to be variants of a single subtype.

The segmented nature of the influenza genome promotes the development of new subtypes of virus. This occurs when a host is simultaneously infected with two subtypes, which can result in replication of both viral types in a single cell. The resulting progeny will possess 1 to 8 genome segments from one parent and the rest from the other parental strain. If the gene segment coding for hemagglutinin is derived from one subtype and the gene segment coding for neuraminidase is derived from the second subtype, an antigenic subtype different from either parent is created. Such a major change is referred to as an antigenic shift. Theoretically, this event could take place in a human coinfected with two different subtypes of influenza A virus. In actuality, greater potential for significant antigenic shift exists when a nonhuman species is simultaneously infected with a subtype endogenous to the particular species and a human subtype. The new recombinant subtypes usually differ significantly from previous human subtypes and may possess the potential to ignite a substantial epidemic. Indeed, this appears to be the case with the virus responsible for the great pandemic of 1918–1919 and the various Asian flu epidemics of more recent years, where viruses with new hemaglutinin (H) specificities appeared. Antigenic characterization of these HA proteins indicates that they are similar to Hs of swine, equine, and duck origin.

Less dramatic antigenic drift results from the mutation of subtypes, with the creation of antigenic variants. Increasing divergence from the original subtype results over time from additional mutations that normally take place.

An individual's first experience with an influenza A virus results in clinical infection and the development of immunity to the particular subtype. This immunity extends to closely related variants, with diminishing effectiveness as the variants diverge from the original protective immunogen. In general, protection does not extend to other subtypes. However, if the second virus shares the same hemagglutinin or neuraminidase subtype, the severity of the illness may be lessened.

Prevention and Treatment

An effective inactivated influenza vaccine is available. Whole virus vaccine is prepared by growing virus in embryonated chicken eggs, followed by purification and inactivation. Split virus vaccines, which are preferred for certain populations, are prepared by dissociating viral particles and purifying the neuraminidase and hemagglutinin subunits. In any given year, the decision on which strains to include in that year's vaccine is determined by an analysis of the strains isolated during the preceding year and an assessment of their potential for producing an epidemic.

Highest priority groups for receiving the vaccine include persons with severe chronic disorders of the cardiovascular or pulmonary systems and residents of nursing homes and other chronic care facilities. Dental care personnel can serve as a source of infection during an epidemic and, therefore, should be immunized. This is particularly true of those who have contact with any of the high-risk patient populations previously described. If sufficient vaccine is available, its administration to populations at a moderately high risk is recommended. These include healthy individuals over 65 years of age and adults as well as children with chronic metabolic disease, renal dysfunction, anemia, or asthma that is severe enough to have required medical attention during the previous year.

The vaccine is available in two forms, a split virus vaccine and a whole virus vaccine, with the split virus vaccine inducing fewer febrile reactions. For this reason, this subunit form of the vaccine is recommended for children under 12 years of age. With adults, a single dose of the vaccine is sufficient to induce immunity, since essentially all adults have had previous exposure to influenza virus and have thus been immunologically primed for an anamnestic response. Children, on the other hand, may not have been exposed previously. Therefore, it is recommended that children under 12 years of age be given two doses of vaccine at least 4 weeks apart. Side effects of the influenza immunization are generally of the mild febrile variety, although anaphylactic reactions can occur in individuals with allergies to egg proteins, traces of which may remain in the vaccine even after the purification procedure. It is recommended that persons with such a medical history not be given this vaccine.

Although not as effective as influenza vaccine in preventing disease, the antiviral agent amantadine hydrochloride has been shown to be 70% to 80% effective in preventing illness caused by type A influenza viruses and, during an outbreak of infections, can be administered prophylactically to individuals who might be allergic to the vaccine. For those individuals for whom vaccination is recommended but who for some reason have not been immunized, short-term protection against influenza A infection during an epidemic can be provided by amantadine and longer-term protection by concurrent administration of the vaccine.

Amantadine therapy also has been shown to reduce the severity of influenza A infections if administered within 24 to 48 hours after the onset of symptoms and continuing for at least 48 hours after the resolution of the illness. This treatment is recommended for all high-risk individuals who manifest signs and symptoms suggestive of influenza regardless of whether they have received the vaccine. It must be noted that this drug is ineffective against influenza B.

PARAMYXOVIRUSES

Viral Structure

Human pathogens in this family include the parainfluenza, mumps, rubeola (measles), and respiratory syncytial viruses. In contrast to the influenza virus, the genomes of all viruses of this group are unsegmented single strands of RNA with a molecular weight of 5 to 6 $\times$ 10^6 daltons, each associated with a helical capsid that is composed of the protein NP. The envelope that surrounds the nucleocapsid consists of lipid derived from host cell plasma membranes and a matrix (M) protein. Like the influenza virus, surface projections on the envelope, called spikes, are observed. However, unlike influenza, only one type is present, which consists of two glycoproteins—the HN, which has hemagglutinin and neuraminidase activities, and the F protein, which induces hemolysis and cell fusion. Although similar in structure and chemical makeup, the various paramyxoviruses differ antigenically.

Parainfluenza Virus

Pathogenesis. Infection with these agents is via the respiratory route, with the first clinical signs appearing after an incubation period of 1 to 6 days. During this time, viral replication usually is limited to the upper respiratory tract, with involvement of the lower respiratory tract in a relatively small number of patients.

The severity of symptoms is to a large degree a function of the extent of viral invasion of the respiratory tract. The disease can range from asymptomatic, particularly in adults or individuals with a prior experience, to a mild respiratory infection, to laryngotracheobronchitis (croup), bronchiolitis, and pneumonia. The last infections are most likely to occur in infants or young children without prior exposure to the virus. However, even in infants, most infections are subclinical.

Epidemiology, Prevention, and Control. These agents are spread primarily by respiratory secretions, either by inhalation of aerosols or by hand contact with contaminated surfaces, followed by transfer to appropriate orifices. Peak occurrence during the colder seasons correlates well with that of other respiratory pathogens.

Protection against infection appears to depend primarily on the presence of secretory IgA antibodies in nasal secretions directed against the F protein. Attempts to develop a vaccine have thus far been unsuccessful.

Preventing transmission of these viruses to high-risk individuals, such as hospitalized infants or young children, is highly desirable and can be facilitated by isolating children with respiratory symptoms. Persons with patient contact should wash their hands often and wear a mask whenever they have respiratory symptoms.

Respiratory Syncytial Virus

Pathogenesis. There are at least three antigenic variants of respiratory syncytial virus (RSV), with a considerable degree of cross-reactivity among all isolates.

Infection appears to occur primarily by the respiratory route via inhalation of aerosolized virus or transmission by hands contaminated with virus. Primary replication of the virus takes place in epithelial cells that line the upper respiratory tract, from which it can spread to the bronchi, bronchioli, and pulmonary parenchyma. First clinical symptoms appear 1 to 4 days after infection, with the specific signs and their severity being largely dependent on the tissues involved. RSV is a major lower respiratory pathogen in infants and children. A primary infection with the virus, particularly in infants less than 6 months old, can lead to a relatively severe bronchiolitis or pneumonia, requiring hospitalization. Most children experience a much milder upper respiratory infection, and infections of adults are generally subclinical.

Severity of infection, in general, is dependent on the immune status of the individual, with those infants whose mothers possess only low levels of immunity to RSV experiencing the most serious infections. Higher levels of passive immunity usually result in limited upper respiratory, common cold symptoms. Protection against reinfection depends on the presence of SIgA antibodies, which are relatively short-lived. Therefore, children and adults are susceptible to numerous reinfections, which in the presence of partial immunity, lead to mild illnesses or an infection without any clinical manifestations.

Epidemiology, Prevention, and Control. Epidemics of RSV infections occur yearly during the winter and spring months, with clinical disease appearing in susceptible infants and children and quite possibly subclinical or mild infection of large numbers of adults. Upward of 30% of all infants are infected during the first year of life, with few if any children not being infected by age 6. The most common source of virus probably is by hand transfer of infectious materials, followed by droplet infection, with aerosols implicated to a far lesser degree. It is most important to prevent the infection of compromised infants, since this carries an increased risk of morbidity and mortality. Numerous reports have appeared on the nosocomial spread of RSV, with up to 45% of infants hospitalized for other reasons being infected during an epidemic. Studies have revealed that reducing the number of beds on a ward and frequent handwashing by staff are the most effective means of lowering infectivity rates among hospitalized children.

At present, there are no vaccines available for RSV. Aerosolized ribavarin has been shown to be effective in reducing the severity of RSV infections and is approved for treatment of severe infections.

Mumps Virus

Pathogenesis. The mumps virus, usually in salivary droplets, enters the body via the respiratory and oral routes, infecting the respiratory tract epithelium and cervical lymph nodes. Following viral replication in cells at these sites, a primary viremia is established that seeds the salivary glands and other organs, which can include the testes, ovaries, pancreas, and meninges. Replication in these tissues and perhaps others results in cellular degeneration and inflammation, together with the production of infectious virus that causes a secondary viremia with an accompanying viruria (Fig 27–2).

The clinical manifestation most commonly associated with mumps is swollen salivary glands, particularly the parotids, which appears 2 to 3 weeks after initial exposure (Fig 27–3). This inflammation, which may be unilateral or bilateral, usually is resolved within 1 week but may be followed by more serious complications.

One complication of mumps is orchitis, a painful inflammation and swelling of the testes, which occurs in approximately 25% of all infections involving postpubertal males. In about 95% of these cases, it is unilateral and has minimal effect if any on fertility.

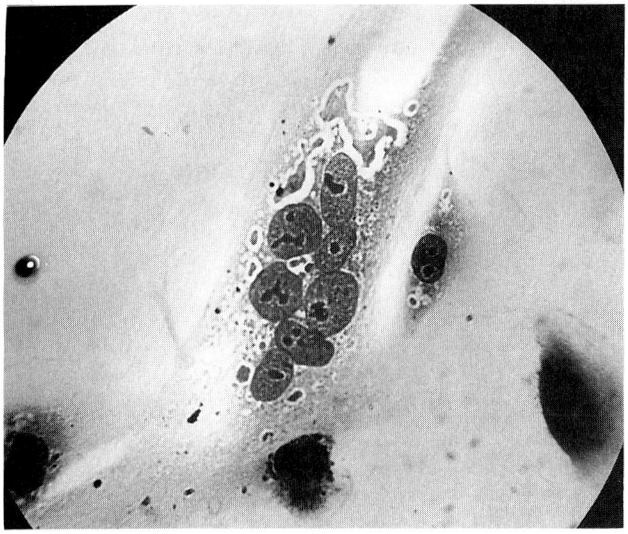

Figure 27–2. Monkey kidney cells 8 days after infection with mumps virus. Note the presence of cytoplasmic inclusions and the formation of giant cells. H&E. ×450. *(From Brandt CD.* Virology. *1961;14:1.)*

However, in those instances where it is bilateral, sterility can result, although it is a rare consequence. CNS involvement may be quite common, although the symptoms are usually inconsequential, with fewer than 0.5% of all cases resulting in meningoencephalitis, which can be fatal. Infection of other tissues may lead to temporary functional abnormalities that are resolved on recovery. It should be noted that many mumps infections are subclinical.

Epidemiology, Prevention, and Control. The mumps virus is present in saliva before the onset of symptoms and continues to be secreted for up to 15 days. Although less infectious than measles and chickenpox, mumps is still quite contagious, resulting in the infection of most nonimmune individuals during childhood in the absence of an immunization program.

A significant reduction in the numbers of cases of mumps reported annually in the United States has resulted from large-scale immunization of children. The vaccine, which is composed of live attenuated virus, is almost 100% effective in inducing protective antibodies in children more than 1 year old. Establishing a primary infection of its own, the vaccine virus provides long-term protection without the viremia and symptoms associated with the wild-type virus. Although fetal infection has not been reported, there is always that possibility with a live virus vaccine. Thus it is recommended that the immunization of pregnant women be avoided.

Nonimmune dental professionals are at increased risk for mumps infections. Anyone practicing dentistry who is unsure of his or her immune status should be tested for antibodies and be immunized if

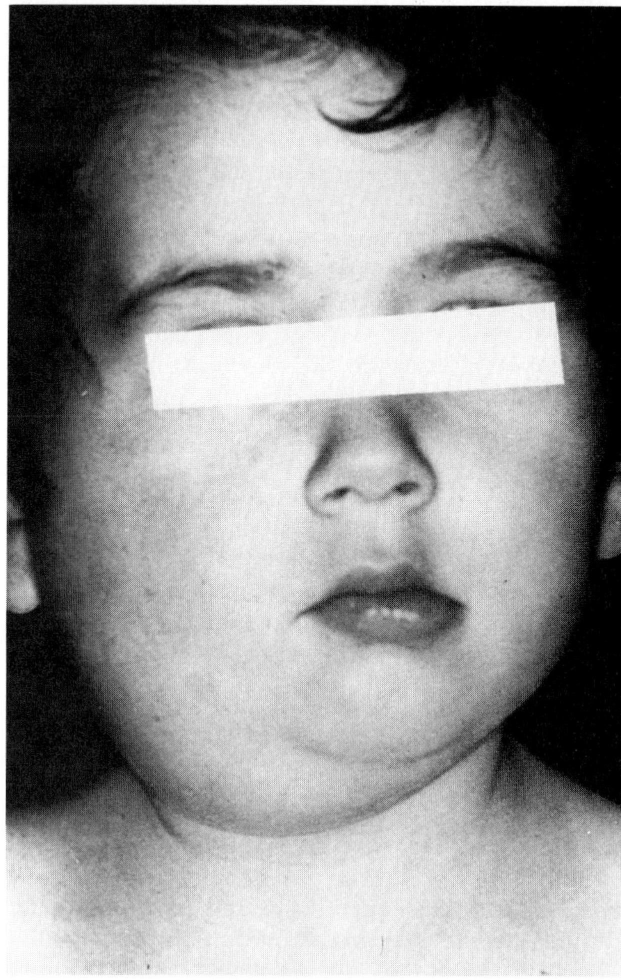

Figure 27–3. Swollen parotid glands. Inflammation of the parotid glands is a hallmark of clinical mumps virus infection. *(From Emond RT.* Color Atlas of Infectious Diseases. *Chicago, Ill: Year Book; 1974.)*

seronegative. Treatment of patients with symptoms of mumps should be avoided unless an emergency situation exists, in which case, gloves and mask should be used. Any nonimmune dentist who is exposed to mumps should consider having mumps hyperimmune globulin administered to reduce the risk of serious complications.

Measles Virus

Pathogenesis. Measles virus, also known as rubeola, is one of the most highly transmissible of all infectious agents. Patients typically experience profuse respiratory secretions that contain virus and are probably the primary source of infectious virus. Infection occurs when virus comes in contact with respiratory tract membranes through direct contact with infectious secretions or droplets. Initial replication takes place in the epithelium of the upper respiratory tract and regional lymphoid tissues, resulting in a viremia that facilitates the spread of virus to more distant sites, including lymphoid tissue. Additional replication takes place at these sites, as evidenced by the presence of virus and multinucleated giant cells, which are characteristic of measles viral replication. A secondary viremia seeds other organs, including the skin, where a characteristic rash appears.

The first symptoms of measles, which appear 10 to 14 days after infection, include a mild fever, coryza, a nonproductive cough, sore throat, conjunctivitis, photophobia, and headache. Koplik's spots, which consist of bright red areas of inflammation, each with a small whitish spot in the center, appear on the buccal mucosa (Fig 27–4). Examination of tissue from these lesions reveals multinucleated giant cells containing the measles virus. Other erythematous diseases are, on occasion, misdiagnosed as measles, and finding Koplik's spots, which are pathognomonic of measles, ensures the accuracy of the diagnosis.

The characteristic measles rash appears 2 to 3 days after the onset of the early symptoms, beginning on the head and spreading to the trunk and extremities over the next 3 days. Erythema is thought to represent a cell-mediated hypersensitivity reaction in which sensitized lymphocytes attack virus-infected cells in the skin. Following onset of the rash, the fever subsides, and subsequently the reddish hue of the erythema fades to a more brownish color, which is followed by a return to normal skin coloration.

Recovery from measles usually is uneventful. Bacterial superinfections, however, can occur and have been implicated in such complications as otitis media, sinusitis, and pneumonia. A much more serious illness, encephalomyelitis, occurs in approximately 1 in 2000 cases. The actual numbers are somewhat lower in healthy children and higher in older children, adults, and children whose health is compromised by malnourishment or other factors. Fatality rates of 10 to 15% have been reported, and tissue damage severe enough to cause long-term physical and mental problems occur in up to 50% of those who survive. A far rarer complication, subacute sclerosing panencephalitis (SSPE), occurs several years after the initial measles infection. Symptoms of the disease include loss of various mental and motor functions. In SSPE, antibodies to the measles virus are found in the cerebrospinal fluid, and the presence of viral antigens and viral RNA can be demonstrated in brain cells.

Epidemiology, Prevention, and Control. The measles virus is a highly infectious agent that is readily transmitted to nonimmune individuals. Virus is present in respiratory secretions, tears, and urine before the onset of clinical illness. Thus, any of these represents a potential source of infection. Measles epidemics generally occur during the winter and spring every 2 to 3 years in the urban setting and less often in rural areas. These dynamics are determined by the numbers of susceptible individuals needed to sustain an epidemic.

Because none of the present antivirals are effective in the treatment of measles, the emphasis is on prevention of infection. Dental treatment of individuals should be postponed until recovery except in emergency situations. A live attenuated virus vaccine is available. It is administered by injection to children over 1 year of age to avoid interference by maternally acquired antibodies. This vaccine has reduced the incidence of measles by more than 90%. Lax enforcement of requirements for vaccination before entering school has resulted in sporadic measles outbreaks in several communities.

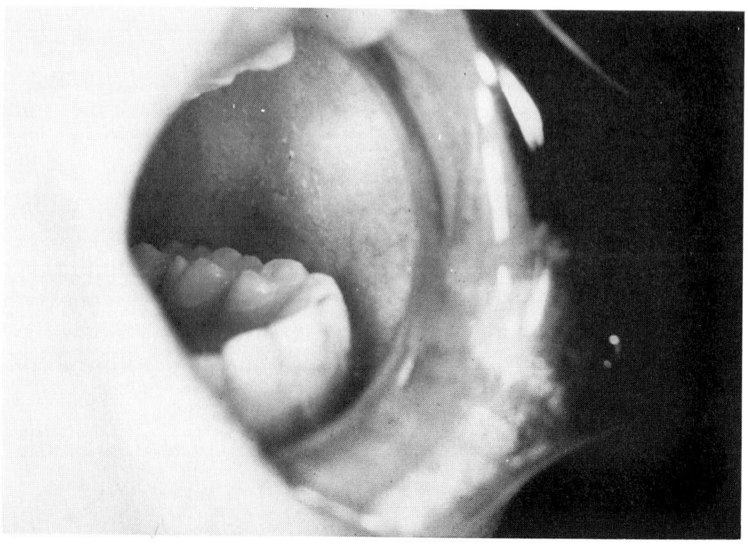

Figure 27–4. Koplik spots. These small grayish white patches on the buccal mucosa are pathognomonic of measles viral infection. *(Courtesy of G. Blozis.)*

ORAL ASPECTS

All of the viruses discussed in this chapter are transmitted either orally or via the respiratory tract. Oral manifestations are evident in two of the infections, Koplik's spots in measles and swollen parotid glands in mumps. Dentists should be aware of the potential that exists for the transmission of influenza in the dental operatory and take appropriate measures to reduce the risk.

SUGGESTED READINGS

Centers for Disease Control. Prevention and control of influenza. *MMWR.* 1984;33:254–266.

Centers for Disease Control. Mumps prevention. *MMWR.* 1989;38:388–400.

Colman PM, Ward CW. Structure and diversity of influenza virus neuraminidase. *Curr Top Microbiol Immunol.* 1985; 114:177–255.

Couch RB, Kasel JA. Immunity to influenza in man. *Annu Rev Microbiol.* 1983;37:529–549.

Douglas RG Jr. Antiviral drugs 1983. *Med Clin North Am.* 1983;67:1163–1175.

Hall CB. The nosocomial spread of respiratory syncytial viral infections. *Annu Rev Med.* 1983;34:311–319.

Hall WW, Choppin PW. Measles virus proteins in the brain tissue of patients with subacute sclerosing panencephalitis. *N Engl J Med.* 1981;304:1152.

Henderson FW, Collier AM, Clyde WA Jr, et al. Respiratory syncytial virus infections, reinfections and immunity: A prospective longitudinal study in young children. *N Engl J Med.* 1979;300:530–534.

Hethcote HW. Measles and rubella in the United States. *Am J Epidemiol.* 1983;117:2–11.

Lamb RA, Choppin PW. The gene structure and replication of influenza virus. *Annu Rev Biochem.* 1983;52:467–506.

Markowitz LE, Preblud SR, Orenstein WA, et al. Patterns of transmission in measles outbreaks in the United States, 1985–1986. *N Engl J Med.* 1989;320:75–81.

Ward CW. Structure of the influenza virus hemagglutinin. *Curr Top Microbiol Immunol.* 1981;94/95:1–74.

CHAPTER 28

Picornaviruses, Coronaviruses, and Reoviruses

Walter K. Long

PICORNAVIRUSES
- General Characteristics
- Poliovirus
- Coxsackievirus
- Echovirus
- Rhinovirus

CORONAVIRUSES
- Pathogenesis
- Epidemiology and Prevention

REOVIRUSES
- Pathogenesis, Epidemiology, and Control

SUGGESTED READINGS

PICORNAVIRUSES

General Characteristics

Picornaviruses include the agent most often implicated in the common cold, and the etiologic agent of poliomyelitis. The control of polio marked one of the great triumphs of medical science, but the search for a cure to the common cold continues to baffle medical scientists.

Picornaviruses can be divided into two groups, the enteroviruses and the rhinoviruses, which infect the intestinal tract and upper respiratory tract, respectively. The enteroviruses are further subdivided into the polioviruses, of which there are 3 serotypes, the coxsackie A viruses, with 23 serotypes, coxsackie B viruses, with 6 serotypes, and echoviruses, with 30 serotypes.

Virions of all of the picornaviruses are quite similar in their physical and chemical characteristics. They are 25 to 30 nm diameter icosahedrons without envelopes (Fig 28–1). Genomes are nonsegmented, single-stranded RNA, with a molecular weight of approximately 2.6×10^6 daltons, which has a positive polarity and thus serves as mRNA during viral replication. Among the most resilient viruses, they are stable at room temperature for an extended period of time and are resistant to the effects of ether and other lipid solvents. The enteroviruses, but not the rhinoviruses, are stable under conditions as acidic as pH 3.

Poliovirus

Pathogenesis. Infection is generally by ingestion of materials that have been contaminated with the virus and is followed by primary virus replication in tissues of the oropharynx and intestines. Much of the virus produced is excreted in the feces, which in turn serve as a major source of infection. Virus also can be found in the throat and saliva at this time. Virus is then taken up by local lymph nodes, subsequently entering the bloodstream. From the blood, virus can enter the CNS, infecting a variety of tissues, with neurologic symptoms ensuing. The anterior horn cells of the spinal cord are most commonly infected, with the

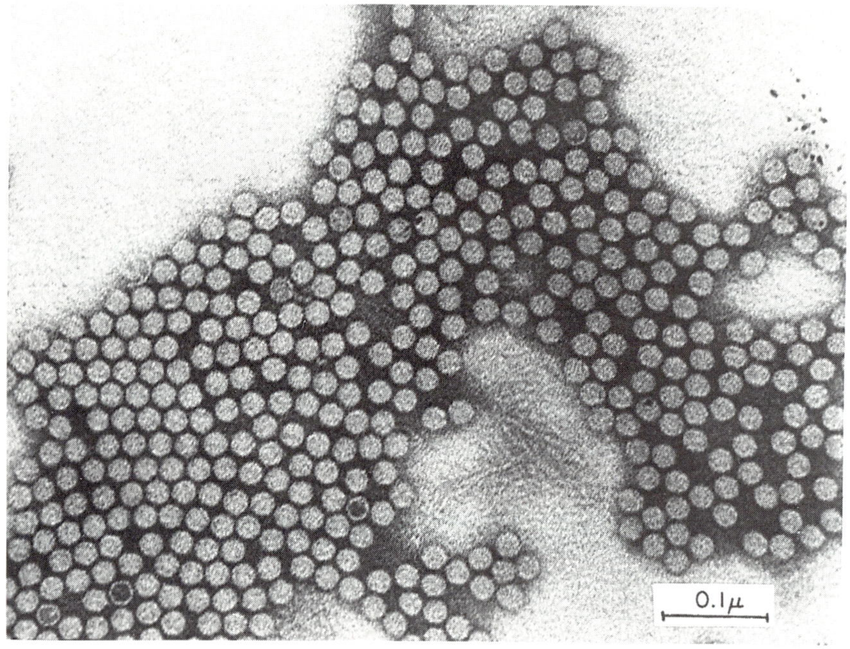

Figure 28–1. Electron micrograph of a purified preparation of poliovirus reveals numerous nonenveloped icosahedral viral particles. Mag. ×150,000. *(Courtesy of H. D. Mayor.)*

medulla, brainstem, and cortex less frequently involved. Paralytic disease is most often associated with infection of anterior horn cells. Most fatalities, however, occur when lesions are present in the medulla or brainstem, where respiratory and cardiac functions are most likely to be affected.

The normal incubation period for poliovirus infections is 7 to 14 days. In greater than 90% of the cases, an asymptomatic or subclinical infection results, as evidenced by virus isolation or the acquisition of antibody in the absence of symptoms. Most of the clinical illnesses that do occur are quite mild, and symptoms most often experienced include fever, malaise, and myalgia. Recovery from this illness is complete and rapid.

In 1 to 4% of all infections, CNS involvement is evident, with severity ranging from a mild aseptic meningitis to fatal paralytic poliomyelitis. Headache and stiffness of the back and neck are neurologic symptoms associated with aseptic meningitis and are accompanied by the fever and malaise noted in the mild illness.

More extensive neurologic involvement can result in paralytic poliomyelitis, the severity of which is determined by which particular cells of the CNS are infected and subsequently destroyed, with resulting loss of muscle function. Paralysis can accompany the impairment of muscle function. Muscular involvement progresses rapidly, reaching its peak within a few days, after which symptoms subside slowly. Most fatalities can be attributed to respiratory or cardiac failure. For those who survive, compensatory hypertrophy of uninvolved muscles results in varying degrees of recovery from paralysis.

Once an individual is infected by a particular serotype of poliovirus, antibodies are induced that provide lifelong immunity against reinfection with homologous virus but only partial protection, if any, to heterologous serotypes.

Epidemiology. Poliovirus can be transmitted via any body secretions that contain the virus. Replication of virus in the oropharynx and intestinal tract results in the presence of virus in saliva and feces, both of which can serve as sources of infection. Transmission via saliva probably is limited to close contacts. Epidemics usually involve fecal contamination of food and water. In the temperate areas of the world, the warmer seasons seem to favor the spread of infection.

Sanitary conditions play an important role in the epidemiology of infections, with poor sanitary conditions facilitating the spread of virus, resulting in the infection of most individuals early in life. The more advanced the sanitary measures, the more sporadic the outbreaks of infection and the greater the likelihood that individuals will be infected later in life. In general, the older an individual is when infected, the more likely it is that paralytic disease will occur—thus, the irony of advances in civilization resulting in more severe disease, spurring the quest for a vaccine.

Prevention. Virus-specific therapy is not available for poliovirus infections. Therefore treatment is limited to alleviation of symptoms and support of vital functions. This is particularly true in the case of respiratory failure, which can prove fatal.

Development of a vaccine to prevent paralytic poliomyelitis was made possible by the work of Enders, Weller, and Robbins, who perfected a way to grow poliovirus in tissue culture. Salk used the 3 antigenic types of the virus propagated in this manner to create a vaccine in which virus was inactivated by the addition of formalin. This trivalent vaccine is given in a series consisting of a primary injection followed by two booster injections within a 6-month period. Immune response to the vaccine is excellent, with the development of IgM followed by IgG antibodies. Although the antibodies produced do not necessarily prevent infection and initial replication of virus, they do block the viremia that precedes CNS involvement, thus precluding paralytic disease. Naturally occurring reinfections stimulate the anamnestic response to maintain effective levels of antibody. In the absence of such antigenic stimuli, antibody levels will decline, making booster injections every 5 years advisable.

In general, attenuated live virus vaccines make better immunogens, providing longer lasting protection than inactivated virus. The Sabin attenuated virus vaccine, consisting of a mixture of all three serotypes, is administered orally, whereupon the viruses replicate. In addition to IgM and IgG responses, a significant SIgA response is manifested. Thus, antibody is present in saliva, where it serves as a first line of protection against viral infection, in addition to affording the same immunity as the Salk vaccine. Excretion of vaccine virus by those thus immunized can result in the subsequent infection and thus immunization of individuals who have not received the vaccine.

The most significant disadvantage of any attenuated virus vaccine is the possibility of back mutation of the virulent type. The fewer the mutations, the more likely this will occur. With the Sabin vaccine, the type 3 virus component is more prone to reversion than are types 1 and 2. Approximately 1 in every 3.6 million persons immunized experiences a vaccine-associated illness, probably related to back mutation. Nonimmune close contacts of the vaccinee are at significantly greater risk. Use of the Salk-killed virus vaccine is advised for those who wish to avoid this risk.

Coxsackievirus

Coxsackieviruses are similar in structure to polioviruses. First discovered in 1948 in fecal material from children in Coxsackie, NY, they are divided into group A and group B based on the pathology they produce when injected into newborn mice. There are 23 group A serotypes and 6 serotypes in group B.

Pathogenesis. Coxsackievirus is believed to be transmitted for the most part by the fecal–oral route, although oral–oral spread also is possible. Replication takes place in the oropharynx and intestinal tract, followed by a viremia, then rarely CNS involvement.

With a few exceptions, coxsackievirus infections are either asymptomatic or characterized by very mild symptoms. Children may suffer many nondescript febrile illnesses and exanthems. In many of these cases, A and B coxsackieviruses have been implicated. Several A serotypes have been shown to cause acute upper respiratory infections, often referred to as summer colds. Several A and B serotypes are capable of producing an aseptic meningitis that may progress to a usually mild paralytic disease. Group B viruses appear to have a predilection for heart tissues, having been implicated in a relatively rare but highly fatal myocarditis of the newborn and pericarditis in children and adults of varying degrees of severity.

Herpangina, the coxsackievirus syndrome most likely to be encountered by dental professionals, is an acute illness characterized by the development of papules on the posterior pharynx and soft palate that progress to vesicles then ulcerate. It is accompanied by fever and a sore throat (Fig 28–2). Several A serotypes have been implicated in this syndrome, which occurs primarily in young children.

Epidemiology and Prevention. The epidemiology of coxsackievirus resembles that of poliovirus. Because there are no vaccines, control is dependent to a large degree on sanitary measures to reduce fecal–oral spread in the general population and on personal hygiene within family groups or other commonly housed populations. If evidence of a coxsackievirus infection is present, dental treatment other than in an emergency situation should be deferred until the patient has recovered from the illness.

Echovirus

Thirty serotypes of echovirus have been identified thus far. The virions are similar in structure to poliovirus.

Pathogenesis. Most echovirus infections are either asymptomatic or very mild, resulting in a variety of clinical syndromes. These include aseptic meningitis, upper respiratory tract infections, a mild febrile illness accompanied by a rash particularly in young children, enteritis, pleurodynia, and myocarditis. Fatal CNS infections have been reported, but they are very rare.

Fecal–oral transmission is believed to be the primary route, with respiratory and oral secretions providing a second means of spread among close contacts. Upon entry, the virus multiplies in the mucosa of the oropharynx and intestines. An ensuing viremia

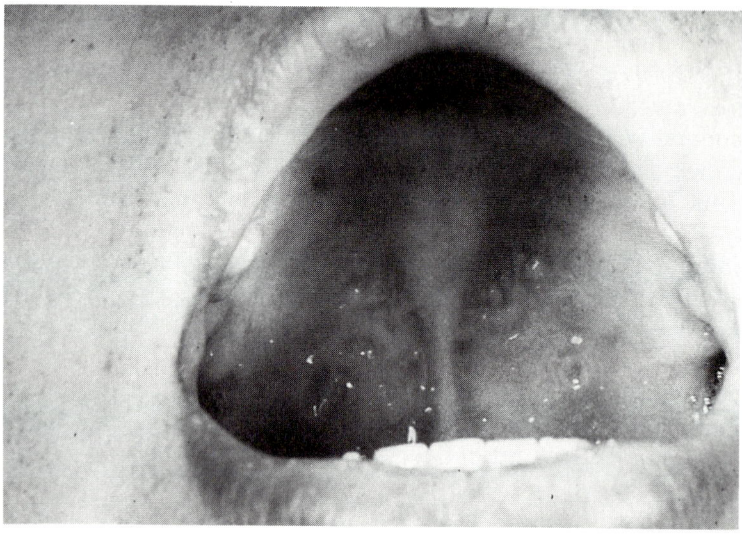

Figure 28–2. Oral vesicular lesions pathognomonic of herpangina, a primary coxsackievirus A infection. *(Courtesy of J. Marquard.)*

can result in dissemination to other organs, resulting in fever and exanthems. If there is CNS involvement, aseptic meningitis can follow.

Epidemiology and Prevention. The epidemiology of echovirus infections closely resembles that of poliovirus, occurring primarily during the warmer seasons, with fecal contamination of water and food serving as the most important source of infectious virus. Spread by respiratory secretions may play an important role with echovirus type 9, which has been implicated in epidemics of respiratory disease. The relatively mild nature of most echovirus infections and the technical difficulties of producing a vaccine to all 30 serotypes have dampened the enthusiasm to develop a vaccine. Specific antiviral chemotherapy is not available for treatment of echovirus infections.

Rhinovirus

The rhinoviruses resemble the enteroviruses but can be differentiated by buoyant density measurements. Rhinoviruses are also more acid labile than are enteroviruses. At the present time, more than 100 serotypes of rhinoviruses have been identified.

Pathogenesis. Infection is usually by inhalation of virus in aerosol or droplets or by hand contact with infectious material and subsequent transfer to the mouth. Virus replication takes place in epithelial cells lining the upper respiratory tract, where damage to these cells results in symptoms we associate with the common cold. These may include increased nasal discharge and blockage of nasal passages, cough, sore throat, and malaise. Lower respiratory tract involvement is a relatively rare event, occurring more often in children than adults. The duration of illness is variable but usually is limited to a week or less, with recovery being accompanied by the appearance of specific IgA and IgG antibodies in nasal secretions. The lack of effective antiviral therapy for rhinoviruses limits its treatment to palliative measures.

Epidemiology and Prevention. In temperate climates, infections occur most frequently during the late fall, winter, and early spring. Several factors have been postulated to account for this observation. It is during these times of the year that people are more apt to be crowded indoors in situations where ventilation is limited, favoring the spread of virus. Cooler air results in lower temperatures over a larger area of the respiratory tract, providing conditions more conducive to virus replication, and the lower humidity levels that often accompany indoor heating tend to dry out the mucous membranes, limiting their effectiveness as barriers to infection.

Vaccine development has been hindered by the large number of serotypes and the observation that natural infection appears to provide relatively short-lived protection. Prevention is primarily dependent on avoiding contact with infected individuals, which admittedly can be rather difficult. Recent studies indicate that hand contact with virus followed by contact with the mouth may be the most efficient and common route of transmission and one that can be reduced to some extent by frequent handwashing.

Much effort has been made to develop drugs capable of preventing these infections, but at present none have been approved for human use. One drug that shows some promise is interferon, and studies are currently underway to determine the feasibility of using intranasally administered interferon for the prophylaxis of infections by a number of respiratory viruses, including rhinovirus.

CORONAVIRUSES

Coronavirus virions possess a single-stranded RNA genome, enclosed in a spherical capsid, which is surrounded by an envelope. Virions are pleomorphic in shape, with a size range from 80 to 160 nm in diameter. There appear to be at least 3 antigenic types of this virus.

Pathogenesis

Infection is apparently via the respiratory and oral routes, with virus replication taking place in epithelial cells, such as those lining the upper respiratory tract. The symptoms, which appear after an incubation period of approximately 3 days, are indistinguishable from those we associate with common colds caused by rhinoviruses. Virus has been isolated from the feces of patients with gastroenteritis, but no causal relationship has been established.

Epidemiology and Prevention

Infections with these agents are most prevalent during the winter and early spring, following the same epidemiologic patterns as the rhinoviruses, and thus should be subject to the same preventive measures. Vaccines for the prevention of these infections are not available.

REOVIRUSES

Reoviruses are uniquely structured, possessing a segmented double-stranded RNA genome with a total molecular weight of 10 to 15 $\times$ 10^6 daltons and a 70 to 80 nm diameter double icosahedral capsid. These virions do not have envelopes.

Pathogenesis, Epidemiology, and Control

Three genera of this virus family, *Reovirus, Orbivirus,* and *Rotavirus,* have been isolated from humans. The ubiquity of these agents has complicated efforts to determine their role in disease processes. Reovirus has been isolated from the feces and respiratory tract of healthy individuals as well as from cases of minor respiratory illness and enteric distress and less commonly from hydrocephalus, encephalitis, hepatitis, lymphoma, and pneumonia.

The etiologic agent in Colorado tick fever is an orbivirus, which is transmitted from rodents to humans through the bite of an infected tick. This usually mild infection is characterized by headache, fever, chills, nausea, and muscle and joint pain. The pathology of this disease is not well understood, but there is evidence of an associated persistent viremia.

Rotavirus has been implicated in a diarrheal illness of young children. Transmission is believed to be primarily by the fecal–oral route and is followed by an incubation period of about 3 days. The illness itself lasts 1 to 2 weeks and is characterized by diarrhea, vomiting, and high fever. For a gastrointestinal pathogen, the epidemiology of these infections is unusual, with peak occurrence during the winter.

The ubiquity of certain of these viruses and the lack of vaccines limit any attempts to control the spread of infection, and the mildness of most of these infections does not appear to warrant the development of vaccines.

SUGGESTED READINGS

Centers for Disease Control. Adult immunization: Recommendations of the immunization practices advisory committee. *MMWR.* 1984;33:No.1S.

Estes MK, Palmer EL, Obijeski JF. Rotaviruses: A review. *Curr Top Microbiol Immunol.* 1983;105:123–184.

Macnaughton MR. The structure and replication of rhinoviruses. *Curr Top Microbiol Immunol.* 1982;97:1–26.

Paul JR. *A History of Poliomyelitis.* New Haven, Conn: Yale University Press; 1971.

Wege H, St Siddel, Ter Meulen V. The biology and pathogenesis of coronaviruses. *Curr Top Microbiol Immunol.* 1982;99:165–200.

Zhaori G, Sun M, Ogra PL. Characteristics of the immune response to poliovirus virion polypeptides after immunization with live or inactivated polio vaccines. *J Infect Dis.* 1988;158:160–165.

CHAPTER 29

Togaviruses and Rhabdoviruses

Walter K. Long

INTRODUCTION

TOGAVIRUSES
Rubella Virus
Arthropod-borne Togaviruses

RHABDOVIRUSES
Rabies

SUGGESTED READINGS

INTRODUCTION

Togaviruses and rhabdoviruses have been implicated in a number of potentially fatal disease states. One of them, rubella, can be transmitted orally, and thus control of its transmission is of some concern to dentists. Although the other agents are not transmitted in the dental setting, all health care professionals should be aware of the severe illnesses they produce and how they are controlled and treated.

TOGAVIRUSES

Early classification schemes often placed viruses in groups based on mode of transmission or type of disease produced. Current methods rely on physical characteristics and chemical composition, a consequence of which has been a reordering of virus classification. Nowhere has this been more apparent than with the creation of the family Togaviridae, into which the arboviruses, so named because they are transmitted to humans by arthropod vectors, were placed along with the etiologic agent of rubella.

Togaviruses are enveloped icosahedral virions with diameters ranging from 40 nm to 75 nm. The genome is a linear single strand of positive polarity RNA (serves as mRNA) between 2.5 and 4.5×10^6 daltons MW. The capsids of each viral type appear to be composed of a single protein, whereas 1 to 3 different proteins are associated with the envelope, with at least one of these being glycosylated and penetrating through the envelope to form spikes that have hemagglutinating activity.

Rubella Virus

Pathogenesis. Infection generally occurs when an individual is exposed via the respiratory or oral route to respiratory secretions containing infectious virus. Initial virus replication is believed to take place in cells of the upper respiratory tract and lymphoid tissue, leading to a viremia where virus undergoes further replication and is transported to other sites, including the placenta of pregnant women, synovial membranes, and rarely to the CNS.

The first symptoms of rubella appear approximately 14 to 21 days after exposure. They usually are mild and can include a fever, malaise, coryza, pharyngitis, and some swelling of the cervical and occipital lymph nodes. These initial signs are followed within 2 days by the appearance of a maculopapular rash, first on the face, spreading to the trunk and extremities, then disappearing within 3 days (Fig 29–1). Rubella infections of children usually are uneventful, with complications usually limited to adults and fetuses. In some adults, particularly women, involvement of the

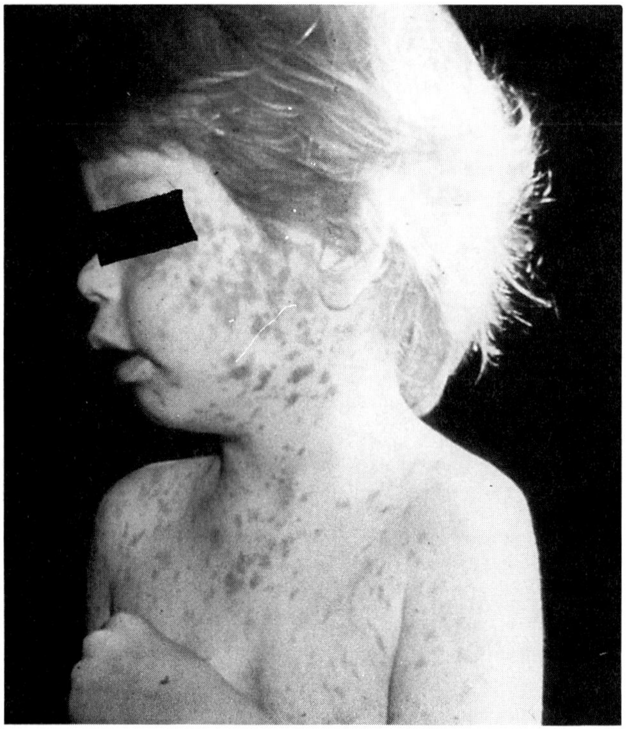

Figure 29–1. Rubella rash. *(Courtesy of Centers for Disease Control, Atlanta, Ga.)*

synovial membrane can result in a transient arthralgia or arthritis.

The most frightening complication of rubella occurs when a nonimmune woman in the first trimester of pregnancy is infected. In these instances, placental infection is common, resulting in infection of the developing fetus, giving rise to congenital rubella syndrome (CRS). The earlier the stage of development at the time of infection, the more severe the damage. Approximately 85% of fetuses infected during the first month of pregnancy show congenital abnormalities. By the third month, the number is down to about 15%. Fetuses infected near term apparently are unaffected. Examination of infected fetuses reveals viral killing of some cells and the induction of chromosomal aberrations in other cells. In the most severe cases, the fetus is killed. Those children who survive may suffer a variety of developmental and neurologic abnormalities, including glaucoma, cataracts, and other anomalies of the eyes, defects of the cardiovascular system, mental retardation, microcephaly, deafness, low birth weight, anemia, interstitial pneumonia, and thrombocytopenic purpura. Infants with CRS may exhibit any one or more of these signs at birth, whereas other children appear to be perfectly normal. Long-term follow-up studies of the latter have revealed that they are predisposed to certain illnesses later in life, such as diabetes mellitus, progressive degenerative panencephalitis, and chronic pneumonitis.

Epidemiology and Prevention. Rubella is a highly contagious disease. Before the development of a vaccine, epidemics occurred every 6 to 8 years with the resulting infection of most nonimmune individuals who were exposed. Many of those infected experienced asymptomatic illnesses. Lifelong protection against clinical disease apparently follows primary infection. Passive immunization with immune globulin has been attempted to protect susceptible individuals exposed to rubella, particularly pregnant women. However, clinical evidence has failed to demonstrate any beneficial effect of this treatment.

A live attenuated virus vaccine is available for the prevention of rubella infection. Nasopharyngeal isolation of virus following immunization indicates that the vaccine virus replicates, however, it does not appear to produce a viremia. Over 95% of the recipients seroconvert. However, the antibody levels are lower than those that result from a natural infection. Immunized subjects, therefore, are more susceptible to reinfection, albeit an asymptomatic infection which serves primarily to boost antibody titers. Side effects are quite common in adult women who receive the vaccine, with approximately one third of them experiencing a mild arthralgia and about 1% arthritis. Other complications which have been observed include fever and a rash. The vaccine virus has been shown to cross the placenta, but there are no reported instances of this leading to CRS. Because there is a remote possibility of CRS, immunization of pregnant women is contraindicated, and it is recommended that women who are immunized take measures to avoid conception for at least 3 months following vaccination. It is desirable that all nonimmune persons in the population be immunized, particularly women before they enter the childbearing years. Because the incidence of asymptomatic infection is so high and such persons can transmit the virus to others, it is strongly advised that dental care providers ensure their own immunity so as to reduce the risk of infecting patient contacts. As with other infectious diseases, dental treatment of an obviously infected patient should be deferred until resolution of the illness, if at all possible. If emergency treatment is required, gloves, goggles, and mask should be worn.

Arthropod-borne Togaviruses

Pathogenesis. The usual route of transmission for viruses of this group to humans is through arthropod vectors. Virus can be maintained in an infectious state in the salivary glands of specific species of arthropods (eg, mosquitoes and ticks) for several months and can be transmitted to the vertebrates on which they feed. Initial virus replication takes place in reticuloendothelial cells of the lymph nodes and spleen, resulting in a viremia. Sites subsequently infected via the blood vary depending on the tissue tropisms of the particular virus.

Encephalitis Viruses. The equine encephalitis viruses, eastern equine encephalitis virus (EEE), western equine encephalitis virus (WEE), Venezuelan equine encephalitis virus (VEE), St. Louis encephalitis virus (SLE), and Japanese B encephalitis virus, are togaviruses that cross the blood–brain barrier and infect tissues of the CNS. Of these, EEE produces the most severe illness, with a high mortality rate and severe damage to the nervous system of most survivors. Histologic examination reveals lesions of the brain and spinal cord, particularly the brainstem and basal ganglia. In contrast, WEE lesions usually are confined to the brain and are less extensive. The disease produced by this virus usually is not as severe, but the fatality rate among infants and young children is high, as are residual effects among survivors. Japanese B encephalitis virus infections are usually mild or asymptomatic. However, there is a fatality rate of about 8% and neurologic effects in another 30%, with most of these severe illnesses primarily confined to young children and the elderly. Although fatalities and residual effects have been reported, VEE and SLE infections usually are inapparent, and the symptoms that do occur usually are limited to fever, chills, and headache.

Other togaviruses may attack a variety of tissues, including blood vessels, skin, muscle, and various internal organs. Dengue fever is an example of a virus that infects skin tissues, producing a macular rash that is accompanied by fever, headache, and muscular aches. Mortality from this disease is rare, and recovery usually is uneventful. Hemorrhagic dengue, on the other hand, is characterized by severe lesions to blood vessels, resulting in internal hemorrhage. Shock and subsequent death are common in untreated patients. Infection of various internal organs, including the heart, kidneys, and liver, occurs with yellow fever. Functioning of the affected organs is impaired, leading to a variety of symptoms, including jaundice, cardiac abnormalities, and bleeding, together with headache and fever. As would be expected, the fatality rate is high, although survivors usually recover completely.

Epidemiology and Prevention. The epidemiology of these infections can be rather complex and is dependent on a number of interrelated factors. The usual vector for transmission is an arthropod. In the diseases previously described, they are various species of mosquitoes. Virus is transmitted by mosquitoes to various vertebrate hosts, where an apparent or inapparent infection can occur, with a transient viremia as one of the consequences of infection. Other mosquitoes become infectious by feeding on the viremic animal and can harbor infectious virus in their salivary glands for an extended period of time. There is evidence that some viruses may be passed vertically to offspring. These viruses are thus maintained by cycling betwen arthropod and vertebrate hosts, with variations in the particular species involved being dependent on the particular etiologic agent.

WEE, EEE, and SLE are cycled in wild and domestic birds, with infection of rodent and mammal populations occurring via infected mosquitoes. Infections of these secondary hosts, which include horses and humans, are referred to as dead-end infections because they do not serve as sources of virus for the mosquitoes. Control measures aimed at interrupting the chain of transmission involve reduction of mosquito populations when there is evidence of infection of reservoir animals or outbreaks of disease in humans or horses.

Humans are more than an incidental dead-end host in yellow fever and dengue—in fact, they are an integral part of the cycle. These particular agents are capable of initiating productive infections in humans and certain subhuman primates. Virus is cycled among primates in the jungle setting and among humans in the urban environment. However, mosquitoes are capable of and do transmit virus from human to monkey and monkey to human, providing a means for introducing the disease into urban areas. The difficulty of controlling yellow fever in the jungle environment has led to the development of a live attenuated virus vaccine, the use of which is recommended for individuals traveling to areas where yellow fever is endemic. Vaccines for EEE, WEE, and VEE are routinely given to horses in areas where the particular disease is prevalent. Administration to humans is restricted to individuals who work with the viruses in laboratories. Medical and dental professionals are not at increased risk for these infections unless their work takes them to areas where yellow fever and dengue are endemic, in which case they should follow the current immunization recommendations for all visitors to these areas.

RHABDOVIRUSES

Rhabdoviruses have single-stranded RNA genomes 3.5 to 4.5×10^6 daltons MW. This RNA is of a negative polarity, necessitating the inclusion of an RNA transcriptase in the virion. Surrounding these molecules is a helical capsid, which is composed entirely of the N protein. During the replication process, the nucleocapsid acquires an envelope, which gives the infectious virion its characteristic bullet shape. Three virus-specified proteins are incorporated into the envelope, the nonglycosylated M_1 and M_2 proteins that serve as the matrix of the envelope and the glycosylated G protein that forms the surface projections which have hemagglutinating activity and function in the attachment of virus to cells. The completed virions are 130 to 240 nm long and 70 to 80 nm in diameter.

Rabies

Pathogenesis. Infection is usually via the bite of an infected animal or, more rarely, by inhalation of virus in bat secretions. Initial virus replication takes place in muscle and connective tissue at the site of exposure, followed by movement of the virus along peripheral nerves to ganglia and subsequently the CNS, where extensive damage to the brain takes place. From the brain, virus travels via efferent nerves to other sites, such as the skin, cornea, and salivary glands, all of which can serve as sources of infection under appropriate circumstances. Histologic examination of the brain of a human or animal with rabies reveals infiltration by monocytes and neuronal destruction. The single most important finding is that of well-defined round eosinophilic inclusions, called Negri bodies, in the cytoplasm of brain cells (Fig 29–2). These inclusion bodies, which consist of viral antigens, are diagnostic for rabies.

The incubation period for this disease is dependent on the site of inoculation and size of the inoculum and may range from 1 week to 1 year. In most instances, however, it is 1 to 2 months. Paresthesia at the site of inoculation and increased irritability are among the early symptoms of the disease, followed by the one clinical characteristic most often associated with rabies, hydrophobia, or fear of water, which results from spasms of the muscles of deglutition, making the swallowing of liquids, even one's own saliva, very painful. With rare exception, the disease progresses to extensive CNS involvement culminating in coma and death.

Prevention, Treatment, and Control. Rabies occurs in mammalian populations throughout the world, in both wild and domestic animals. Because of human proximity to them, domestic animals, particularly dogs, represent the single greatest source of human infection. Programs to remove stray and unwanted dogs and to immunize all other dogs have led to a dramatic reduction in the incidence of dog rabies in the United States. However, this is not the case in all parts of the world. Currently, cat rabies exceeds that of dogs in this country, and it is recommended that all cats also be immunized. Foxes, skunks, bats, and raccoons experience high rates of infection, with the adaptation of raccoons to human surroundings making them a potential source of human infection.

Caution is advised in handling any animal that has not been immunized against rabies, particularly one that appears ill. If a person is bitten by an animal, the particular species of animal involved and the circumstances should be ascertained to determine if postexposure prophylaxis is advisable. A bite by a

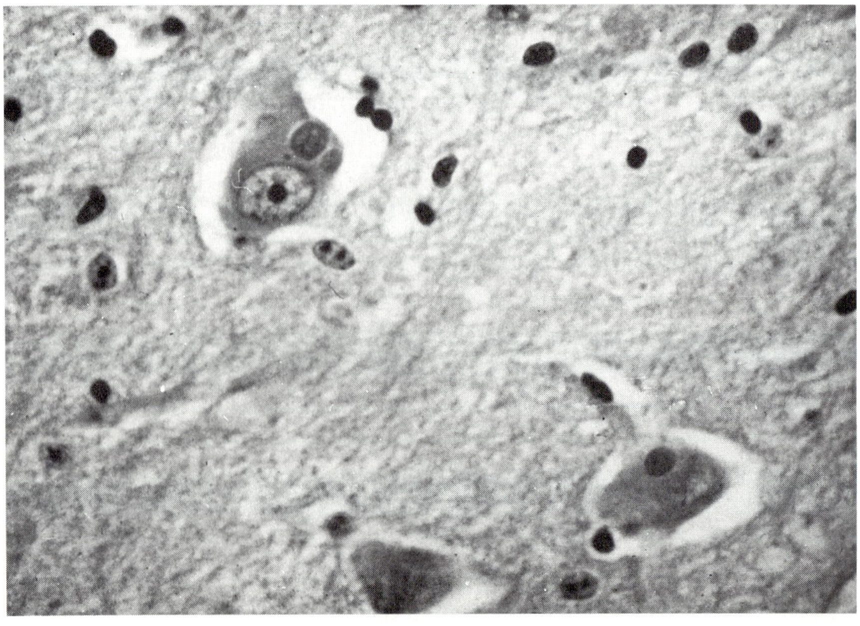

Figure 29–2. Negri bodies, cytoplasmic inclusion bodies in brain cells of a dog infected with rabies. They are believed to represent sites of viral replication. *(Courtesy of J. Fantasia.)*

domestic dog or cat would not warrant further consideration if the animal had a current vaccination. In cases where the animal was not immunized, it should be observed for a period of 10 days by a veterinarian for signs of illness. If any illness develops that possibly could be rabies, the animal should be humanely killed as soon as possible and the brain examined for Negri bodies. Skunks, bats, foxes, coyotes, raccoons, bobcats, and other carnivores are considered infected unless proof to the contrary is available. Whenever possible, any one of these animals that bites an individual should be killed, and the brain should be examined. If this cannot be done, the person bitten is treated as if he or she has been exposed to rabies. Another consideration is whether the attack was provoked, since studies have shown that rabid animals are more likely to attack without provocation. Bites by livestock and rodents are not deemed to merit prophylaxis unless there is evidence of current infection in these populations.

Immediately following any bite, the wound should be cleansed with soap and water regardless of the source of exposure. If it is determined that postexposure prophylaxis is necessary, it should be initiated as soon as possible and should include antibody and vaccine. The antibody preparation consists of rabies immune globulin (RIG) obtained from individuals who have been immunized. It is administered in one dose, half used to infiltrate the site of the wound and half administered intramuscularly. Rabies virus grown in human cell cultures is inactivated to make a rabies vaccine, which is given intramuscularly in a series of five to six doses. On subsequent exposure to the virus, anyone previously immunized should be given two booster doses of the vaccine.

SUGGESTED READINGS

Centers for Disease Control. Field evaluations of preexposure use of human diploid cell rabies vaccine. *MMWR.* 1983;32:601–603.

Centers for Disease Control. Rabies prevention—United States, 1984. *MMWR.* 1984;33:393–408.

Centers for Disease Control. Rubella prevention. *MMWR.* 1984;33:301–318.

Centers for Disease Control. Viral hemorrhagic fever: Initial management of suspected and confirmed cases. *MMWR.* 1983;32:No. 2S.

Hatwick MAW. Human rabies. *Public Health Rev.* 1974; 3:229–274.

Horstman DM. Controlling rubella: Problems and perspectives. *Ann Intern Med.* 1975;83:412–417.

Miller E, Cradock-Watson JE, Pollock TM. Consequences of confirmed maternal rubella at successive stages of pregnancy. *Lancet.* 1982;2:781–784.

Monath TP. Arthropod-borne encephalitides in the Americas. *Bull WHO.* 1979;57:513–533.

Wiktor TJ, Plotkin SA, Koprowski H. Development and clinical trials of the new human rabies vaccine of tissue culture (human diploid cell) origin. *Dev Biol Stand.* 1978; 40:3–9.

CHAPTER 30

Hepatitis Viruses

Walter K. Long

INTRODUCTION
HEPATITIS A
Structure and Morphology
Pathogenesis
Epidemiology
Laboratory Diagnosis
Prevention and Control
HEPATITIS B
Structure and Morphology
Pathogenesis
Epidemiology
Serologic Markers and Laboratory Diagnosis
Prevention and Control
DELTA AGENT
NON A, NON B HEPATITIS
ORAL ASPECTS
SUGGESTED READINGS

INTRODUCTION

Examination of the earliest written descriptions of illnesses indicates that hepatitis has afflicted mankind for thousands of years. We now know that the symptoms of this disease are due to liver inflammation, which can result from exposure to certain toxic substances or infection with a number of different etiologic agents. Although a variety of bacteria, protozoa, and viruses have been implicated as causative agents, classic epidemic hepatitis follows infection with specific viruses that have a predilection for hepatic tissue. Epidemiologic and serologic findings have confirmed that dental professionals are at increased risk for infection with certain of these agents.

Current evidence indicates that there are at least 6 different hepatitis viruses. These etiologic agents of viral hepatitis differ markedly, but the clinical diseases they produce (Table 30–1) are virtually indistinguishable without the aid of serologic tests. Hepatitis viruses apparently can be transmitted by several different routes, with a proclivity for one mode of transmission over another based on differences in pathogenesis that exist among the various etiologic agents. None of these agents are capable of traversing intact skin. Infection, therefore, occurs through breaks in the skin or mucous membranes and congenitally. Morbidity and mortality are largely determined by route of infection and host factors. As many as half of all hepatitis infections result in inapparent or subclinical illnesses, and the remaining symptomatic infections are, for the most part, acute and self-limiting. Common symptoms include abdominal pain, fever, chills, loss of appetite, nausea, and malaise, accompanied by an enlarged liver and spleen. Jaundice, historically the symptom most commonly associated with hepatitis, actually appears in only about half of all cases with clinical symptoms. When jaundice does occur, it usually lasts less than 6 weeks. Hepatic dysfunction, hepatic enlargement and tenderness, and fatigue generally last 2 to 3 months, with resolution of the illness following. The onset of symptoms can be quite rapid, particularly with hepatitis A virus (HAV), or of a more insidious nature with hepatitis B virus (HBV).

A minority of patients experience a more protracted illness, which may be acute or chronic. In-

TABLE 30–1. COMPARISON OF TYPES OF HEPATITIS

	Hepatitis A	Hepatitis B	NANB	Hepatitis C	Delta
Etiologic agent	HAV	HBV	Several viruses	HCV	Delta agent
Incubation period	15–50 days	50–180 days	Variable	Unknown	Unknown
Carrier state	No	Yes	Yes	Yes	Unknown
Transmission	Fecal–oral	Parenteral Sexual Vertical	Parenteral Fecal–oral	Parenteral	Parenteral

creased hepatic necrosis leads to the acute form, in which symptoms are more pronounced and there is more severe hepatic impairment. A few of these patients recover completely after varying periods of time, but most progress to cirrhosis. Between 1% and 5% of all clinical cases of hepatitis become fulminant infections, characterized by massive hepatic necrosis, often accompanied by rapid mental deterioration and subsequent death of most victims.

HEPATITIS A

Structure and Morphology

Hepatitis A virus (HAV) is the etiologic agent of a disease often referred to as infectious hepatitis. HAV resembles poliovirus with respect to physical characteristics and epidemiology. The virion consists of a single-stranded RNA genome enclosed in a 27 nm diameter capsid with helical symmetry. Like poliovirus, it is relatively resistant to physical and chemical methods of inactivation, including treatment with ether and exposure to conditions of acidity as low as pH 3.0. Infectivity can be destroyed by boiling for 5 minutes, standard steam sterilization (121°C for 15 minutes), and by formalin treatment for 3 days.

Pathogenesis

HAV is transmitted orally and has an incubation period of approximately 2 weeks to 2 months. Virus replicates first in the intestinal epithelium and mesenteric lymph nodes. The resulting viremia seeds various internal organs, including the liver. As a result of infection, the liver becomes enlarged. Histologic examination reveals necrosis of hepatocytes, which is characterized by cellular degeneration and ballooning and by the appearance of acidophilic bodies and monocyte infiltration.

Epidemiology

The mode of transmission of HAV is to a large degree determined by its pathogenesis and physical characteristics. HAV is excreted in the feces for approximately 1 month, beginning 2 weeks before the onset of symptoms. It is accompanied by a viremia of similar duration. Such a transient viremia means that the blood is infectious for a relatively short period of time and is thus not a significant source of infection. On the other hand, fecal contamination of water and foodstuffs by a virus resistant to chemical and physical inactivation provides a means of infecting large numbers of individuals. HAV epidemics have resulted from the consumption of HAV-contaminated water and food, with uncooked shellfish from contaminated waters being involved in a number of outbreaks.

Laboratory Diagnosis

HAV infection is characterized by the presence of hepatitis A antigen (HAAg) in the blood and feces before the onset of symptoms through the acute phase of the infection, followed by the appearance of IgM antibodies, then IgG antibodies, both to HAAg.

Prevention and Control

A vaccine is not yet available. Immune serum globulin can be used to prevent infection if administered within 1 to 2 weeks of exposure. Modern sanitation measures undoubtedly reduce the size of and numbers of outbreaks, as do restrictions on harvesting shellfish from contaminated waters.

HEPATITIS B

Structure and Morphology

Hepatitis B virus (HBV) is both structurally and antigenically distinct from HAV. The complete virion, also called the Dane particle, is a 42 nm diameter double-shelled structure with a double-stranded DNA genome. Hepatitis B surface antigen (HBsAg) comprises the outer shell, and the inner structure is composed of core antigen (HBcAg) (Fig 30–1). Two other, noninfectious structural forms found in conjunction with the Dane particle, 22 nm diameter spheroids and tubules, are made entirely of HBsAg (Fig 30–2).

Pathogenesis

Clinical signs of HBV first appear 50 to 180 days after infection. Both the route of transmission and the size

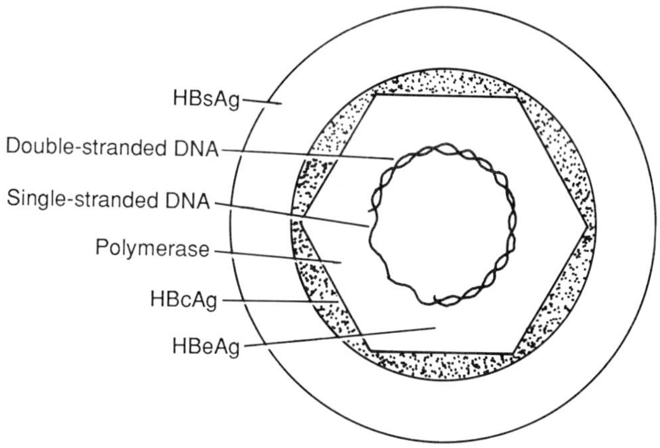

Figure 30–1. Structure of hepatitis B virus (HBV). One characteristic that sets HBV apart from other viruses is that its core contains a double-stranded DNA that includes a single-stranded region. In contrast to most DNA viruses, HBV carries its own DNA polymerase. Another component of the viral inner core is the hepatitis B core antigen (HBcAg). The hepatitis B e antigen (HBeAg) is associated with viral particles. The outermost structure of the virus is composed of the hepatitis B surface antigen (HBsAg). This protein also forms noninfectious aggregates seen in the blood of infected individuals. *(Reproduced with the permission of Merck, Sharp & Dohme, division of Merck & Co., Inc.)*

of the inoculum influence the length of the incubation period. Acquisition of virus by the parenteral route may provide a more direct means of infecting the host, resulting in incubation times at the short end of the spectrum. Nonparenteral infection provides for a more protracted interval. Increasing the numbers of infectious viral particles in an inoculum appears to shorten the incubation period.

The severity of HBV may range from inapparent to a fulminating type of disease. Approximately 90% of the cases are of the milder form and do not persist longer than 8 to 10 weeks. Resolution of acute hepatitis usually is followed by a return of normal liver pathology. In striking contrast, more extensive hepatocyte destruction and a more intense inflammatory response, with infiltration of plasma cells in addition to monocytes, characterize fulminant hepatitis, which occurs in less than 1% of HBV infections.

Chronic hepatitis, which follows approximately 10% of HBV infections, is characterized by the persistence of biochemical markers of hepatitis and antigenic markers of HBV. Over 70% of these cases are classified as chronic benign hepatitis and the remainder as chronic aggressive hepatitis. In both instances, the patient is typically asymptomatic during the early phases of chronicity, with differentiation requiring histologic examination. Chronic benign hepatitis carries with it a good prognosis. On the other hand, the extreme liver necrosis evident in chronic aggressive hepatitis makes the development of cirrhosis a likely outcome and the increased risk of hepatocellular carcinoma a possibility. Chronic hepatitis most often fol-

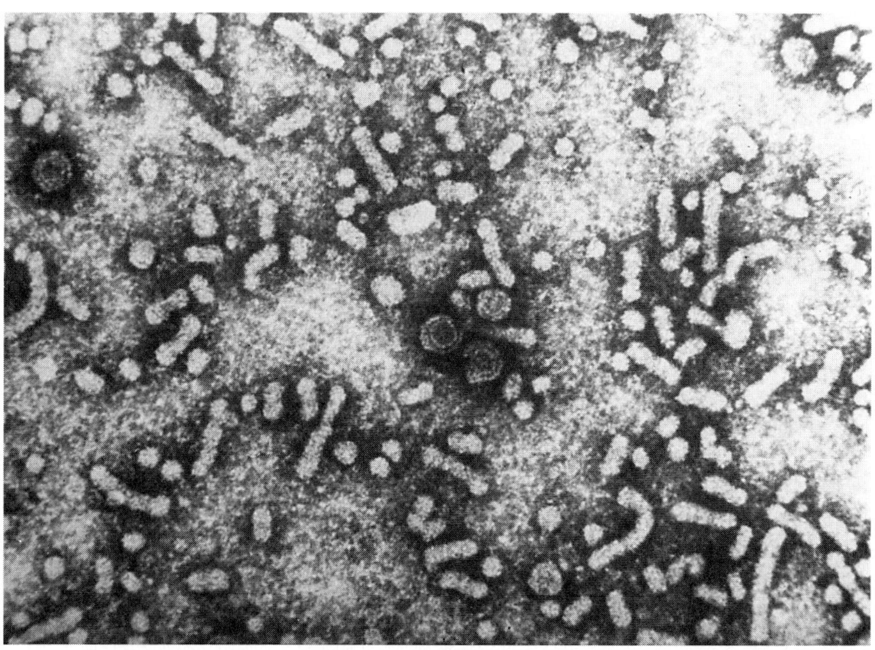

Figure 30–2. Electron micrograph of HBV in the blood of a chronic carrier. When a serum sample containing HBV is examined under the electron microscope, three morphologic forms can be seen. The few large spherical structures are intact viral particles. The numerous smaller spheres and long tubules are aggregates of HBsAg. *(Reproduced with the permission of Merck, Sharpe & Dohme, division of Merck & Co., Inc.)*

lows asymptomatic or mild clinical infections, usually escaping detection until symptoms become evident in cases of aggressive disease.

Epidemiology

The epidemiology of HBV is very different from that of HAV, with fecal–oral spread being either rare or nonexistent. The feature that facilitates the spread of this virus is its ability to establish persistent infections, in which virus may be found in the blood and other secretions over an extended number of years. Virus is found in highest concentrations in the blood and in lesser amounts in the feces and a number of body secretions, including saliva, urine, tears, semen, and genital secretions. At one time, the transfusion of blood or the administration of products derived from human blood was responsible for a major portion of HBV infections. The advent of testing for HBsAg has reduced dramatically the infection rate of individuals receiving these products. Blood, however, still represents a major source of infection. This is particularly evident in the high infectivity rates of intravenous drug abusers who often share needles. Dental personnel are exposed to blood during routine procedures, and any needlestick, cut, or abrasion of the skin can facilitate viral entry.

Studies carried out on institutionalized children have demonstrated spread of the virus to cohorts, in which instance, HBV is most probably spread via various body secretions. Male homosexuals are among the highest risk groups, experiencing infective rates as high as 70 to 80% in some urban areas, suggesting that certain sexual practices unique to this group may provide an efficient means of transmitting the virus. Female prostitutes are at a moderately increased risk for developing HBV infections, as are other promiscuous heterosexuals.

In some parts of the world, particularly Asia and Africa, vertical transmission from mother to offspring is very common, with congenital and neonatal routes of infection both believed to play a role. This situation is exacerbated by the fact that infections of infants result in carrier rates of over 30%, creating a situation where there are a large number of carriers in the population ensuring a continued high rate of infection.

Epidemiologic studies have revealed a correlation between HBV infection and the development of primary hepatocellular carcinoma (PHC). Persons with PHC are 5 to 70 times more likely to have been infected with HBV than PHC-negative individuals, and chronic HBV carries a 250-fold increased risk of PHC. The mechanisms of oncogenesis are not known, but continual hepatic injury and regeneration may serve to promote the activation of oncogenes.

Serologic Markers and Laboratory Diagnosis

Much of our knowledge concerning the course of HBV infections has been made possible by the development of serologic tests to detect viral antigens and antibodies (Table 30–2).

Multiple antigen and antibody systems have been described for HBV, the use of which provide an excellent means of determining the course of infection. The hepatitis B surface antigen (HBsAg) appears in blood and other body fluids 2 to 5 weeks before the onset of symptoms, reaching highest levels shortly after their onset (Fig 30–3A). HBsAg usually disappears in another 1 to 5 months but can persist for years, even decades in the 5 to 10% who become chronic carriers (Fig 30–3B). Its presence indicates that an individual is possibly infectious. Screening blood for this particular antigen has significantly reduced the incidence of posttransfusion HBV hepatitis. Antibody to HBsAg (HBsAb), first of the IgM then the IgG class, appears following the disappearance of HBsAg and indicates that complete recovery from the infection has taken place. It has been determined that HBsAb is a neutralizing antibody providing protection against reinfection with homologous virus.

HBeAg, which is derived from the core of HBV, can be detected at the peak of HBsAg expression, and its presence correlates with a high degree of infectivity. The disappearance of HBeAg and the subse-

TABLE 30–2. COMMON SEROLOGIC TESTS FOR HBV AND THEIR INTERPRETATION

Positive Tests	Interpretation
HBsAg (surface antigen)	Active hepatitis B infection, either acute or chronic
Anti-HBs (in absence of HBsAg)	Protection against reinfection (immunity); remains for years
Anti-HBc (in absence of anti-HBs)	Active HBV infection cannot be excluded; a recent HBV infection can be confirmed by examining the sample for high titers of IgM anti-HBc
HBeAg[a]	Active hepatitis infection, acute or chronic; found in presence of HBsAg; indicates specimens that exhibit potential for enhanced infectivity
Anti-HBe	When present in HBsAg carrier, blood is potentially less infectious

[a]Other HBV serologic markers that may be present at the same time include HBV (Dane particles), observable by electron microscopy. Core antigen and viral DNA polymerase can be measured by disrupting HBV.

From Jawetz E, Melnick JL, and Adelberg EA. Review of Medical Microbiology. *17th ed. E Norwalk, Conn: Appleton & Lange; 1987.*

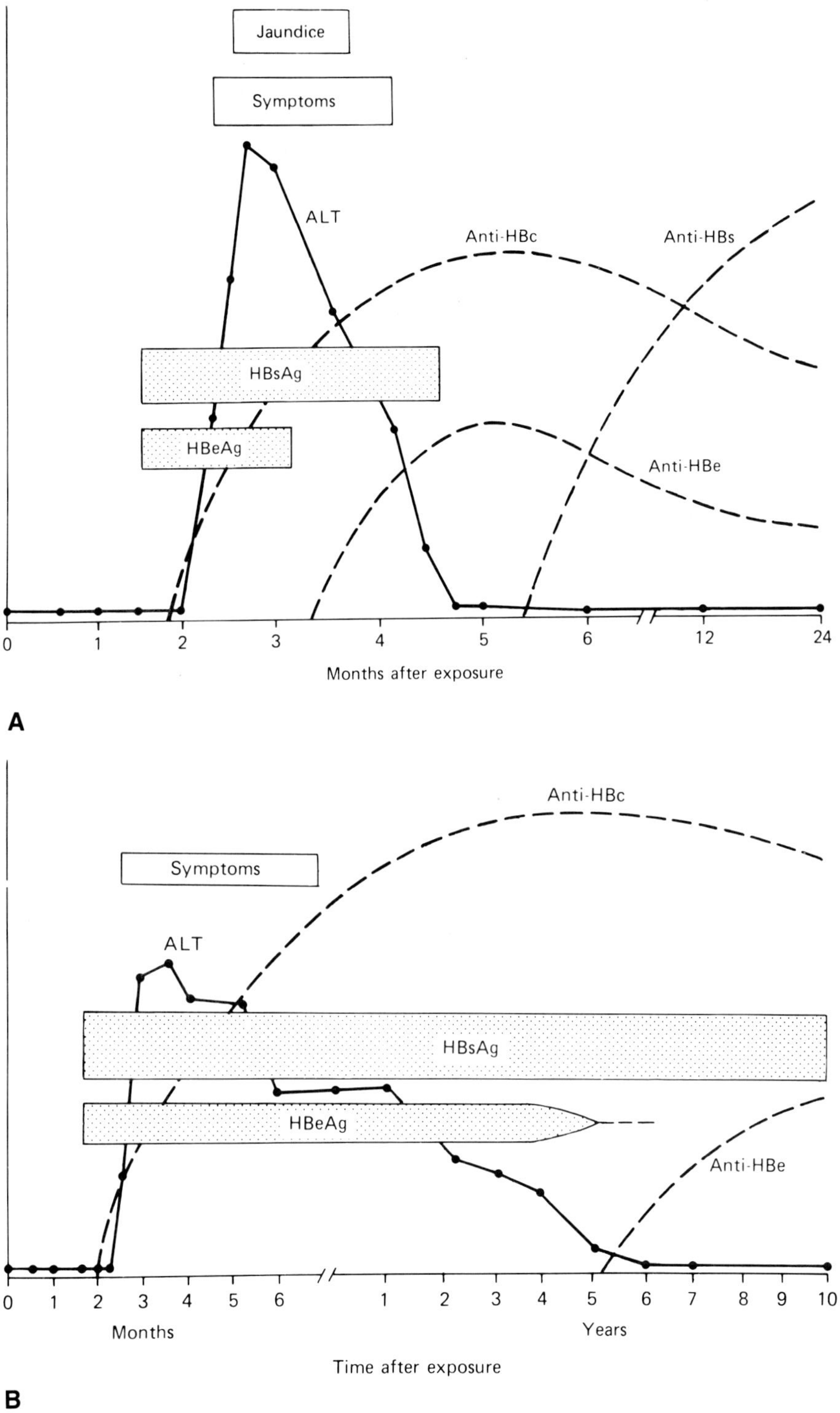

Figure 30–3. The serologic events associated with the typical course of acute type B hepatitis (A) and the development of the chronic hepatitis B virus carrier state (B). HBsAg, hepatitis B surface antigen; HBeAg, hepatitis B e antigen; ALT, alanine aminotransferase; anti-HBs, antibody to HBsAg; anti-HBc, antibody to hepatitis B core antigen; anti-HBe, antibody to HBeAg. *(From Hoofnagle JH.* Annu Rev Med. *1981;32:1–11.)*

quent appearance of antibody (HBeAb) usually signal the end of clinical illness.

Antibody to hepatitis B core antigen (HBcAb) can first be detected shortly after the appearance of HBsAg and persists for several years. It indicates present or past infection and is most useful in the absence of other markers, a situation that, for example, exists for a short period of time after the waning of HBsAg and before the appearance of HBsAb.

At the present time, there are no antiviral drugs approved for the treatment of hepatitis B. With current therapy limited to supportive measures, the prevention of hepatitis assumes increased importance.

Two basic approaches are available, physical interruption of viral transmission and immunization of potential victims. Passive immunization is available for HBV. The administration of hepatitis B immune globulin (HBIG) is indicated when an HBsAb-negative dentist or auxiliary is exposed, particularly through needlesticks or cuts, to the blood or saliva of an

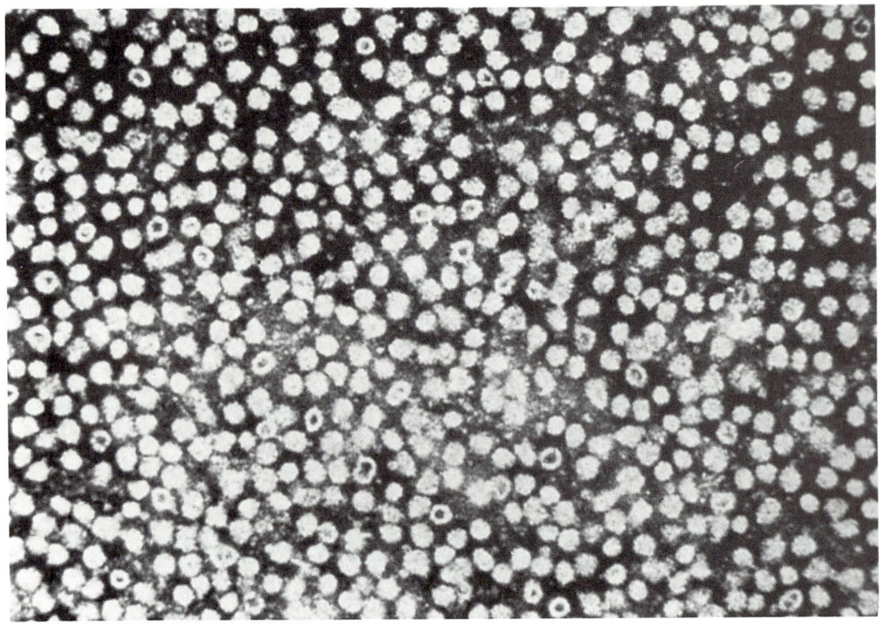

Figure 30–4. Electron micrograph of HBV vaccine. Vaccine consists of purified hepatitis B surface antigen. It contains no intact virus, no e antigen, and no DNA polymerase. *(Reproduced with permission of Merck, Sharpe & Dohme, division of Merck & Co., Inc.)*

HBsAg-positive or, even worse, an HBeAg-positive patient. Globulin should be administered within 24 hours of the exposure and repeated after 1 month.

Two vaccines are available for active immunization against HBV. Both are composed of purified HBsAg. In the first instance, it is purified from the blood of carriers as the immunogen (Fig 30–4). Noninfectivity of the vaccine is ensured by inactivation with urea, pepsin, and formalin, and purification is accomplished by ultracentrifugation and biochemical procedures. The second vaccine is a result of recombinant DNA technology. The gene coding for HBsAg has been cloned into yeast, where it is expressed and subsequently purified for use in the vaccine.

The same regimen is followed for the administration of both vaccines. An initial intramuscular deltoid injection followed by boosters at 1 and 6 months results in the induction of protective HBsAb in over 95% of those immunized. Vaccination of those who already possess HBsAb will only serve to boost antibody levels. Unfortunately, HBsAg carriers are not cured by this vaccine; on the other hand, they do not suffer any deleterious effects. HBIG and the initial injection of hepatitis B vaccine can be administered simultaneously, albeit at different sites, without any adverse effects on the efficacy of the vaccine. Thus, this combination should be considered whenever HBIG is indicated. It would ensure long-term protection and alleviate any future need for passive HBV immunization.

DELTA AGENT

The delta agent, discovered in 1977, is a replication defective virus. This virus requires the presence of HBV in order to replicate. It possesses an RNA genome in a 35 nm diameter capsid.

Although the delta agent was first described in 1977, several lots of immune serum globulin prepared from pooled blood serum collected as early as 1944 were found to contain antibody to the delta agent, indicating that this was not a new etiologic agent. Beginning in 1972, all blood collected in the United States was screened routinely for HBsAg to eliminate the risk of HBV transmission in blood or blood products. Since delta replicates only in the presence of HBV, elimination of blood containing HBV has resulted also in the elimination of delta agent from the same pools.

Delta agent and antibody have been detected in individuals infected with the delta agent. In all cases, markers of present or past HBV infection also are found. Delta agent can infect simultaneously with HBV and, according to some studies, promotes the chronicity of HBV infection. Infection of chronic carriers of HBV, on the other hand, tends to result in acute disease.

Transmission is believed to occur primarily by contact with unscreened blood, as would be the case with intravenous drug abusers who share needles and medical and dental personnel who suffer needlesticks or other cuts or abrasions to the skin and the nature of whose profession results in exposure to blood from numerous individuals.

HEPATITIS C AND NON A, NON B HEPATITIS

Epidemiologic and serologic evidence indicates that many cases of viral hepatitis cannot be attributed to HAV, HBV, or the delta agent. Pending more definitive characterization, these etiologic agents have been designated as non A, non B hepatitis viruses (NANB). Recently, one of these, a positive-stranded RNA virus, was cloned and has been designated hepatitis C virus (HCV).

More than 90% of transfusion-associated hepatitis in the United States is currently attributed to NANB, and it appears that a majority of these cases have a HCV etiology. Indications are that these agents are transmitted via blood and that they probably establish a long-term carrier state. These, of course, are characteristics also of HBV.

In one study, antibody to HCV was detected in 0.9% to 1.4% of volunteer blood donors in the greater New York area. This serologic test for antibody is now used to screen blood. Additionally, the Red Cross is using tests for antibody to HBV core antigen and alanine aminotransferase (ALT) to ascertain the risk for NANB. Since similar risk factors exist for infection with HBV and NANB, an individual infected with HBV would be considered to be at increased risk for infection with NANB, while high ALT levels are indicative of liver disease. Blood carrying any of these markers is not used for transfusions.

Current data that indicate HCV and NANB transmission profiles similar to HBV suggest that dentists are at increased risk for these infections.

At least one NANB agent, responsible for outbreaks in India, has produced epidemics similar to epidemics caused by HAV and presumably is transmitted by the fecal–oral route.

ORAL ASPECTS

It cannot be emphasized too strongly that although the hepatitis B vaccine is very effective in preventing HBV infections and indirectly prevents infections by the delta agent, it does not appear to have any effect on infections by NANB or any other etiologic agents.

HBV, the delta agent, and NANB may be present in blood or saliva for an extended period of time, providing potential for transmission in the dental operatory. The absence of symptoms in up to half of all cases of hepatitis severely limits the value of a medical history in determining the risk posed by an individual patient. Serologic markers are quite useful for HBV and delta but less so for NANB. However, most patients are not routinely tested for these markers. The safest course of action is to treat all patients as if they are infectious.

Patient-to-patient spread can largely be eliminated by proper sterilization of all instruments and disinfection of appropriate items in the operatory. The dentist can be protected from infection by the patient through barrier techniques, which shield potential viral entry sites, such as the mouth, nose, eyes, and cuts and abrasions of the hands, from exposure to blood and saliva. To this end, routine use of gloves, mask, and glasses and goggles provides a significant degree of protection to the dental operator. Transmission of virus from dentist to patient occurs at a much lower frequency. Nevertheless, it has been documented. In these instances, cuts or abrasions on the dentist's hands are probably the sources of infectious virus, making gloving the most effective method of preventing transmission.

SUGGESTED READINGS

Alward W, McMahon B, Hall D, Heyward W, Francis D, Bender T. The long-term serological course of asymptomatic hepatitis B virus carriers and the development of hepatocellular carcinoma. *J Infect Dis.* 1985;151:604–609.

Centers for Disease Control. Postexposure prophylaxis of hepatitis B. *MMWR.* 1984;33:285–290.

Choo Q-L, Kuo G, Weiner AJ, Overby LR, Bradley DW, Houghton M. Isolation of a cDNA clone derived from a blood borne non-A, non-B viral hepatitis genome. *Science.* 1989;244:359–362.

Dienstag JR. Non A, non B hepatitis. II. Experimental transmission, putative virus agents and markers, and prevention. *Gastroenterology.* 1983;85:743–768.

Farci P, Smedile A, Lavarini C, et al. Delta hepatitis in inapparent carriers of hepatitis B surface antigen: A disease simulating acute hepatitis B progressive to chronicity. *Gastroenterology.* 1983;85:669–673.

Gitnick G. Non A, Non B hepatitis, etiology and clinical course. *Annu Rev Med.* 1984;35:265–268.

Hilleman M. Prevention of human hepatitis. *Perspect Biol Med.* 1984;27:543–557.

Hoofnagle JH. Serologic markers of hepatitis B virus infection. *Annu Rev Med.* 1981;32:1–11.

Kane M, Lettau L. Transmission of HBV from dental personnel to patients. *J Am Dent Assoc.* 1985;634–636.

Krugman S, Davidson M. Hepatitis B vaccine: Prospects for duration of immunity. *Yale J Biol Med.* 1987;60:333–338.

Mori M. Status of viral hepatitis in the world community: Its incidence among dentists and other health personnel. *Int Dent J.* 1984;34:115–121.

Ponzetto A, Hoofnagle JH, Seeff LB. Antibody to the hepatitis B virus-associated delta-agent in immune serum globulins. *Gastroenterology.* 1984;87:1213–1216.

Stevens CE, Taylor PE, Pindyck J, et al. Epidemiology of hepatitis C virus: A preliminary study in volunteer blood donors. *JAMA.* 1990;263:49–53.

CHAPTER 31

Tumor Viruses, Human Immunodeficiency Virus, and Slow Viruses

Walter K. Long

INTRODUCTION
TUMOR VIRUSES
Mechanisms of Carcinogenesis
RNA Tumor Viruses
DNA Tumor Viruses
HUMAN IMMUNODEFICIENCY VIRUS
Clinical Disease and Pathogenesis
Epidemiology
Laboratory Diagnosis
Prevention and Treatment
Oral Aspects
SLOW VIRUS DISEASES
SUGGESTED READINGS

INTRODUCTION

In the preceding chapters, we have been concerned primarily with acute viral infections. However, there are a number of viral agents that do not follow this pattern. The disease states for which these agents are responsible are characterized by lengthy incubation periods of 1 year or longer. Illnesses falling in this category include cancers with a viral etiology, the neurotropic slow virus syndromes, and acquired immunodeficiency syndrome (AIDS).

TUMOR VIRUSES

Since the initial observation in 1911 by Peyton Rous that certain sarcomas of chickens were of a viral etiology, numerous tumor viruses have been described in a variety of species. The types of tumors include sarcomas, lymphomas, leukemias, and mammary tumors. Resemblance of these cancers to human malignancies prompted a concerted effort to identify human cancer viruses. Although this undertaking was a disappointment in its failure to conclusively identify human cancer viruses, in the process much was learned about viral and eukaryotic gene regulation.

Mechanisms of Viral Carcinogenesis

Much of our current knowledge concerning mechanisms of carcinogenesis has its roots in tumor virology. Viruses that transform normal cells into malignant cells in culture have proven particularly useful. The transformed cells can be differentiated from their normal counterparts by changes in cellular morphology and altered growth characteristics. Through the use of viral mutants, oncogenes have been identified that are responsible for these changes. DNA hybridization analysis revealed homologs of the viral oncogenes in normal cells, which are referred to as cellular oncogenes. This finding, combined with the fact that retroviruses lacking a functional oncogene replicate normally, indicates a probable cellular origin for these genes.

The proteins encoded by oncogenes include, protein kinases, GTP binding proteins, growth factors, nuclear proteins, and hormone receptors. It has been postulated that at least some of these genes are actively transcribed during fetal development, perhaps playing a role in cellular differentiation. The genes are either silent or expressed at very low levels in differentiated cells. Transformation of cells requires a particular level of oncogene expression. This can be achieved in one of several ways. Infection of a cell by an oncogene-carrying virus is one way. Integration of a viral genome into cellular DNA adjacent to a normally silent cellular oncogene can result in concomitant expression of the viral genome and cellular oncogene. Mutation of a cellular oncogene may also alter its expression. For example, a single base change leading to a single amino acid was the only difference noted between an inactive and a highly oncogenic form of one human oncogene. Some cancers are characterized by chromosomal translocations whereby an oncogene is placed adjacent to an active gene promoter.

RNA Tumor Viruses

Retroviruses have been shown to cause cancer in laboratory strains of chickens, mice, and other species. In the 1960s, feline leukemia virus was found to produce leukemia as well as immune deficiencies in cats, and the virus was shown to be transmitted between cats in household settings.

It was not until 1978 that the first human retrovirus was identified. This virus, now designated human T cell lymphotropic virus (HTLV-I), has been implicated in adult T cell leukemia. A second related virus, HTLV-II, was isolated from a man who had a T cell variant of the disease known as hairy-cell leukemia. Although both of these are relatively rare diseases, it must be emphasized that the associated retroviruses were isolated only after the application of sophisticated biochemical and cell culture techniques. With the rapid advances being made in molecular biology, the distinct possibility exists that viruses will be found to be associated with other, more common malignancies.

DNA Tumor Viruses

These viruses differ from those with RNA genomes in at least one significant aspect. Replication of virus leads to cell death. Transformation takes place when a defective virion infects a cell or when a virus capable of inducing a latent infection infects a cell.

The most extensively studied of these is the Epstein-Barr virus (EBV), the causative agent of infectious mononucleosis, a self-limiting lymphoproliferative disease. This virus also has been shown to be associated with Burkitt's lymphoma and nasopharyngeal carcinoma. Burkitt's lymphoma occurs primarily in parts of Africa and New Guinea. These lymphomas usually are located in the jaw and abdomen and consist of undifferentiated lymphocytes. EBV antigens and DNA can be detected in most of these tumors, and those afflicted have high EBV antibody titers. Similar tumors occur at a much lower frequency in other parts of the world, and these are usually EBV negative. A two-step carcinogenesis process has been proposed, with EBV inducing rapid cell proliferation, providing a target population of cells that are subject to mutagenesis by various environmental agents, such as dietary nitrosamines. Lending support to this hypothesis are the chromosomal translocations that have been noted in Burkitt's lymphoma. In the rearranged chromosomes, cellular oncogenes are placed downstream from the promoter region of immunoglobulin genes. Such a location would presumably lead to increased expression of the oncogenes.

Evidence exists for a causal relationship between EBV and nasopharyngeal carcinoma. It is the only human carcinoma that has been shown to be regularly associated with a virus. This condition, which is rare in the western world, is the most common cancer in southern China and of Chinese in Singapore and Malaysia. Virtually all of the tumor cells express EBV antigens and carry the EBV genome, and the victims have high IgA antibody titers to EBV. Other cancers also may have an EBV etiology, particularly the B cell lymphomas that have been associated with AIDS and other immunosuppressive states.

The correlation between sexual promiscuity and cervical carcinoma has been known for many years, and medical researchers have postulated an infectious origin for a long time. One of the viruses linked through seroepidemiology is herpes simplex virus type 2 (HSV-2). Although this virus has the ability to transform cells in culture, it has not been possible to detect it in most cases of this cancer. A recent prospective study of over 7000 women aged 25 to 35 in Czechoslovakia revealed no correlation between HSV-2 infection and the subsequent development of cervical carcinoma when populations were matched for a number of factors, including lifestyle. Instead, it may act as a cofactor, since the effects of HSV-2 infection appear similar to those of chemical carcinogens.

The etiologic role of human papillomaviruses (HPV) in the development of benign warts has been known for a long time. It now appears that these same agents are involved in human malignancies. One line of evidence comes from studies of epidermodysplasia verruciformis (EV), a disease characterized by the development of skin lesions that resemble flat warts, beginning at about age 6. These lesions persist throughout life, and by the third decade as many as one third of these individuals develop squamous cell carcinomas. HPV DNA can be detected in both the warts and the carcinomas. HPV also has been implicated as the etiologic agent in papillomas of the genitalia, known as condyloma acuminatum. This condition is transmissible, as indicated by the development of condyloma in about 60% of sexual partners of infected individuals after a 4 to 6 week incubation period. Condyloma acuminatum predisposes to the development of cervical dysplasia and cervical carcinoma. HPV has been found in numerous cervical carcinomas, with types 16 and 18 being particularly common. Male sexual partners of infected women are at increased risk of developing penile intraepithelial neoplasia. Papillomas of the oral cavity also have an HPV etiology, and the virus has been found in several oral cancers of squamous cell origin.

A correlation between chronic hepatitis B infection and primary hepatocellular carcinoma has been established (Chapter 30). The resulting tumors carry copies of the hepatitis B virus genome integrated into the cellular genome. At present, it is not known whether the hepatitis B virus codes for an oncogene or whether its integration affects the expression of cellular oncogenes.

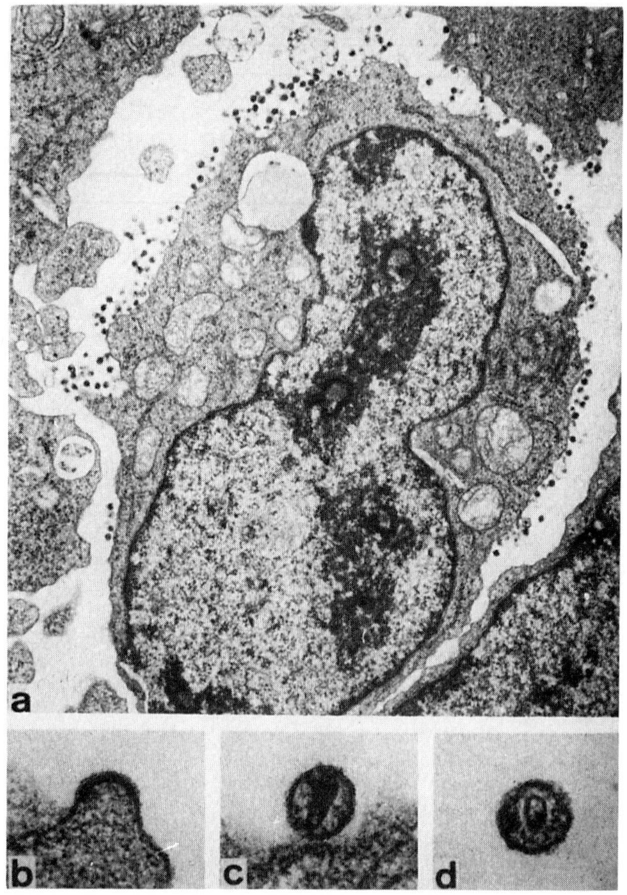

Figure 31–1. Electron micrograph of HIV-infected cells obtained from saliva. **A.** Leukocyte-expressing HIV. ×10,000. **B.** Budding virus. ×150,000. c, d. Mature virus particles. ×150,000. *(From Groopman JE, et al.* Science. *1984;226:448.)*

HUMAN IMMUNODEFICIENCY VIRUS

Reports first appeared in 1981 describing opportunistic infections and a malignancy, Kaposi's sarcoma, in young homosexual males. These particular syndromes usually are associated with immunodeficiency that results from disease, immunosuppression, or advanced age. However, in these cases, none of these factors were present. The term acquired immunodeficiency syndrome (AIDS) was coined to describe this condition. A concerted search for the etiologic agent led to the discovery of the human immunodeficiency virus (HIV).

HIV is a retrovirus that is related to HTLV-I (Fig 31–1). It does, however, possess some unique characteristics not seen in other retroviruses. In addition to the usual genes coding for core proteins, envelope proteins, and reverse transcriptase, there are four new genes designated *tat, trs, sor,* and *3'orf,* which encode proteins involved in the regulation of viral gene expression. Variants of HIV exist, as evidenced by differences at the nucleotide level and antigenic specificity.

Clinical Disease and Pathogenesis

HIV is the etiologic agent in a protracted illness that culminates in the syndrome known as AIDS. Virus is transmitted through intimate sexual contact or by direct exposure to infected blood. HIV infects and replicates in cells bearing the CD4 antigen. The CD4 molecule is found on the surfaces of all helper T lymphocytes, approximately 40% of monocytes and macrophages, and 5% of B lymphocytes. At approximately 2 to 6 weeks after infection, at least some individuals experience symptoms resembling infectious mononucleosis or influenza. Some of the symptoms reported include fever, dysuria, hematuria, dysphagia, rash, cough, sore throat, diarrhea, diffuse arthralgias, and myalgias.

Following either asymptomatic infection or resolution of this primary illness, antibodies to the virus can be detected. This usually is the first definitive evidence of HIV infection, and for purposes of staging the infection, it is regarded as the first stage.

Within 6 months to 1 year, patients enter the second stage of infection, which is characterized by the development of chronic lymphadenopathy. This stage lasts 3 to 5 years. Patients eventually experience the constellation of symptoms formerly called the AIDS-related complex (ARC). These include persistent fever, night sweats, chronic diarrhea, and weight loss. The next clinically evident stage of infection includes skin and mucous membrane manifestations, which reflect a suppression of cell-mediated immunity. These infections are usually of a fungal or viral etiology. They include oral thrush and vaginal infections, both caused by *Candida albicans,* and chronic oral and genital infections with herpes simplex virus. One of the most common lesions at this stage of the disease is hairy leukoplakia, a lesion of the tongue that appears as adherent, fuzzy, white patches (Fig 31–2). Epstein-Barr virus and human papillomavirus have been detected in a majority of lesions examined.

AIDS represents the final stage of infection. It is characterized by severe systemic immunodeficiency and is accompanied by a variety of infections, many of them potentially fatal (Table 31–1). In addition, many patients experience AIDS dementia, which can leave them unable to walk or think clearly.

Currently, the prognosis for individuals infected with HIV is not good. Statistics indicate that 10 to 30% will develop AIDS within 5 years of infection. Moreover, incubation periods of at least 7 years have been reported, and undoubtedly this figure will be extended. Based on the analysis of longitudinal studies, it appears that almost all, if not all, of those infected will eventually develop AIDS in the absence of effective chemotherapy. Diagnosed AIDS has a 5-year mortality rate exceeding 90%.

The definition of AIDS has changed somewhat since its initial description. With the development of laboratory tests for detection of HIV antibody and antigen, it is now possible to diagnose the disease at a much earlier stage. The Centers for Disease Control has established a Case Definition for Acquired Immunodeficiency Syndrome. A case of AIDS is defined as an illness characterized by one or more "indicator" diseases (Table 31–1), with laboratory evidence of HIV infection. Several of these diseases have oral manifestations, which may first be recognized by the dental professional. Among these are oral candidiasis, Kaposi's sarcoma (Fig 31–3), and oral lymphomas. Additionally, a positive correlation has been demonstrated between development of hairy leukoplakia and progression to AIDS.

The pathogenesis of HIV is dictated by the types of cells infected by HIV. Viral replication in helper T lymphocytes results in cell death, a fact that is reflected by a dramatic decrease in numbers of these cells in AIDS victims. Destruction of a cell population that plays such a central role in both cell-mediated and antibody-mediated immunity has a significant impact on immune competence. As a result, infection with a normally innocuous organism can lead to a life-threatening illness. Particularly prominent are infections with viral, fungal, and protozoal organisms and the development of tumors, all of which are to a large degree held in check by the cell-mediated immune system (Table 31–1).

Neurologic dysfunctions have been reported in about 60% of AIDS cases. In some instances, these problems can be attributed to toxoplasmosis, cryptococcosis, or a lymphoma of the central nervous system. However, in other cases of what is referred to as AIDS dementia, HIV appears to be solely involved. Examination of the brains of afflicted individuals has revealed HIV-infected monocytes and macrophages. Virus apparently crosses the blood–

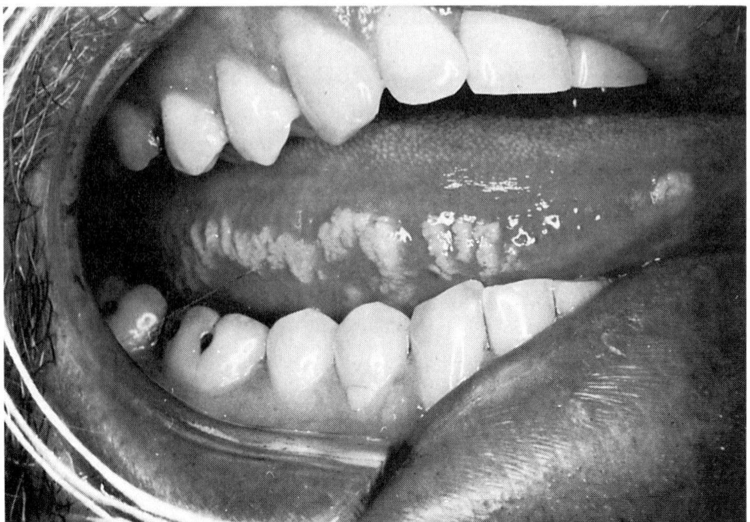

Figure 31–2. Hairy leukoplakia of the tongue. These white patches, which appear on the tongue, cannot be rubbed off. Their appearance precedes the development of AIDS and is an indicator of possible HIV infection. *(Courtesy of D. Greenspan.)*

TABLE 31–1. DISEASES INDICATING AIDS WITH LABORATORY EVIDENCE FOR HIV INFECTION

Protozoal Infections
Pneumocystis carinii pneumonia
Cryptosporidiosis with diarrhea persisting > 1 month
Toxoplasmosis of the brain affecting a patient > 1 month of age
Fungal infections
Candidiasis of the esophagus, trachea, bronchi, or lungs
Extrapulmonary cryptococcosis
Disseminated coccidioidomycosis
Disseminated histoplasmosis
Viral infections
Cytomegalovirus disease of an organ other than liver, spleen, or lymph nodes in a patient > 1 month of age
Herpes simplex virus infection causing a mucocutaneous ulcer that persists longer than 1 month
HIV encephalopathy
HIV wasting syndrome
Bacterial infections
Disseminated *Mycobacterium avium* or *Mycobacterium kansasii* disease
Cancers
Kaposi's sarcoma
Primary brain lymphoma
Non-Hodgkins B cell lymphoma

brain barrier in these cells. HIV replication results in the release of monokines and proteolytic enzymes and infiltration by inflammatory cells. These actions adversely affect neurons and glial cells, leading to neurologic dysfunction

Epidemiology

Over 90% of AIDS in the United States has occurred in homosexual males and intravenous drug users. A significant number of infections also were attributed to the transfusion of blood or blood products. Identification of the etiologic agent has led to the development of serologic tests for the virus and its antibody. Screening of blood was made possible by these tests and thus has largely eliminated this source of infection. Based on these tests, it is estimated that between 1 and 1.5 million individuals in the United States are infected and perhaps as many as 5 million worldwide. The virus is transmitted through both heterosexual and homosexual contact, with receptive anal intercourse and multiple sexual partners significantly increasing the risk of infection. Other sexually transmitted diseases that produce genital lesions are believed to facilitate the sexual transmission of HIV. The high rates of infection among users of injectable drugs results from the sharing of HIV-contaminated needles and syringes. Vertical transmission has also been demonstrated, with children born to HIV-positive mothers being congenitally or perinatally infected. Extensive studies have failed to reveal transmission by other routes. This is evidenced by the lack of transmission to other members of the same household, even when contact included kissing and even sharing the same toothbrush in some instances.

Laboratory Diagnosis

Diagnosis of AIDS usually involves the identification of markers of HIV infection in the presence of indicator diseases (Table 31–1). The two types of markers are HIV antigens and HIV antibodies. Antigen appears before antibody and may be present for years. The persistence of HIV antigenemia indicates a poor clinical prognosis. An ELISA test is most commonly used to detect antigen.

Antibody appears later than antigen, generally 6 to 12 weeks after infection. When it does appear, it is present at higher levels than antigen and is much easier to detect. For these reasons, it is the antibody tests that are in standard use for the determination of HIV status. Generally, a combination of two tests is

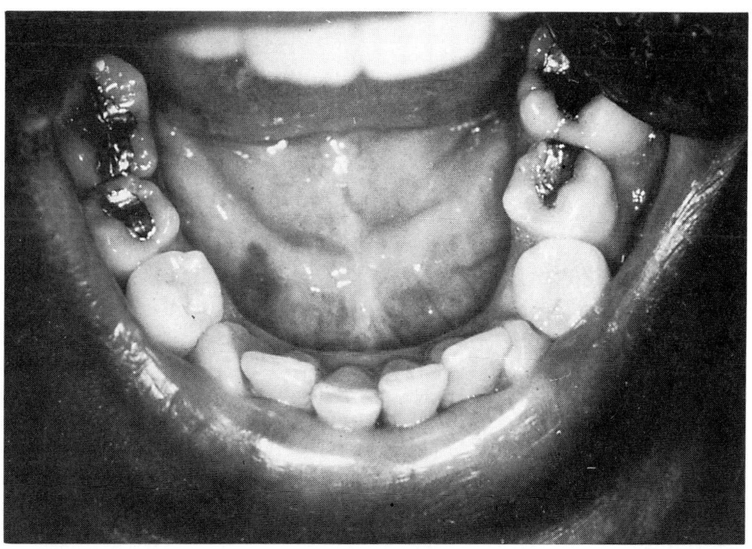

Figure 31–3. Oral lesions of Kaposi's sarcoma. *(Courtesy of Centers for Disease Control, Atlanta, Ga.)*

used to ascertain HIV antibody status. The first of these is an ELISA screening test that uses HIV-infected cells as a source of antigen. It is a sensitive and relatively inexpensive test but does give a small number of false positives. Positive sera are subjected to confirmation by Western blot analysis, a far more tedious and expensive test to perform. A serum is considered positive only when it reacts with at least two different HIV antigens on the Western blot. Improved tests should be available in the very near future. Various HIV genes have been cloned in bacteria and yeast, providing a relatively inexpensive source for large quantities of purified antigens. Preliminary tests using selected antigens in ELISA tests are quite promising. Under these conditions, all of the advantages of the ELISA test are retained, and the problem of false positives is eliminated.

Prevention and Treatment

At present, there is no cure for AIDS. Present strategy is focused on the prevention of transmission of HIV. Much of the focus on the prevention of AIDS has centered on programs to inform the public as a whole and high-risk groups in particular about the measures that can be taken to prevent HIV transmission. It has been demonstrated that condoms reduce the risk of sexual transmission of virus, and their use is recommended in any instance where HIV infection is possible. Attempts are being made to discourage the other major source of infection, the shared use of needles and syringes by intravenous drug users.

The quest for an AIDS treatment has been focused on two areas. One of these involves reconstitution of immune competence via immunomodulators. In this regard, trials were conducted with interleukin 2, but they were inconclusive.

A second approach has concentrated on antiviral therapy. Literally all antivirals currently available have been screened for in vitro activity against HIV. Clinical trials have been conducted on a number of those that showed activity. At present, only one of these, Azidothymidine (AZT) has been approved by the FDA for the treatment of AIDS. It does not cure AIDS or completely eliminate the virus. AZT does, however, prolong the lives of AIDS victims. The mode of action of AZT is similar to that of other nucleoside analogs (Chapter 24). It both acts as a competitive inhibitor of reverse transcriptase and is incorporated into DNA, where it acts as a chain terminator.

Oral Aspects

Dental professionals are not considered to be at high risk for acquiring AIDS. However, transmission of virus by accidental needlestick or other exposure of cuts or openings in the skin to contaminated blood during the administration of health care has been documented, with at least one case involving a dentist. As more members of society are infected with this virus, an increasingly large number of dentists will be exposed. Although transmission in this manner has occurred only rarely, it is prudent to avoid any unnecessary risk. Measures that have proven successful in preventing hepatitis virus infections should certainly suffice for HIV. These include the use of gloves, face mask, and eye protection in the treatment of all patients, with gloves being the single most important item. Although virus has been demonstrated in saliva, transmission by saliva appears unlikely, based on the results of studies of household contacts previously described. As with hepatitis B, blood is the most important body fluid for the dentist to consider. The Centers for Disease Control has developed specific recommendations designed to protect health care professionals from occupation-related HIV infection (Chapter 4). These recommendations are based on the fact that medical history and examination cannot reliably identify all patients with HIV or other blood-borne pathogens. Therefore, blood and body fluid precautions should be consistently used for all patients, especially those in emergency care settings in which the risk of blood exposure is increased and the infection status of the patient usually is unknown. Furthermore, the CDC states that blood, saliva, and gingival fluid from all dental patients should be considered infective and that special emphasis should be placed on following precautions for preventing transmission of blood-borne pathogens in dental practice in both institutional and noninstitutional settings.

Dental professionals can play an important role in the diagnosis of AIDS. Many of the indicator diseases of HIV infection have oral manifestations that might well first come to the attention of the dentist.

The most common of these infections is candidiasis, which is present at some stage of the infection in up to 90% of all AIDS patients. This disease has a tendency to be more severe in HIV-positive patients, with the possibility of esophageal and tracheal involvement. Mucocutaneous herpes is also more prevalent and more severe in this group. The previously described hairy leukoplakia has so far been seen only in HIV-positive patients, with most of these progressing to AIDS within 3 years.

Kaposi's sarcoma appears in approximately 20% of all AIDS patients. Lesions may be present both orally and on the body, and in some cases only oral lesions are seen.

Another manifestation of advanced AIDS is an acute periodontal syndrome marked by rapid tissue destruction and intense pain.

SLOW VIRUS DISEASES

A number of progressive degenerative diseases of the CNS have been described that are infectious in origin and are characterized by lengthy incubation periods encompassing several years. The etiologic agents in these infections are viruses or subviral particles called prions. Diseases that fall into this category include subacute sclerosing panencephalitis (SSPE), progressive multifocal leukoencephalopathy (PML), progressive rubella panencephalitis, kuru, and Creutzfeld-Jakob disease (CJD).

An altered form of the measles virus has been implicated in SSPE. Virus appears to enter the CNS via infected lymphocytes, after which it undergoes mutations that enable it to escape eradication by the immune system. Viral replication and the inflammatory response to it result in the destruction of neural cells.

Two related viruses, JC and SV40, are associated with PML. In these infections, viral antigens are expressed. However, there appears to be an underlying immunodeficiency. Reduced immune responses that occur during pregnancy and with immunosuppressive therapy for organ transplantation are correlated with development of this disease.

In rare instances, rubella virus produces a panencephalitis 10 or more years after the initial infection. Infectious virus can be recovered from brain tissue, but viral antigens cannot be detected in the CNS.

A great deal of controversy exists as to the nature of the etiologic agents in kuru and CJD. They have been referred to as prions. These agents, which consist of protein and possibly a very small genome, are quite resistant to the effects of proteases and nucleases, which commonly inactivate viruses. Kuru is one of the most extensively studied of the so-called slow virus diseases. It was first described in Aborigines in New Guinea. Transmission of the disease was traced eventually to the practice of ritual cannibalism, in which the brains of the deceased were consumed by women and children of the tribe. In this manner, a normally noninfectious agent was transmitted from those who died of kuru to others, perpetuating this endemic disease. The tribe's people did not associate the disease with such practices, since the illness occurred after a lengthy incubation period of several years and progressed over an extended period of time, eventually leading to complete incoordination and dementia.

CJD generally is not evident until the sixth decade of life, at which time it first occurs as ataxia, finally progressing to dementia. Transmission has been traced to corneal transplants from a victim and to contaminated electroencephalographic electrodes.

At present, evidence does not exist to indicate that these diseases are transmitted in the dental operatory. What is known about them does, however, serve to emphasize the importance of properly sterilizing instruments, being aware that infectious agents exist that are resistant to many of the methods of disinfection commonly used.

SUGGESTED READINGS

AIDS: A single topic issue. *Sci Am.* 1988;259:40–134.

Barr CE, Marder MZ. *AIDS: A Guide for Dental Practice.* Chicago: Quintessence Publishing Co; 1987.

CDC. Revision of the CDC surveillance case definition for acquired immunodeficiency syndrome. *MMWR.* 1987; 36:Suppl 1S.

Croce CM, Klein G. Chromosome translocations and human cancer. *Sci Am.* 1985;252:54–60.

Fauci A. The human immunodeficiency virus: Infectivity and mechanisms of pathogenesis. *Science.* 1988;239:617–622.

Gluckman JC, Klatzman D, Montagnier L. Lymphadenopathy-associated virus infection and acquired immunodeficiency syndrome. *Annu Rev Immunol.* 1986; 4:97–117.

Greenspan JS, Greenspan D, Lennette ET, et al. Replication of Epstein-Barr virus within the epithelial cells of oral "hairy" leukoplakia, an AIDS-associated lesion. *N Engl J Med.* 1985;313:1564–1571.

Hirsch MS, Kaplan JC. Treatment of human immunodeficiency virus infections. *Antimicrob Agents Chemother.* 1987;31:839–843.

Ho DD, Pomerantz RJ, Kaplan JC. Pathogenesis of infection with human immunodeficiency virus. *N Engl J Med.* 1987; 317:278–286.

Pfister H. Human papillomavirus and genital cancer. *Adv Cancer Res.* 1987;48:113–147.

Prusiner SB. Prions: Novel infectious pathogens. *Adv Virus Res.* 1984;29:1–56.

Vonka V, Kanka J, Roth Z. Herpes simplex type 2 virus and cervical neoplasia. *Adv Cancer Res.* 1987;48:149–191.

CHAPTER 32

Oral Microflora

Samuel Rosen and Memory Elvin-Lewis

INTRODUCTION
METHODS OF STUDY
Sampling for Oral Bacteria
Media Selection, Cultivation, and Identification
FACTORS THAT AFFECT THE NORMAL ORAL MICROFLORA
BACTERIAL CHANGES FROM BIRTH TO DEATH
MECHANISMS OF ORAL MICROBIAL ADHERENCE, COLONIZATION, AND AGGREGATION
DENTAL PLAQUE
Development of Dental Plaque
Microbial Composition of Plaque
Changes in Microbial Composition of Plaque
Chemical Composition of Plaque
Adherence and Colonization Mechanisms
Dental Calculus
Plaque Control
ORAL MICROBIAL ECOLOGY
PATHOGENIC POTENTIAL OF THE NORMAL ORAL FLORA
SUMMARY
SUGGESTED READINGS

INTRODUCTION

The oral cavity harbors a large and diverse microbial population, with billions of bacteria present in a healthy individual's mouth. The oral cavity is analogous to a continuous culture system. Nutrients are supplied in the form of saliva, gingival fluid, and desquamated epithelial cells, and the oral cavity is an initial depository for incoming nutrients and microorganisms. The mouth has ideal conditions for supporting the growth of diverse microorganisms, including aerobic as well as anaerobic bacteria. It is moist, warm (35 to 36°C) and has an optimum pH (6.8 to 7.2) for most bacteria. The oral cavity has hard tissue surfaces and a variety of soft tissue surfaces that serve as optimal areas for adherence and colonization of a variety of microbial forms. The oral flora have been considered either harmless or having a low order of virulence. However, under suitable conditions, numbers of certain species of the oral flora increase to cause dental caries and periodontal disease. Furthermore, this flora has the pathogenic potential for causing systemic infections, such as infectious endocarditis, actinomycosis, candidiasis, and mixed anaerobic infections. This chapter presents (1) methods for the study of oral flora, (2) its composition, (3) changes in flora from birth to death, (4) a discussion of the factors that influence adherence and colonization of the oral flora, (5) plaque flora, (6) oral ecology, and (7) pathogenic potential of the oral flora.

METHODS OF STUDY

Sampling for Oral Bacteria

There are no standardized procedures for sampling plaque, saliva, gingival crevice, or soft tissue areas. For example, the type of organisms that will be recovered from the sample of plaque depends on the site, since organisms that colonize the smooth surfaces of the teeth vary from those found interproximally, subgingivally, or on occlusal surfaces. Likewise, both qualitative and quantitative differences have been found when stimulated, unstimulated, or cannulated saliva samples were compared. Variations are related also to host factors, such as immunologic status, age, salivary flow, and food intake. Specific antibodies (IgA and IgG levels), adolescence, and xerostomia should be considered when determinations are made of the oral flora. The kinds of foods consumed must be considered; for example, refraining from eating any refined carbohydrates usually results in lower levels of salivary lactobacilli. Also, bacterial counts decrease after brushing and eating, gradually increase before meals, and reach their highest values after the long overnight incubation period.

The use of strict anaerobic techniques for sampling and cultivation is often necessary for the maintenance of viability and growth of oral microorganisms, since many are strict anaerobes. A guide to the type of technique used should be related to the area sampled. The study of fastidious anaerobes requires anaerobic sampling techniques. Material from gingival sulci has been removed under nitrogen gas to retain anaerobic conditions. Organisms deep within the gingival sulcus, the pulp, or carious lesions are more likely to be obligate anaerobes than those inhabiting the exposed areas of the tongue or buccal mucosa, where the oxidation-reduction potentials are considerably higher.

Organisms such as spirochetes and other oral flora difficult to cultivate can be visualized in the living state by phase contrast or darkfield microscopy. This may provide a rapid assessment of oral microbial health by the clinician without the necessity of microbiologic techniques necessary for isolation and cultivation. In addition, phase or darkfield microscopy may be the only means of identifying, at least on a morphologic basis, these organisms that are unable to be cultivated because of stringent biochemical and biophysical requirements. On the other hand, cultivation, although time consuming, is necessary for definitive identification as well as for studying biochemical and immunologic parameters that may influence the host-parasite relationship in the oral cavity.

Media Selection, Cultivation, and Identification

In attempting to isolate and identify microflora from the oral cavity, selective or nonselective media may be used. The advantage of selective media is that you can more easily isolate an organism that you are seeking. Selective media have been developed for the isolation of streptococci, yeasts, lactobacilli, actinomyces, *Campylobacter,* treponemes, and *Mycoplasma.* For example, Mitis-Salivarius agar (MSA) is selective because it contains crystal violet and potassium tellurite, which inhibit most microorganisms except certain streptococci. Sucrose in the medium promotes the production of extracellular polysaccharides that confer upon the oral streptococcal species a distinctive colony shape and consistency that aid in their identification. Through the addition of bacitracin, further selectivity is achieved, since this antibiotic inhibits oral streptococci except for most *Streptococcus mutans.* The disadvantage of selective media is that they will not permit enumeration and identification of all varieties of microorganisms found in the mouth, and often they inhibit the species sought, thus leading to inaccuracy in enumeration. For this purpose, a nonselective medium such as brain-heart infusion blood agar may be used. Even the use of nonselective media has its limitations because a single medium will not support growth of all microorganisms:

In order to study oral microflora, both aerobic and anaerobic cultivation techniques are used. Since the microorganisms to be studied come from a source at body temperature, the temperature of incubation is usually 35°C to 37°C. Some oral microorganisms grow quickly and others slowly. The incubation time varies from 1 to 9 days.

Identification of oral microorganisms generally proceeds according to standard techniques and tests. Included among these are biochemical reactions, use of differential media, immunologic assays, and DNA probes. Fermentation of sorbitol and mannitol are useful in identifying *S. mutans* because these streptococci generally ferment these sugal alcohols, whereas only a few other microorganisms, such as *Streptococcus faecalis,* are able to ferment them. Species of *Antinomyces* can be identified by fluorescent antibody staining. Other species of oral bacteria require more extensive tests for identification. A cultural protocol used to identify bacteria associated with periodontal disease is shown in Fig 32–1.

FACTORS THAT AFFECT THE NORMAL ORAL MICROFLORA

The normal oral flora are those organisms present that are permanent inhabitants of the oral cavity in

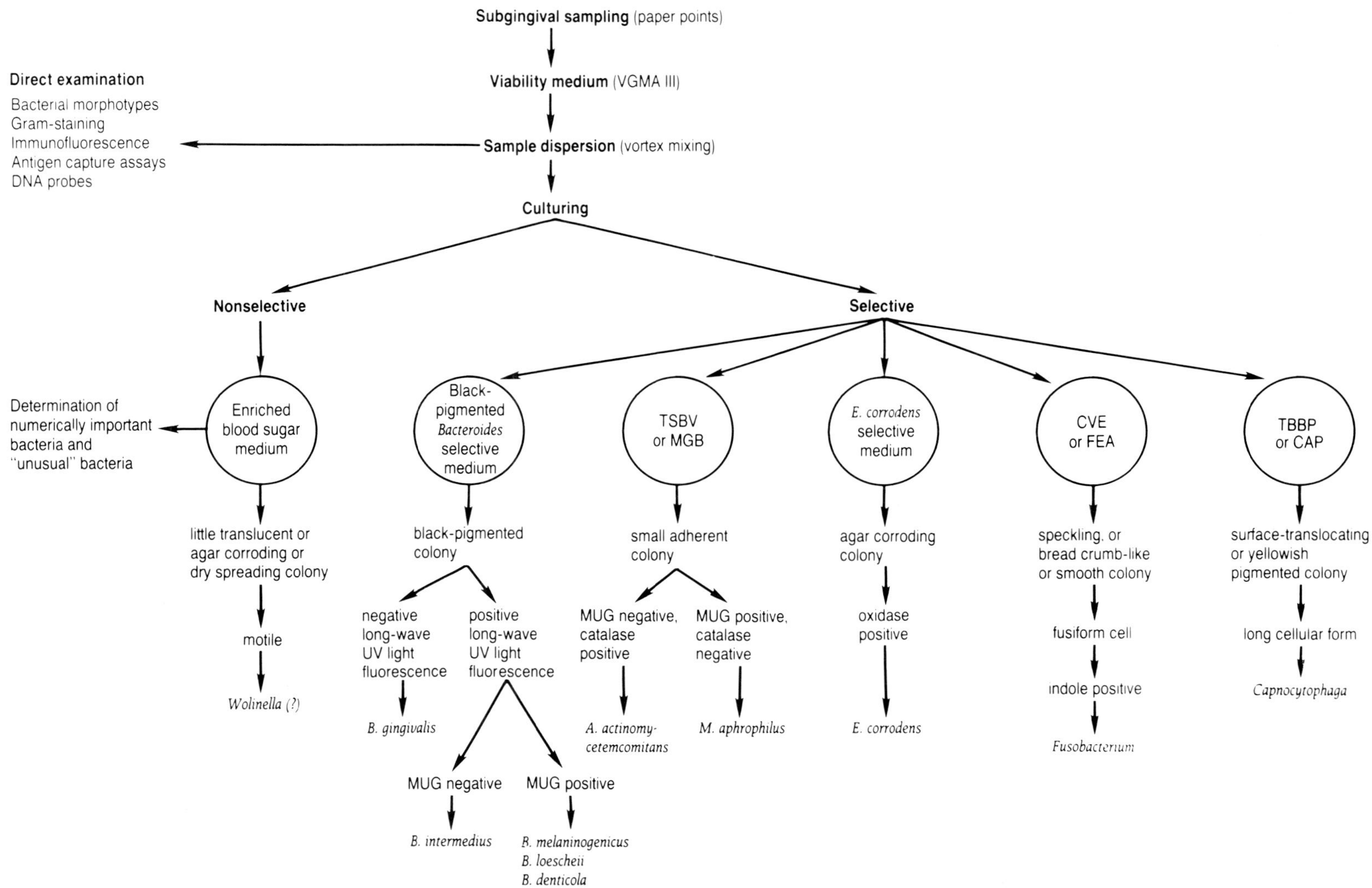

Figure 32–1. Flow chart for rapid presumptive identification of important periodontal organisms. *(From Slots J.* Oral Microbiol Immunol. *1986; 1:48–55.)*

TABLE 32–1. BACTERIAL GENERA COMMONLY ISOLATED FROM THE NORMAL HUMAN MOUTH

Gram-positive bacteria	Gram-negative bacteria
Actinomyces	*Actinobacillus*
Arachnia	*Bacteroides*
Bacterionema	*Branhamella*
Bifidobacterium	*Capnocytophaga*
Eubacterium	*Eikenella*
Lactobacillus	*Fusobacterium*
Micrococcus	*Peptostreptococcus*
Neisseria	*Haemophilus*
Propionibacterium	*Leptotrichia*
Rothia	*Selenomonas*
Streptococcus	*Simonsiella*
	Treponema
	Veillonella
	Wolinella

From *March PO, Martin M.* Oral Microbiology. *2nd ed. Washington, DC: American Society for Microbiology; 1984.*

dentulous individuals. These consist of a wide range of viruses, yeasts, protozoa, and bacteria. More than 300 species inhabit the oral cavity. Of these about 30 are found routinely and account for the majority of the cultivable strains.

This chapter concentrates on the bacteria found in the mouth, since these constitute the majority of the microorganisms. The bacterial genera commonly isolated from the mouth are shown in Table 32–1.

Various factors contribute to oral microbial composition. The site in the oral cavity makes a difference as to the types of bacteria. The approximate intraoral proportion distribution of some of the more common oral bacteria is given in Table 32–2. *Streptococcus salivarius* preferentially colonizes the tongue; *Streptococcus mitior* colonizes both soft and hard tissues, and *Streptococcus sanguis* and *S. mutans* are found in highest proportions on the surfaces of teeth. *Bacteroides,* vibrios, and spirochetes show a preference for the gingival crevice. This selectivity results from complex, dynamic relationships involving host, microbial and environmental factors.

Certain microorganisms tend to support each other (commensal activity) by the production of nutritional factors that influence the proportions of microorganisms present in the oral cavity. For example, the metabolite, para-aminobenzoic acid is produced by *S. sanguis* and used by *S. mutans,* and *Bacteroides gingivalis* is dependent on other bacteria to produce vitamin K (Table 32–3). Consumption of sucrose tends to increase the numbers of *S. mutans* and of lactobacilli.

As oral disease develops, the composition of the microflora changes due to changes in environment, such as plaque buildup, oxygen tension, and morphologic changes in teeth as caries progresses. Numbers of *S. mutans* and lactobacilli increase with the develop-

TABLE 32–2. INTRAORAL DISTRIBUTION OF BACTERIA[a]

	Ecologic Niches				
Normal Oral Flora	***Gingival Crevice***	***Coronal Plaque***	***Tongue Dorsum***	***Buccal Mucosa***	***Saliva***
Gram-positive cocci					
Streptococcus salivarius	<1	<1	20	11	20
S. mitior (mitis)	8	15	8	60	20
S. sanguis	8	15	4	11	8
S. mutans	?[b]	0–50	<1	<1	<1
Enterococci	0–10	<1	<1	<1	<1
Gram-positive filaments					
Actinomyces, Nocardia, Rothia, Corynebacterium, Bacterionema, Leptotrichia	35	42	20	?	15
Gram-positive rods					
Lactobacilli	<1	<1	<1	<1	<1
Gram-negative cocci					
Veillonella sp.	10	2	12	1	10
Neisseria	<1	<1	<1	<1	<1
Gram-negative rods					
Bacteroides oralis	5	5	4	?	?
B. melaninogenicus	6	<1	<1	<1	<1
Vibrio sputorum	5	1	<1	<1	<1
Fusobacterium	3	4	1		<1
Spirochetes					
Treponema, Borrelia sp.	2	<1	<1	<1	<1

[a]Data are expressed as a percent of the total flora cultivable on anaerobically incubated blood agar.
[b]Unknown or not determined.
Adapted from Gibbons RJ, van Houte J. Annu Rev Microbiol. *1975;29:19–44.*

TABLE 32–3. COMMENSAL ACTIVITY OF THE ORAL FLORA

Product	Produced by	Used by
Levan, amylopectin	*Streptococcus salivarius* *Neisseria*	Streptococci and lactobacilli
Glucan	Streptococci	*Streptococcus mutans* *Streptococcus mitior* *Streptococcus salivarius* *Actinomyces israelii* *Capnocytophaga ochraceus*
Para-aminobenzoic acid	*Streptococcus sanguis*	*Streptococcus mutans*
Isobutyrate, putrescine, spermine	Fusobacteria	Oral spirochetes
Succinate	Gram-positive rods	Oral spirochetes
Hydrogen, formate	Fusobacteria, Bacteroides	*Vibrio*
Vitamin K	Various bacteria	*Bacteroides gingivalis*
Lactate	Oral streptococci	*Veillonella* *Neisseria* *Bacterionema*

ment of dental caries. Gram-negative anaerobic bacteria increase during the development of periodontal disease.

The presence of natural teeth or dentures favors an anaerobic flora. This is due to a buildup of microflora that use oxygen, resulting in a lowering of the oxidation-reduction potential (Eh). Outer layers of bacteria in dental plaque tend to be aerobic and use oxygen, permitting anaerobic bacteria to proliferate in the deeper layers. The environment in the gingival sulcus is different from that of other oral econiches. The Eh is low, allowing the growth of anaerobic species. There is a direct relationship between the decrease in plaque Eh and the increase in the numbers of anaerobic bacteria observed as plaque ages (Fig 2–1). Such subgingival microflora shifts are associated with the onset of disease.

A low pH at a particular site in the mouth due to production of acid by bacteria metabolizing carbohydrates would deter the development of nonaciduric microorganisms. A low pH is due to the presence of large numbers of acidogenic microorganisms, such as lactobacilli and certain streptococci, which degrade fermentable carbohydrates to acid. Low salivary flow could also contribute to a low pH. This occurs at sites of incipient caries.

Any deviation from the normal state may predispose to changes in the oral flora. For example, ill-fitting dentures and broad-spectrum antibiotic therapy may allow opportunistic microbes such as *Candida albicans* to increase in number. Certain malignancies and immunosuppressive therapy may predispose to enhanced growth of many fungi and bacteria that are absent or found in low, harmless numbers in the normal individual.

BACTERIAL CHANGES FROM BIRTH TO DEATH

Detectable organisms rapidly increase in 6 to 20 hours after birth and are mainly aerobic and facultatively anaerobic. The source of these organisms may be from the parents or other persons kissing or handling the infant or through fomites (substances, such as clothing or baby rattles, capable of transmitting a disease). *Streptococcus salivarius* usually is detected between 10 and 24 hours after birth. Other indigenous organisms, such as *Neisseria, Staphylococcus, Lactobacillus, Fusobacterium, Nocardia,* certain *Actinomyces,* and *Veillonella,* are found with increasing regularity in infants within their first year of age and tend to be present thereafter. *Streptococcus mitior, S. mutans, S. sanguis,* and *Actinomyces viscosus* are not found until teeth erupt. Anaerobes appear as soon as teeth erupt and then increase even more at puberty. Organisms such as *Bacteroides* and spirochetes are more frequently isolated, especially in the gingival crevices. If periodontal disease occurs, the population of anaerobes and pyogenic (pus-forming) organisms increases at the expense of facultative bacteria (such as streptococci). The microflora in edentulous mouths, like the infant, are primarily aerobic, but with dentures, the anaerobic and facultative flora is restored once again because there is plaque buildup on dentures. However, evidence for this is not complete.

MECHANISMS OF ORAL MICROBIAL ADHERENCE, COLONIZATION, AND AGGREGATION

As exogenous microorganisms enter the mouth, they first make contact with the saliva and then may make contact with the oral soft tissues, oral appliances, and teeth. In order to join the community of oral microflora, a microorganism must be able to colonize some fixed surface within the oral cavity. Otherwise, it will be washed away in the saliva that is constantly swallowed. Some microorganisms, such as lactobacilli, have no adherent mechanism and must be retained by entrapment, especially in pits and fissures. Other microorganisms, such as spirochetes and *Bacteroides,* are retained in the gingival crevice of the periodontal pocket. They have little avidity for either mucosal or tooth surface but can survive in a suitable

TABLE 32–4. RELATION BETWEEN THE EXPERIMENTALLY OBSERVED ADHERENCE OF BACTERIA AND THEIR PROPORTIONS PRESENT NATURALLY ON ORAL SURFACES

	Approximate Proportions Found Naturally[a]				Experimentally Observed Adherence		
Organism	*Saliva*	*Coronal Plaque*	*Tongue Dorsum*	*Buccal Mucosa*	*Coronal Tooth Surfaces*	*Tongue Dorsum*	*Buccal Mucosa*
Streptococcus salivarius	20	<1	20	11	Low	High	Moderate
Streptococcus sanguis	8	15	4	11	High	Moderate	Moderate
Streptococcus mitior	20	15	8	60	High	Moderate	High
Streptococcus mutans	<1	0–50[b]	<1	<1	Low	Low	Low
Veillonella sp.	10	2	12	1	Low	High	Low
Lactobacillus sp.	<1	<1	<1	<1	Low	Low	Low

[a]Data expressed as a percentage of the total cultivable flora on blood agar plates.
[b]Proportions vary with dietary sucrose intake.
Adapted from Gibbons RJ. J Dent Res. *1984;63:378–385.*

environment. However, *Bacteroides* may be retained in the plaque as a result of coaggregation with *Actinomyces.* Before bacteria can adhere to an oral tissue, they must first contact that tissue's surface with a certain degree of frequency and numbers. It has been shown experimentally that about 10^4 cells per milliliter of saliva is required for a single cell of *S. sanguis* to become attached to a tooth surface. For *S. mutans,* the concentration is about 10-fold higher. Explanations for why these levels of microorganisms are needed would be speculative. Oral bacteria have been used to test for specificity of adherence by in vitro techniques. Adsorption of these bacteria was evaluated using buccal epithelial cells and saliva-coated hydroxyapatite surfaces. When compared to in vitro findings, there was a striking similarity of the proportions of bacteria found naturally adhering to specific oral tissues (Table 32–4). Thus, the bacterial cell surface must contain an adherence system that enables it to interact with specific different components on buccal or tongue epithelial cells or teeth. Therefore, the relative resistance or susceptibility of a particular oral tissue to colonization by a specific microorganism is usually dependent on the ability of that microorganism to attach to the tissue.

The high degree of specificity of bacterial attachment to oral tissues indicates that there is a complex interaction system. It is now known that certain bacteria possess adherent surface molecules known as adhesins. Polysaccharide-binding lectins are examples of adhesins that can specifically bind to complementary substrate molecules or ligands found on the surfaces of prokaryotic or eukaryotic cells. These adhesins may be associated with the bacterial cell as surface binding proteins.

Adherence properties also are associated with the glucosyltransferases and glucans of *S. mutans.* This is due to the enzyme's attachment to fibrils on the exterior of the cell. Glucan is bound to the enzyme as polymerization of the glucose moiety of sucrose occurs. Thus, the glucans are cell-associated and can bind to the tooth surface or to other bacteria. Moreover, certain oral bacteria possess proteins that allow them to adhere to glucans in the plaque matrix or to those associated with other oral bacteria. Several binding sites or only one binding site may be used for adherence. A multiple binding site, as shown for species B in Fig 32–2, is indicative of stronger binding activity than the single binding site of species A and is more likely to be retained on the oral surface. Strepto-

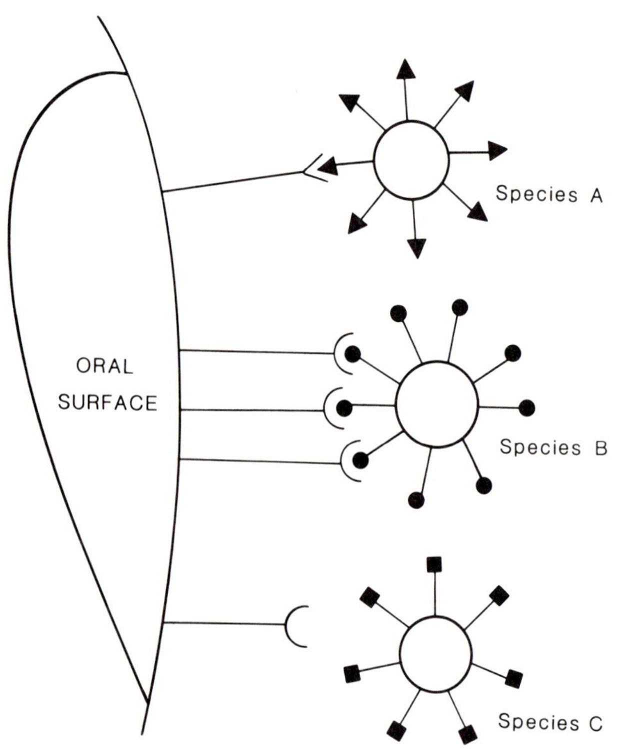

Figure 32–2. Complementary receptor site hypothesis. Diagram shows oral surface (teeth or soft tissues) with complementary receptors specific for two bacterial species, A and B, and with noncomplementary receptors for one bacterial species, C. Note that single or multiple binding sites may be available.

cocci have a number of other components associated with their adherence properties that include lipoteichoic acids on their surface and fibrillae that bind to all eukaryotic cells and to a ubiquitous surface glycoprotein called fibronectin (found in plasma). These compounds are located on cell surfaces and in extracellular matrixes, such as pellicle, and to salivary agglutinins. Adhesins are also found as components of filamentous structures, called fimbriae, or on fine, hairy, irregular structures, called fuzz or fibrillae (Fig 32–3). (The term pili is now restricted to those fimbriae that are used for sexual conjugation among certain prokaryotic species.)

Since adhesins often are found on the fibrillar appendages of microorganisms, the presence or absence of these appendages may be a factor in adherence and subsequent disease. It has been shown that *A. viscosus* strain T14Vi causes severe bone loss in rats, whereas *A. viscosus* strain T14Av causes no damage. Examination of the cell surfaces of each strain revealed that T14Vi had more surface fibrils than did strain T14Av. In addition, the fibrils that were present on strain T14Av were embedded in a cell-associated microcapsule (Fig 32–4).

In addition to initial attachment of bacteria to cell surfaces mediated by adhesins binding to complementary receptor sites, electrostatic interaction may be involved in initial bacterial cell to oral surface adherence (Fig 32–5). In this interaction, initial attachment is mediated by calcium ions, hydrogen bonding, or hydrophobic bonding, which serves as a bridge between the negative charges on the oral surface and lipoteichoic acid on the bacterial surface. Evidence to support the theory of electrostatic interaction comes from the finding that chelators remove calcium ions and dissolve newly developed plaque. In addition, the antiplaque agents, chlorhexidine and quaternary ammonium compounds will reduce the affinity between the oral cell surface and the bacterial cell surface due to their binding to carboxyl, phosphate, and sulfate groups.

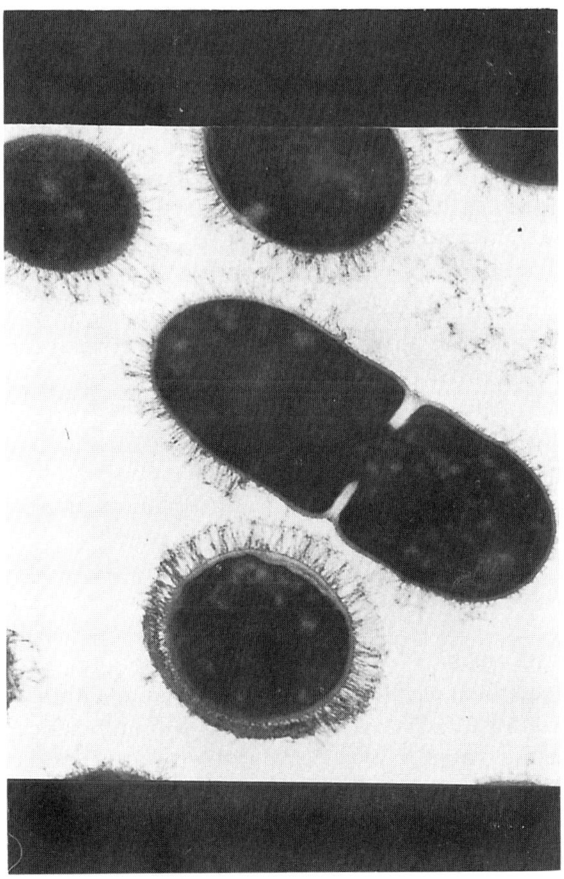

Figure 32–3. Electron micrograph of *Streptococcus salivarius* (strain 9652) and *Streptococcus mitior* (strain RE-7). Immunoelectron microscopic identification and localization of *Streptococcus sanguis* with peroxidase-labeled antibody showing hairlike processes (fibrillae) on periphery of cell that are believed to be associated with adherence of these organisms to oral epithelial cells. *(From Lai C, et al.* Infect Immun. *1975;11:197.)*

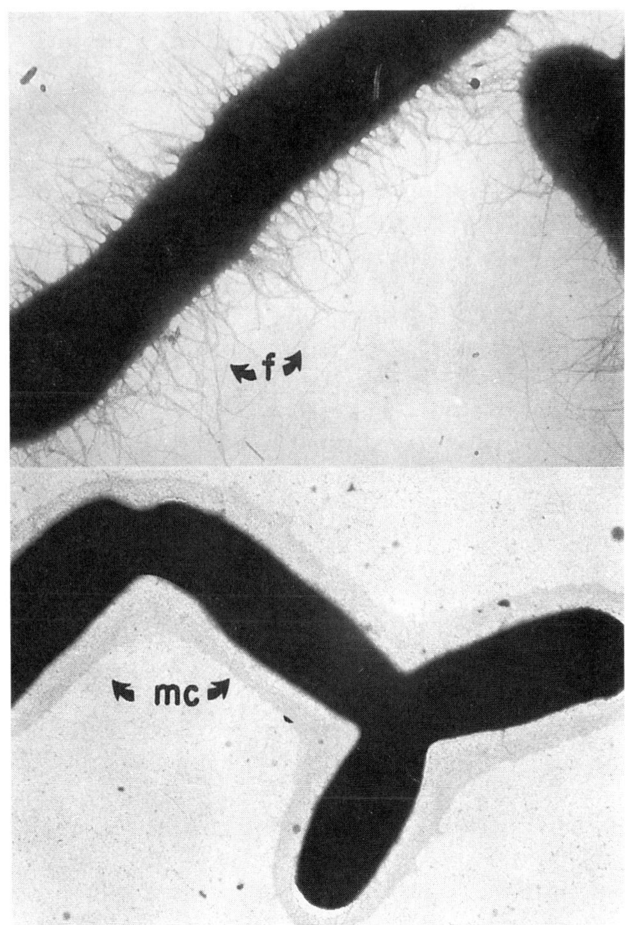

Figure 32–4. Transmission electron photomicrographs of *Actinomyces viscosus*. **Top.** Virulent *A. viscosus* strain T14Vi with numerous surface appendages, f. **Bottom.** Avirulent *A. viscosus* strain T14Av enclosed in a cell-associated microcapsule, mc. *(Courtesy of Dr. D.C. Birdsell, University of Washington, Seattle.)*

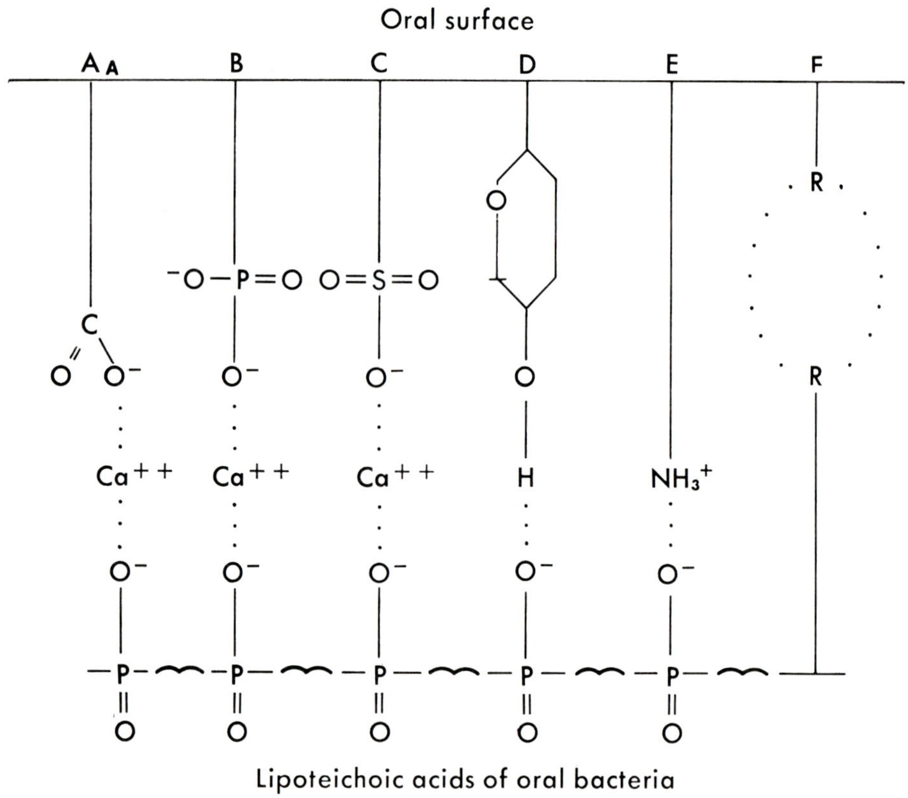

Figure 32–5. Electrostatic interaction hypothesis. Diagram shows some of the functional groups of host macromolecules with which bacterial lipoteichoic acids may interact during adherence. A, B, and C. Examples of interactions mediated by divalent cations. D. Hydrogen bonding. E. An ionic interaction. F. Hydrophobic bonding. *(Adapted from Rolla G, Bonesvoll, Opermann R. Interactions between oral streptococci and salivary proteins.* Microbiol Abstr. *1979;(Suppl.):227–241.)*

Bacteria may aggregate (clump with themselves, as in the case of *S. mutans* with dextran or glucan) or they may coaggregate (one species adheres to another species, as in Fig 32–6). These processes may be mediated by specific salivary antibodies and nonspecific glycoprotein factors. Aggregation and coaggregation can be part of the colonization process, or these phenomena may act as a host defense mechanism. In the latter case, when the clumps become large enough, they would be susceptible to mechanical cleansing by shear forces and by salivary flow. When coaggregation occurs between a coccus and a rod, a corncob formation is seen (Fig 32–6B). An example of this formation occurs between *Actinomyces* and *Veillonella.* Other examples of oral bacteria that coaggregate are *Bacteroides* with *Capnocytophaga*, *Actinomyces* with *Fusobacterium*, and *Streptococcus* with *Actinomyces.*

Once the bacteria have found their econiche whether by an adhesive or nonadhesive mechanism, the process of colonization begins. Bacteria begin to multiply provided that the appropriate biochemical and biophysical conditions are present.

DENTAL PLAQUE

The tooth's surface is covered by several layers of organic material. The innermost layer is the acquired enamel pellicle, an adherent organic coating of the tooth derived from saliva. The next layer is dental plaque, which is a dense, noncalcified bacterial mass so firmly attached to the tooth surface that it resists removal by washing action of saliva or physiologic movement of soft tissue. The outermost layer is called material alba, a covering of loosely adherent material, consisting largely of ingested food, which can be dislodged by physiologic movements of soft tissues. Calculus may be formed within dental plaque. It is the hard mineral substance strongly adherent to tooth structure due to dental plaque that has become calcified.

Development of Dental Plaque

Supragingival Plaque. Bacteria in the oral cavity rarely come into contact with the enamel. Within seconds after a tooth surface is cleaned by efficient hygiene measures, salivary glycoproteins are adsorbed, forming the acquired pellicle. The attachment of the pellicle to the tooth surface is not fully understood, but in the initial phase, phosphate and sulfate groups attach to the apatite surface by ion displacement through direct ionic and hydrophobic interaction. In a second phase, additional glycoproteins are adsorbed due to intraction involving hydrogen bonding and van der Waal's forces. The pellicle contains antibodies, specific aggregating factors, and blood group reactive substances in addition to a variety of glycoproteins.

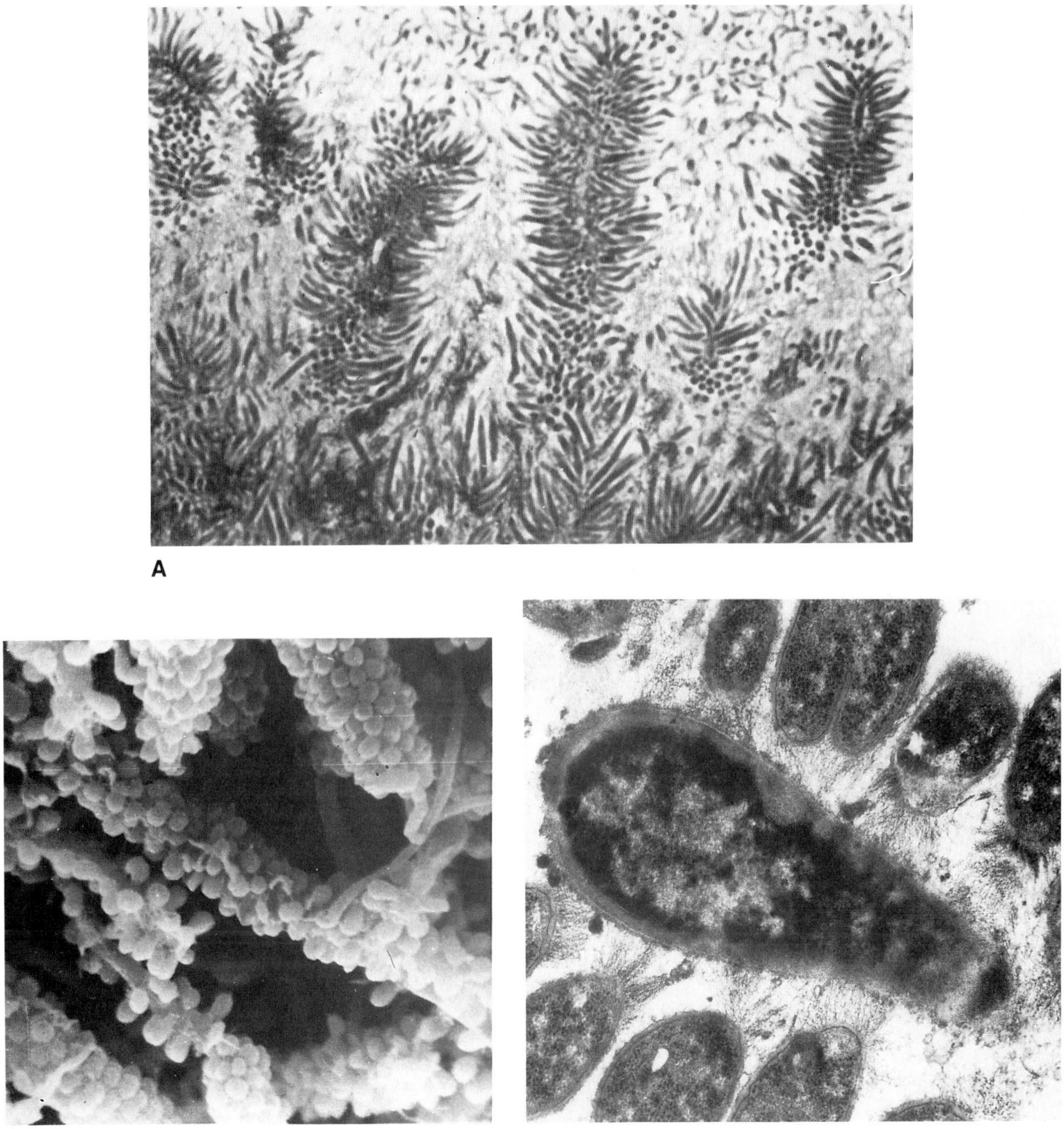

A

B

C

Figure 32–6. Interbacterial associations in dental plaque. A. Transmission electron photomicrograph of longitudinal section through test tube brush formations found in subgingival plaque. ×2200. B. Scanning electron photomicrograph of corncob formations found in supragingival plaque. ×4500. C. Transmission electron photomicrograph of oblique section through corncob formation. Note fibrous attachments between core and surrounding organisms. ×67,000. *(A. From Listgarten MA.* J Periodontol. *1976; 47:1–18. B. Courtesy of Z. Skobe. Reproduced with permission from Grant DA, Stern IB, Everett FG.* Periodontics. *6th ed. St. Louis: CV Mosby; 1988. C. From Kelstrup J, Theilade E.* J Clin Periodontol. *1974;1:15–35.)*

Specific proteins in saliva have been reported that contribute to the adhesion of certain strains of *Streptococcus mutans* to hydroxyapatite. A substance from parotid saliva is known as acidic proline-rich protein. An unidentified substance from submandibular-sublingual saliva that is distinct from secretory immunoglobulin, fibronectin, and mucin has also been described. The pellicle continues to form for about 2 hours, at which time it is about 10 μm thick. The first bacteria to come into contact with the pellicle are cocci. These include *Neisseria* and streptococci, predominantly *S. sanguis*. Streptococci can comprise up to 95% of the total cultivable flora after 24 hours accumulation. These early populations multiply, forming microcolonies that become embedded in material, primarily bacterial extracellular polysaccharides and additional layers of adsorbed salivary glycoproteins. Growth of individual microcolonies eventually results in a confluent film of organisms. Few gram-positive rods are found in the early stages of plaque development, although strains of lactobacilli, actinomycetes, and *Rothia dentocariosa* have been isolated. Other than *Veillonella*, anaerobic species do not appear until the later stages of plaque development. In vivo plaque development is demonstrated in Fig 32–7.

Cross-sections of dental plaque grown in vivo on epoxy resin crowns show morphologically homogeneous bacterial colonies growing perpendicular to the tooth surface (Fig 32–8A). These homogeneous areas may correspond to microcolonies. At higher magnifications, individual bacteria are seen embedded in the plaque matrix (Fig 32–8B).

A higher proportion of aerobic bacteria appear in early plaque. Therefore, the availability of oxygen must exert a considerable influence on the bacterial succession seen during dental plaque formation. Since air in saliva is believed to be the main source of oxygen in the oral cavity, access of saliva to a dentition site could be a major factor determining the extent to which a particular plaque microflora will be aerobic. As the plaque thickens, access of saliva to the deeper bacteria is diminished, and sufficient bacteria are present in the outer layers to remove all of the oxygen entering the plaque. Hence, the plaque oxygen will reach very low levels and ensure conditions in the deeper layers that will sustain an anaerobic flora. Obviously, where saliva access is poor, such as in the approximal sites, the anaerobic state will be easier to achieve.

Subgingival Plaque. Plaque below the gingival margin is associated with the accumulation of supragingival plaque. As certain microflora at the gingival margin produce inflammatory changes in the

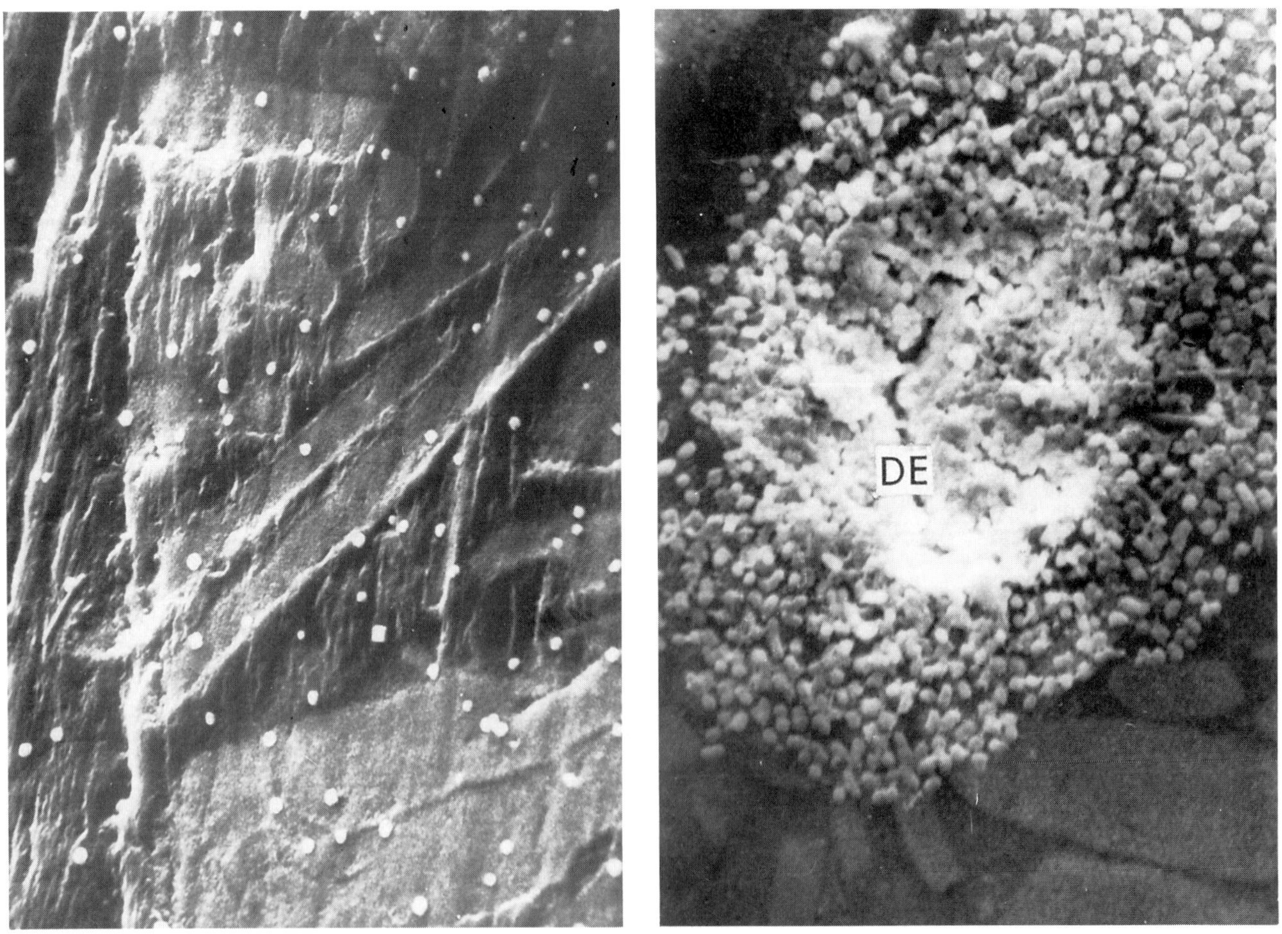

A B

Figure 32–7. In vivo growth of dental plaque on hydroxyapatite splints. **A.** Scattered bacterial cells attached to splint surface 6 hours after implantation. ×1600. **B.** Bacterial colony resulting from colonization of small defect (DE) in splint surface (24-hour specimen). ×1900.

gingiva, the susceptibility of subgingival space for bacterial accumulation increases. Once bacteria have gained access to this space, they are protected from the usual cleansing mechanisms of brushing and flossing. Bacteria that gain access to this space tend to be fastidious anaerobes. The supragingival plaque contributes to the low Eh because it acts as a coating for the subgingival plaque and a consumer of oxygen. The mechanism of initial adherence (or first colonizers) of bacteria in subgingival plaque is not known. It is known that subgingival plaque associated with cementum is different from that associated with the soft tissues. Plaque associated with the cementum is similar to supragingival plaque, with gram-positive rods, cocci, and filamentous bacteria dominating. These microorganisms are associated with root caries and calculus formation. Subgingival plaque associated with the gingival epithelium is dominated by gram-negative rods and cocci and spirochetes. These bacteria are associated with periodontal disease. Further details of subgingival plaque are given in Chapter 34.

Microbial Composition of Plaque

Dental plaque has a diverse population. Approximately 200 to 300 species of bacteria reside as part of the dental plaque community. For each milligram of plaque (wet weight) there are about 10^8 bacteria. Because an average individual's mouth contains from 20 to 100 mg of plaque, there can be as many as 10^{10} bacteria (10 billion) in the plaque of a single individual.

The distribution of organisms within plaque has not been adequately determined. This is due to the technical difficulties of sample preparation and identification of bacteria on the tooth surface in situ. Yet such spatial arrangements are of obvious importance, particularly in pathogenicity. For example, if *S. mutans* exists as microcolonies at the plaque–tooth interface, it is more likely to cause caries than if *S. mutans* exists as small clumps at the middle or outer layers of plaque.

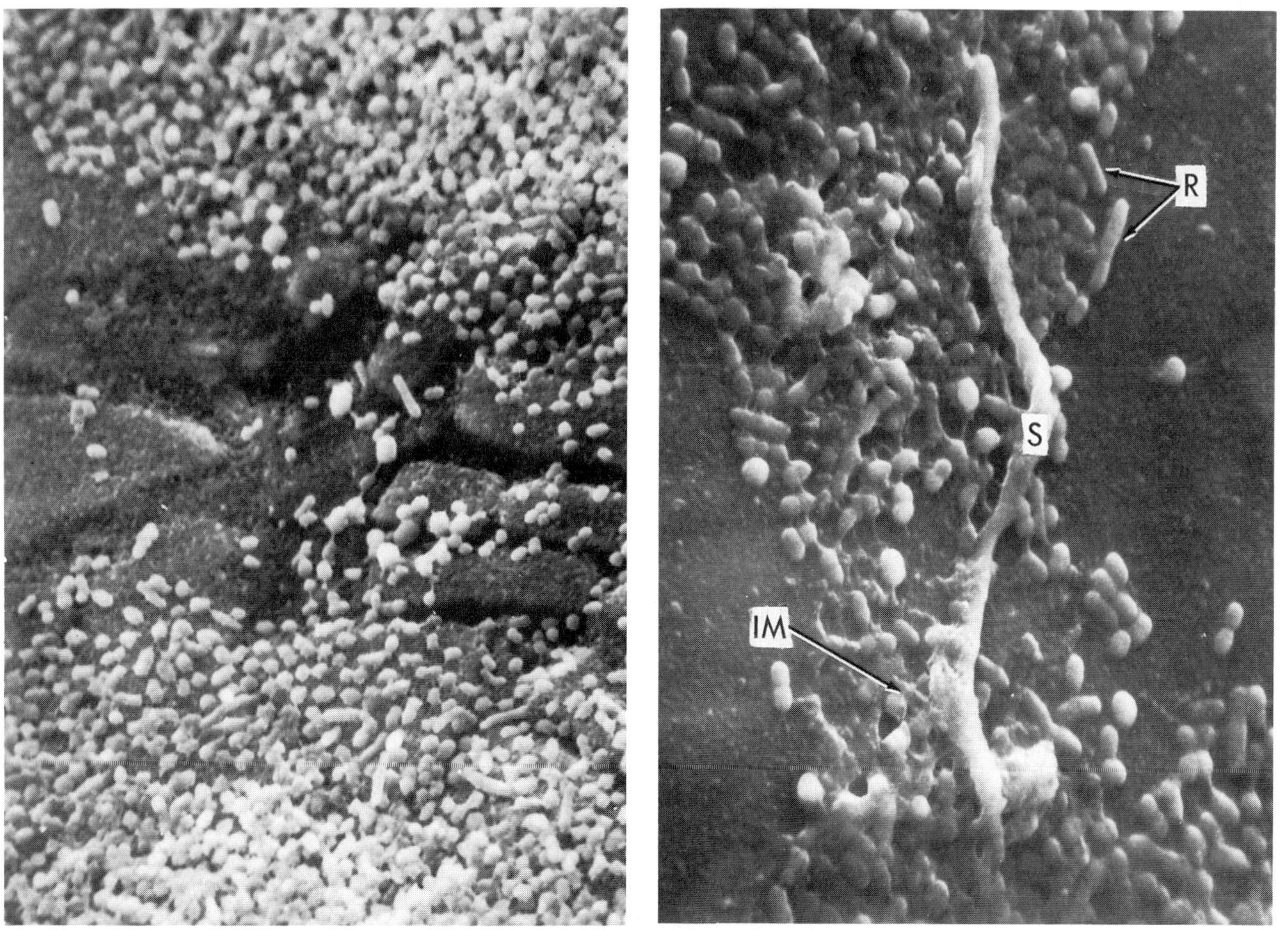

C D

(Figure 32–7, Continued) C. Bacteria from two separate colonies about to coalesce (24-hour specimen). ×2000. **D.** Higher magnification of growing plaque. ×4000. Note intercellular materia (IM), which may anchor bacteria to surface. Spirochete-like organism (S) is attached to layer composed of cocci and a few small rods (R) (48-hour specimen). *(From Lie T.* J Periodont Res. *1977;12:73–89.)*

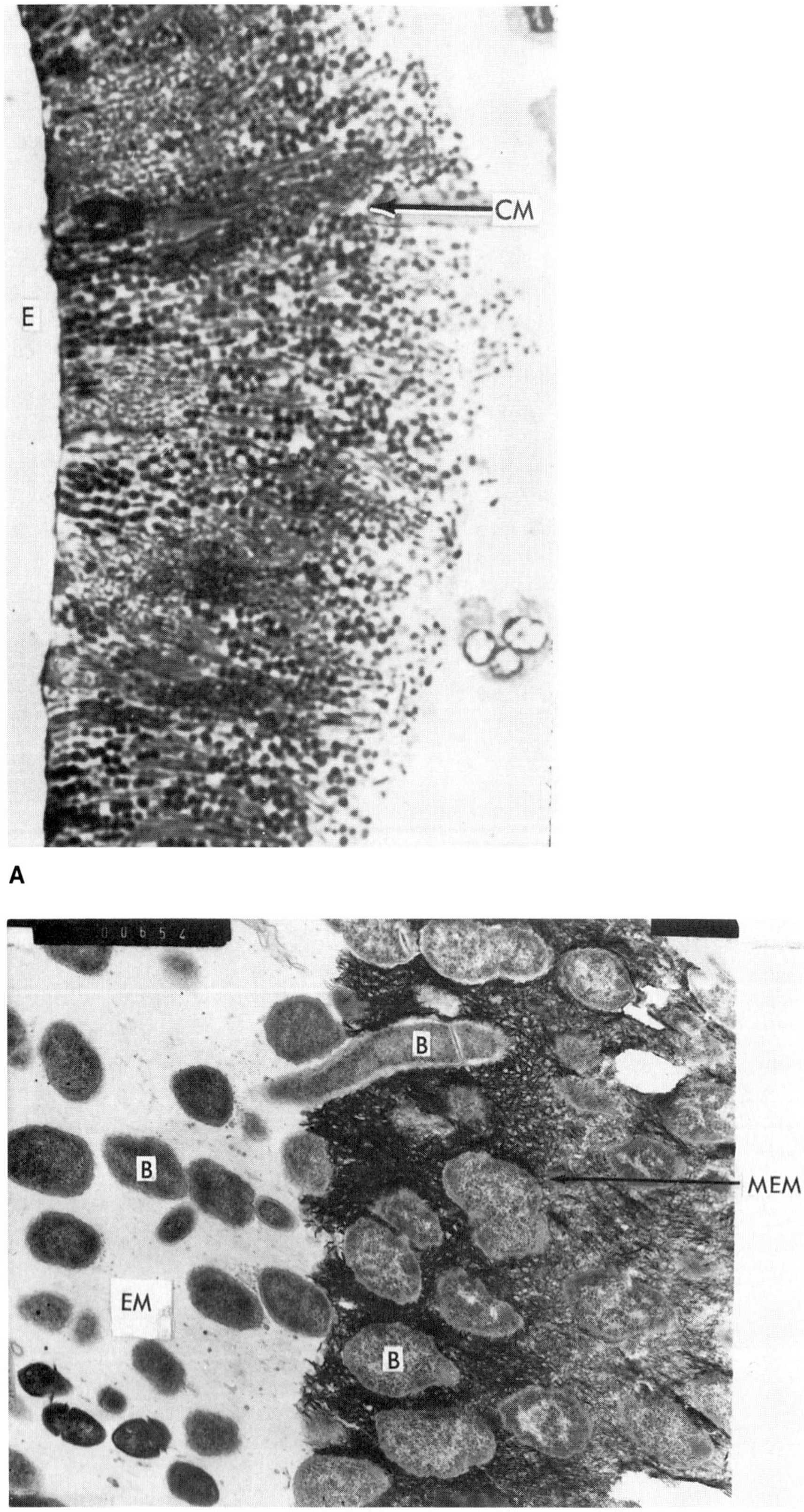

A

B

Figure 32–8. A. Relation of growing bacterial plaque to tooth surface. Transmission electron photomicrograph of predominantly coccoid plaque microflora growing at right angles to enamel surface. E, enamel space; CM, columnar microcolony. ×1324. **B.** Bacteria embedded in plaque matrix. Electron photomicrograph of individual bacteria (B) surrounded by extracellular matrix (EM) of plaque or by mineralized extracellular matrix (MEM) in adjacent calcified area. ×15,000. *(From Listgarten MA.* J Periodontol. *1976; 47:139–147.)*

At best, only rough estimates of microbial plaque composition can be made. Each study tends to yield slightly different results. Even repetitive studies by the same laboratory on the same individuals show variation. There can be variations at different sites on the same tooth, at the same site but in a different individual, right side versus left side, and there could be variations with time.

One report of the composition of coronal plaque and gingival crevice microflora is given in Table 32–2, which indicates a high level of gram-positive filamentous rods and streptococci in the coronal plaque. There are fewer of these organisms in the gingival crevice, which has a higher percentage of gram-negative anaerobic rods, anaerobic cocci (*Veillonella*), and spirochetes.

Plaque streptococci are discussed in detail in Chapter 33.

Gram-positive filamentous rods are discussed in Chapters 19 and 34. Of special interest is the organism *R. dentocariosa*. This organism was isolated and characterized by Genevieve Roth. It is found normally in plaque and root caries and produces gingival inflammation in rodents. It is aerobic and pleomorphic and produces lactic, acetic, and succinic acids from carbohydrates. It is not considered an etiologic agent for oral disease but exists as an opportunist.

Recent studies have revealed the presence of certain gram-negative rods as a significant part of the dental plaque. These include members of the genera *Haemophilus, Eikenella, Capnocytophaga,* and *Wolinella.* Except for *Wolinella,* these genera require or are enhanced by additional CO_2 (more CO_2 than is in the atmosphere) for growth. *Wolinella* does not require CO_2 but is anaerobic (some strains will grow in the presence of 5% oxygen). *Haemophilus, Eikenella,* and *Capnocytophaga* are facultative anaerobes.

Haemophilus. *Haemophilus* species are regularly present in dental plaque and saliva and on soft tissue surfaces. Good growth usually is obtained on chocolate agar plates. The species most commonly isolated from the mouth are *Haemophilus parainfluenzae, Haemophilus paraphrophilus,* and *Haemophilus segnis. Haemophilus aphrophilus* also is found occasionally in dental plaque. *Haemophilus segnis* is a recently described species from dental plaque. It forms smooth or granular, high convex, grayish white colonies up to 0.5 mm in diameter on chocolate agar and is nonhemolytic on blood-containing media. The cells are pleomorphic, nonmotile, and noncapsulated, forming mainly irregular filaments with a few bacillary forms. Colonies of some strains of *H. parainfluenzae* are surrounded by zones of hemolysis on blood agar, and many resemble those of β-hemolytic streptococci.

Eikenella corrodens. This species is a facultatively anaerobic organism that characteristically corrodes or causes pitting of the surface of agar. Several other bacterial species also produce similar corroding colonies, and this property has caused some confusion in the past. In particular, *E. corrodens* has been confused with the obligately anaerobic organism *Bacteroides corrodens* (now designated *Bacteroides ureolyticus*), although it is known that they differ in several important respects, including DNA base ratio.

The cells of *E. corrodens* are small, nonsporeforming, nonencapsulated, nonmotile, microaerophilic, gram-negative coccobacilli. The organism grows on blood or chocolate agar and is enhanced by the presence of 3 to 10% CO_2. This organism can be recovered from active periodontal pockets in humans and has been shown to induce periodontal disease in gnotobiotic rats.

Capnocytophaga. *Capnocytophaga* is the genus name that has been proposed for a group of fastidious, CO_2-requiring, gram-negative, fusiform rods isolated from the oral cavity. The capnophilic organisms characteristically are described as gliding or surface translocating bacteria. Colonies tend to have a spreading, fringelike edge and may be gray-white, pink, or yellow in color. Some strains produce pitting of the agar surface. Three species have been described within the new genus, *Capnocytophaga ochracea, Capnocytophaga sputigena* and *Capnocytophaga gingivalis.* These can be distinguished on the basis of lactose and galactose fermentation and nitrate reduction. Although the names are new, *C. ochracea* was previously known by various other names (including *Fusiformis nucleatus* var. *ochraceus* and *Bacteroides ochraceus*). Isolates of *Capnocytophaga* are clearly differentiated from both *Fusobacterium* and *Bacteroides* on the basis of their ability to grow in air plus CO_2, fermentation of carbohydrates, end products of glucose metabolism, and DNA base composition. These organisms are associated with juvenile periodontitis and possibly other forms of destructive periodontal disease.

Wolinella. This genus name has been proposed recently to accommodate organisms previously called *Vibrio succinogenes* (renamed *Wolinella succinogenes*) and a new group of similar bacteria isolated from periodontal pockets, *Wolinella recta.*

Cells of this genus are helical, curved, or straight, 0.5 to 1.0 $\times$ 2.0 to 6.0 μm, with round or tapered ends. They have a single, polar flagellum and display a rapid, darting motility when examined in wet films. They neither require nor ferment carbohydrates, but growth is stimulated in fluid cultures by the presence of formate and fumarate. Hydrogen and formate can be used as energy sources, formate being oxidized to hydrogen and carbon dioxide.

The two species, *W. succinogenes* and *W. recta,* differ from one another in cellular and ultrastructural morphology, antigenic structure, and their susceptibility to dyes and antibiotics. *Wolinella recta* is found in the human gingival crevice, but its pathogenicity is unknown. *Wolinella succinogenes* has been isolated from a variety of sources. Of interest to oral microbiologists is its presence in dental abscesses and root canals.

Eubacterium. This genus contains a variety of anaerobic filamentous bacteria that are gram-variable. Two species, *Eubacterium alactolyticum* and *Eubacterium saburreum,* are regularly isolated from dental plaque. *Eubacterium alacolyticum* also has been isolated from necrotic dental pulp and carious dentine. Dideoxyhexose is an immunodominant sugar from the cell wall of *E. saburreum.* This was the first demonstration of this compound in a gram-positive organism. *Eubacterium ingens* has been proposed for a new species isolated from dental plaque. These organisms have an unusual colonial morphology, and in fluid medium, they produce a slime composed predominantly of carbohydrate.

Lactobacillus. Lactobacilli are gram-positive nonsporulating rods. Some species produce mainly lactic acid as an end product of metabolism (homofermentative), and others produce a variety of organic acids and gases as end products (heterofermentative).

The heterofermentative species include *Lactobacillus fermentum, Lactobacillus cellobiosus, Lactobacillus brevi,* and *Lactobacillus buchneri.* Lactobacilli are commonly found in low numbers in dental plaque, usually comprising less than 1% of the total cultivable flora. The homofermentative species include *Lactobacillus acidophilus* and *Lactobacillus casei.* The latter are acidogenic organisms, and early work implicated these lactobacilli in the initiation of dental caries. Subsequent research has shown that they are associated more with carious dentine and the advancing front of carious lesions than with the initiation of the disease. However, lactobacilli should not be ruled out as primary etiologic agents (Chapter 33).

Fusobacterium. Members of the genus *Fusobacterium* are obligately anaerobic, gram-negative, nonsporeforming rods. The classification and nomenclature of the fusiform bacteria have changed considerably in recent years, and various species have had a variety of names and designations at various times. Therefore, those bearing a particular name may not be the same organism as originally described and given that designation. *Fusobacterium nucleatum* is designated as the type species and has been isolated from the oral cavity. It produces small translucent colonies on horse blood agar and is usually nonhemolytic and nonmotile. *Fusobacterium nucleatum* has been isolated from infections of the upper respiratory tract and pleural cavity, as well as the oral cavity.

Considerable impetus was given to the role of fusiform bacteria in the etiology of oral gangrenous lesions when they were associated with spirochetes in acute ulcerative gingivitis. The fusobacteria and spirochetes greatly increase in inflammatory periodontal disease and decrease with the abatement of the disease.

Peptostreptococcus. Peptostreptococci are among the most common organisms isolated in anaerobic infections. These include a diverse array of organisms within the genus *Peptostreptococcus* (anaerobic streptococci). The most common clinical isolates of *Peptostreptococcus* are *Peptostreptococcus anaerobius, Peptostreptococcus micros,* and *Peptostreptococcus intermedius.* The last species is actually microaerophilic and, although historically classified as an anaerobe, has now been more properly reclassified as *Streptococcus intermedius.*

Various species seldom produce pathologic lesions when inoculated as pure cultures. However, studies involving mixed infections show anaerobic streptococci to be necessary for synergistic infections. For example, anaerobic streptococci are indispensable components of the inoculum of other oral anaerobes used to produce lung abscesses. More relevant to dental infections are the studies of bacteria isolated from necrotic tooth pulp, which were tested for their capacity to induce abscesses on subcutaneous injection in guinea pigs.

Actinobacillus. Only one of five known species of the genus, *Actinobacillus, Actinobacillus actinomycetemcomitans,* is found as a regular inhabitant of the oral cavity. It frequently has been reported from cases of actinomycosis, usually in association with *Actinomyces israelii.* This organism has been isolated from various abscesses and from patients with infective endocarditis. *Actinobacillus actinomycetemcomitans* is a small, gram-negative, coccoid or coccobacillary organism. As with other facultative gram-negative rods, growth on solid medium, such as blood agar, is enhanced by an atmosphere with 5 to 10% CO_2. *Actinobacillus actinomycetemcomitans* is commonly isolated from patients with juvenile periodontitis, less frequently from adult periodontitis, and only occasionally from children and adults with a healthy periodontium.

A concise listing of the aforementioned bacteria with the oral and systemic diseases they cause is given in Table 32–5.

Oral Protozoa. Protozoa do not usually colonize the healthy oral cavity. Two protozoans, *Entamoeba gingivalis* and *Trichonomas tenax,* frequently are found in the plaque and saliva in which oral hygiene is ne-

TABLE 32–5. EXAMPLES OF ORAL AND SYSTEMIC DISEASES ASSOCIATED WITH ORAL BACTERIA

Genus	Oral Disease	Systemic Disease
Lactobacillus	Dental caries	Pleuropulmonary infections (rare) Cystitis (rare)
Fusobacterium	Ulcerative gingivitis	Human bite wounds Bacteremia Upper respiratory infections
Actinobacillus	Juvenile periodontitis	Infective endocarditis Actinomycosis
Peptostreptococcus	Periodontal disease Pulpitis	Pulmonary abscess Brain abscess
Eubacterium	Periodontitis Pulpitis	None
Haemophilus	Acute bacterial epiglottitis	Pneumonia Sinusitis Meningitis
Eikenella	Periodontal disease	Soft tissue infections (human bites, infected needles of drug abusers)
Capnocytophaga	Juvenile periodontitis	Pneumonia Infective endocarditis
Wolinella	Dental abscesses	Abdominal infections

glected. Although they often are associated with certain disease states, neither is believed to be pathogenic in the oral cavity.

Trichomonas tenax is a member of the subphylum Mastigophora, the flagellated protozoans, and it is the only flagellate found in the mouth. *Trichomonas tenax* is a pear-shaped organism that ranges from 5 to 16 μm (7 μm average) in length and 2 to 15 μm in width. It is enclosed in a form-retaining pellicle and possesses a rigid axostyle that lies along the longitudinal axis of the cell. It carries four flagella that are extended anteriorly and a fifth that is associated with an undulating membrane.

Trichomonas tenax is found in the oral cavity of about 10% of the population, usually in areas of poor oral hygiene. It is often found in gingival crevices or pockets of individuals with gingivitis, necrotizing ulcerative gingivitis, adult periodontitis, and localized juvenile periodontitis. Early investigators who noted the association between the periodontal diseases and the presence of *T. tenax* suggested that this protozoan might be an etiologic agent of disease. However, it is believed currently that the organism is simply a nonpathogenic parasite.

Trichomonas tenax is not known to cause disease in any area of the body, but it has been associated with a small number of pneumonias. It is suspected that aspirates from the oral cavity are the source of the lung infection, but there is no definitive evidence that this protozoan actually causes disease.

Entamoeba gingivalis is a member of the subphylum Sarcodina. Like *T. tenax*, it is frequently found in diseased areas of the mouth but has not been shown to actually cause disease.

Entamoeba gingivalis is an amoeboid cell that ranges from 5 to 35 μm in diameter. It possesses an extremely flexible membrane that permits it to move and to ingest food by means of pseudopodia. It apparently exists only as a trophozoite because no cysts have been associated with this organism.

This incidence of *E. gingivalis* in the human oral cavity reportedly ranges from 5 to 30% in subjects with good oral hygiene to as much as 100% in subjects with advanced periodontitis. It also is found with gingivitis, necrotizing ulcerative gingivitis, and failing dental implants, but it has not been shown to be responsible for the injury associated with any of these conditions. Thus, despite its frequent appearance in these diseased areas, it is still believed to be nonpathogenic.

Changes in Microbial Composition of Plaque

At a given site in dental plaque, there is an ecologic balance in which the indigenous populations are held at a steady dynamic state (homeostatic). This occurs even though many different species are in close contact with each other. Certain species can react with each other in ways in which one species may benefit another (commensalism) (Table 32–3), or one species may act as an antagonist (antibiosis). Furthermore, if there is a temporary change in amounts of plaque or composition, there is a tendency to revert back to the original composition. An example of this is that if plaque is allowed to accumulate without taking oral hygiene measures (ie, teeth are not brushed), it has been observed that at the gingival margin, coccal and small rod forms predominate at first, after 3 to 4 days, filamentous forms appear, and after 5 to 6 days, vibrios and spirochetes are observed (Fig 32–9). When oral hygiene is resumed, the microbial forms are significantly decreased in the reverse order in which they appeared. Changes in microbial composition may result when dietary regimens change (eg, an increase in sucrose consumption results in higher levels of *S. mutans* and lactobacilli), when oral disease occurs (eg, more lactobacilli have been detected as caries progresses), and when antibiotic therapy is instituted (eg, tetracycline reduces levels of spirochetes and motile rods in gingival crevice areas in individuals with periodontal disease). Other factors that may contribute to changes in microbial composition of dental plaque are systemic diseases, aging of the individual, age of plaque, food and liquid consumption, and smoking.

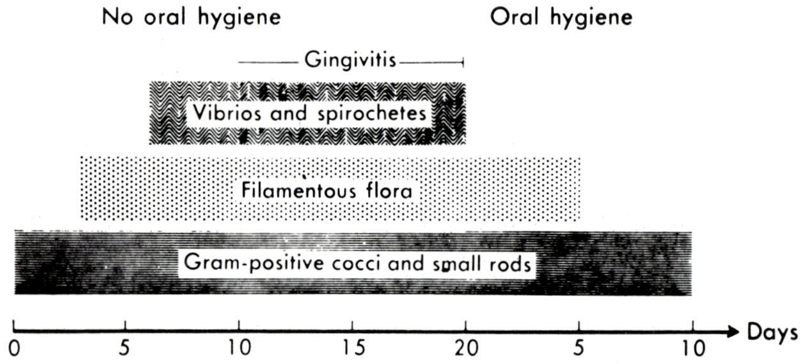

Figure 32–9. Changes in the microflora of the gingival margin during periods or no oral hygiene (20 days) and oral hygiene (10 days). *(From Loe H et al. Experimental gingivitis in man.* J Periodontol. *1965; 36:184.)*

Chemical Composition of Plaque

Gross chemical analyses indicate that 20% of pooled, mostly supragingival plaque scrapings are solid and the remaining 80% is water. Of the solid material, protein, carbohydrate, and lipid content has been approximated to be 45%, 15%, and 12%, respectively (Table 32–6). Inorganic compounds (5 to 10%) are also present. About 20% of the dry weight of plaque has not been determined.

Proteins are a major component of dental plaque. They come from bacteria, saliva, and gingival crevice fluid. Although bacteria contribute most of the protein in dental plaque, salivary proteins, such as amylase, lysozyme, lactoferrin, lactoperoxidase, salivary immunoglobulins (SIgA), and various proteases, have been demonstrated in supragingival plaque. Albumin and IgG that probably originate in the gingival fluid also are found in dental plaque. Bacterial enzymes, such as hyaluronidase, collagenase, and glucosyltransferase, also can be demonstrated in plaque.

Carbohydrates, in the form of polysaccharides, are constituents of plaque. These polysaccharides are heteropolysaccharides and homopolysaccharides (Table 32–7). Most heteropolysaccharides found in plaque are cell wall components, such as polysaccharides, teichoic acids, and lipopolysaccharides. Certain species of *Actinomyces* and *Lactobacillus* synthesize capsular, extracellular polymers containing hexosamines, uronic acids, and hexoses other than glucose. The glucans and fructans are synthesized by plaque bacteria primarily as extracellular polymers and make up a large portion of the plaque matrix. The chemical structures of these homopolysaccharides consist of polymers of either glucose or fructose. Glucans are either dextrans having 1,6-α linkages or mutans having 1,3-α linkages (Fig 32–10). *Streptococcus mutans* produces both kinds of glucans, but more 1,3-α linkages. In general, solubility in water is inversely proportional to the number of 1,3-α linkages. Therefore, mutans are less soluble in water and may serve in plaque as matrix substances. Fructans are polymers of fructose. Levans (fructans) are found also as part of the plaque matrix and can be used as a nutrient by oral streptococci.

Plaque microorganisms are known to produce an intracellular storage product similar to glycogen or amylopectin during periods of carbohydrate excess. This material often has been referred to as intracellular polysaccharide (IPS) and is characterized by its ability to bind iodine (ie, iodophilic). This property enables the organism to be recognized easily when it grows as a colony in agar. IPS may be related to caries development because the bacteria may metabolize this material during fasting periods (overnight), resulting in the extended production of acid.

Lipids in plaque are phospholipids derived from either the host or from gram-negative microorganisms. These may play a role in the mineralization of

TABLE 32–6. CHEMICAL COMPOSITION OF DENTAL PLAQUE

Component	Wet Weight (%)	Dry Weight (%)
Water	80	
Solids	20	
Protein		40–50
Carbohydrate		13–18
Lipid		10–14
Inorganic		5–10

Adapted from Sharma ML, Newburn E. J Dent Res. *1974;54:482–486.*

TABLE 32–7. EXTRACELLULAR POLYSACCHARIDES SYNTHESIZED BY SELECTED PLAQUE BACTERIA

Organism	Homopolysaccharides		Heteropoly-saccharides
	Glucans	*Fructans (Levans)*	
Streptococcus sanguis	+		
Streptococcus mutans	+	+	
Streptococcus salivarius	+	+	
Lactobacillus casei	+		+
Lactobacillus acidophilus	+		
Neisseria sp.			
Actinomyces viscosus		+	+

Adapted from Marsh PO, Martin M. Oral Microbiology. *2nd ed. Washington, DC: American Society for Microbiology; 1984.*

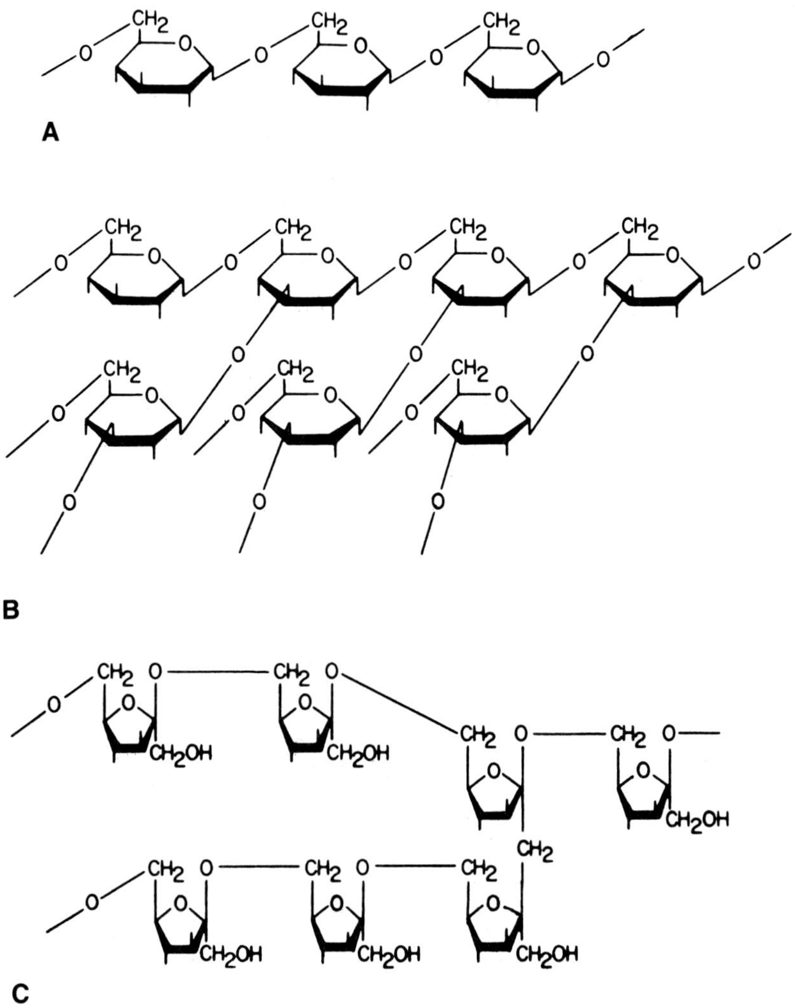

Figure 32–10. Chemical structure of dextran **(A)**, mutan **(B)**, and levan **(C)**. *(From McGhee J, Michalek S, Cassel G, eds.* Dental Microbiology. *New York: Harper & Row; 1982.)*

plaque (calculus) due to their affinity to bind calcium and phosphate ions.

Plaque also contains inorganic ions, such as phosphate, calcium, magnesium, carbonate, and fluoride, which may occur in a bound or free form.

Adherence and Colonization Mechanisms

Initial adherence mechanisms are basically the same for hard tissues as for soft tissues. Complementary receptors on oral epithelial cells are required for specific adhesins on bacterial cells. With teeth, the specific receptors are those found in glycoproteins, constituents of the acquired salivary pellicle. Dense plaque does not build up on oral soft tissue because of continual shedding of epithelial cells. Cohesive plaque accumulates on teeth because adherent bacteria are able to multiply and secrete sticky polysaccharides and may aggregate or coaggregate. A model for plaque accumulation due to polysaccharide synthesis is the organism *S. mutans,* which produces glucosyltransferase (GTF). This enzyme requires an intact molecule of sucrose to carry out the reaction.

$$\text{Sucrose} \xrightarrow{\text{GTF}} (\text{glucose})_n + \text{fructose}$$

GTF catalyzes the reaction to produce certain polymers of glucose, known as glucans. The glucans may be dextran (1,6-α linkage) or mutan (1,3-α linkage).

Such a mechanism for using bacterial polysaccharides to foster accumulation of dental plaque seems to be unique to *S. mutans.* Although several species of bacteria from dental plaque can synthesize extracellular polysaccharides from sucrose (and other carbohydrates), only *S. mutans* has been shown to aggregate into larger masses via this adhesive mechanism.

Dental Calculus

Dental calculus is the calcified deposit that forms on teeth, dentures, or other hard structures in the mouth. Mature calculus consists of 80% (dry weight) mineralized materials and 20% organic constituents. The latter include bacteria and their products. The crystalline (calcium phosphate) structure and the organic composition of calculus vary with the age of the deposit, the location of the tooth, and the individual (Fig 32–11).

Calculus is found both subgingivally and supragingivally. Subgingival calculus is harder and

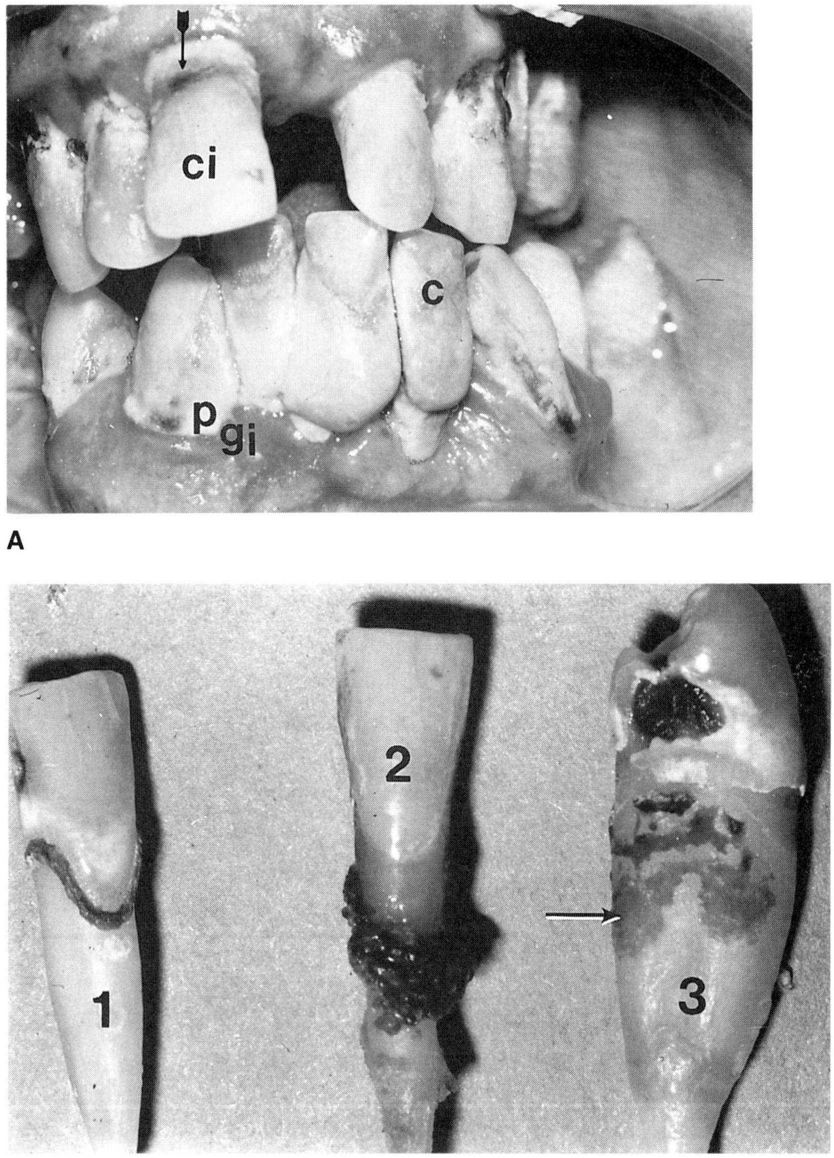

Figure 32–11. A. Two examples of calculus. The lower teeth have extensive supragingival calculus (c). Plaque (p) overlies the calculus at the gingival margin. Gingival inflammation (gi) is apparent. The right maxillary central incisor (ci) shows dark calculus that was formed subgingivally but, due to gingival recession, appears at and coronal to the gingival line (arrow). **B.** Examples of different types of subgingival calculus on root surfaces. Teeth were extracted due to periodontal disease. 1. Ringlike calculus near the cement–enamel junction. 2. Crusty-modular calculus. 3. Thin, veneerlike deposit. These deposits are tenacious and require removal of root structure by scaling following initial debridement. *(Courtesy of Dr. Lew Claman, Ohio State University.)*

denser than supragingival calculus and often is pigmented. The differences in composition are dependent on the relative contributions of saliva, gingival fluid, host cellular components, and variations in the bacterial populations in the areas in which each is formed.

The bacterial flora associated with calculus is complex. As many as 22 different species of bacteria have been isolated from a single calculus sample. The flora reflects the bacterial composition of the dental plaque with which it is associated. Early calculus (2 days) contains primarily streptococci, as does early plaque. As the calculus and plaque age, gram-positive and gram-negative rods become more numerous. A similar relationship is found when comparing subgingival and supragingival calculus. Subgingival calculus has more gram-negative bacteria, and supragingival calculus has more gram-positive bacteria.

There is reason to believe that bacteria may be the initiators of the mineralization resulting in the calculus. However, no one bacterial species has been shown to be individually associated with calculus formation. In fact, there is much evidence that many different oral bacteria may be involved in the mineralization process leading to calculus formation.

Calculus also may form in germ-free animals, indicating that microorganisms are not the only elements that become mineralized. However, animals reared in a conventional environment form less calculus if given penicillin, indicating that plaque bacteria are associated with the accumulation of calculus.

Calculus can appear shortly after dental plaque forms on the surface of the teeth. Minute foci of calcification have been demonstrated within hours after the deposition of pellicle or plaque. The earliest formed calculus has a poorly defined crystalline structure that becomes more crystalline with age. Calcium and phosphate ions, necessary for the process of calcification, are derived from saliva and diet. In the case of subgingival plaque, the source of calcium and phosphate ions is gingival fluid.

The mechanism by which calculus formation is initiated is unknown, but the most popular concept is the epitactic mechanism. This theory states that calcium phosphate crystals are formed with the assistance of organic compounds. These organic compounds provide sites for the deposition and alignment of the calcium and phosphate ions, which leads to crystal formation. This initial crystal then serves as a nidus for further crystal formation. The mineral form of mature calculus is mostly hydroxyapatite, the same mineral structure that makes up the bulk of the mineral substance in enamel. Other crystallized minerals in saliva include whitlockite, octacalcium phosphate, and brushite.

Calculus is porous, and bacterial products may be absorbed into and adsorbed onto this rough deposit. Although the bacteria within calculus die, the bacteria on the surface are alive and may continue to multiply and produce toxic products. The rough surface of calculus facilitates plaque retention and makes removal difficult.

Plaque bacteria also can sequester themselves within the porous structure of calculus following cleaning of the teeth or some other periodontal procedure. The calculus, if it is not removed, can serve as a source of bacteria to repopulate the gingival crevice. The fact that calculus can serve as a source of toxic compounds or of bacteria is a major reason that it must be completely removed from the tooth's surface to enhance the possibility of complete healing from periodontal disease.

Plaque Control

Strong efforts have been made to prevent dental plaque formation and to remove plaque once it is formed. Studies have shown that diligent and efficient removal of plaque can prevent both dental caries and gingivitis. An alternate approach developed recently has been to control the specific pathogens of dental plaque rather than total plaque control. This procedure includes the use of vaccines, antimicrobial agents, and implantation of nonpathogenic bacteria. Each of the following has been considered as a measure for controlling dental plaque.

1. Brushing and flossing. Careful and thorough removal of plaque through these mechanical methods has been effective in inhibiting dental caries and periodontal disease. Dentifrices contain abrasives and detergents to help remove plaque.
2. Oral irrigators. This device uses a strong force of water to remove subgingival plaque, and may be deleterious, especially in individuals with periodontal disease, because it may force bacteria into the bloodstream.
3. Chewing. The chewing of gum and fibrous food such as apples and celery may remove soft deposits (materia alba) but will not reduce plaque score. Individuals in some Asian countries use chewing sticks to clean teeth.
4. Diet. Less frequent consumption of foods containing sucrose will retard formation of dental plaque.
5. Rinsing with water. Oral rinsing will remove soluble constituents of dental plaque, such as sugars and soft deposits, but will not reduce levels of adherent plaque.
6. Enzymes. The use of enzymes such as dextranase in humans has been of questionable value. Some have reported that it can reduce plaque, whereas others have said it is ineffective. Unfortunately, many sticky polymers exist in plaque, and one enzyme is insufficient.
7. Fluoride. Stannous fluoride has been of value in inhibiting plaque development and in suppressing cariogenic bacteria. The stannous ion has antimicrobial properties; other fluorides are not as effective.
8. Antibiotics. Several antibiotics, such as vancomycin, kanamycin, tetracycline, and minocycline, reduce plaque formation as well as inhibit periodontal diseases. These are useful in treating handicapped individuals. These and other antibiotics must be used with caution because of possible allergic reactions and creating resistant strains of bacteria.
9. Metronidazole. This chemotherapeutic agent is effective against anaerobic bacteria, including periodontopathic organisms.
10. Quaternary ammonium compounds. These compounds (eg, cetyl pyridinium chloride) have been incorporated into mouthwashes, and a reduction in plaque accumulation has been reported for 1 to 4 hours.
11. Chlorhexidine. This compound is an effective compound because of its ability to adhere to the tooth surface and its antimicrobial activity. The objectionable features of this compound are that it may cause soreness of the oral mucosa, it has a bitter taste, and it discolors teeth. The discoloration is not permanent, but it will take professional prophylaxis to remove the brown stain.
12. Sanguinarine. This compound is a benzophenanthradine alkaloid obtained by the alcoholic extraction of the bloodroot plant,

Sanguinaria canadensis. Like chlorhexidine, it has antiplaque activity and is retained in plaque for several hours after rinsing.

13. Soluble pyrophosphate. A compound such as tetrasodium pyrophosphate has been incorporated into tarter control dentifrices. These compounds interrupt the transformation of amorphous $Ca_3(PO_4)_2$ into crystalline dental calculus.
14. Low caloric sweeteners. Substances, such as cyclamate and saccharin, have antibacterial properties.

ORAL MICROBIAL ECOLOGY

Many factors are involved in successful establishment and maintenance of the normal oral flora. These involve interrelationships among various microorganisms and between microorganism and the host. Relationships may be antagonistic, synergistic, or commensal. Factors such as the lowering of the Eh favor anaerobes but not aerobes. The ingestion of sucrose accelerates a buildup of dental plaque, and more plaque favors anaerobes in the deeper layers. Reduction in pH favors aciduric bacteria such as lactobacilli, but would be antagonistic to nonaciduric bacteria. Certain nutrients are supplied by the host, which include saliva, crevicular fluid, and desquamated cells. In addition, bacteria provide nutrients for other microorganisms in the mouth. A partial list is given in Table 32–3.

Antagonistic factors in the oral ecosystem include the flow of saliva or crevicular fluid to remove bacteria and dietary substances. Tongue and cheek movements also contribute to cleansing action. Desquamation of epithelial cells and swallowing are additional physical factors limiting the numbers of the normal oral microflora. Secretory IgA and IgG present in saliva, which react with bacterial surface antigens, inhibit the attachment of bacteria to epithelial cells. This event, coupled with desquamation, could lead to elimination of a particular species from the oral cavity.

Certain constituents in saliva exert an antagonistic effect on the oral flora. In addition to the antibodies discussed previously, saliva contains lysozyme, lactoperoxidase, and lactoferrin. The normal oral flora is resistant to lysozyme alone, but when lysozyme is combined with certain immunoglobulins, or complement, some bacteria are lysed. Lysozyme may prevent transient sensitive organisms from becoming oral residents. The lactoperoxidase system is active against oral microorganisms such as *S. mutans*, *S. sanguis*, *S. mitior*, *A. viscosus*, and lactobacilli. Lactoferrin is a substance that ties up iron, which is required by many microorganisms, including *S. mutans*.

Normal oral microorganisms produce substances antagonistic against other indigenous bacteria. These substances include nonvolatile organic acids, volatile fatty acids, hydrogen peroxide, and bacteriocins. Bacteriocins are large, complex molecules synthesized by bacteria that can inhibit the growth of similar or closely related species. The effectiveness of bacteriocins in vivo is questionable, since both bacteriocin-sensitive and bacteriocin-producing strains have been isolated from human dental plaque. Certain streptococcal bacteriocins are inactivated by proteases present in dental plaque, which suggests that bacteriocins may be inactivated in the mouth. On the other hand, there is evidence for an in vivo role for bacteriocin acting as an inhibitor. It has been shown in gnotobiotic rats that a bacteriocin-producing strain of *S. mutans* can inhibit the colonization of bacteriocin-sensitive strains of *A. viscosus* and *S. mutans*.

PATHOGENIC POTENTIAL OF THE NORMAL ORAL FLORA

The primary pathogenic potential of the normal oral flora is the causation of periodontal diseases, caries, and abscesses. However, the flora indigenous to the oral cavity also are capable of causing systemic infections. This can be due to translocation of an organism from one part of the body to another, a weakening of the body's immune system, or a shift in microbial ecology.

Organisms may enter the bloodstream from the oral cavity during dental procedures that involve bleeding (eg, surgical procedures such as tooth extraction and gingivectomy).

Certain microorganisms that enter the bloodstream from the oral cavity can cause oral infections through a process known as anachoresis (localization of organisms in the bloodstream tends to occur at an oral site that has been injured). In addition to surgical procedures, bacteria may enter the bloodstream from deep carious lesions, the infected periodontal pocket, and by way of a fractured tooth.

The body's immune system is weakened when treated with immunosuppressants, which occurs in certain cancers and transplant surgery. Under these conditions, normal flora may cause disease. Oral organisms, such as *C. albicans*, need to be controlled to prevent serious infections.

There are many bacteria present as normal oral flora that occasionally cause overt disease in other parts of the body. They have been mentioned previously in this chapter (Table 32–5).

SUMMARY

The oral microflora consist of a large number of diverse species for one anatomic site. Diversity consists of a multitude of morphologic types, anaerobes and aerobes as well as facultative organisms, potential pathogens and nonpathogens, and adherent and nonadherent bacteria. Although there are about 1 trillion microorganisms in the mouth, not every known species is represented. Of the thousands of known species, only a few species from 30 genera have been characterized from the oral cavity. The oral environment, like any other environment, presents forces that are friendly to some species and hostile to others. Flora can be protective by inhibiting colonization of potential pathogens. For example, *C. albicans* is held in check by the indigenous flora. When certain antibiotics, such as tetracycline, are taken, *C. albicans* increase in numbers because this yeast is unaffected by tetracycline. As long as some oral hygiene is maintained, there is a balance in host–parasite relationship and no disease. The balance within the oral cavity can be tilted to disease by poor oral hygiene, immunosuppressive drugs, or systemic diseases that decrease local resistance. This can lead to caries and periodontal disease or various other oral lesions, such as candidiasis. Oral flora can also cause infections in other parts of the body. A few examples are *Haemophilus* causing pneumonia, streptococci causing infective endocarditis, and *Eikenella* causing skin infections.

From a clinical standpoint, control of dental plaque is of utmost importance. For most individuals, this would reduce dental caries and periodontal disease significantly.

SUGGESTED READINGS

Carranza FA. *Glickman's Clinical Periodontology.* 6th ed. Philadelphia: WB Saunders; 1984:391–426.

Christensen GD, Simpson WA, Beachey EH. Microbial adherence in infection. In: Mandell GL, Douglas GR, Bennett JE, eds. *Principles and Practice of Infectious Diseases.* 2nd ed. New York: Wiley Medical Publication; 1985:6–23.

Gibbons RJ. Microbial ecology: Adherent interactions which may affect microbial ecology in the mouth. *J Dent Res.* 1984;63:378–385.

Gibbons RJ, Hay DI, Adsorbed salivary acidic proline-rich proteins contribute to the adhesion of *Streptococcus mutans* JBP to apatitie surfaces. *J Dent Res.* 1989;68:1303–1307.

Kishimoto E, Hay DI, Gibbons RJ. A human salivary protein which promotes adhesion of *Streptococcus mutans* serotype C strains to hydroxyapatite. *Infect Immun.* 1989;57:3702–3707.

Kolenbrander PE. Intergeneric coaggregation among human oral bacteria and ecology of dental plaque. *Annu Rev Microbiol.* 1988;42:627–656.

Lillich T. Oral microbiology. In: Roth GI, Calmes R, eds. *Oral Biology.* St. Louis: CV Mosby; 1981:307–339.

Listgarten MA. Nature of periodontal diseases: Pathogenic mechanisms. *J Periodontal Res.* 1987;22:172–178.

Marsh PD, Martin M. *Oral Microbiology.* 2nd ed. Washington, DC: American Society for Microbiology; 1984.

Mergenhagen SE, Rosan B. *Molecular Basis of Oral Microbial Adhesion.* Washington, DC: American Society for Microbiology; 1985.

Rosen S. Microbiology, plaque, caries, and oral defense mechanisms. In: Di Orio LP, ed. *Clinical Preventive Dentistry.* E Norwalk, Conn: Appleton-Century-Crofts; 1983: 121–176.

Slots J. Rapid identification of important periodontal microorganisms by cultivation. *Oral Microbiol Immunol.* 1986; 1:48–55.

Socransky SS, Maganiello AD. The oral microbiota of man from birth to senility. *J Periodontol.* 1971;42:485–494.

CHAPTER 33

Dental Caries

Samuel Rosen

INTRODUCTION

THEORIES OF CARIES DEVELOPMENT

THE CARIOUS LESION

INTERRELATIONSHIP AMONG HOST, DIET, AND BACTERIA
- Host Factors
- Dietary Factors
- Bacteria

ROOT SURFACE CARIES

ROLE OF LACTIC AND OTHER ACIDS

PREVENTION

DECLINING PREVALENCE OF DENTAL CARIES

CARIES ACTIVITY TESTS

SUMMARY

SUGGESTED READINGS

INTRODUCTION

Dental caries is a bacterial disease of the dental hard tissues, characterized by a localized, progressive, molecular disintegration of tooth structure. It is a worldwide disease known since antiquity. In 1962, distribution worldwide varied from one country to another (Fig 33–1). Industrialized nations tended to have higher levels of caries than underdeveloped nations, and intranational variation was considerable. Within the United States, there was in 1970 significantly more dental caries in the north than in the south. Prolonged major disasters, such as wars, alter a population's experiences with dental caries. For example, Norway had less dental caries during the latter part of and immediately after World War II. Explanations for this event include the import of less sugar and flour and increased dependence on native foods. Many industrialized areas have less caries today than in 1962. Caries rates are declining. In 1951, the average 13-year-old person in Massachusetts had 12 decayed, missing, or filled teeth (DMFT), and in 1981 a 13-year-old had 4.5 DMFT. However, regions exist where caries rates are high. This occurs in low income groups in Western nations and in developing countries. The phenomenon of declining caries rates is discussed in this chapter.

Caries occurs in our younger population (under age 20). These individuals are dependent on others for appropriate care of their oral health. Therefore, prevention of caries is an important consideration.

Another consideration for prevention is the cost. The cost in 1978 for dental caries alone was estimated to be about \$6 billion. Considering that fluoridated water reduces dental decay by 60%, this figure could have been extrapolated to \$15 billion without fluoridation. In addition, dental problems result in lost work hours due to dental appointments or discomfort. In 1978, there were over 21 million days of restricted activity caused by acute dental conditions. This wage loss or fringe benefit cost to the yearly dental bill increases the total actual cost of dental care.

In spite of the many advances made in caries research, the multifactorial etiology makes this dis-

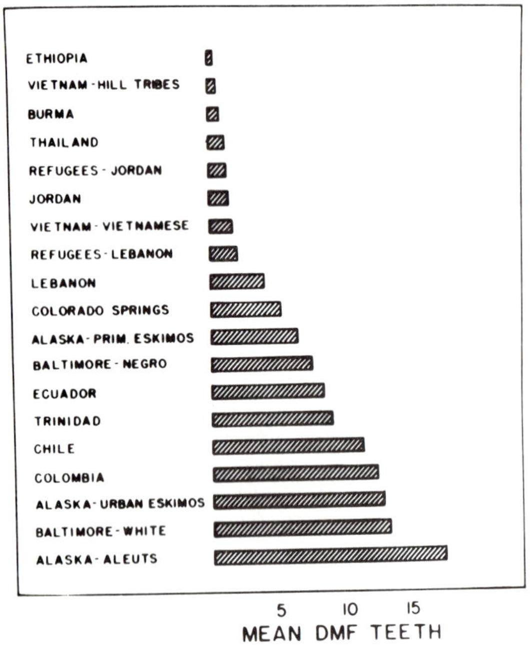

Figure 33–1. The mean number of decayed, missing, and filled (DMF) teeth is shown for various contemporary population groups. *(From Russell AL. World epidemiology and oral health. In: Kreshover SJ, McClure FJ, eds.* Environmental Variables in Oral Disease. *Publication 81. Washington, DC: AAAS; 1966:312.)*

ease complex and a challenge for scientists to uncover its many facets. Host factors (eg, saliva), microbial factors (eg, specific vs. nonspecific microbial etiology), and dietary factors (eg, which foods contribute to dental caries) are a few samples of the intricate etiologic network.

THEORIES OF CARIES DEVELOPMENT

W.D. Miller, in 1890, is given credit for the chemoparasitic theory, which stated that any oral microorganism capable of producing acid from a variety of carbohydrates would cause dental caries. He showed that bacteria from saliva could produce acid from a mixture of bread and saliva. A tooth immersed in this mixture underwent decalcification. This observation let to the statement that microorganisms acting on a fermentable carbohydrate to produce acid would cause caries. Specificity of microorganisms and carbohydrates was not considered until later. A few years later, Williams observed dental plaque on the enamel surface and considered plaque to be the means by which organic acids formed by microorganisms are localized on the tooth surface.

Although the weight of evidence favors acceptance of the chemoparasitic theory, others have been proposed. These are the proteolytic, proteolytic chelation, and phosphate sequestration theories. The proteolytic theory states that the protein fraction of enamel is initially attacked by bacteria and that destruction of the mineral fraction of teeth follows. An extension of this theory was that chelation is the mechanism by which calcium is removed from enamel after the organic portion of the enamel is destroyed. The chelators of the oral cavity would be lactate or citrate, which could remove calcium from enamel in either an acid or neutral environment. The phosphate sequestration theory was developed after the cariostatic properties of phosphate were discovered. This theory states that as bacteria take up phosphate from the saliva and plaque, inorganic phosphate is removed from enamel. If phosphate is removed, teeth become more susceptible to decalcification by acid.

THE CARIOUS LESION

Dental caries can occur on the occlusal surfaces, interproximal surfaces, smooth surfaces, and root surfaces of teeth. Deep fissures are highly susceptible to caries because they are inaccessible to toothbrushes and other oral hygiene devices (Fig 33–2). Interproximal areas require careful flossing for adequate removal of plaque. Root surface caries occurs usually in older individuals as the gingival margin recedes secondary to periodontal disease and root surfaces are exposed. Caries also may occur around leaky restorations and orthodontic wires.

Severe caries results in infants bottle-fed with carbohydrate-containing fluids for long or frequent periods of time. The anterior maxillary teeth generally are involved. Young individuals consuming refined carbohydrates frequently tend to suffer from rampant caries.

As plaque accumulates at a site, acid is formed by specific bacteria that metabolize refined carbohydrates. The acid at the plaque–tooth interface decalcifies the enamel at a discrete location. When decalcification has proceeded to the dentin–enamel junction, there is a lateral spread of the decalcified areas, and bacteria such as streptococci and lactobacilli begin to invade the dentinal tubules (Fig 33–3). As the carious process proceeds, there is a disintegration of the enamel and dentin structure.

INTERRELATIONSHIP AMONG HOST, DIET, AND BACTERIA

The causation of dental caries is extremely complex. However, it has been shown that there is an interrelationship among host, diet, and bacteria (Fig 33–4). The teeth of the host must be susceptible (eg, low in fluoride). Specific cariogenic microorganisms must be

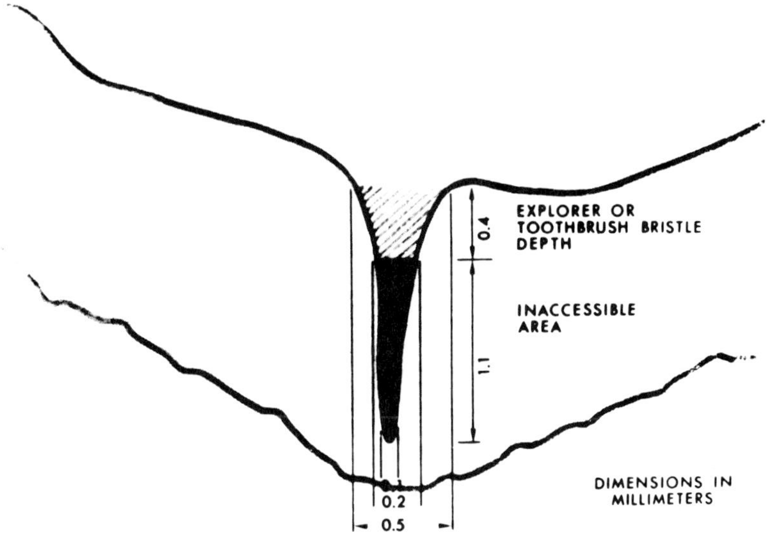

Figure 33–2. Cross-section of an occlusal fissure showing the inability of an explorer or toothbrush bristle to reach the base. *(From Newbrun E. Microflora. In: Newbrun E, ed.* Cariology. *3rd ed. Chicago: Quintessence Publishing Company; 1989.)*

present. Substrate for the bacteria must be introduced from external sources as part of the host's diet. The food consumed should reach the cariogenic bacteria on the teeth. The interlocking circles in Fig 33–4 indicate that all three factors must be present for caries to occur: susceptible host, specific, bacteria, and appropriate diet.

Host Factors

Variation in host susceptibility may be due to genetic factors, age of the tooth, tooth composition, salivary flow and composition, and immune status.

Genetics has been shown to be a factor in caries etiology by animal and human studies. Two strains of rats have been developed that differ in caries susceptibility. When these strains were crossbred, using reciprocal matings (male resistant × female susceptible and male susceptible × female resistant), the offspring of caries-resistant and caries-susceptible strains did not differ in caries experience. This indicated that genes influence caries experience and not the microflora transmitted by the nursing mother. A comparison of fraternal with identical human twins showed that the intrapair difference in caries experience was higher with fraternal than with identical twins, indicating that there are inheritable factors that influence caries. It is not known what these inheritable factors are, but those that have been considered are tooth form and spacing, pit and fissure shape and depth, tooth composition, saliva volume and composition, and immune status.

Another host factor that has an effect on caries

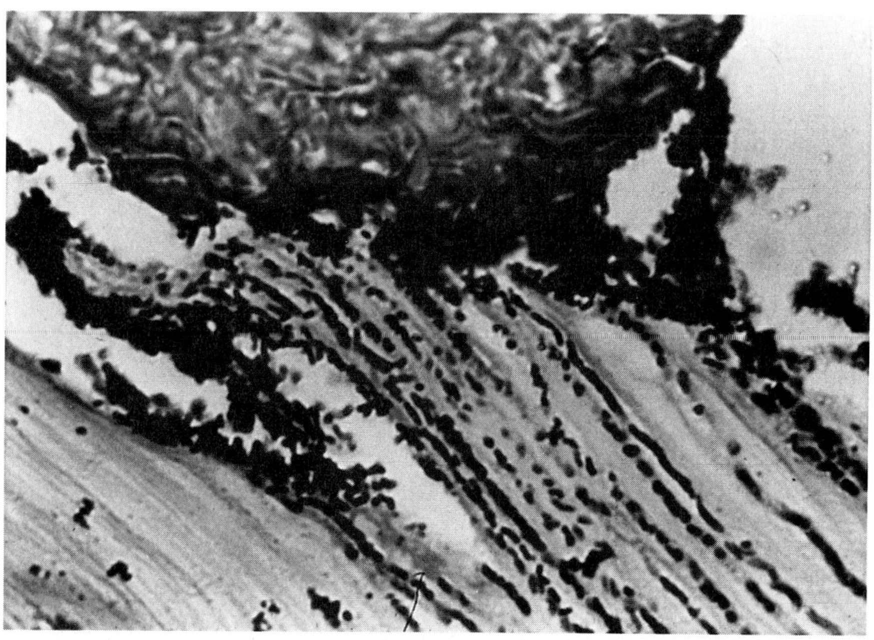

Figure 33–3. Penetration of lactobacilli into the dentinal tubules in a gnotobiotic rat. ×400. *(From Rosen S, Lenney WS, O'Malley JE.* J Dent Res. *1968; 47:358.)*

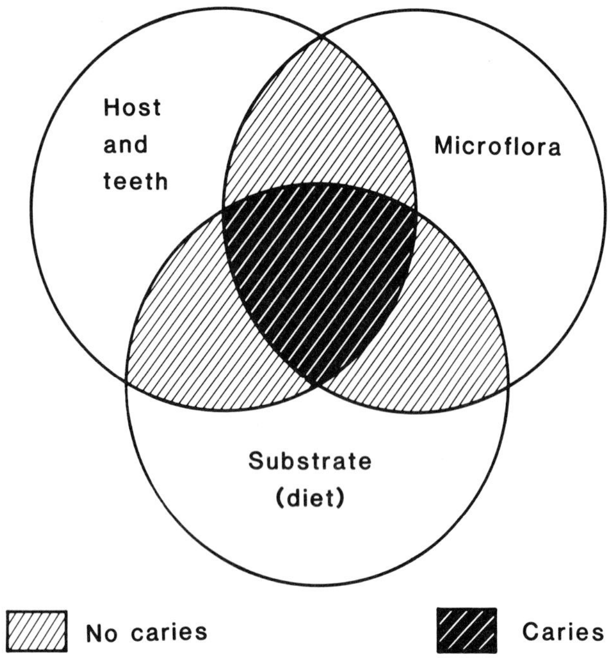

Figure 33–4. Host–parasitic–dietary relation to the initiation of dental caries. Caries occurs when there is a critical combination of the three variables shown. Prevention consists of modifying these factorial areas so that the critical combination does not occur. *(From Keyes PH, Jordan HV. Factors influencing the initiation, transmission, and inhibition of dental caries. In: Sognnaes RF.* Mechanism of Hard Tissue Destruction. *Washington, DC: AAAS; 1963:263.)*

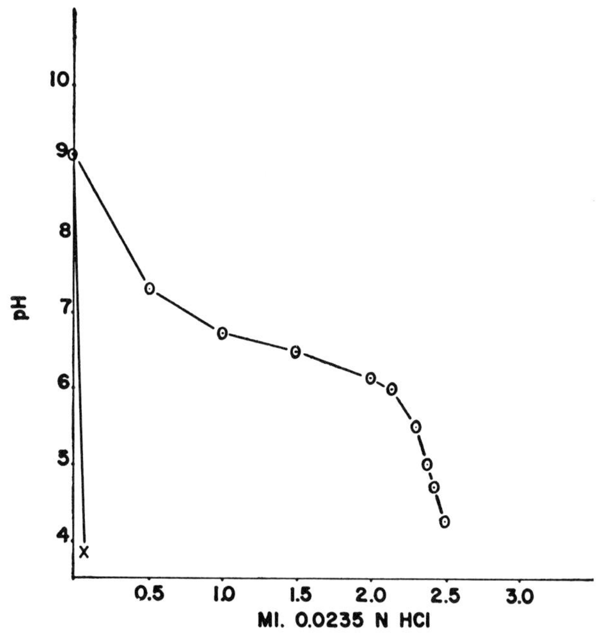

Figure 33–5. Typical curve illustrating buffering capacity of diluted rat saliva compared with that of distilled water. 0-0, 1 ml rat saliva + 4 ml distilled water; 0-X, 4 ml distilled water adjusted to pH 9.1 with sodium hydroxide. *(From Sylvester CJ, et al.* J Dent Res. *1964; 43:528.)*

etiology is the age of the tooth. In humans, caries is primarily a disease of children, indicating that the tooth is more resistant in older individuals. With experimental animals, the longer one takes to provide them with a cariogenic challenge (cariogenic bacteria and a high sucrose diet), the more resistant they are to caries. In both humans and animals the age factor appears to be one of enamel maturation, in which calcium salts from saliva are incorporated into the tooth structure, resulting in increased calcification.

Another important factor affecting tooth composition is exposure of the tooth to fluoride. Both ingestion of fluoride and its topical application increase the fluoride content of the tooth and confer marked resistance to dental caries.

The amount of saliva also is relevant. Animals that have had their salivary glands removed are more susceptible to caries. Humans who have undergone oropharyngeal irradiation therapy for cancer, resulting in diminished salivary flow, rapidly develop extensive carious lesions. Saliva also contains antibacterial factors (Chapter 32), buffers (Fig 33–5), and antibodies that may affect the development of caries.

Dietary Factors

Dietary factors that contribute to the development of dental caries are centered primarily about various sugars, especially sucrose. Sucrose, a disaccharide of fructose and glucose molecules, is refined from sugar cane and sugar beets. It is the most common sugar used in baking and confectioneries. Most studies support the statement that sugar is the most important dietary factor leading to the development of caries. Findings of these studies include

1. Certain cultural groups, such as Eskimos, African Masai, and natives of Tristan da Cunha (an island off the coast of Portugal where the natives consumed mostly fish), developed caries only after refined foods that included sugar were added to their diets.
2. Caries rates decreased in most countries deprived of sugar imports during wars.
3. In a longitudinal study in Vipeholm, Sweden, it was found that sugar consumed between meals and sticky sugar products, such as toffees and caramels, consumed with meals increased caries (Fig 33–6).
4. Individuals suffering from hereditary fructose intolerance (HFI) are unable to consume foods containing fructose or sucrose, which contains fructose. HFI is a rare, autosomal recessive disorder of fructose metabolism. Intolerance to fructose results from reduced activity of fructose 1-phosphate aldolase in the liver and small intestine. This enzyme splits fructose 1-phosphate into two 3-carbon frag-

ments that are subsequently metabolized by the Embden-Meyerhof pathway. After intake of fructose, persons with HFI become nauseated, vomit, and sweat excessively. Most of these symptoms can be attributed to a secondary hypoglucosemia resulting from a block in glycogenolysis. The numbers of decayed, missing, or filled teeth (DMF) of HFI patients were considerably less than those for normal individuals. Members of the same family not afflicted by HFI show a usual degree of caries development.

There is, however, evidence challenging the etiology of sugar in caries.

1. Although sugar cane chewers have a higher incidence of caries in Cuba and Jamaica, a similar correlation does not exist in South Africa.
2. Although dental caries incidence fell in many countries in World War II when dietary changes included a fall in sugar intake, the caries incidence also fell in Germany, where the sugar intake rose during the war.
3. Studies on four ethnic groups of South African adolescents revealed no significant differences in the DMF index between those consuming high quantities and low quantities of sugar.

The preponderance of evidence favors sugar, but other dietary factors should be considered. The frequency of eating also is an important consideration.

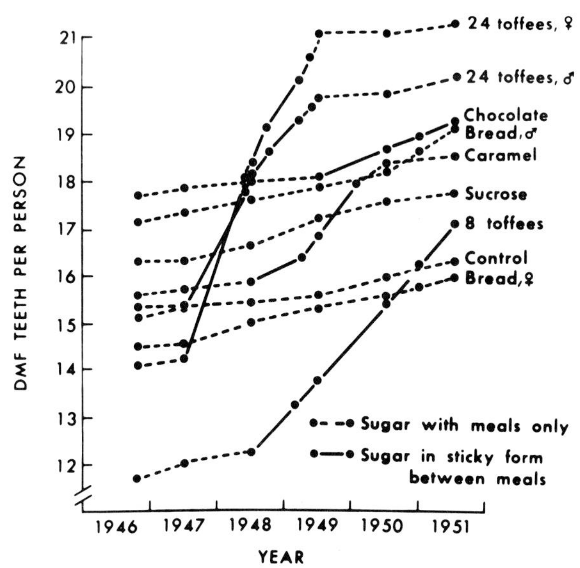

Figure 33–6. Results of the Vipeholm dental caries study. Sugar in various forms was given either between or with meals over several years, and the rate of caries increase was studied. The caries increment was much lower when sugar was given with meals compared with sugar between meals. DMF, decayed, missing, filled teeth. *(From Gustafsson B, et al.* Acta Odontol Scand. *1954;11:254.)*

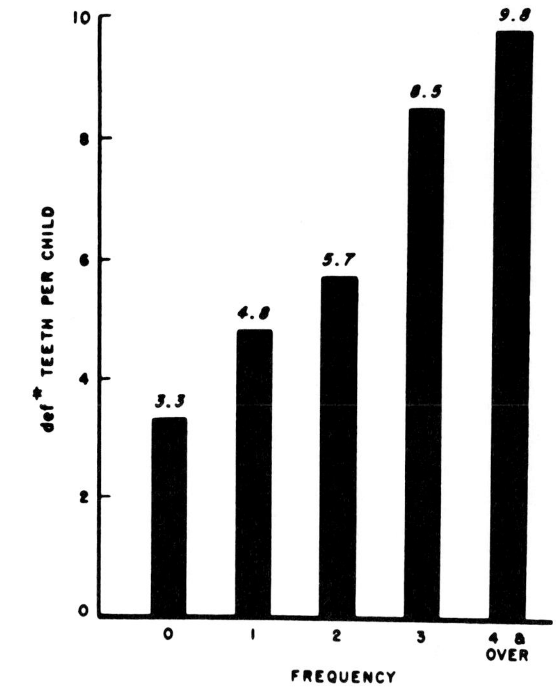

Figure 33–7. The effect of between-meal eating on caries activity in 5- to 6-year-old children. The more snacks children eat, the higher is the caries increment. DEF, decayed, extracted, filled teeth. *(From Weiss RL, Trithart AH. Between meal eating habits and dental caries experience in preschool children.* Am J Public Health. *1960;50:1097.)*

Snacking is a pastime of many individuals, and many snacks contain a high proportion of sugar. The more snacks consumed, the greater the caries activity (Fig 33–7).

A study has confirmed that foods containing sugar are cariogenic in rats (Table 33–1). In this study, a programmed feeder was used to deliver a single food item at specific intervals over a 24-hour period. This study not only reinforced that sucrose is an etiologic factor for caries but also demonstrated several other concepts about the cariogenicity of foods. This study showed that cereals containing 8%, 14%, or 60% sucrose were equally cariogenic. Also, it has been shown that more frequent feedings of sucrose with short intervals between feeding yielded higher caries activity.

Bacteria

Caries as an Infectious Disease. Although dental plaque is composed of a variety of microorganisms, only certain specific bacteria are known to cause dental caries. In order to prove whether or not a particular bacterium caused caries, it was necessary to apply Koch's postulates. This was difficult to do because of the numerous species of microflora in the oral cavity. Bacteria were isolated from individuals with caries.

TABLE 33–1. CARIOGENICITY OF FOODS IN RATS EXPRESSED AS A RATIO OF THE CARIOGENICITY OF SUCROSE (LESIONS IN THE SULCUS OF THE OCCLUSAL SURFACE ONLY)

Food	Cariogenic Potential Index (CPI)
Sucrose	1
Chocolate cookie with soft filling	1.4
Fortified cereal (14% sucrose)	1.06
14 meals of sucrose	0.99
Cereal (8% sucrose)	0.96
Presweetened cereal (60% sucrose)	0.94
Sugar-coated chocolate candy	0.91
Potato chips	0.84
Caramel	0.73
Chocolate bar	0.72
11 meals of sugar	0.59
Unsweetened cereal (2% sucrose)	0.45
Starch	0.45
Sugar and 7.5% calcium phosphate	0.42
8 meals of sugar	0.36
3 meals of sugar	0.14
0 meals by mouth	0

From Bowen WH, et al. A method to assess cariogenic potential of foodstuffs. J Am Dent Assoc. *1980; 100:677.*

Pure cultures of each microorganism were obtained and were used to infect germ-free rats, and an appropriate dietary challenge (usually a diet containing 56% sucrose) was given. Certain microorganisms caused caries, whereas others did not. Until about 1955, it was suspected that only certain lactobacilli could cause caries. Since then, certain species of streptococci and lactobacilli have been known to cause coronal caries, which resembles human coronal caries.

In the 1960s, it was shown in animal experiments that caries was a transmissible disease. Animals that appeared to be immune to caries developed this disease when caged with animals who had caries.

Establishing an etiologic spectrum of bacteria was not limited to the use of germ-free rats. It was not possible to establish a germ-free hamster, but administration of antibiotics to conventional hamsters and rats depressed the indigenous cariogenic flora. The animals were then infected with a microorganism suspected of being able to cause caries. As with germ-free rats, it was found that only certain microorganisms were able to cause caries.

Specific Versus Nonspecific Hypothesis. An area of importance in caries etiology, which is still controversial, is whether the microbial etiologic component is specific or nonspecific. Specific etiology means that a single microorganism causes dental caries. Nonspecific etiology means that several microorganisms cause dental caries. If a specific etiology could be established, certain preventive or treatment modalities could be carried out with greater efficiency (eg, vaccine or antimicrobial agent). Cross-sectional and longitudinal studies in humans have shown that *Streptococcus mutans* is associated with dental caries, but in a smaller but significant number of cases, this organism was not detected when caries was present (or was not detected before the occurrence of an incipient lesion). Conversely, *S. mutans* was found on tooth surfaces when caries did not occur. Proponents of the nonspecific hypothesis contend that any acidogenic microorganism in dental plaque contributes to the causation of dental caries.

Evidence for* Streptococcus mutans *as an Etiologic Agent. In 1924, Clarke identified a coccus from a carious lesion, which he named *S. mutans*. Clarke believed this organism was a mutant and had no knowledge that it produced the polysaccharide, mutan, from sucrose. The organism was adherent, acidogenic, and present in high numbers in the lesion.

The facts that indicate that streptococci, especially *S. mutans*, are etiologic agents are as follows. Certain streptococci, especially *S. mutans*, have been isolated from human carious lesions and from plaques of individuals with high caries activity. In people with low caries activity, *S. mutans* is found less frequently and in lower numbers. Cross-sectional and longitudinal epidemiologic surveys have implicated *S. mutans* in the etiology of human caries.

When preventive measures were used to reduce *S. mutans* in mothers of infants, there was a decrease of *S. mutans* in both mothers and infants when compared to controls (no preventive measures used). Less caries was observed in these infants when they became 3 years old, provided that *S. mutans* was not present. Also, if a child had *S. mutans* at 15 months of age, he or she had caries at 3 years of age.

Streptococcus mutans causes caries in experimental animals. Studies of an experimental caries vaccine in animals have shown that a vaccine derived from *S. mutans* reduces caries.

Streptococcus mutans produces insoluble extracellular polysaccharides from sucrose that allow it to stick to the teeth and form larger amounts of plaque. Other oral bacteria do not produce these polysaccharides. *Streptococcus mutans* adheres to saliva-coated hydroxyapatite, indicating that it could form the innermost layer of dental plaque. *Streptococcus mutans* is more active than other plaque bacteria in its ability to convert sucrose to acids and reserve polysaccharides.

pH levels of 5.0 or lower may persist in caries-active plaques for several hours. This indicates that the microbial acid production is maintained in the presence of plaque and salivary buffer systems. The plaque continues to produce acid at these low pH levels. Certain plaque species, such as *Actinomyces viscosus, Streptococcus sanguis, Streptococcus salivarius,* and *Streptococcus mitior,* are unable to produce acid from sucrose at pH 5.0, but *S. mutans* and certain lactobacilli (eg, *Lactobacillus casei*) continue to be active. In fact, *S. mutans* is more active at pH 5.0 than at pH 7.0, which suggests that it is the principal acid producer in vivo when plaque pH is buffered at pH 5.0. Thus, the frequent ingestion of sucrose could lead to the selection of a microbe that because of its aciduricity (capable of tolerating acid) is most competitive at pH levels that both solubilize the tooth mineral and discriminate against other plaque species.

Characterization of Streptococcus mutans. The possible role of other bacteria as etiologic agents is minor compared to that of *S. mutans. Streptococcus mutans* can be distinguished from other oral streptococci by its ability to ferment sorbitol and mannitol (except for about 4%), its colonial appearance, and its ability to produce mutan, dextran, and fructan (Table 33–2).

Table 33–3 summarizes some basic differences in the mutans group of streptococci. The antigenic composition of this species has been studied in considerable detail because of the possibility of immunizing humans with *S. mutans* as a protective measure against dental caries and the use of serologic techniques for the rapid identification of fresh isolates. *Streptococcus mutans* does not belong to any of the Lancefeld serotypes except that serotype e cross reacts with Lancefeld's group E. However, this organism has been divided into the species *S. mutans, Streptococcus rattus, Streptococcus sobrinus, Streptococcus critecus,* and *Streptococcus ferus,* which are related to their serotypes (ie, *S. mutans* is c,e or f, *S. rattus* is b, and so on) (Table 33–3). *Streptococcus mutans* can be subdivided into 8 serotypes (a through h) on the basis of carbohydrate antigens associated with the cell wall. Although these carbohydrate antigens are serotype specific, they can be responsible for cross-reactions among some of the other serotypes. The 8 serologic divisions are supported by cell wall analysis and DNA base content (% guanine and cytosine). Immunodominant sugars (ie, that part of a molecule recognized for the immune response) have been characterized for most of the serotypes.

Geographic differences occur in the prevalence of serotypes of *S. mutans.* Serotypes c and d are the most common in Europe and the United States. Serotypes a and b were found in samples from Egypt. The reasons for these variations are not known. Physiologic differences also are associated with some of these serotypes. Thus, many serotype d strains do not ferment sorbitol, and serotype b strains characteristically hydrolyze arginine. In addition to carbohydrates, lipoteichoic acids associated with the membranes and cell walls of *S. mutans* (and other streptococcal species) are highly antigenic and cause wide serologic cross-reactions throughout the streptococci. Lipoteichoic acids may play a role in the adherence of oral streptococci to the tooth surface.

Evidence for Other Bacteria as Etiologic Agents. Although most investigators believe that *S. mutans* is the primary etiologic microorganism for typical coronal caries, lactobacilli should not be ignored. They certainly should be considered to have a secondary or opportunistic role.

The implication of lactobacilli as etiologic agents is supported by both experimental evidence and clinical observation. (1) Lactobacilli caused rampant dental caries in germ-free rats. (2) Artificial caries in human teeth was induced by lactobacilli. (3) When carious areas were restored in humans or if there was a spontaneous regression of caries, lactobacilli were no longer observed. (4) A longitudinal study in humans has shown that lactobacilli are present at a sound, susceptible site before the clinical observation of caries. In addition, homolactic lactobacilli, such as *Lactobacillus acidophilus* and *L. casei,* which produce only lactic acid as

TABLE 33–2. *STREPTOCOCCUS MUTANS* IN RELATION TO OTHER STREPTOCOCCI

Species	Fermentation of		Ammonia from arginine	Hydrolysis of esculin	Acetoin production (VP test)	H_2O_2 Production	Colonial appearance on sucrose agar	Chemical nature of polysaccharide from sucrose
	Mannitol	*Sorbitol*						
S. mutans	+	+	–	+	+	–	Hard	Mutan Dextran Fructan
S. sanguis	–	–	+	+	–	+	Hard	Glucan
S. mitior	–	–	–	–	±	+	Hard or soft	Glucan
S. milleri	–	–	+	+	+	–	Soft	—
S. salivarius	–	–	–	+	–	–	Mucoid	Fructan

+, majority of strains give a positive reaction.
–, majority of strains give a negative reaction.
±, variable reaction.

Adapted from Marsh PO, Martin M. Oral Microbiology. *2nd ed. Washington, DC: American Society for Microbiology; 1984.*

TABLE 33–3. SUMMARY OF SOME BASIC DIFFERENCES WITHIN THE MUTANS GROUP OF STREPTOCOCCI

Species	mutans			rattus	sobrinus			critecus	ferus
Serovar	c	e	f	b	d	g	h	a	c
Genotype mol/100 mL G + C[a]		36–38		42–43		44–45		43–44	44
Antigenic serovar determinant	Glucose-(α) (1–4)glucose	Glucose-(β) (1–4)glucose	Glucose-(α) (1–6)glucose	(α)galactose	Galactose-(β) (1–6) glucose	(β)galactose	ND[c]	Glucose-(β) (1–6)glucose	ND
Cell wall carbohydrate		Glucose, rhamnose		Galactose, rhamnose		Glucose, galactose, rhamnose		Glucose, galactose, rhamnose	Glucose, rhamnose
Fermentation									
Mannitol	+	+	+	+	+	+	+	+	+
Sorbitol	+	+	+	+	±	±	−	+	+
Raffinose	+	+	+	+	−	−	−	+	−
Melibiose	+	±	+	+	−	−	+	+	N.D.
NH_3 from arginine	−	−	−	+	−	−	−	−	−
Growth in bacitracin[b]	+	+	−	+	−	+	−	−	−

[a]G + C guanosine + cytosine.
[b]β 0.2 U/ml
[c]ND, not determined.
From Newbrun E. Cariology. *3rd ed. Chicago: Quintessence Publishing Co; 1989.*

an end product of carbohydrate metabolism, are more cariogenic than heterolactic lactobacilli. Heterolactic strains produce end products other than lactic acid, such as formic acid and CO_2. Lactobacilli are aciduric, which means that they can tolerate acid. This feature allows this organism to survive in dental plaque and carious areas and to continue to damage tooth structure as fermentable carbohydrates are consumed by the host.

Lactobacilli, however, are now considered by some to be opportunistic in the development of dental caries. Their population in dental plaque is 10 to 100-fold less than streptococci. They have no obvious adherence mechanisms. Furthermore, they do not cause caries in hamsters, an animal whose molar tooth topography does not readily allow for impaction of food and bacteria. Only acidogenic bacteria with adherent properties causes caries in hamsters. Certain epidemiologic studies indicate that lactobacilli increase in population only after caries is initiated.

Bacteria other than lactobacilli and *S. mutans* display a degree of selectivity as to which tooth area they will attack. Table 33–4 is a list of sites susceptible to decay, along with a list of microorganisms and their possible significance in human disease as judged by animal experiments.

Species of stretptococcus other than *S. mutans* (eg, *S. salivarius* and *S. sanguis*) have been reported as being cariogenic by some and as noncariogenic by others. This is one reason why they are considered as not being too significant in human caries (Table 33–4). *Streptococcus mutans,* because of its adherent nature, tends to cause caries on smooth surfaces, whereas other streptococci as well as *S. mutans* and lactobacilli cause caries in pits and fissures. Species of *Actinomyces* cause caries usually only on root surface.

ROOT SURFACE CARIES

As progress continues in biomedicine, the life span of our population is increasing to a point where periodontal disease causes a resorption of alveolar bone, thereby exposing the root surfaces of teeth. Root surfaces caries has been found in 60% to 70% of individuals between 60 and 70 years old (Fig 33–8). An example of this disease is shown in Fig 33–9. In experimental animal root caries was reduced by treatment with fluoride but alveolar bone loss was not affected significantly. (Fig 33–10).

Strains of *S. mutans, S. sanguis, Arthrobacter* sp., *Veillonella, Rothia dentocariosa, A. viscosus,* and *Actinomyces naeslundii* have been isolated from human cemental lesions root caries.

Recent studies with humans indicate a questionable etiology for *Actinomyces* in root surface caries because it has been shown that *Actinomyces* is found on sound root surfaces in the same concentration as is found on carious root surfaces.

TABLE 33–4. TYPES OF DENTAL CARIES IN ANIMAL MODEL SYSTEM

Type of Caries	Etiologic Organism	Possible Significance in Human Disease
Pit and fissure	*Streptococcus mutans*	Very significant
	Streptococcus sanguis	Not very significant
	Other streptococci	Not very significant
	Lactobacillus sp.	Very significant
	Actinomyces sp.	May be significant
Smooth surface	*Streptococcus mutans*	Very significant
	Streptococcus salivarius	Probably not significant
Root surface	*Actinomyces viscosus*	Very significant
	Actinomyces naeslundii	Very significant
	Other filamentous rods	Very significant
	Streptococcus mutans	Significant
	Streptococcus sanguis	May be significant
	Streptococcus salivarius	Probably not significant
Deep dentinal caries	*Lactobacillus* sp.	Very significant
	Actinomyces naeslundii	Very significant
	Actinomyces viscosus	Significant
	Other filamentous rods	Very significant
	Streptococcus mutans	May be significant

From Newbrun E, Cariology. *3rd ed. Chicago: Quintessence Publishing Co; 1989.*

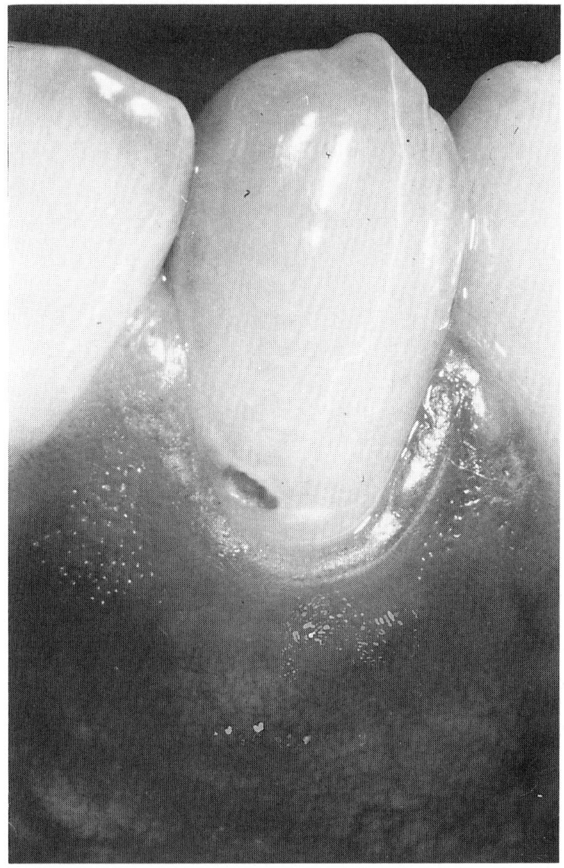

Figure 33–9. Root surface caries in a human. *(Courtesy of Dr. Lew Claman, Ohio State University.)*

ROLE OF LACTIC AND OTHER ACIDS

Lactic acid bacteria (lactobacilli and streptococci) derive their energy from glycolytic pathways, with the end product being lactic acid. Other organic acids are formed in dental plaque, but lactic acid has been the most studied and is the dominant cause of enamel decalcification. More lactic acid is produced from sucrose metabolism by plaque from carious sites than plaque from noncarious sites (Fig 33–11).

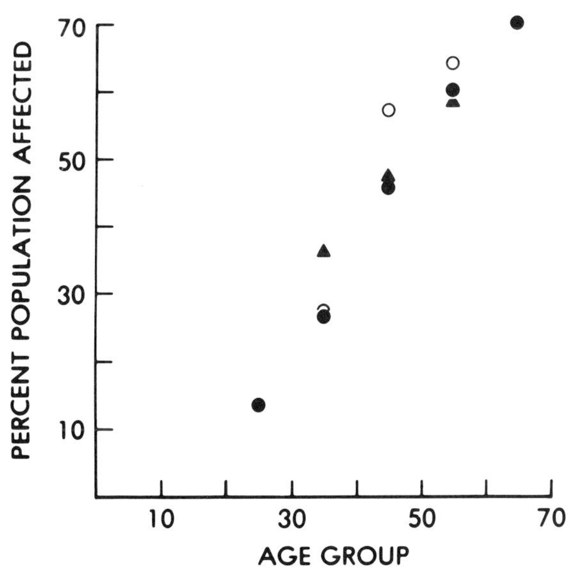

Figure 33–8. Prevalence of root caries in selected contemporary populations by age groups. O, V.A. Hospital patients and staff; ▶ insurance company employees; ●, Coast Guard base residents. *(From Newbrun E, ed.* Cariology. *3rd ed. Chicago: Quintessence Publishing Co., 1989.)*

Figure 33–12 shows how dietary carbohydrates are metabolized by plaque bacteria, leading to the production of lactic acid and subsequent enamel dissolution. Dietary carbohydrates, such as starch, lactose, sucrose, glucose, and fructose, are available for enzyme activity on the tooth surface, which leads to enamel dissolution. Except for starch, carbohydrates are metabolized by plaque bacteria to lactic and other acids (eg, pyruvic and formic) that contribute to enamel dissolution. Formic and pyruvic acid are not as powerful as lactic acid in their abilities to liberate the hydrogen ion. Therefore, it is considered by some that the presence of *Veillonella* and other bacteria that produce these acids may retard caries by producing weaker acids from carbohydrates. Starch that remains on the tooth surface may be converted into maltose by the salivary enzyme, amylase, thus also contributing to the development of acids. Glucan and fructan are sticky extracellular polysaccharides formed by the ac-

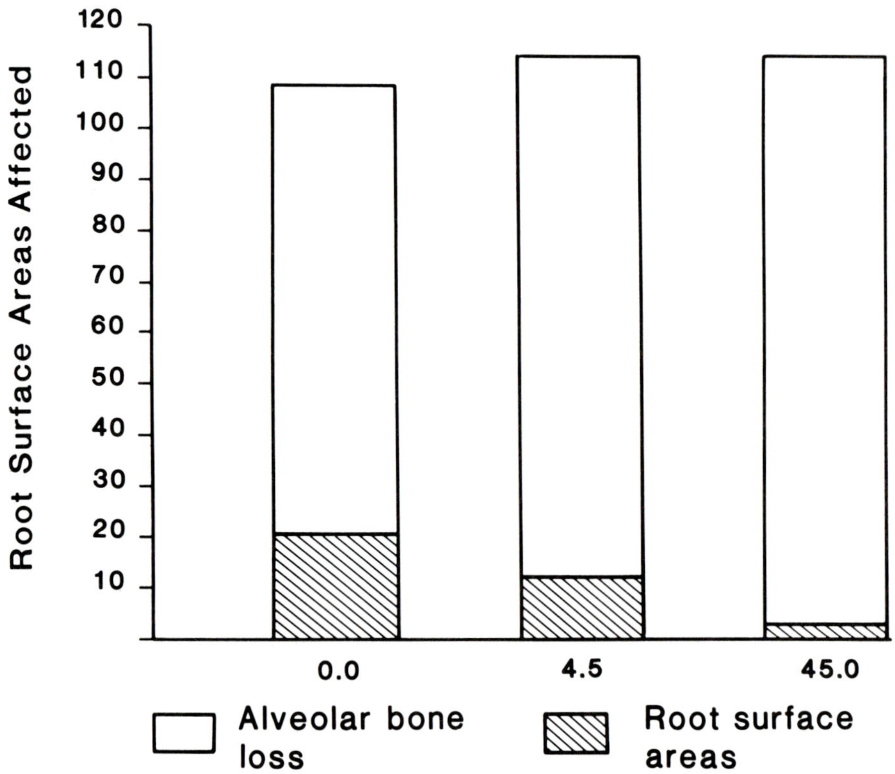

Figure 33–10. Effect of 0.0, 4.5, and 45 ppm fluoride on alveolar bone loss and root surface caries in rats. Bone loss was measured by length of root exposure, and root caries was measured by the area of the root showing caries. *(Adapted from Rotilie JA, et al.* J Dent Res. *1977; 56:1408.)*

tion of *S. mutans* cell-associated enzymes (Chapter 32) on sucrose. They are important parts of the dental plaque matrix. Various plaque bacteria store iodophilic polysaccharides (dextrins) intracellularly. Dextrins are starch breakdown products of sufficient molecular weight to be stained by iodine. During starvation, dextrins are converted slowly into acids. Thus, the caries process continues between meals and very likely goes on during sleep.

Acid in dental plaque is responsible for the carious lesion. At a certain critical pH, 5.5, decalcification of enamel accelerates. With increasing concentration of hydrogen ions in the plaque, more phosphate ions (in the form of HPO_4^{2-} and $H_2PO^-_4$ will leave the solid apatite phase.

$$\text{Apatite} - PO_4 \underset{-\,H^+}{\overset{+\,H^+}{\rightleftharpoons}} HPO_4^{2-} \underset{-H^+}{\overset{H^+}{\rightleftharpoons}} H_2PO_4^-$$

The concentration of calcium and phosphate influences the apatite dissolution rate by the law of mass action. Calcium is the cation associated with phosphates and in part of the apatite crystal structure. As the concentrations of calcium and phosphate are in-

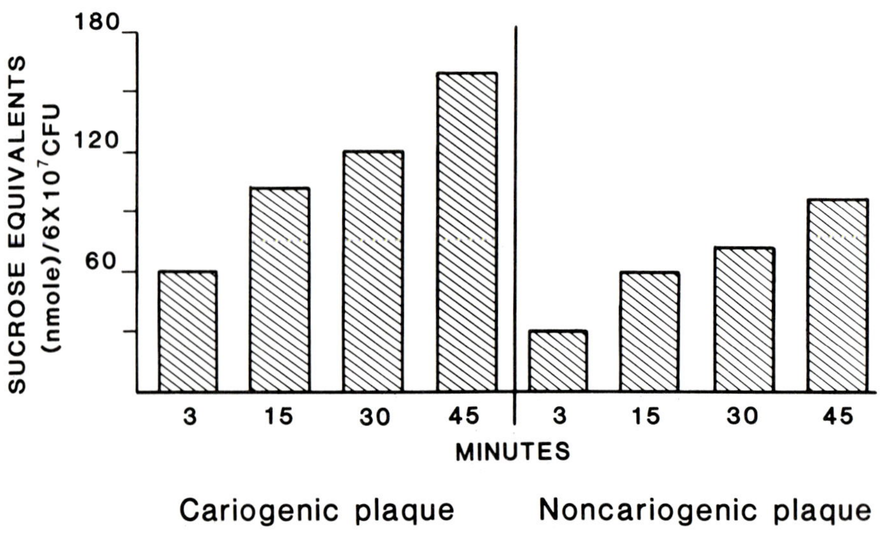

Figure 33–11. Lactic acid produced from sucrose metabolism by cariogenic and noncariogenic plaque. Sucrose equivalent is the amount of sucrose that was converted into lactic acid and other products. *(Adapted from Minah GE, Loesche WJ.* Infect Immun. *1977;17:43–54.)*

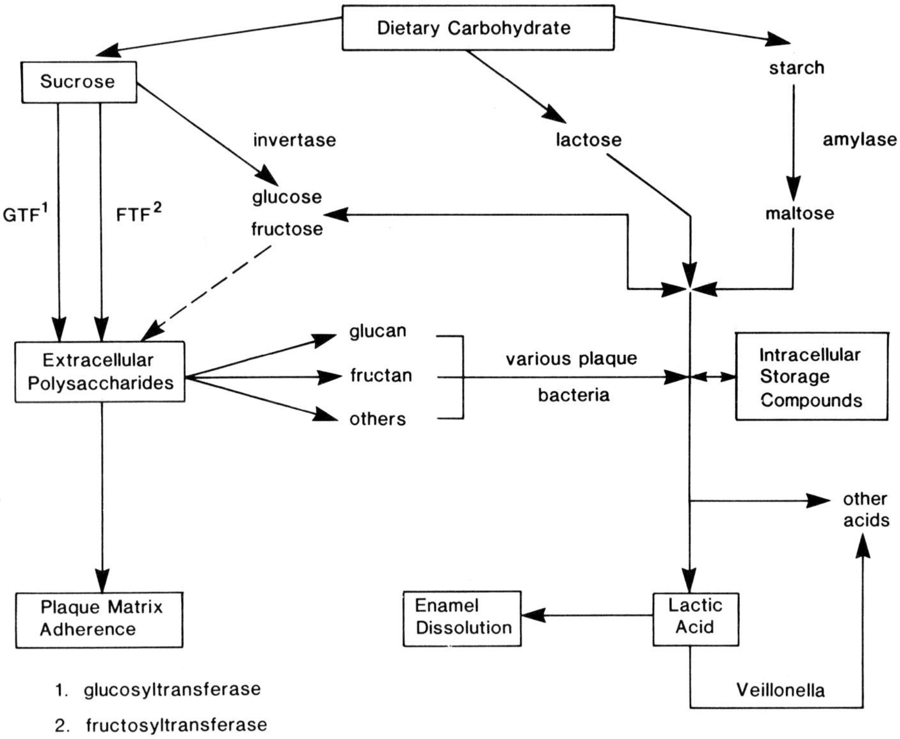

Figure 33–12. Simple diagram to show the possible fate of dietary carbohydrates. Some metabolic interactions involving plaque bacteria also are indicated. Factors relating to the pathogenesis of dental caries are boxed. *(Adapted from Marsh PD.* Oral Microbiology. *Washington, DC: American Society of Microbiology; 1980.)*

creased in the system, the reaction is driven to the left.

It is reasonable to assume that microorganisms adhering to teeth or packed into pits and fissures cause caries because bacteria have the enzymes to catalyze sugars to acids. If acid is the harmful material, it should be possible to demonstrate acidity on a tooth surface. Using an antimony electrode, Stephan was able to measure the pH of dental plaque before and after a sugar rinse. He did this in five groups of subjects ranging from caries-free to caries-rampant (Fig 33–13). He showed that acid forms on the tooth surface within seconds after a sugar rinse, as judged by a drop in pH. The low pH remains for about 20 to 30 minutes and then gradually returns to the original ph after about 60 minutes. The study by Stephan also showed that the resting (zero time) plaque pH was lowest in individuals with high caries activity, and their plaques reached lower pH levels after challenge, suggesting that these individuals had an active acidogenic plaque microflora. It is interesting to note that plaques of only the more caries-prone groups attain pH values below 5.5 on topical glucose challenge. This information is used by the government of Switzerland, which permits food manufacturers to label their food "Friendly to the teeth" if it does not reduce the pH of plaque below 5.7 within 10 minutes.

The effect of different carbohydrates on plaque pH is shown in Fig 33–14. The greatest drop in pH is seen when glucose, fructose, or sucrose is applied to dental plaque. When sorbitol, a low-caloric sweetening agent, is used, there is only a slight drop in pH. Sorbitol is fermented slowly compared to the rate of glucose, fructose, or sucrose. This allows the buffering activity of saliva to keep the pH high when sorbitol contacts dental plaque. The drop in pH and its duration are influenced by the amount of plaque, the kinds of plaque bacteria, the type and concentration of the substrate, and the accessibility of saliva to the plaque. If saliva is restricted (eg, by blocking flow with cotton rolls or in patients with xerostomia), the pH of plaque does not return to its initial value (Fig 33–15). The pH also will remain low if sugars are applied to the plaque for long periods of time.

PREVENTION

Methods used to control dental caries include mechanical removal of plaque, sealants, dietary measures, and fluoridation. Consideration has been given to the use of a vaccine.

Brushing and flossing, if practiced diligently and performed by professionally trained individuals, will result in marked reduction of oral disease. Biweekly administration of a dental prophylaxis by professionals to children in schools has resulted in virtual elimination of dental disease. It has not been demonstrated that good oral hygiene practices by individuals reduce dental caries.

Removal of plaque by mechanical means from deep, narrow pits, as shown in Fig 33–2 is impossi-

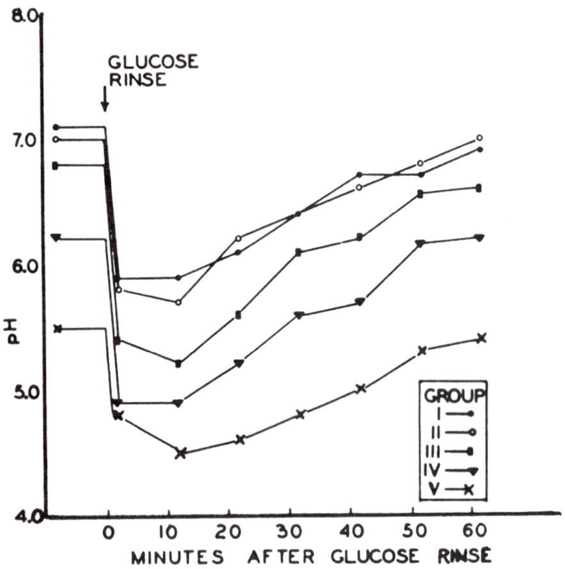

Figure 33–13. pH of dental plaques measured in situ in individuals of varying caries activity before and after rinsing the mouth with 5% glucose solution. Group 1, caries-free; group 2, no active lesions; group 3, a few active lesions; group 4, several active lesions; group 5, rampant decay. Note that the resting plaque pH differed among groups; groups with highest caries activity had lower resting pH values. Following the glucose rinse, the pH of all plaques dropped. In individuals of high caries activity, acidities of pH 5 or below were evident. Note also that the pH of the plaques returned slowly to their starting levels. *(From Stephan RH. Intraoral hydrogen ion concentration associated with dental caries activity.* J Dent Res. *1944; 23:257.)*

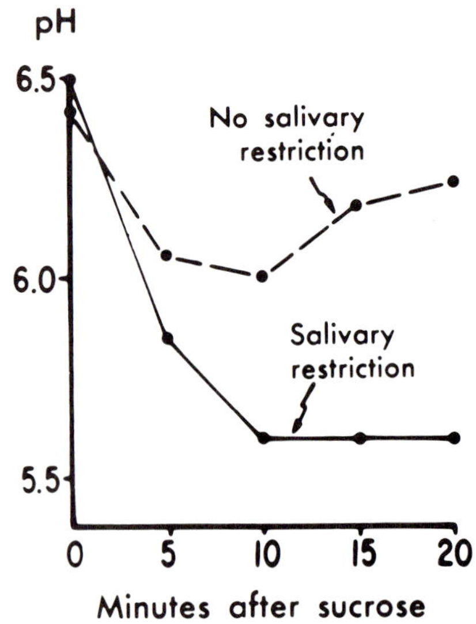

Figure 33–15. Effect of salivary restriction on the pH of dental plaque in situ after rinsing with a sucrose solution. The curves are the results for 50 persons. *(From Kleinberg I. Dental caries. In: Nolte W, ed.* Oral Microbiology. *4th ed. St. Louis: CV Mosby Co; 1982.)*

ble. Additional measures for prevention should be taken.

Polymers have been used to coat the enamel surface to prevent exposure to the demineralizing acids produced by plaque. The most effective contain the epoxy resin, bisphenol, A-glycidal methacrylate (Bis-GMA). These plastics are effective as occlusal sealants but are less effective on smooth surfaces.

Dietary restriction of refined carbohydrates is an effective measure to control dental caries. It is particularly useful in individuals with rampant caries. However, proof is lacking that certain foods are cariogenic in humans. Reduction of between-meal snacks would allow for remineralization of enamel and reduce the duration of exposure to acidic conditions that cause demineralization. Noncaloric sweeteners, such as xylitol and sorbitol, are used as substitutes for sucrose in many foods. These sugar alcohols are fermented slowly so that acid can be neutralized by salivary buffers before the enamel is decalcified. Although some adaptation of human oral microflora to continuous use of sorbitol as the only carbohydrate consumed has been reported, it is unlikely that the human population would use sorbitol as a sole source of carbohydrate.

The use of 1 ppm fluoride in public water supplies is gradually being accepted worldwide. There is no need to exceed the 1 ppm concentration, since communities having higher natural fluoride do not show a greater decrease in dental caries experience (Fig 33–16). Increasing fluoride concentration beyond 1 ppm also increases the risk of dental fluorosis (mottled enamel). Fluoride has been used as a topical application in dental offices, in dentifrices, in oral rinses in schools, and in mouthpiece gels. Fluoride prevents dissolution of enamel, inhibits bacterial acid production, and enhances remineralization. Whether it is given systemically or topically, fluoride is incorporated into the mineral structure of enamel. Fluor-

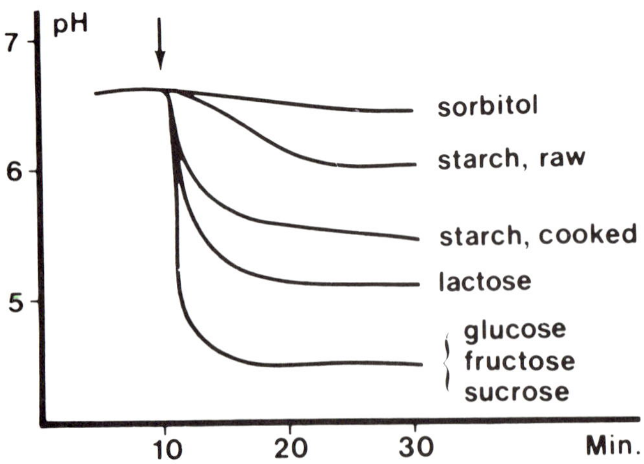

Figure 33–14. pH changes in plaque following application of different carbohydrate solutions. Time of application is indicated by arrow (Stephan curve). *(Modified from Newbrun E, ed.* Cariology. *3rd ed. Chicago: Quintessence Publishing Co; 1989.)*

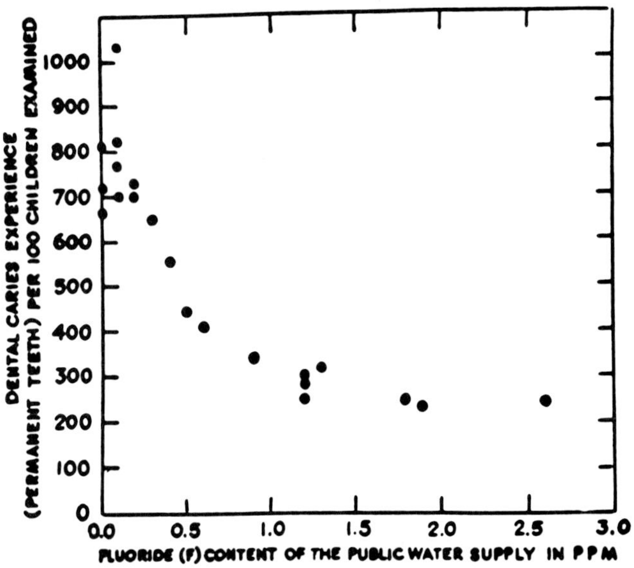

Figure 33–16. The accumulated lifetime dental caries experience for the permanent teeth of 7257 children from 21 cities in four states is plotted against the fluoride content of the public water supply in those cities. Note the low plateau in dental caries experience attained with between 1.0 and 1.5 ppm of fluoride in public water supplies. *(From Dean HT, et al.* Public Health Rep. *1942;57:1155.)*

apatite replaces some of the hydroxyapatite, which is more resistant to dissolution by acid. Incipient carious lesions are repaired by a natural remineralization process. This is believed to be due in part to soluble calcium phosphates in saliva. When fluoride is added to a synthetic calcifying solution, there is a significant increase in remineralization. Synthetic calcifying solutions are used in patients with little or no salivary flow. Enzymes important in the metabolism of carbohydrates to lactic acid are sensitive to fluoride. Phosphatase and enolase, key enzymes in glycolysis, an important energy mechanism for lactobacilli and streptococci, are inhibited by fluoride.

The production of caries by specific bacteria has stimulated the search for a vaccine capable of inhibiting this disease. Success was first achieved with the organism *Streptococcus faecalis* in gnotobiotic rats. However, when the vaccine was tested in conventional rats, it was unsuccessful.

Salivary antibody effective in inhibiting dental caries is secretory immunoglobulin A (sIgA). When the oral–gastric route was used to administer a vaccine, induction of these antibodies occurred in B cells in the Peyer's patches of the small intestine. Plasma cells became sensitized to oral bacteria. These cells migrated to the salivary gland, which produced sIgA.

Another approach to the development of a vaccine for dental caries has been to immunize animals with glucosyltransferase (GTF). This enzyme, which catalyzes the conversion of sucrose to glucans, is found on the surface of many cariogenic streptococci. Glucans are sticky polymers of glucose essential to dental plaque development. The rationale is to block the organism's capacity to synthesize glucans. Reports on the success of this approach have been conflicting, depending on the animal used. It has been more successful in rodents than in primates.

Whole cells and cell walls of *S. mutans* have been used to vaccinate animals, with moderate success. The oral–gastric route has been used to immunize animals. These studies were done in gnotobiotic rats in which sIgA correlated with a reduction in caries. If administered by other than the oral–gastric route, hypersensitivity may develop. This method has been more successful in reducing caries on smooth surfaces than in fissures.

To avoid systemic side effects, a novel immunization procedure was to apply a low molecular weight (3.8 K) streptococcal antigen (SA) topically to the gingival crevices of monkeys. After a year, there was a lower incidence of dental caries and colonization with *S. mutans* when compared with sham-immunized controls. Also, there was an increase in gingival crevicular IgG and salivary IgA anti-SA antibodies, but there was no change in serum SA antibodies. Apparently, numbers of *S. mutans* are reduced by induction of sIgA antibodies, which prevents adherence of *S. mutans* to teeth, and by IgG, which enhances phagocytosis by the local neutrophils.

Following vaccination with *S. mutans* or GTF, there is an increase of the immunoglobulin sIgA directed against *S. mutans* in the saliva of animals. Some studies have shown a reduction of *S. mutans* that correlates with increased levels of salivary IgA and protection against caries.

Although some success has been achieved with a vaccine for dental caries, there are certain problems associated with this immunization process.

1. Dental caries is initiated on the external surfaces of enamel, where the standard immune responses are not elicited as effectively as they would be to a systemic infection.
2. The rodent model may be infected with *S. mutans* before administration of a vaccine. There may be a need to immunize early (ie, before caries develops). Therefore, the immune system may not be fully developed. If immunization is delayed, teeth develop resistance.
3. There is uncertainty about *S. mutans* as the only causative agent in humans. Even with *S. mutans,* antigenic properties may change (drift), which would render immunity less effective.
4. Caries is not a life-threatening disease, and a vaccine may result in more harm than good.

Streptococci, including *S. mutans,* have antigenic components shared with heart muscle. This could result in the induction of humoral antibodies that damage the heart tissue.

5. The disease is in a state of decline in most western countries.

DECLINING PREVALENCE OF DENTAL CARIES

Caries rates are declining in more developed areas of the world. An example is given in Fig 33–17, which shows the relationship of DMFT to age in Massachusetts schoolchildren. Caries prevalence in 1979–1981 declined by about one half since 1951. More recent data show that the decline is still continuing but at a much lower rate. In a 1986–87 survey conducted by the National Institute for Dental Research, half the children aged 6 to 17 were totally free of caries. The decline has occurred in areas both with and without organized preventive programs or fluoridation of water supplies. However, since fluoride is available in dentifrices, in dental offices applied professionally, in systemic fluoride supplements professionally prescribed, and in school programs, a logical explanation for the decreased prevalence of caries is that declining caries rates correlate with fluoride usage.

Another explanation is that there has been more restorative care, which is preventive because open lesions serve as foci for the spread of infection.

An increase in the use of antibiotics also could be a factor in explaining the decline in prevalence of dental caries. Children receiving antibiotics for streptococcal pharyngitis occasionally experience a marked and prolonged suppression of *S. mutans.* An inverse relationship between caries experience and antibiotics usage has been reported. The last generation of children has been exposed to more antibiotics than any previous generation.

A change in the pattern of sugar consumption from sucrose to glucose or fructose began in 1973 in certain countries following a sharp increase in the price of refined cane and beet sugar (sucrose). Sweeteners such as corn syrup (an enzymatically produced glucose–fructose mixture from corn starch), were cheaper and equally efficient in many cases. Since sucrose is more cariogenic than glucose or fructose, it follows that this change in sugar consumption could be an additional factor in explaining the decline in caries rate.

CARIES ACTIVITY TESTS

Accurate caries activity tests could be of value to the clinician to aid in the prognosis of future carious lesions. Most caries activity tests assume that specific microorganisms cause caries. Thus, the rationale has been to look for these microorganisms and to correlate their levels with current and future caries. Initially, it was believed that the chief etiologic agents were lactobacilli, so tests were developed to assay for numbers of these bacteria in saliva.

A common medium used for this purpose in the microbiology laboratory is Rogosa's SL agar. This me-

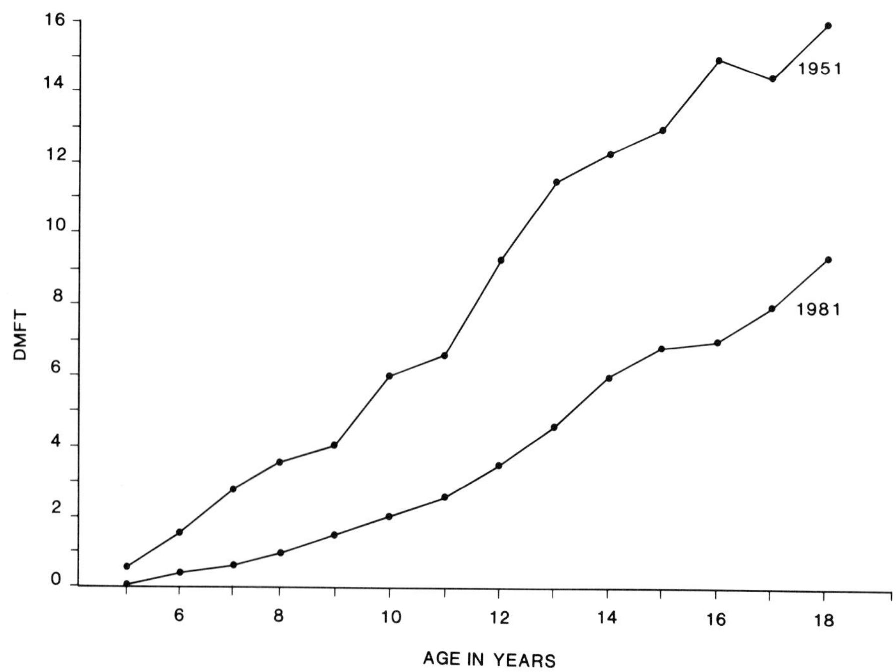

Figure 33–17. DMFT by age: 1951 vs 1979 to 1981, all phases. *(From DePaola PF, et al. J Dent Res. 1982; 61:1356–1360.)*

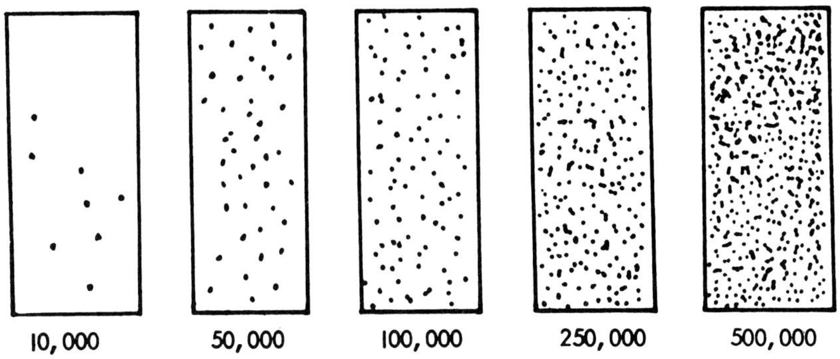

Figure 33–18. Cariescreen SM colony density comparator chart. Each dot represents a colony. The numbers below indicate the number of colonies per milliliter of saliva. *(From Jordan HV, et al.* J Dent Res. *1987; 66:57–61.)*

dium relies on a low pH (5.4) and a high content of acetate to select lactobacilli.

Snyder developed a differential, low pH agar that contains a pH indicator. As organisms grew in the agar, acid was produced, and the color of the medium changed from green to yellow. There was a good correlation of the rapidity of the change with salivary *Lactobacillus* count.

These tests showed that groups of individuals with active caries showed greater numbers of lactobacilli than individuals without caries or with inactive caries. The results were not considered accurate on an individual basis, nor were they considered accurate enough to predict future caries activity. Such tests have been reported to be an appropriate indicator of patient cooperation as far as adherence to a low cariogenic diet. Thus, effective dietary counseling, together with patient motivation, can result in reduced *Lactobacillus* counts and reduced initiation and progression of dental caries. The microbiologic tests can aid in patient motivation by acting as a diet monitor.

Several selective media exist for the isolation and enumeration of *S. mutans.* A commonly used medium for the microbiology laboratory is mitis-salivarius agar to which bacitracin and additional sucrose have been added. A recent development has been for a patient to spit into a vial containing a buffer and bacitracin. After a few minutes, a slide coated with mitis-salivarius agar is dipped into the vial, removed, and incubated. The colony-forming units per milliliter of saliva is determined from a density comparator chart (Fig 33–18). Each dot on the chart represents a colony and the value below each slide indicates the number of colonies per milliliter of saliva.

Krasse has assembled a series of procedures for caries risk assessment that include salivary counts for lactobacilli and *S. mutans,* salivary secretion rate and buffer capacity, and nutritional counseling. For *S. mutans,* if 1,000,000 or more CFUs/mL are present or, for lactobacilli, if 100,000 or more CFUs/ml are present, the patient is considered to be at high risk. The normal salivary secretion rate in adults using paraffin stimulation is 1 to 2 ml per minute with less than 0.7 ml per minute considered a low rate. The buffer capacity of saliva is determined by the addition of acid to saliva. Low buffer capacity increases caries risk. Diet assessment is of value in the determination of frequency of caries-accelerating snacks.

SUMMARY

Although dental caries is in a state of decline, the disease is still important from many points of view. Evidence exists that *S. mutans* and lactobacilli are human ondontopathogens; that is, dental caries is a diagnosable and treatable infection. Aside from pain, patients who are afflicted with dental caries are concerned with their appearance, costs, and occlusion. Many individuals go to the dentist only when they have pain, so caries remains untreated. Pockets of high caries prevalence are associated with low-income groups. Caries has a multifactorial etiology. The host must be susceptible, a cariogenic diet must be consumed, and bacteria with the appropriate virulence factors must be present on the tooth. These factors include acidogenicity, aciduricity, and ability to adhere.

Whether or not *S. mutans* is the only microbial agent that initiates dental caries (specific plaque hypothesis) is still not clear. Some investigators believe that any acidogenic bacterium in the plaque can initiate and promote dental caries. Colonization of *S. mutans* occurs after tooth eruption, and if the deepest part of the fissures become colonized with this organism, decay is inevitable. However, if this colonization is delayed until the fissure depth is occupied by other bacteria, there is the possibility that decay will not occur or its occurrence will be greatly reduced. Caries can be treated by restorative procedures and can be prevented by several measures. Treatment with fluoride, use of good dental hygiene measures, less frequent consumption of snacks, and use of sealants all contribute to caries prevention.

SUGGESTED READINGS

DiOrio LP. *Clinical Preventive Dentistry.* Norwalk, Conn: Appleton-Century-Crofts; 1983.

Grenby TH. *Developments in Sweeteners.* London: Elsevier Applied Science; 1987, vol. 3.

Jordan HV, Laraway R, Snirch R, Marmel M. A simplified diagnostic system for cultural detection and enumeration of *Streptococcus mutans. J Dent Res.* 1987;66:57–61.

Kohler B, Andreen I, Jonsson B. The effect of caries-preventive measures in mothers on dental caries and the oral presence of the bacteria *Streptococcus mutans* and lactobacilli in their children. *Arch Oral Biol.* 1984;20:879–884.

Krasse B. *Caries Risk.* Chicago: Quintessence Books; 1985.

Lehner T, Mahlert A, Caldwell J. Local active gingival immunization by a 3800-molecular-weight streptococcal antigen in protection against dental caries. *Infect Immun.* 1986;52:682–687.

Linke HAB. Sugar alcohols and dental health. *World Rev Nutr Dietetics.* 1986;47:134–162.

Loesche WL. Role of *Streptococcus mutans* in human dental decay. *Microbiol Rev.* 1986;50:353–380.

Marsh PO, Martin M. *Oral Microbiology.* 2nd ed. Washington, DC: American Society for Microbiology; 1984.

Newburn E. *Cariology.* 3d ed. Chicago: Quintessence Books; 1989.

Russell RRB, Johnson NW. The prospects for vaccination against dental caries. *Br Dent J.* 1987;16:29–34.

Stiles HM, Loesche WJ, O'Brien TC. Microbial aspects of dental caries. *Microbiol Abstr.* 1976;V1–3.

Thylstrup A, Fejerskov O. *Textbook of Cariology.* Copenhagen: Munksgard; 1986.

CHAPTER 34

Periodontal Microbiology

Chris H. Miller

INTRODUCTION
THE DISEASE SITE
MICROBIAL ETIOLOGY
VIRULENCE FACTORS
- Colonization of Subgingival Sites
- Toxins
- Enzymes
- Bacterial Metabolites
- Bone-Resorbing Factors
- Antigens Causing Adverse Immunologic Reactions
- Bacterial Substances That Activate the Complement System
- Immunosuppressive Factors

POTENTIAL VIRULENCE OF SPECIFIC BACTERIA
- Gram-Positive Bacteria
- Gram-Negative Bacteria

HOST REACTIONS IN PERIODONTAL DISEASE
- PMN Response
- The Immune Response

TYPES OF INFLAMMATORY PERIODONTAL DISEASES
- Healthy Gingiva
- Chronic Gingivitis
- Acute Necrotizing Ulcerative Gingivitis
- Adult Periodontitis
- Juvenile Periodontitis
- Rapidly Progressive Periodontitis
- Prepubertal Periodontitis
- Refractory Adult Periodontitis
- Other Forms of Periodontitis

PERIODONTAL DISEASE AND ROOT CARIES
MICROBIOLOGY AND THE DIAGNOSIS OF PERIODONTAL DISEASES
TREATMENT OF PERIODONTAL DISEASES
PREVENTION OF PERIODONTAL DISEASES
SUGGESTED READINGS

INTRODUCTION

Although gingivitis and periodontitis had been recognized for a long time, it was not until the 1900s that their cause was clearly related to oral bacteria. Since then, both clinical and basic science research in dentistry have generated a great deal of information on the cause, prevention, and treatment of these diseases. This chapter presents the current understanding of the role of microorganisms in the initiation of the diseases, the related potential virulence factors of the organisms involved, the role played by host defense mechanisms, and approaches for the prevention and control of these diseases.

The periodontium can exhibit various pathologic states. This has resulted in the development of sev-

TABLE 34–1. INFLAMMATORY PERIODONTAL DISEASES

Gingivitis
Chronic
Acute necrotizing ulcerative
Periodontitis
Adult
Juvenile
Rapidly progessive
Prepubertal

eral disease classification schemes based on histopathology, etiology, or the course of the disease, and possible predisposing factors. This chapter discusses the inflammatory periodontal diseases listed in Table 34–1.

THE DISEASE SITE

The information given here describes the relationship between the physical, microbiologic, and immunologic aspects of the periodontium. Figure 34–1 is a schematic representation of the periodontal tissues. The gingival sulcus is the furrow between the detached gingival tissue and the surface of the tooth. The normal gingival sulcus is protected from the physical cleansing action of the tip of the tongue and musculature of the cheeks and is one of the so-called nonself-cleansing areas of the mouth. These areas (which also include pits and fissures on the occlusal tooth surface and approximal tooth surfaces) are particularly susceptible to bacterial plaque accumulation. The apical part of the sulcular epithelium merges with the junctional epithelium that joins the connective tissue of the gingiva to the tooth surface. The junctional epthelium is not keratinized and is more susceptible to penetration by potentially harmful microbial products than is the keratinized oral epithelium.

Pathologic conditions resulting from an accumulation of plaque in the sulcular space may cause a loss of attachment of the junctional epithelium, forming a periodontal pocket. The pocket provides additional protection for the plaque bacteria from the natural self-cleansing action in the mouth and permits only limited access by the bristles of a toothbrush or by dental floss.

The gingival connective tissue consists mainly of cells (fibroblasts, undifferentiated mesenchymal cells, mast cells, and macrophages), collagen fibers and bundles, and blood vessels embedded in an amorphous ground substance. The supraalveolar connective tissue contains collagenous bundles that anchor the gingival tissue to the alveolar bone and tooth cementum. Other fibers encircle the tooth, and some run interproximally between the cementum of adjacent teeth. The dense connective tissue between the alveolar bone and tooth cementum is termed the periodontal ligament. The collagenous fibers in this area attach the tooth to the bone.

During disease, fiber collagen may be suscepti-

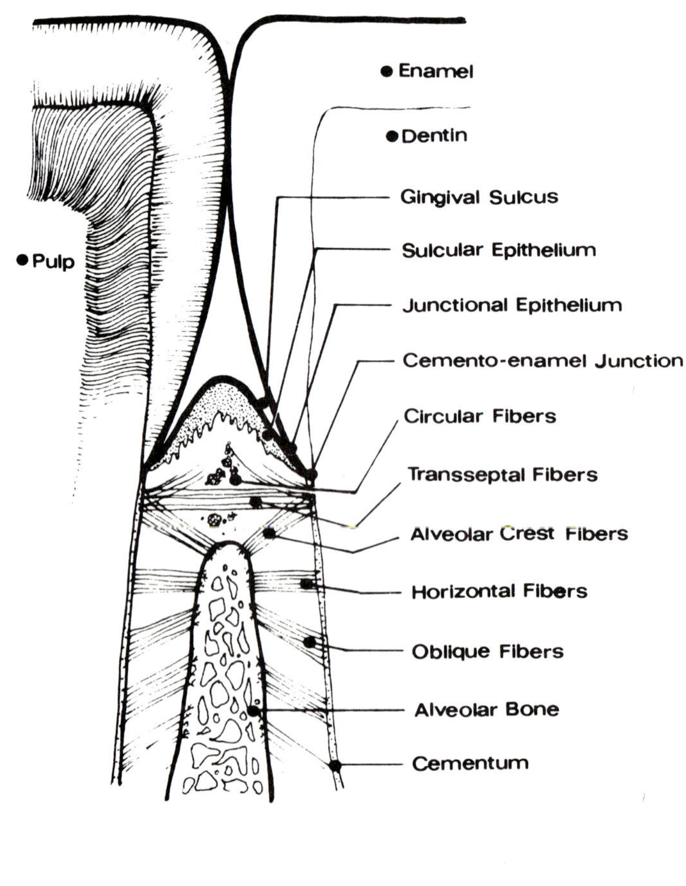

Figure 34–1. A schematic drawing of the periodontal tissues.

ble to degradation by intrinsic and microbial collagenases. The mucopolysaccharides (hyaluronic acid, chondroitin) in the ground substance of connective tissue also may be degraded by microbial hyaluronidase and chondroitinases. Protein components of ground substance also may serve as substrate for microbial enzymes. Enzymatic degradation of these supporting structures in gingival connective tissue is likely an important aspect of the progression of periodontal disease. Bacterial endotoxin may be directly cytotoxic and, along with many other antigens in plaque, can induce immunobiologic reactions that damage the tissues through complement activation, lymphokine production, and cytotoxicity. Bone resorption may be induced directly by plaque products or indirectly after stimulation of intrinsic factors.

MICROBIAL ETIOLOGY

Gingivitis and periodontitis are infectious diseases in that microorganisms are the primary extrinsic cause of the diseases (Table 34–2). The initial definitive evidence for this came in 1965, when it was shown that withdrawal of all measures of oral hygiene in healthy persons with clinically normal gingivae resulted in dental plaque formation and development of gingivitis within 10 to 21 days (*see* Fig. 32–9). When oral hygiene measures were reinstituted, the gingival tissue returned to its normal healthy state. This demonstrated that dental plaque was a cause of gingivitis and not a result of the disease. Numerous investigators have since used this approach to experimentally induce gingivitis, so that various aspects of the disease can be studied under controlled conditions. The occurrence of gingivitis has been associated clearly with the presence of microorganisms at the disease site, and the histologic nature of the tissues involved is indicative of an inflammatory response induced by microorganisms. Additional evidence for the microbial etiology of periodontal disease is that numerous antimicrobial agents are effective in reducing plaque accumulation and periodontal diseases. Also, certain strains of bacteria isolated from periodontal disease sites in humans can induce periodontal destruction as monocontaminants in gnotobiotic animals.

TABLE 34–2. EVIDENCE FOR A BACTERIAL ETIOLOGY OF PERIODONTAL DISEASE

Gingivitis develops with increasing plaque accumulation
The inflamed tissue in gingivitis is restored to its healthy state by plaque removal
Certain antibacterial agents prevent gingivitis and may aid in treatment of periodontitis
Laboratory animals infected experimentally with specific oral bacteria develop periodontal disease
Laboratory animals maintained in a bacteria-free environment do not develop periodontal disease

Although it is clear that inflammatory periodontal diseases are caused by microorganisms, it is also clear that these diseases differ from most other infectious diseases in that gingival and periodontal disease sites are associated with large numbers of different microorganisms. This has resulted in the development of two hypotheses related to the microbial etiology. The nonspecific plaque hypothesis suggests that periodontal disease is caused by a quantitative increase in the amount of plaque rather than by the presence of certain microorganisms in the plaque. The specific plaque hypothesis suggests that periodontal disease is caused by the presence or the concentration of a specific microorganism(s) in plaque. Intensive research continues in the field of periodontal microbiology to determine if specific species or groups of organisms are responsible for these diseases. The general approaches to study this hypothesis are to consider species that are frequently encountered or are predominant at the disease sites, to consider differences in the microbiota present at healthy vs. diseased sites, to consider periodontal species that also are common pathogens at other sites in the body, and to consider species whose numbers or proportions are reduced during successful treatment of the disease.

Culturing and identification of organisms from healthy, diseased, and treated periodontal sites is of major importance in determining the exact role of specific bacteria in periodontal diseases. These types of studies are very difficult to perform in a definitive way for a variety of reasons. First, the microbial composition of gingival sulcus plaque and periodontal pocket debris differs among individuals in both healthy and diseased states. Furthermore, this composition may differ among sites within the same mouth, and the composition of material within a single periodontal pocket will vary according to the specific site within the pocket. For example, the bacteria on the tooth side of the pocket have been described as those that form attached plaque and contain high numbers of gram-positive species, including streptococci and actinomycetes. On the gingival tissue side, or at the apex of the pocket, the subgingival material may consist of high numbers of less adherent organisms, a high proportion of which are gram-negative species. Thus, supragingival and subgingival plaque are not homogeneous mixtures of organisms. They are populations of several microbial communities interacting within the same environment (Fig 34–2).

In addition to the variability in microbial composition, other aspects of the subgingival microbiota make culturing studies difficult. Some organisms (eg,

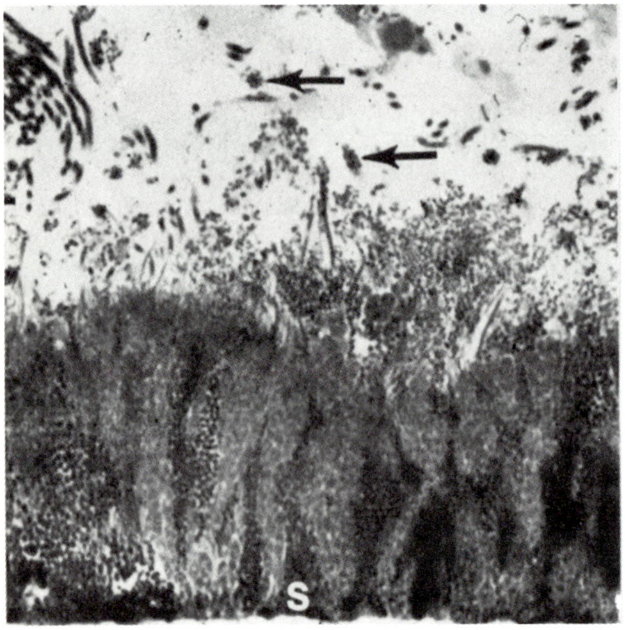

Figure 34–2. Three-day plaque allowed to develop in the human mouth on an epoxy resin crown. The bulk of the plaque consists of densely packed bacteria arranged into well-defined, columnar microcolonies extending from the crown surface(s). Some filamentous forms extend beyond the densely packed bacterial mass. They may be associated with cocci in corncob formations (arrows). ×1050. *(From Listgarten MA, Mayo HE, Tremblay R.* J Periodontol. *1975; 46:16.)*

certain spirochetes) in the gingival sulcus or periodontal pocket are difficult, if not impossible, to culture. This results from a combination of the strict anaerobic nature, high motility, and unknown nutritional requirements of the organisms. Some organisms that can be cultured do not fit into any previously described classification scheme. Also, some organisms cannot be separated from each other during culturing, and separation into a pure culture is required for identification. Organisms may influence the growth of other organisms, and when isolation techniques are applied for identification, the organisms may not grow. Another problem is in actually measuring the amount of plaque removed from the pocket so that the composition of the plaque can be quantitatively compared to other samples. The amount of plaque removed frequently is too small to weigh. It is also difficult to know if a plaque sample removed from a pocket is representative of all the organisms present because the microbial composition varies in different portions of the pocket (eg, apical vs. more coronal, tooth side vs. soft tissue side of the pocket). Because plaque is an adhesive mass, the microorganisms within the mass must first be separated from each other (dispersed) before the sample can be quantitatively cultured on agar. Common dispersion methods include sonic oscillation, vortexing with glass beads, or expelling through a small-gauge syringe needle. None of these methods will totally disperse the plaque without destroying some cells.

Even though culturing the oral flora is difficult, about 20 new species of bacteria isolated from periodontal pockets have been described within the last 10 years. It is now known that over 300 to 400 subtypes of bacteria are potential inhabitants of periodontal disease sites. Meeting the challenges of isolating and identifying the periodontal microbiota actually has resulted in advances in many areas of microbial culturing and taxonomy. Improved anaerobic techniques, uniquely designed sample collection devices, and the development of new taxonomic schema have resulted in continuous growth in our ability to describe the microbiota from various ecologic sites.

VIRULENCE FACTORS

Microbial factors in the development of an infectious disease include colonization of the host (frequently a specific site), growth of the organism, penetration of tissues by the microorganism or products of the microorganism, and direct bacterial or immunologically induced damage to the tissue.

Colonization of Subgingival Sites

Adherence Factors. The initiation and subsequent accumulation of supragingival dental plaque has been described in earlier chapters. *Streptococcus sanguis* and *Actinomyces viscosus* apparently play important roles as very early colonizers of the previously cleaned tooth surface. These, as well as other attached cells, proliferate, and the resulting chemical and physical changes with the developing plaque influence attachment and proliferation of similar or additional types of bacteria. These changes include the production of growth-enhancing or inhibitory substances and the amount of specific cell surface structures that may be involved in adhesive interaction (coaggregation) with other bacteria. Sucrose appears to favor the accumulation of *S. mutans* in plaque, as described in Chapter 33. In addition, glucans synthesized from sucrose may bind to species of *Actinomyces* and enhance their accumulation in plaque.

The natural environment of subgingival (sulcular) sites differs from that of supragingival sites on the teeth. Subgingival sites have less exposure to saliva and dietary components and are protected from the self-cleansing actions of the tip of the tongue and cheek musculature. The components of gingival crevice fluid may be more concentrated in the subgingival sites, and the exposed tooth surface in deepened sulci is cementum rather than enamel.

All of these differences might affect the types and numbers of organisms that colonize subgingival sites. Unfortunately, little is yet known about these specific influences. Nevertheless, colonization of subgingival sites by organisms that may directly or indirectly cause damage to the periodontium is a requirement for disease development.

Although gram-negative bacteria have been more often related to the cause of periodontal diseases than gram-positive bacteria, the latter also play potentially important roles. Colonization of the pellicle-coated tooth surface by gram-positive bacteria is an initial step in plaque formation. As the plaque bacteria proliferate, the microbial mass extends in all directions, including into the gingival sulcus. This predominantly gram-positive plaque, if allowed to remain, can cause gingival inflammation that may result in further extension of the microbial mass into subgingival sites. Besides being responsible for the early plaque development, certain species of *Streptococcus* and *Actinomyces* can undergo coaggregation and bind gram-negative organisms. For example, *Actinomyces* species can bind *Fusobacterium nucleatum, Eikenella corrodens, Veillonella parvula, Capnocytophaga ochracea, Bacteroides gingivalis, Bacteroides intermedius,* and *Bacteroides melaninogenicus.* Since gram-negative bacteria do not usually adhere to the tooth surface or gingival tissue, their binding to gram-positive organisms is thought to be their primary mechanism for colonization of subgingival sites. Once organisms become established in subgingival sites, they are no longer subjected to natural oral cleansing actions. This permits their accumulation under conditions where selective adherence is less important. This suggested progression of subgingival colonization correlates well with the physical arrangement of the microbiota in some periodontal pockets. As mentioned earlier, the gingival side of the pocket contains a less adherent mass, a high proportion of which are gram-negative organisms. Thus, colonization of the gingival sulcus involving specific host–bacteria and interbacterial adherence mechanisms is a major factor in determining the subgingival microbiota associated with periodontal disease.

Growth and Penetration of Tissues. In most bacterial diseases, the causative bacteria must multiply after colonization to a harmful level that overwhelms natural body defenses. This level will vary among individuals, depending on the original dose of the pathogen and the resistance of the host. In periodontal disease, growth of bacteria resulting in the accumulation of subgingival plaque, or the accumulation of specific organisms within the subgingival site, also is important in the disease process. As the bacteria grow, the relative amounts of antigens, irritants, toxic metabolic products, or tissue-destroying enzymes increase, resulting in damage to the host. Treatment of bacterial diseases is aimed at decreasing the level of a specific toxic product or decreasing the numbers of viable cells to a level that will permit natural body defenses to eliminate the pathogens and toxic substances or reduce them to harmless levels.

Bacterial penetration of the periodontal tissues has long been thought to occur only in acute necrotizing ulcerative gingivitis (ANUG). Massive invasion of spirochetes was clearly demonstrated within the diseased tissue of ANUG in 1965. There had been less convincing reports of bacteria detected within gingival tissues during other periodontal diseases, and these results have been considered unreliable. However, within the last few years, several studies using improved techniques have demonstrated the presence of some bacteria within the tissues during adult periodontitis and juvenile periodontitis.

Since in these latter studies, bacteria did not occur in great numbers within tissues, their significance to the disease process is uncertain. It has been hypothesized that they may serve as a reservoir for reinfection of the gingival sulcus or pocket following therapy. Thus, the tissue destruction that occurs in periodontal diseases is due not only to harmful extracellular products of plaque bacteria but also to potentially harmful antigens or endotoxins in the cell walls of the bacterial cells.

Toxins

Exotoxins. Many bacteria produce extracellular substances that are toxic to certain cells or tissues of the body. These include botulinum, tetanus, diphtheria, erythrogenic toxins, leukotoxin, and several enterotoxins.

The only exotoxin thus far thought to be related to periodontal disease is the leukotoxin (LT) produced by *Actinobacillus actinomycetemcomitans* (Table 34–3). LT apparently is released into the extracellular environment through membrane vesicles, and it has been shown to kill PMNs and monocytes from blood and PMNs from the gingival crevice. Since *A. actinomycetemcomitans* is thought to be important in juvenile periodontitis, its LT may play a role as a virulence factor in that disease.

Endotoxins. An important virulence property common to all gram-negative bacteria is the presence of biologically active endotoxin or lipopolysaccharide (LPS) (Table 34–3). Unlike bacterial exotoxins, LPS is an integral part of the outer membrane of gram-negative bacteria. As described in Chapter 9, endotoxin once released from the cell may exert a variety of

TABLE 34–3. BACTERIAL SUBSTANCES THAT MAY DAMAGE PERIODONTAL TISSUE OR PROMOTE TISSUE INVASION

Substance	Source	Potential Effect
Enzymes		
Hyaluronidase	*Streptococcus mitis,* *Bacteroides fragilis* Some gram-positive rods	Increases tissue permeability
Collagenase	*Bacteroides gingivalis,* *Bacillus* sp., *Actinobacillus actinomycetemcomitans*	Disrupts connective tissue
Protease	*Bacteroides* Some fusobacteria	Damages cell membranes
Phospholipase A	*Bacteroides gingivalis* *Bacteroides intermedius*	Damages cell membranes, induces prostaglandin-mediated bone resorption
Lecithinase	*Eubacterium tenue*	Damages cells membranes
Nuclease	*Fusobacterium nucleatum* Some streptococci	Degrades nucleic acid
Phosphatase	*F. nucleatum* *B. gingivalis* *B. intermedius* *A. actinomycetemcomitans* *Capnocytophaga*	Damages cell membranes
Neuraminidase	*Actinomyces*	Membrane damage to PMNs
IgA/IgG Proteases	*B. gingivalis* *B. intermedius* *Capnocytophaga*	Degrades immunoglobulins
Catalase	*Actinomyces viscosus* *A. actinomycetemcomitans*	Decreases PMN peroxidase killing
Fibrolysin	*B. gingivalis* Some spirochetes	Destroys fibrin barrier
Metabolic end products		
Mercaptans	*B. gingivalis* *B. intermedius*	Cytotoxicity
Hydrogen sulfide	*F. nucleatum* *B. gingivalis* *B. intermedius* *Wolinella*	Cytotoxicity
Butyrate, propionate	*B. gingivalis*	Cytotoxicity
Ammonia	Some bacteroides some peptostreptococci	Cytotoxicity
Acids	Streptococci, actinomycetes *F. nucleatum,* others	Cytotoxicity
Indole	*F. nucleatum* *B. gingivalis* *B. intermedius*	Cytotoxicity
Others		
Endotoxins	All gram-negative organisms	Cytotoxicity, bone resorption, complement activation
Leukotoxin	*A. actinomycetemcomitans*	Leukocyte toxicity
Immunosuppressive factors	*A. actinomycetemcomitans* *Treponema denticola* *F. nucleatum* *Treponema socranskii* *Centipeda periodontii*	Inhibits proliferation of lymphocytes
Lipoteichoic acid	Several gram-positive organisms	Bone resorption
Polysaccharides (dextran, levan)	*Streptococcus mutans, Streptococcus sanguis,* *A. viscosus*	Complement activation
Cell wall material	*A. viscosus*	Bone resorption, hypersensitivity
Sonic extract	*A. actinomycetemcomitans,* *T. denticola*	Inhibits proliferation of endothelial cells
Epitheliotoxin	*B. gingivalis,* *B. intermedius,* *Capnocytophaga,* *A. actinomycetemcomitans*	Epithelial cell toxicity
Superoxide inhibitors	Oral treponemes	Decreases PMN killing
Chemotaxis inhibitors	*B. gingivalis*	Decreases PMN defense
Capsules	Many	Decreases phagocytosis

biologic activities that promote tissue damage. Examples of the activities of LPS from various oral bacteria are described in later sections of this chapter. They include cytotoxicity, complement activation, and bone resorption through direct or indirect mechanisms. However, it should be noted that LPS isolated from different bacteria express different degrees of biologic activity. Of general importance is that gram-negative bacteria are abundant at periodontal disease sites, and their increase in concentration at these sites is positively correlated with increased severity of disease. An increase in endotoxin-like material in fluid collected from the gingival crevice area has been shown to occur within the first 7 days of experimentally induced gingivitis in humans. Thus, the association of gram-negative bacteria with destruction of periodontal tissue focuses attention on the possible important role of LPS as a virulence factor in these diseases.

LPS also may be related to posttreatment healing in periodontitis. There is some evidence that endotoxin-like material may be adsorbed onto the cementum of the tooth during periodontitis, and if not thoroughly removed through mechanical debridement of the root surface during periodontal therapy, it may interfere with fibroblast-mediated reattachment, an ultimate objective of therapy.

Enzymes

Oral bacteria possess many types of enzymes. Some of these are extracellular, and others are within the cells but can be released when the cell dies. In some cases, components of mammalian cell surfaces, intracellular substance, connective tissue fibers, or ground substance may serve as substrates for these enzymes, resulting in damage to cells or loss of tissue integrity (Table 34–3). Determining the exact role of microbial enzymes in tissue destruction is difficult because tissues themselves, or cells such as PMNs or macrophages, may have similar enzymes that aid in regulating tissue turnover or have some other function in maintaining tissue quality.

Collagenase. In periodontal disease, a large amount of the connective tissue collagen is destroyed, at least part of which is assumed to occur by the action of collagenase. Although collagenase has been detected in gingival tissue, alveolar bone, PMNs, macrophages, and fibroblasts, certain strains of periodontal bacteria (eg, *B. gingivalis, A. actinomycetemcomitans*) also have collagenases (Table 34–3). Since these bacteria have been found in high concentrations in periodontal disease sites, it is possible that several of their potentially harmful products, including collagenase, may contribute to the marked reduction in gingival collagen fibers. Nevertheless, the respective roles of the mammalian and bacterial collagenolytic systems in periodontal diseases have not been established.

Hyaluronidase. Hyaluronic acid is a mucopolysaccharide that serves as an intercellular cement in gingival epithelium and as part of the ground substance in connective tissue. Hyaluronidase breaks down this polymer, decreasing its viscosity and facilitating tissue penetration of the bacterium or nearby substances. Externally applied hyaluronidase increases permeability of animal gingival tissue. The fluid collected from the gingival crevice has about an eightfold higher concentration of hyaluronidase at moderately inflamed sites than at healthy sites. In fact, most healthy sites have no hyaluronidase activity. As with collagenase, there is confusion about the role of mammalian and microbial hyaluronidases in periodontal disease. Hyaluronidase has been detected in inflamed gingival tissue, neutrophils, and macrophages, as well as from oral bacteria, such as *Streptococcus mitis*, some other streptococci, *Bacteroides fragilis*, and uncharacterized gram-positive rods (Table 34–3).

Other Enzymes. Table 34–3 lists other enzymes of oral bacteria that may have the potential to participate in destruction of periodontal tissue. These include phospholipase A, lecithinase, phosphatase, proteases, and neuraminidase, all of which could damage mammalian cell membranes. Some proteases also can destroy IgA and IgG and interfere with mucosal immunologic defense.

Bacterial Metabolites

As bacteria grow, they produce many low molecular weight waste products (Table 34–3). The metabolites from crude extracts of dental plaque have been shown to cause direct cell damage and to inhibit growth of human fibroblasts. Hydrogen sulfide and ammonia are highly toxic to cells, and these, along with various organic acids, have been detected in periodontal pockets or plaque.

Bone-Resorbing Factors

Healthy bone in a nongrowing individual undergoes constant deposition and resorption without any net change in the bone mass. Periodontitis is characterized by a decrease in alveolar bone mass, and this loss of bone may result from increased bone resorption, decreased bone deposition, or an uncoupling of these processes. A variety of laboratory studies suggests that both cell-mediated and antibody-mediated immunity, as well as nonimmunologic reactions, may contribute to the resorption of bone. However, the actual contribution of these reactions to the bone loss observed during periodontal disease in humans is as yet unknown.

Much of the laboratory evidence for bone-resorbing activity of a given agent comes from quantitatively measuring release of previously incorporated radioactive calcium (^{45}Ca) from fetal rat bones in organ culture. Using the fetal rat bone culture system, it has been shown that activated complement and the lymphokine osteoclast-activating factor (OAF) stimulate bone resorption. Since many plaque bacteria and their components or products can activate complement and induce formation of OAF, these bone resorptive processes may indeed be active during periodontal diseases. Production of type E prostaglandins (PGE) is involved in both of these resorption mechanisms, and elevated levels of prostaglandins occur in inflamed gingival tissue.

PGE has a direct resorptive effect on bone and is produced by a cellular component of bone after exposure to antibody specific for a cell surface antigen and complement. The osteoclast presumably is the cell that responds to these components. Macrophages also synthesize and secrete prostaglandins when cultured with antibodies and complement. PGE from macrophages causes stimulated lymphocytes to produce OAF that, in turn, resorbs bone by a prostaglandin-independent mechanism.

Several other agents have been shown to mediate bone loss in the fetal rat bone model. These include LPS from *B. gingivalis* and *A. actinomycetemcomitans,* lipoteichoic acid from gram-positive bacteria, soluble plaque extracts, and components from *A. viscosus* (Table 34–3). LPS in combination with PGE or with OAF also acts synergistically in stimulating more bone destruction than the sum of that observed with the individual components. Thus, bone destruction in periodontal disease may result from direct or indirect microbial or host-related mechanisms.

Antigens Causing Adverse Immunologic Reactions

Bacterial antigens that gain entrance into gingival tissues may initiate immune responses that lead to tissue destruction in periodontal disease. Such antigens would originate from the subgingival bacteria and might include extracellular products, such as enzymes, structural components, such as LPS, protein, polysaccharide, glycoprotein, or lipoprotein from the cell envelope, polysaccharide from the cell capsule, or protein from flagella, and cell contents, such as proteins and nucleoproteins.

The destructive immune mechanisms that might be stimulated by bacterial antigens are described in a later section and involve anaphylactic, cytotoxic, immune complex, and cell-mediated hypersensitivities.

Bacterial Substances That Activate the Complement System

As discussed in Chapters 6 and 8, some of the biologically active fragments released on activation of the complement system may cause more damage than good. Antigen–antibody complexes activate complement through the classic pathway, but many bacterial substances also can activate complement through the alternate pathway involving the properdin system. Bacterial substances with this activity include LPS, dextran, levan, teichoic acid from cell walls, and some proteases. Thus, both gram-negative and gram-positive bacteria may be involved in the complement-mediated inflammatory events in periodontal diseases (Table 34–3).

Immunosuppressive Factors

An important virulence property of some microorganisms is their ability to suppress the immune response. A prime example of this occurs in the acquired immunodeficiency syndrome (AIDS), where the human immunodeficiency virus (HIV) destroys a subpopulation of T lymphocytes. Many other microorganisms, including other viruses as well as some bacteria and fungi, have immunosuppressive properties that might include activation of T suppressor cells or suppressor monocytes, inhibition of T helper cells, inhibition of bone marrow stem cells, or interference with lymphocyte recirculation.

As mentioned in Chapter 9, some suspected periodontopathogens are capable of suppressing lymphocyte responses. Inhibition of antigen-induced or mitogen-induced proliferation of lymphocytes occurs with products from *A. actinomycetemcomitans, Treponema denticola, Treponema socranskii, F. nucleatum, Centipeda periodontii,* and *C. ochracea.* The immunosuppression by *A. actinomycetemcomitans* appears to function by activing T suppressor cells, whereas that by *T. denticola* apparently results from activation of suppressor monocytes. Periodontal infection with immunosuppressive organisms could establish an immunologically compromised site that would be particularly susceptible to the damaging properties of the pathogens present. Since many periodontally diseased patients do develop a detectable antibody or cell-mediated immune response to certain periodontal pathogens, the extent of such immunosuppression may be of short duration. Nevertheless, temporary immunosuppression could be very important during disease onset or reactivation of a previously diseased site.

POTENTIAL VIRULENCE OF SPECIFIC BACTERIA

Gram-Positive Bacteria

Actinomyces. Frequently detected oral strains of *Actinomyces* include *A. viscosus, Actinomyces naeslundii, Actinomyces israelii,* and *Actinomyces odontolyticus,* although others also may be present in the mouth (eg, *Actinomyces meyeri*). The high concentrations of *Actinomyces* in early supragingival plaque and in the human gingival sulcus and their high frequency of occurrence in human periodontal pockets suggest very efficient mechanisms for colonization of supragingival or subgingival sites. In addition, the *Actinomyces* may be important in serving as plaque binding sites for gram-negative and other gram-positive bacteria. *Actinomyces* species have been shown to bind to *S. sanguis, S. mitis,* and several gram-negative species as described earlier.

Besides their apparent importance in microbial colonization of subgingival sites, *Actinomyces* species are capable of inducing destruction of periodontal tissues in animal models. Studies with hamsters and with monocontaminated gnotobiotic rats have demonstrated clearly the ability of *A. viscosus* and *A. naeslundii* to form plaque (in the presence or absence of sucrose), to induce destruction of periodontal tissues, including bone loss, and to cause root surface caries. Potential mechanisms of tissue destruction by *Actinomyces* (as demonstrated in vitro or in laboratory animals) include production of substances that induce an inflammatory response, that are chemotactic for PMNs, that stimulate the release of enzymes from PMN lysosomes, that serve as a B cell mitogen, and that stimulate bone resorption. *Actinomyces viscosus* and *A. naeslundii* also produce extracellular neuraminidase that aids in their attachment to certain host cells. In addition, neuraminidase has been shown to induce membrane damage to PMNs.

In summary, given members of the genus *Actinomyces* commonly are present in supragingival and subgingival plaque, and they might aid other bacteria in colonizing subgingival sites. Their proportions in plaque have been associated specifically with the development of gingivitis, and they can damage periodontal tissues in laboratory animals. Also, they have been associated with extraperiodontal pathosis in humans, and they produce substances that have a potential to promote tissue destruction. For these reasons, oral *Actinomyces* are considered as significant periodontal organisms.

Other Gram-Positive Bacteria. Streptococci are present in subgingival plaque, and like the *Actinomyces,* some species (eg, *S. sanguis, S. mitis*) can bind to several gram-negative and other gram-positive organisms to influence total colonization of subgingival sites. Although some streptococci can produce some potentially histolytic (tissue-destroying) enzymes and cytotoxic substances (hyaluronidase, protease, organic acids), this group of organisms is considered to be much more important in dental caries than in periodontal diseases.

Members of the genera *Peptostreptococcus* (anaerobic streptococci), *Eubacterium,* and *Propionibacterium* (gram-positive rods) commonly are present at periodontal disease sites and have been isolated from mixed culture wound infections, dental or other abscesses, or infections of the tonsils, appendix, and sinuses. Unfortunately, little is known about their true pathogenic potential or about their possible virulence properties, although all produce organic acids that might be cytotoxic or induce an inflammatory reaction.

Gram-Negative Bacteria

Actinobacillus. *Actinobacillus actinomycetemcomitans* is a gram-negative, capnophilic (requires CO_2), rod-shaped organism with a capsule. In vitro studies have demonstrated that this organism (microbiologically and immunologically related to juvenile periodontitis) produces a leukotoxin (LT) that kills PMNs or monocytes and, thus, might alter the subgingival host defense (Table 34–3). Strains of *A. actinomycetemcomitans* also produce PMN chemotaxis inhibitors and can stimulate PMN lysosome release. The LPS isolated from oral strains of this bacterium induces bone resorption, macrophage cytotoxicity, and platelet aggregation, as demonstrated by in vitro assays. The release of LPS and LT from this organism and their availability for possible penetration into periodontal tissues is apparently mediated through outer membrane vesicles (blebs) released into the extracellular environments during growth that not only contain LPS and LT but also other bone-resorption factors. Soluble extracts from *A. actinomycetemcomitans* have been shown to inhibit the proliferative response of human peripheral blood B cells and T cells, likely through activation of T suppressor cells.

Actinobacillus actinomycetemcomitans has been shown to produce periodontal damage with massive bone destruction when orally inoculated as a monocontaminant in gnotobiotic rats. In addition, this organism has been recovered from several extraoral disease sites in humans and has been implicated as a cause of infective endocarditis in 37 reported cases. This information clearly suggests an important pathogenic potential for this organism.

Bacteroides. Black-pigmented *Bacteroides* (BPBs) is a very complex group of anaerobic organisms. As described in Chapter 17, they were originally named *Bacteroides melaninogenicus* and were later divided into three subspecies and then into the oral species, including, *B. gingivalis, B. intermedius, B. melaninogenicus, Bacteroides loescheii, Bacteroides denticola, Bacteroides levii, Bacteroides endodontalis,* and *Bacteroides forsythus.*

The BPBs usually are present in higher proportions in the periodontal pockets in most adults with severe periodontitis than in those with gingivitis, early periodontitis, or healthy gingiva. Thus, these organisms are thought to be associated with the development, progression, or at least the presence of advanced periodontitis. *Bacteroides* also are isolated frequently from mixed anaerobic wound infections and abscesses in various body tissues. Although *Bacteroides* species may produce several substances that have the potential to damage human tissues (Table 34–3), not all strains induce experimental harmful infections in laboratory animals when used in pure culture. On the other hand, the addition of some of these *Bacteroides* strains to mixtures of avirulent oral bacteria can make the total bacterial complex virulent, causing abscess formation in experimental animals. It is probable that growth of *Bacteroides* species in the body with subsequent expression of pathogenic properties requires, or at least is enhanced by, specific *Bacteroides* growth factors produced by other bacteria at the same body site.

Bacteroides gingivalis has been shown to induce a harmful infection in pure culture. Oral inoculation of the organism as a monocontaminant into gnotobiotic rats produces alveolar bone resorption. *Bacteroides gingivalis* exhibits collagenolytic activity, erythrocyte hemagglutinating activity, and several other proteolytic activities that degrade IgA and IgG and fibrin and induce secretion and subsequent activation of host procollagenase. This *Bacteroides* also produces butyrate and propionate that have cytotoxic activity and, along with *B. intermedius*, produces other cytotoxins, such as indole, ammonia, and the volatile sulfur compounds hydrogen sulfide and dimethylmercaptan and methylmercaptan.

Bacteroides gingivalis and *B. intermedius* express LPS-induced bone resportion, produce chemotaxis inhibitors, and exhibit resistance to phagocytosis, intracellular killing, and complement-mediated killing.

All BPBs produce IgA protease and, with the exception of *B. melaninogenicus*, produce IgG protease. The BPBs also elaborate polyclonal B cell activators and produce phospholipase A that may provide prostaglandin precursors and thereby help initiate prostaglandin-mediated bone resorption. In addition, LPS isolated from *B. gingivalis* (as well as from other gram-negative bacteria) stimulates resorption of bone in vitro. Strains of *B. melaninogenicus* and *B. intermedius* have been shown to produce a phospholipase A that causes damage to the membranes of hamster cheek pouch epithelial cells.

Capnocytophaga. This genus of organisms is characterized as a group of flexible rods with gliding motility and a requirement for CO_2. The three species are *C. ochracea* (formerly *Bacteroides ochraceus*), *Capnocytophaga gingivalis*, and *Capnocytophaga sputigena*. The cultivable microflora in subgingival periodontal lesions of patients with juvenile or insulin-dependent diabetes mellitus is predominated by *Capnocytophaga* along with anaerobic vibrios. *Capnocytophaga* also are present at high levels in periodontal pockets of children with prepubertal periodontitis. *Capnocytophaga sputigena* produces rapid and massive destruction of the periodontium of monocontaminated gnotobiotic rats, and it liberates a substance that inhibits proliferation of human fibroblasts. Sonic extracts and culture fluids of this species contain one or more substances that cause defects in the functioning or morphology of PMNs, which, if active during disease conditions, might interfere with PMN-mediated host defense. Purified LPS from *C. ochracea* has bone-resorbing activity when tested in vitro. *Capnocytophaga* also produces chemotaxis inhibitors, IgA and IgG proteases, and polyclonal B cell activators (Table 34–3).

Fusobacterium. *Fusobacterium nucleatum* is one of the most frequently occurring anaerobic bacteria in diseased periodontal sites. This bacterium can destroy the periodontium in monocontaminated gnotobiotic rats and produces proteases and organic acids that at least have the potential to damage mammalian cells (Table 34–3). LPS from *F. nucleatum* has bone-resorbing activity when tested in the laboratory.

Other Gram-Negative Bacteria. Additional bacteria isolated from periodontally diseased sites include *Eikenella* and *Wolinella*. *Eikenella corrodens* and *Wolinella recta* induce periodontal disease with bone destruction as monocontaminants in gnotobiotic rats, and both contain LPS and other potentially damaging substances (Table 34–3).

HOST REACTIONS IN PERIODONTAL DISEASES

Within the last 10 years a tremendous amount of information has been generated relating the response of the host tissues to the microbial assault in periodontal diseases. It is likely that many products from the subgingival microbiota cause direct damage to the periodontal tissues through enzymatic degradation of cells or extracellular material and direct cytotoxicity by bacterial metabolites. These microbial products also may cause indirect damage to periodontal tissues as a result of initiating inflammatory and immune responses. Although these responses are commonly noted as host defense mechanisms against infectious disease agents, tissue damage may result from their chronic, or at least frequently intermittent, stimulation by organisms that are allowed to remain at subgingival sites. Thus, the host response may influence the course of pathogenesis of periodontal disease depending on the extent to which protective or harmful reactions occur (Fig. 34–3).

PMN Response

As described in earlier chapters, migration of polymorphonuclear neutrophilic granulocytes (PMNs) to sites of infection in the body is a major early line of nonspecific host defense. These phagocytic cells are chemotactically attracted to sites of injury and infection and engulf and digest microorganisms, antigen–antibody complexes, and cellular debris. Microbial accumulation near the gingival tissue enhances migration of PMNs from the gingival vessels into the gingival sulcus. The PMNs accumulate at the gingival surface of the microbial mass and are active in engulfing and digesting bacteria in attempts to block microbial damage to the tissue.

PMNs have a capacity to cause tissue destruction. This is classically demonstrated in the Arthus reaction, which involves antigen–antibody complexes, complement, and PMNs. Hydrolytic enzymes and other products within phagocyte granules may

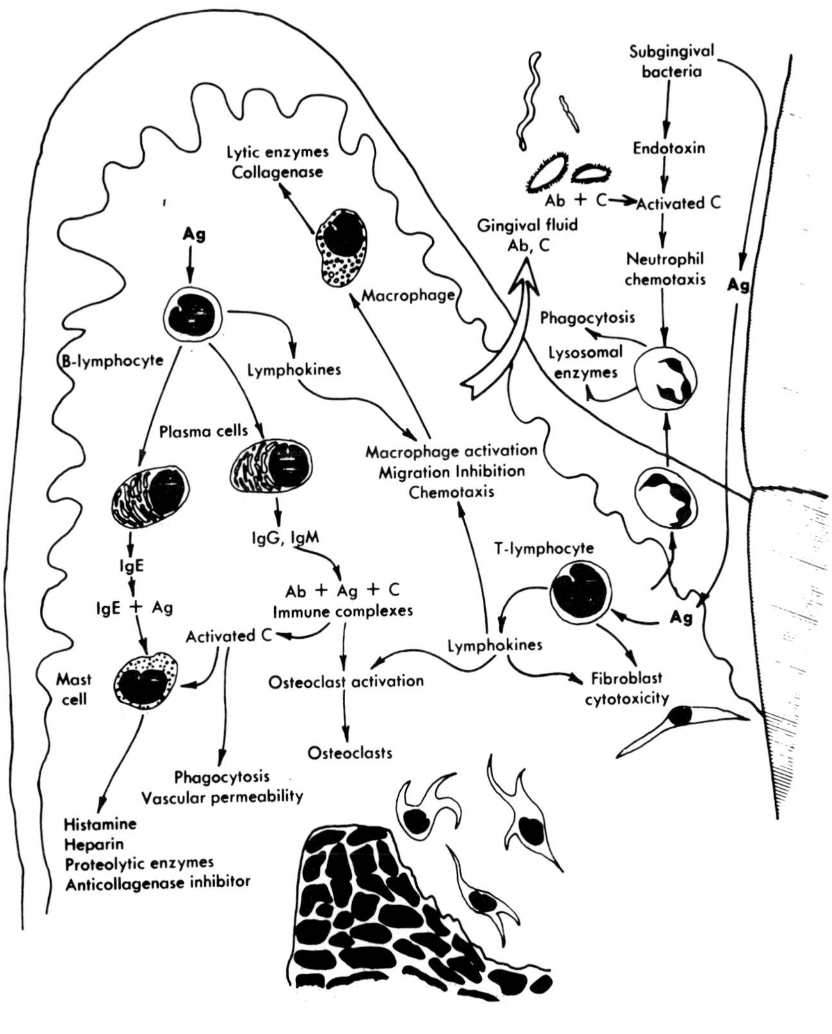

Figure 34–3. Potential host response in periodontal disease that may lead to protective or harmful results. The diagram describes how plaque components directly or indirectly stimulate the neutrophil defense system and immunologic reactions mediated by B lymphocytes and T lymphocytes. *(Adapted from Nisengard RF.* J Periodontol. *1977; 48:505.)*

leak out of the phagocytes or be released on death of these cells. For example, PMNs contain collagenase and prostaglandins that might destroy collagen and induce bone resorption, respectively. On stimulation of the phagocyte by engulfment of a microbe or by one of several soluble mediators, the harmful oxygen products formed in the phagocytic cell may be released into the external environment. Besides possibly damaging tissue cells, these oxygen products also may play some role in activating or suppressing tissue responses to infection. Evidence is beginning to accumulate that these oxygen products are interconnected with the activities of several substances (cyclic nucleotides, prostaglandins, divalent cations, lymphokines) that control various cellular mechanisms.

Although PMNs may cause tissue damage in periodontal disease, they also have a beneficial role. Defects in the neutrophil defense system can predispose many to bacteria-mediated destruction of the periodontium. Patients with chronic benign agranulocytopenia, drug-induced secondary agranulocytosis, cyclic neutropenia, Chediak-Higashi syndrome, and the lazy leukocyte syndrome often have severe periodontal disease that has been attributed to leukocyte defects. The fact that most patients with localized juvenile periodontitis and prepubertal periodontitis have depressed neutrophil chemotaxis and, possibly, impaired phagocytosis provides further evidence for an important protective role of neutrophils in periodontal disease. As mentioned earlier, *C. sputigena* and *A. actinomycetemcomitans* are associated with localized juvenile periodontitis and produce substances that might interfere with neutrophil functions in the periodontal pocket.

The Immune Response

As discussed in Chapters 6 and 7, stimulation of a specific immune response to an infectious disease agent or its products involves the interaction of immunogens and mitogens with macrophages and the appropriate subpopulations of B and T lymphocytes. The immune responses result in proliferation of selected B and T cells, with subsequent differentiation into cells that are cytotoxic and produce lymphokines and antibodies. The activities of these cellular and soluble products of the immune response, along with activation of the complement system, result in protection against the original disease agent or in tissue damage from hypersensitivity reactions.

Presence of Immune Components in Gingival Area

Antigens. Several studies have shown that a variety of immunogens (eg, ovalalbumin, human albumin, collagenase, peroxidase, dextrans) can penetrate the gingival tissues of laboratory animals. Although comparable studies in humans have not or cannot be performed, indirect information demonstrates that substances from the subgingival microbiota apparently do penetrate gingival tissues to initiate inflammatory and immune responses. The junctional epithelium is a permeable tissue, and substances with molecular weights of up to probably 700 000 may pass through the intercellular spaces from the sulcus to the connective tissues. Such substances from subgingival plaque would include extracellular enzymes, polysaccharides, and other products, as well as antigenic components released from the bacterial cell on death or autolysis. The last might include intracellular materials and cell wall components, such as LPS. Dextrans, levans, LPS, and lipoteichoic acid may serve as immunosuppressive or immunopotentiating agents. Some penetration of human gingival tissue by whole bacterial cells occurs in some periodontal diseases, and this can provide a multitude of available antigens in the tissues.

Cellular Components. In normal gingival tissue, few lymphocytes are seen, but as gingivitis occurs, the gingival inflammatory infiltrate exhibits an increasing concentration of lymphocytes. In early gingivitis, the lymphoid cell population is predominantly T cells with some B cells. As the disease progresses to chronic gingivitis or periodontitis, there is a shift to a predominance of B cells and plasma cells. Analyses of the gingival tissue lymphoid cell population in periodontitis patients who have undergone treatment by oral hygiene control and subgingival scaling have shown an apparent shift back to T cell predominance. The mixed lymphocytes isolated from diseased gingival tissue are capable of producing lymphotoxin and other lymphokines, and the B lymphocytes extracted are actively secreting immunoglobulins. Thus, there is a definite lymphoid cell response in periodontal disease, and the gingival lymphocytes appear to be at least activated to produce lymphokines and immunoglobulins.

Support for a systemic immune response in periodontal disease has come from studies demonstrating the ability of peripheral blood lymphocytes to undergo blastogenesis in response to several oral bacteria or their products or components. Although conflicting results have arisen from this rapidly advancing field of study, it appears, in general, that oral bacteria stimulate both B and T lymphocytes from peripheral blood.

Immunologic Molecules

IMMUNOGLOBULINS. Serum antibodies to many oral microorganisms have been detected in subjects with a normal or diseased periodontium. Although the presence of some of these antibodies apparently is not related to any particular stage or form of periodontal disease, others may indeed have such a relationship. For example, a serum antibody response to *A. actinomycetemcomitans* occurs in most juvenile periodontitis patients, and this response is correlated with the presence of *A. actinomycetemcomitans* in periodontal lesions. Many patients with adult periodontitis or a more generalized, rapidly destructive form of the disease have elevated serum antibody responses to *B. gingivalis*. Patients with acute necrotizing ulcerative gingivitis exhibit higher serum IgG and IgM titers to intermediate-sized spirochetes and higher IgG titers to *B. intermedius* than do patients with gingivitis or healthy patients. Attempts to further delineate the systemic antibody response in periodontal disease have involved comparing serum antibody levels to several periodontopathic bacteria with the presence of homologous bacteria in disease-active subgingival sites. The findings support the hypothesis that elevated systemic antibodies to periodontopathic bacteria are reflective of subgingival colonization and occur as a response to a bacterial infection at disease-active sites.

As described in the previous section on the cellular components of gingival tissue, a local antibody response occurs during periodontal disease. The extent and bacterial specificity of this response have not been fully determined, but elevated antibody levels to *A. actinomycetemcomitans, B. gingivalis,* and *B. intermedius* have been detected in gingival tissue and gingival crevice fluid from some periodontal diseased sites.

Of particular importance to this discussion of the antibody response in periodontal disease is the demonstrated ability of several oral bacteria and bacterial components (LPS, dextran, levan) to act as mitogens and induce a polyclonal B cell response. For example, *F. nucleatum* can act as a potent polyclonal B cell activator of cultured human peripheral blood lymphocytes. At low concentrations of the bacterium, IgM antibody specific for *F. nucleatum* is produced by the stimulated lymphocytes. At higher concentrations, IgM antibodies specific for each of three test oral organisms (*A. viscosus, B. gingivalis,* and *S. sanguis*), in addition to those specific for *F. nucleatum,* are produced. These results suggest that some of the subgingival microorganisms in periodontal disease may stimulate the formation of an array of antibodies, some of which are specific for the inducing microorganism and others which are specific for antigenic determinant sites on other periodontal microorganisms.

Since a systemic antibody response to at least some oral bacteria occurs during periodontal disease and since antibodies have been detected in gingival fluid of serumal origin, specific antigen–antibody reactions should occur in the gingival sulcus or pocket. This has been confirmed by the detection of immunoglobulin-coated bacteria in the subgingival flora. It is possible also that antigen–antibody reactions may occur within the diseased gingival tissues. These tissues exhibit an increased concentration of B lymphocytes and plasma cells as the severity of periodontal disease increases. Most of the plasma cells present synthesize IgG, but some produce IgA, and few produce IgM and IgE. Most of the these cells appear to produce nonspecific immunoglobulins, possibly resulting from polyclonal B cell responses. However, there is evidence that some of the plasma cells may produce antibodies specific for plaque antigens. For example, normal and diseased gingival tissue has been examined histologically, using immunofluorescence techniques to detect antigens and antibodies related to *A. viscosus, A. naeslundii, B. gingivalis,* and *B. intermedius.* All of these bacteria or their antigens were demonstrated within various diseased gingival tissue samples and were complexed with specific antibodies. Diseased tissue also contained antigens of the two actinomycetes and of *B. gingivalis* complexed with complement components. Plasma cells and T cells also were detected in some of these tissues. Neither bacteria, bacterial antigens, nor immune complexes were found within healthy gingival tissue.

COMPLEMENT. Complement components have been detected within inflamed gingival tissue. The increased vascular permeability that occurs in the inflammatory response results in leaking of serum proteins (such as complement components) and cells from the capillaries into the surrounding connective tissue. Components C3, C4, C5, and C3 proactivator have been detected in gingival crevice fluid, which is of serumal origin. In addition, IgG and IgM are present in gingival crevice fluid, and if a portion of these immunoglobulins are specific for plaque antigens, resulting immune complexes can activate complement through the classical pathway. Many different bacteria and several substances (LPS, dextran) that are capable of activating complement through the alternate pathway are present in subgingival plaque.

LYMPHOKINES. Antigen-activated T cells release a variety of soluble substances collectively referred to as lymphokines. These lymphokines influence the activities of several types of cells, including macrophages, PMNs, basophils, eosinophils, and lymphocytes.

Immunogen or mitogen-stimulated B lymphocytes (in addition to differentiation into antibody-producing plasma cells) also can produce lymphokines (eg, monocyte chemotactic factor, macrophage-activating factor, osteoclast-activating factor). Thus, production of lymphokines as one part of the cell-mediated immune response can involve both T lymphocytes and

B lymphocytes. Since B cells predominate in diseased periodontal tissues, B cell lymphokine production coupled with antibody from B cell-derived plasma cells could mediate several major adverse reactions in the tissues.

Studies of the cell-mediated immune response in periodontal disease have involved detecting blastogenesis (cell transformation) and lymphokine production by peripheral blood lymphocytes (PBLs) after stimulation with oral bacteria. PBLs from patients with periodontal disease can be transformed by incubation with dental plaque, *Veillonella alcalescens, A. viscosus, F. nucleatum, Bacteroides* species, and other oral bacteria. Some studies have suggested that the lymphocytes from periodontally diseased patients are more responsive to plaque antigens (or mitogens) than are those from nondiseased subjects. PBLs from patients with periodontal disease have been shown in vitro to produce lymphotoxin, osteoclast-activating factor, and monocyte chemotactic factor after stimulation with plaque or pure culture bacterium-derived antigens. Lymphocytes extracted from gingival tissue also produce lymphotoxin and are cytotoxic for gingival fibroblasts.

Immune Protection in Periodontal Disease. Although immunopathologic reactions have great potential to cause a part or all of the tissue destruction seen in periodontal disease, immunoprotective reactions also may occur. Examples of protective reactions involving antigen–antibody complexes include complement-mediated chemotaxis of PMNs and macrophages, enhanced phagocytosis through opsonization or complement-mediated immune adherence, neutralization or inactivation of bacterial antigenic toxins or histolytic enzymes, and complement-mediated lysis of susceptible gram-negative bacteria.

A few animal studies have suggested a partially protective component of the immune response in periodontal disease. During the development of experimental gingivitis in dogs, those animals previously immunized with dog plaque exhibited a less pronounced degree of gingival exudate and size of the gingival connective tissue lesion compared to those of nonimmunized dogs. Immunization of gnotobiotic rats with *S. mutans* or *A. naeslundii,* followed by challenge with the same organisms, resulted in one study in definite trends toward reductions in periodontal bone loss. How these results in animals might relate to a protective aspect of immunity in human periodontal disease is not known. Some comparisons in humans have shown that immunosuppressed individuals show greater tendency to oral, including gingival, infections. Other studies have suggested the opposite. The discrepancies could be explained on the basis of a balance between protective and harmful immunity. Mild immune suppression may aid in preventing immune injury. However, when the suppression is such that it allows opportunists to cause disease, the suppression would appear to be injurious.

The possible importance of the protective nature of the immune response has been suggested by the fact that patients with systemic neutrophil defects often have severe periodontal disease and that most patients with localized juvenile or prepubertal periodontitis have defective neutrophils. However, neutrophils may involve nonspecific rather than specific host defense mechanisms.

Immunologic Injury in Periodontal Disease. There are multiple immunologic reactions that may occur during periodontal disease, and the disease itself may be the ultimate result of these reactions. The four types of hypersensitivity reactions that may be involved in the immunopathogenesis of periodontal disease are described in detail in Chapters 7 and 8. It should be remembered that although there is evidence of their involvement in the disease, the true biologic significance of these reactions in periodontal disease is not known.

Type I reactions (anaphylactic or immediate hypersensitivity) involve IgE-mediated release of pharmacologically active substances from mast cells and basophils. Gingival tissues contain both IgE and mast cells, and histamine concentrations are reported to be elevated in inflamed gingiva. Skin testing has demonstrated that immediate hypersensitivity to *A. viscosus,* a prominent plaque bacterium, occurs with a significantly greater incidence in periodontitis patients than in healthy subjects or patients with gingivitis. Immediate hypersensitivity also has been demonstrated by passive cutaneous anaphylaxis in monkeys using subgingival plaque and sera from some patients with periodontitis.

Type II reactions (cytotoxic hypersensitivity) involve interaction of antibodies with antigens on cell surfaces, followed by destruction of cells from phagocytosis, antibody-dependent T cell cytotoxicity, or complement activation. For these reactions to be involved in periodontal disease, surface components on cells in the periodontal tissue would have to be recognized as foreign antigens. This would initiate an autoimmune type of response. There is no evidence for the participation of type II reactions in periodontal disease. However, it is possible that cellular antigens in periodontal tissue may be changed by the action of bacterial or lysosomal enzymes. Additionally, cross-reacting antibodies may be produced that recognize a cellular antigen with a structural similarity to an inducing bacterial antigen.

Type III reactions (immune complex hypersensitivity) involves the formation of antigen–antibody complexes, followed by complement activation and release of biologically active complement fragments. The necessary components for type III reactions (antigen, antibody, complement, neutrophils) are present in diseased gingival tissue. Immune complexes have been demonstrated in diseased gingival tissue. Activation of complement by an immune complex will induce increased vascular permeability, platelet aggregation, chemotaxis of phagocytes, immune adherence, and phagocytosis. This is related to release of lysosomal enzymes from PMNs and macrophages that may damage the tissue. Complement activation also may cause bone resorption mediated by prostaglandins and can produce a C3b fragment that binds to lymphocytes, stimulating release of lymphokines. Activation of the alternate complement pathway by LPS, cell wall components, or bacterial polysaccharides may result in reactions similar to those induced by immune complexes activating the classical pathway.

Type IV reactions (cell-mediated hypersensitivity) result in the release of lymphokines that have the potential to contribute to periodontal tissue damage. Lymphokines may be released from stimulated T and B cells. Type IV reactions have been classically related to lymphokine production from T cells. However, B cells also produce lymphokines, and since B cells are so dominant in diseased periodontal tissues, it is likely that B cells play a major role in these reactions. Of particular importance is their activation by polyclonal B cell mitogens that cause release of lymphokines that mediate inflammatory injury.

Diseased gingival tissue contains lymphocytes that are capable of performing immune functions that can result in tissue damage. These tissue lymphocytes (presumably activated by exposure to bacterial antigens during the disease) are cytotoxic to gingival fibroblasts and produce lymphotoxin, a lymphokine that is cytotoxic to a variety of cells. The gingival tissue lymphocytes extracted from more severely diseased tissue have a greater capacity to kill fibroblasts and produce lymphotoxin than do the lymphocytes extracted from the normal or less diseased tissue.

TYPES OF INFLAMMATORY PERIODONTAL DISEASE

Healthy Gingiva

Clinically healthy gingiva has a pink color, a shallow sulcus with an intact junctional epithelium, does not easily bleed on probing, and is not swollen.

Electron microscopic observations of undisturbed subgingival plaque on the surfaces of extracted teeth from healthy periodontal sites reveal a thin layer of mainly gram-positive coccobacillary cells

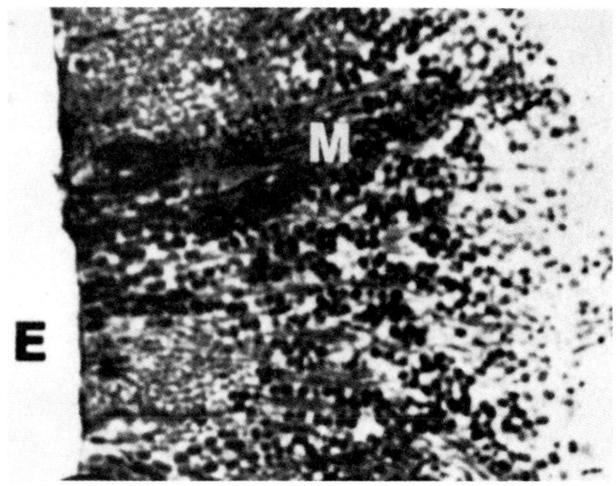

Figure 34–4. Relatively thin, predominantly coccoid flora on the enamel surface associated with nondiseased gingival tissue. E, enamel space; M, columnar microcolony. ×1325. *(From Listgarten MA.* J Periodontal. *1976; 47:3.)*

(Fig 34–4). Flagellated cells and spirochetes are only rarely present, and gram-negative and filamentous cells, present in low numbers, tend to be more predominant in the outer aspects of the microbial mass rather than at the tooth surface area. Filamentous forms may be more prevalent in the microbial mass closer to the epithelium attachment site. Light microscopic observation of crevicular material from healthy gingiva also shows a predominance of coccoid cells (Table 34–4).

Culturing, identifying, and comparing the microorganisms from healthy and diseased periodontal sites are important approaches in establishing which microorganisms might be associated with a given periodontal disease. The complexity of the microbial flora present at all of these sites and the variability in the concentrations of individual species from site to site in the same mouth and from person to person have made this approach difficult but no less important. Thus far, no individual bacterial species has been identified as the single cause of any form of periodontal disease. On the other hand, comparing the microorganisms present at healthy and diseased periodontal sites is beginning to identify a select group of species, the individuals of which may occur more frequently or in higher concentrations during many instances of different periodontal diseases. These comparisons are shown in Tables 34–5 and 34–6. Associations of the microorganisms listed with different forms of periodontal disease are described subsequently.

Culturing has revealed that the microbiota present in the sulcus of healthy gingival tissue consists mainly of gram-positive cocci and rods and is predominated by species of *Streptoccocus, Actinomyces,* and *Veillonella* (Tables 34–5, 34–6). *Bacteroides, Fusobac-*

TABLE 34–4. MEAN PERCENTAGES OF DARKFIELD GROUPS OBSERVED IN SAMPLES FROM HEALTHY SULCI AND DISEASED SITES OF GINGIVITIS, ADULT, AND JUVENILE PERIODONTITIS SUBJECTS

	Healthy	Gingivitis	Adult Periodontitis	Juvenile Periodontitis
Small spirochetes	2.1 ± 1.2	13.1 ± 3.1[a]	31.9 ± 4.9[b]	25.8 ± 5.6[c]
Medium spirochetes	0.0 ± 0.0	2.9 ± 1.3	8.4 ± 3.8[b]	5.2 ± 1.7[c]
Large spirochetes	0.0 ± 0.0	0.8 ± 0.4	1.7 ± 0.9	1.0 ± 0.4
Small motile rods	0.5 ± 0.4	0.9 ± 0.7	6.6 ± 2.4[b,d]	10.3 ± 1.5[c,d,f]
Large motile rods	0.4 ± 0.4	2.2 ± 0.8	2.9 ± 1.3	1.9 ± 0.5[c]
Curved motile rods	0.7 ± 0.5	5.1 ± 1.3	15.9 ± 3.5[b,d]	10.9 ± 2.0[c]
Filaments	3.6 ± 1.7	3.5 ± 1.1	1.7 ± 0.7	3.5 ± 1.1
Fusiforms	6.9 ± 2.7	17.1 ± 2.6[a,d]	9.0 ± 2.2	10.9 ± 1.5
Small nonmotile rods	17.9 ± 6.3	37.9 ± 3.9[a,d,e]	13.1 ± 2.2	19.4 ± 4.2
Cocci	66.2 ± 8.9[a,b,c]	14.5 ± 3.5[d,e]	3.9 ± 1.4	4.3 ± 2.2
Other nonmotile rods	1.7 ± 1.2	2.0 ± 1.6	4.9 ± 3.6	6.8 ± 5.9

Significantly elevated proportions at $p < 0.05$
[a]Health vs. gingivitis.
[b]Health vs. adult periodontitis.
[c]Health vs. juvenile periodontitis.
[d]Gingivitis vs. adult periodontitis.
[e]Gingivitis vs. juvenile periodontitis.
[f]Adult periodontitis vs. juvenile periodontitis.
From Savitt ED, Socransky SS. J Periodont Res. *1984; 9:111–123.*

terium, Capnocytophaga, Eikenella, Selenomonas, and spirochetes, among others, also may be present in low numbers.

Chronic Gingivitis

Chronic gingivitis is a naturally occurring inflammation of the gingival tissue without involvement of the alveolar bone or periodontal ligament. The inflammation results from an accumulation of dentogingival plaque that in some sites may mineralize to form calculus. Clinical features of the diseased gingiva may vary but tend to include swelling (Fig 34–5), discoloration from pink to bluish red, bleeding, and visible inflammatory exudate.

The plaque-induced inflammation may have a rapid onset (acute gingivitis), it may recur (recurrent gingivitis), or it may have a slow onset and be of long duration (chronic gingivitis). The inflammation may be localized and confined to a single tooth or groups of teeth, or it may involve the entire mouth, depending on the distribution of accumulated plaque and calculus and on host resistance. Chronic gingivitis is the most common form of the gingival diseases and is widespread in occurrence, affecting most adults and many children.

Gingivitis is unique among the infectious diseases of humans, since it can be induced experimentally and then eliminated without permanent damage to the tissues. The disease that develops is called experimental gingivitis (in contrast to natural or chronic gingivitis),

TABLE 34–5. PREDOMINANT CULTIVABLE BACTERIAL TYPES ASSOCIATED WITH VARIOUS PERIODONTAL DISEASES

Bacterial Type	Health (%)[a]	Chronic Gingivitis (%)[a]	Advanced Periodontitis (%)[a]	Juvenile Periodontitis (%)[a]
Gram-positive				
Facultative cocci	39.6	26.8	6.2	10.2
Anaerobic cocci	0.8	3.0	ND[b]	6.1
Facultative rods	35.1	16.9	3.9	3.1
Anaerobic rods	9.5	9.2	15.1	15.3
Gram-negative				
Facultative cocci	0.3	ND	ND	ND
Anaerobic cocci	2.0	4.3	0.6	1.8
Facultative rods	ND	14.8	ND	4.5
Anaerobic rods	12.7	25.0	74.3	59.3

[a]Percent of total cultivable flora.
[b]ND, Not detected.
Adapted from Slots J. J Clin Periodontol. *1979; 6:351.*

TABLE 34–6. PREDOMINANT CULTIVABLE SUBGINGIVAL MICROORGANISMS ASSOCIATED WITH PERIODONTAL DISEASES

Health
- *Streptococcus mutans*
- *Streptococcus mitis*
- *Actinomyces viscosus*
- *Actinomyces naeslundii*

Naturally occurring gingivitis
- *Fusobacterium nucleatum*
- *Bacteroides intermedius*
- *Capnocytophaga gingivalis*
- *Actinomyces viscosus*
- *Actinomyces naeslundii*
- *Actinomyces israelii*
- *Streptococcus sanguis*
- *Streptococcus mitis*

Necrotizing ulcerative gingivitis
- *Fusobacterium*
- *Bacteroides intermedius*[a]
- Spirochetes[a,b]

Adult periodontitis
- *Bacteroides gingivalis*
- *Bacteroides intermedius*
- Other *Bacteroides*
- *Fusobacterium nucleatum*[a]
- *Eikenella corrodens*
- *Wolinella recta*[a]
- *Eubacterium* species
- *Actinobacillus actinomycetemcomitans*
- *Peptostreptococcus micros*
- *Treponema denticola*[a,c]
- Other spirochetes

Rapidly progressive periodontitis
- *Bacteroides gingivalis*
- Other *Bacteroides*
- *Actinobacillus actinomycetemcomitans*[a]
- *Wolinella recta*[a]
- *Eikenella corrodens*

Juvenile periodontitis
- *Actinobacillus actinomycetemcomitans*[a]
- *Fusobacterium nucleatum*

Prepubertal periodontitis
- *Bacteroides intermedius*
- *Actinobacillus actinomycetemcomitans*
- *Capnocytophaga*
- *Eikenella corrodens*

Refractory adult periodontitis
- *Actinobacillus actinomycetemcomitans*
- *Bacteroides gingivalis*
- *Bacteroides intermedius*

[a]Also induces serum antibody response.
[b]By microscopic observation of plaque.
[c]By quantitative ELISA with monoclonal antibody.

and this approach has been used to study many characteristics of the disease in its early stages. The original studies of experimental human gingivitis by Löe et al. in 1965 actually proved the microbial etiology of the disease. They demonstrated beyond doubt that accumulations of microbial plaque result in the development of gingivitis and that its removal and control result in resolution of the lesions. Test subjects with healthy gingiva receive a dental prophylaxis to remove all previously existing plaque and calculus. They then refrain from subsequent oral hygiene. Supragingival and subgingival plaque accumulate, and the subjects develop marginal gingivitis within 2 days to 3 to 4 weeks. Reinstitution of oral hygiene brings the tissues back to normal. (*see* Fig 32-9).

Histologic Characteristics. Since bacteria and their products normally are found in the gingival crevice, it is sometimes difficult to distinguish between normal and pathologic tissue reactions. Even when the gingiva is clinically healthy as a result of maintaining a relatively plaque-free state, slight inflammatory signs within the gingival tissue can be microscopically detected. Histologic evidence for inflammation usually is apparent within 1 to 4 days of plaque accumulation. The initial histologic sign is that of an acute inflammatory response, beginning with dilatation of the blood vessels subjacent to the junctional epithelium. There is adherence of leukocytes to the luminal walls of the vessels, and PMNs are present in the extravascular connective tissue and begin to increase in number in the junctional epithelium.

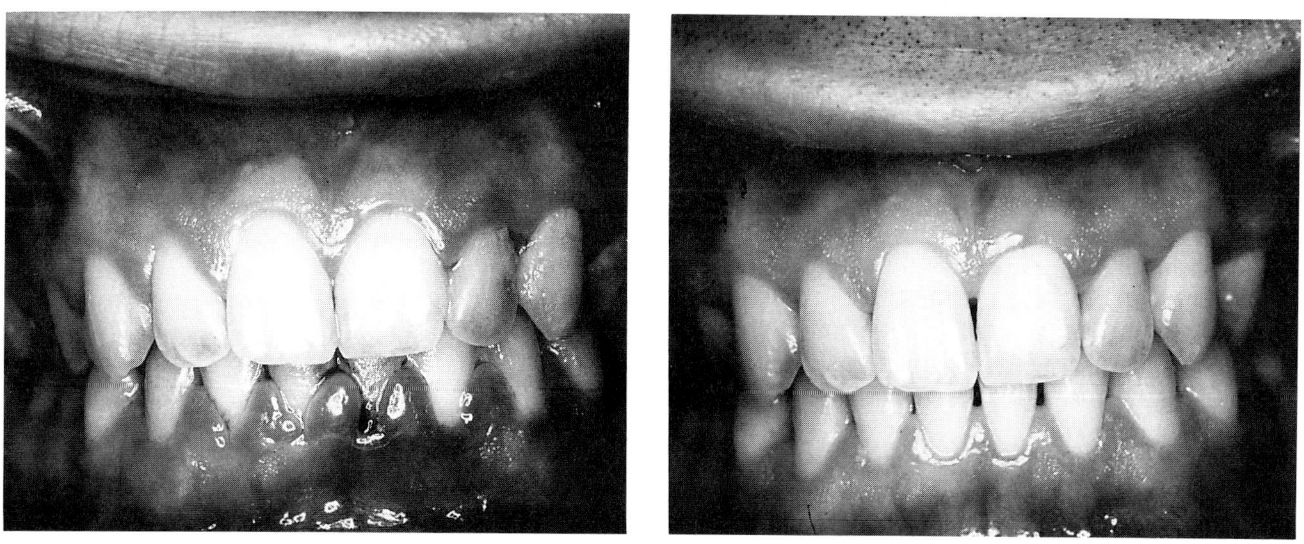

A B

Figure 34–5. A. Clinical signs of severe gingivitis superimposed on a slight periodontitis in an adult. **B.** Same patient, 7 days after gross debridement by scaling and root planing followed by oral hygiene instruction. *(Courtesy of Dr. Timothy J. O'Leary, Indiana University, Indianapolis.)*

Within 4 to 7 days of plaque accumulation, a dense lymphoid cell infiltration develops below the junctional epithelium, with lymphocytes constituting about 75% of the leukocytes. Although most of the lymphocytes are T cells, a few B cells are present. Leukocyte infiltration of the junctional epithelium increases, and alterations in fibroblasts and collagen fibers are evident.

Within 2 to 3 weeks of plaque accumulation, the predominant feature is a dramatic increase in the concentration of B cells and plasma cells in the connective tissue adjacent to the junctional epithelium. Plasma cells are found also around blood vessels and collagen fibers. Most of the plasma cells produce IgG, and extravascular immunoglobulins are present in connective tissue and junctional epithelium. Destruction of the collagen fibers just below the junctional epithelium occurs, causing loss of tissue attachment. The junctional epithelium proliferates and migrates apically to cover the denuded tooth surface. This gingival lesion may persist for a long time, as in chronic gingivitis. It also may progress into the advanced lesion of periodontitis.

Microscopic Observations of Plaque. Microbial masses involved with natural gingivitis exhibit a thick, dense layer of cells containing a wide variety of cell types, including both coccoidal and filamentous forms, with gram-positive and gram-negative cell wall patterns (Fig 34–6). Filamentous bacteria are more numerous than in the microbial mass from nondiseased sites, and flagellated cells and spirochetes may be found.

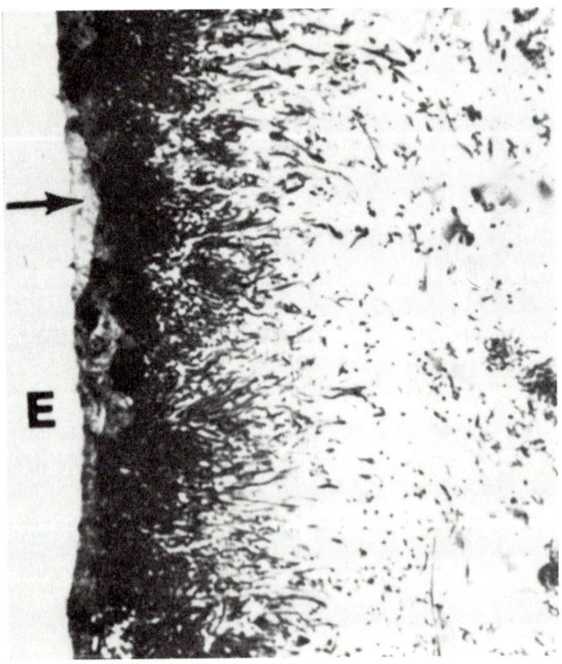

Figure 34–6. Dense, predominantly filamentous bacterial mass on enamel surface associated with gingivitis. E, enamel space. Arrow denotes an area of calcification. ×650. *(From Listgarten MA.* J Periodontol. *1976; 47:4.*

Predominant Microorganisms

Darkfield Microscopy. Darkfield microscopic observation of samples collected from sulcular or diseased subgingival sites permits a morphologic classification of the different microbes inhabiting the site. For example, analysis of disease sites in patients with gingivitis shows a significant increase in the concentration of small spirochetes, fusiform bacteria, and small nonmotile rods and a decrease in coccoid cells when compared to healthy sulci (Table 34–4). The frequency of detection of several morphologic types also increases in gingivitis sites compared to healthy sites. The most significant of these increases are those for small nonmotile rods, small spirochetes, and curved motile rods.

Cultivable Bacterial Types. Subgingival material from individuals with naturally occurring chronic gingivitis contains a greater percentage of gram-negative microorganisms than does material from healthy sites (Table 34–5). One study has shown that chronic gingivitis plaque may contain about 44% gram-negative bacteria, whereas healthy gingival sulci contain about 15% gram-negative types. Most of the gram-negative bacteria in chronic gingivitis are anaerobic rods. The concentrations of gram-positive facultative cocci and rods are decreased in chronic gingivitis (compared to the healthy sulcus) but still make up about 44% of total flora. There is an overall increase in the concentration of subgingival gram-negative bacteria during the development of experimental gingivitis.

Specific Cultivable Bacteria in Naturally Occurring Gingivitis (Table 34–6).

FUSOBACTERIUM. *Fusobacterium nucleatum* may be one of the most predominant gram-negative rods in sites from both healthy tissues and all forms of inflammatory periodontal diseases. Its mean percentage of all cultivable organisms present and its frequency of detection at gingivitis sites are significantly increased over those at healthy gingival sites. It causes periodontal destruction when inoculated into gnotobiotic animals, and its potential tissue-destroying properties include nuclease, phosphatase, acids, indole, and LPS (Table 34–3).

BACTEROIDES. Numerous *Bacteroides* species have been isolated from gingivitis sites, and *B. intermedius* usually appears as the predominant species. Its percentage of the total cultivable bacteria at gingivitis sites is significantly increased over that at healthy sites. *Bacteroides intermedius* produces many substances that might damage host tissues and, like all other gram-negative bacteria, contains LPS, which has the potential to activate complement and induce bone resorption (Table 34–3).

OTHER BACTERIA. *Streptococcus mitis, S. sanguis, A. viscosus, A. naeslundii,* and *A. israelii* constitute about half of the cultivable subgingival bacteria in gingivitis. These gram-positive species may provide sites for colonization of gram-negative species, and they produce acids that may damage host cells. *Streptococcus sanguis* and *A. viscosus* also produce polysaccharides that can activate complement by the alternate pathway, and actinomycetes are capable of inducing periodontal disease destruction as monocontaminants in gnotobiotic rats. *Haemophilus parainfluenzae* and other *Haemophilus* species have been found in high concentrations at some gingivitis sites. Some gingivitis sites also contain *C. gingivalis* in a higher incidence and concentration than in healthy sulcus material.

Specific Cultivable Bacteria in Experimental Gingivitis. Analysis of all of the plaque (both supragingival and subgingival) at developing gingivitis sites indicates a shift from a *Streptococcus*-dominated plaque to an *Actinomyces*-dominated plaque with increasing time of plaque accumulation. An analysis of only the subgingival material (that is most closely associated with the tissue) in experimental gingivitis has identified several bacteria that increased in concentration, were at least 1% of the total flora present, and were present in all patients tested. There were several strains of *A. naeslundii* and *A. odontolyticus,* and *F. nucleatum,* a lactobacillus, *P. micros, Streptococcus anginosus, S. mitis, V. parvula,* and a treponeme.

Acute Necrotizing Ulcerative Gingivitis

Acute necrotizing ulcerative gingivitis (ANUG) is an acute inflammation of the gingiva that is also known as trench mouth, Vincent's infection, or fusospirochetal infection (Fig 34–7). This disease apparently was recognized about 24 centuries ago and was described by Vincent in 1896 as a disease related to the presence of fusiform bacteria and spirochetes.

ANUG is characterized by a sudden onset, resulting in ulceration and necrosis of the interdental papillae. The lesions commonly are described as punched out papillae or craterlike lesions. The marginal gingiva also may be involved. The affected tissue frequently is covered with a gray pseudomembrane and has a high bleeding tendency. The affected areas usually are very painful, and the patients usually have a putrid mouth odor. The inflammation may be localized most commonly around anterior teeth but can occur throughout the mouth.

The onset of ANUG has been related to many possible predisposing factors, including nutritional deficiencies, debilitating diseases, emotional and physical stress, poor oral hygiene, smoking, and preexisting gingival disease. ANUG can occur in any age group but is most prevalent between the ages of 15 and 30. This disease is not contagious.

Plaque present during ANUG was first described as containing a fusospirochetal component over 50 years ago. Electron micrographic examination of ANUG lesions has shown that spirochetes actually penetrate the tissue (Figs 34–8, 34–9) and that the lesion has four zones, all of which include spirochetes.

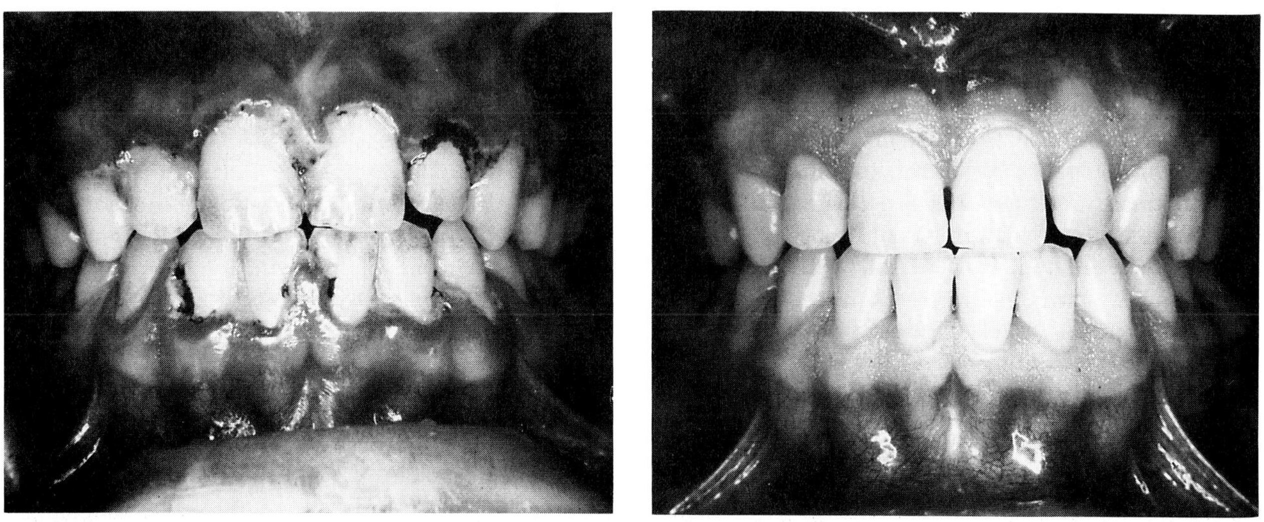

A B

Figure 34–7. A. Acute necrotizing ulcerative gingivitis. **B.** Same patient, 45 days after gross debridement by scaling and root planing followed by oral hygiene instruction. *(Courtesy of Dr. Timothy J. O'Leary, Indiana University, Indianapolis.)*

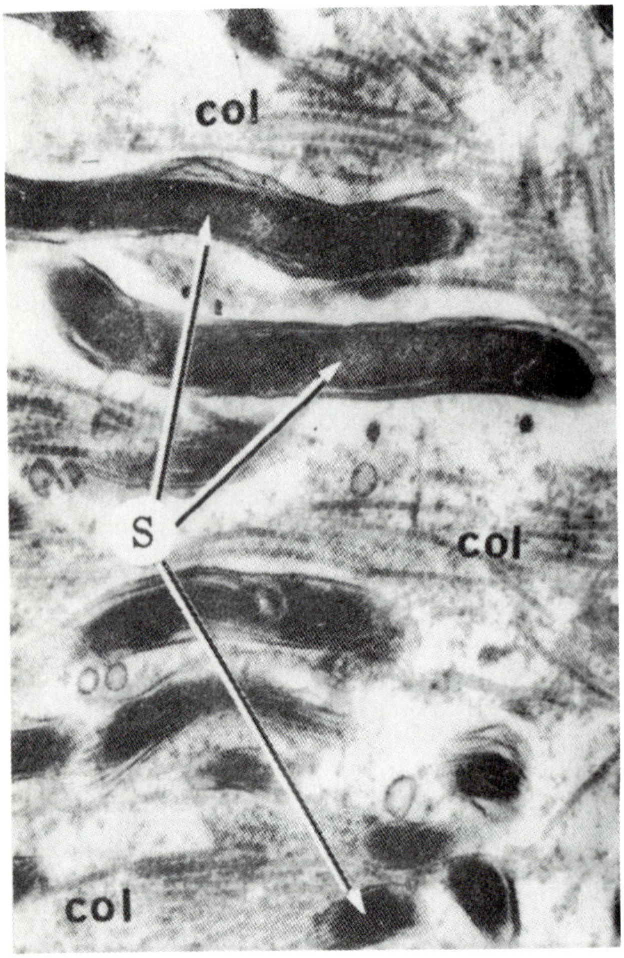

Figure 34–8. Spirochetes (S) infiltrating the connective tissue beneath the ulcerated lesion in ANUG. col, collagen fibrils. ×24,000. *(From Listgarten MA.* J Periodontol. *1965; 36:68.)*

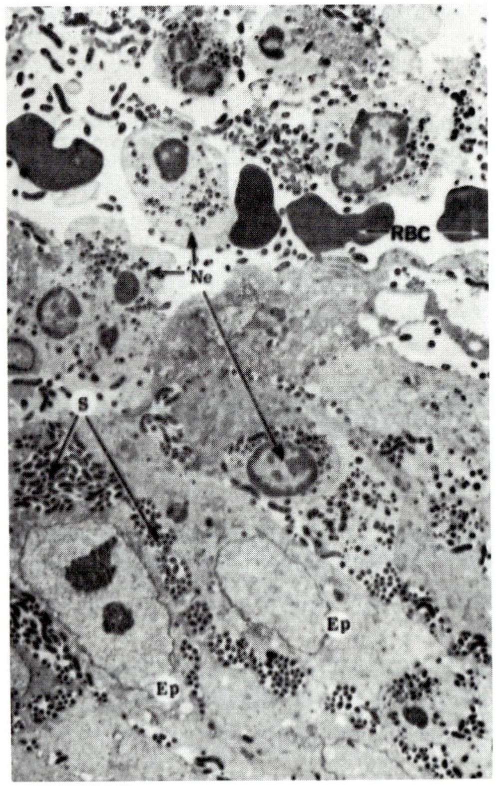

Figure 34–9. Spirochetes within the intercellular spaces of epithelium adjacent to the ulcer in ANUG. S, spirochetes; RBC, red blood cell; Ne, neutrophils; Ep, epithelial cell. ×3500. *(From Listgarten MA.* J Periodontol. *1965; 36:68.*

1. The bacterial zone is the most superficial and contains bacteria of different morphology, including a few spirochetes (Fig 34–8).
2. The neutrophil-rich zone also contains many spirochetes and some other microorganisms.
3. The necrotic zone contains many spirochetes and fusiform-shaped bacteria among the disintegrating tissue cells (Fig 34–9).
4. The zone of spirochetal infiltration is nonnecrotic tissue that has been infiltrated with spirochetes.

Thus, ANUG is one periodontal disease in which there is obvious microbial invasion of the tissues, lending considerable credence to the idea that the invading spirochetes are causing most, if not all, of the injury.

Predominant Microorganisms (Table 34–6). Recent culturing, immunofluorescent, and microscopic observations of material collected from ANUG sites has redocumented the presence of fusobacteria and spirochetes. The mean percentage of spirochetes in 22 patients ranged from about 13% to 30% of the total microscopic cell count at the diseased sites. *Fusobacterium* sp. made up about 3% of the total cultivable bacteria at diseased sites. *Bacteroides intermedius* averaged from 8% to 24% of the total viable bacteria at ANUG sites and may be another contributor to, or indicator of, this disease. Both *B. gingivalis* and *Fusobacterium* sp. were detected at disease sites in all of the patients studied.

Adult Periodontitis

Adult periodontitis is the most common form of periodontitis. It is a localized or generalized chronic disease of the periodontium, with over 80% of the cases occurring in those over age 35. The plaque-induced inflammatory process proceeds at a slow rate, continuing to involve deeper tissues. Apical migration of the junctional epithelium causes the formation of a periodontal pocket that contains the subgingival microbiota. As the disease process continues, the periodontal ligament and alveolar bone are slowly destroyed, culminating in loss of tooth support and exfoliation (Fig 34–10). The entire pro-

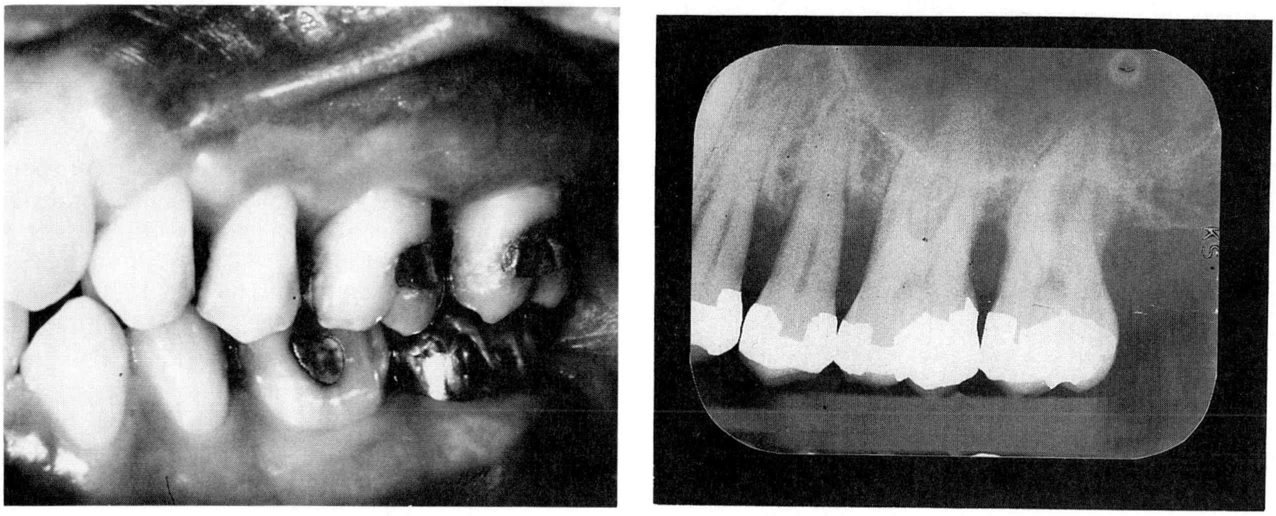

A B

Figure 34–10. **A.** Adult periodontitis. **B.** Radiograph of the left maxillary molar area. Arrow shows approximate normal bone level. *(Courtesy of Dr. Timothy J. O'Leary, Indiana University, Indianapolis.)*

cess may occur with periods of inactivity over a time span of 20 or more years.

Microscopic Observations of Plaque. The overall structure of supragingival periodontitis plaque is similar to that of gingivitis plaque (Fig 34–11). The subgingival microbial mass in periodontitis may exhibit a different structure in the most apical portion, with fewer of the large filamentous forms that commonly predominate in the supragingival plaque. The subgingival flora in the periodontal pocket has been shown to contain many flagellated forms and spiral organisms. In some cases, this loosely packed population of apparently motile microbes has been shown to overlie the densely packed tooth-adherent plaque (Fig 34–12). At other times, the loosely packed mass may predominate even at the tooth surface, with little adherent plaque.

Predominant Microorganisms

Darkfield Microscopy. Microscopic observation of dispersed subgingival microbial masses has indicated that differences occur in the microbiota that populate healthy and diseased periodontal sites. When the morphologic nature of the periodontal flora from healthy sites and adult periodontitis sites is compared, clear differences are observed (Table 34–4). Coccoid cells are more predominant at healthy sites, whereas motile rods and spirochetes are more predominant at diseased sites. The ratio of nonmotile/motile forms may be about 40:1 at healthy sites and about 1:1 at diseased sites. In addition, mechanical debridement of root surfaces of periodontitis patients is associated with subsequent clinical improvement and a decrease in the proportions of spirochetes and motile rods and an increase in the proportions of coccoid cells.

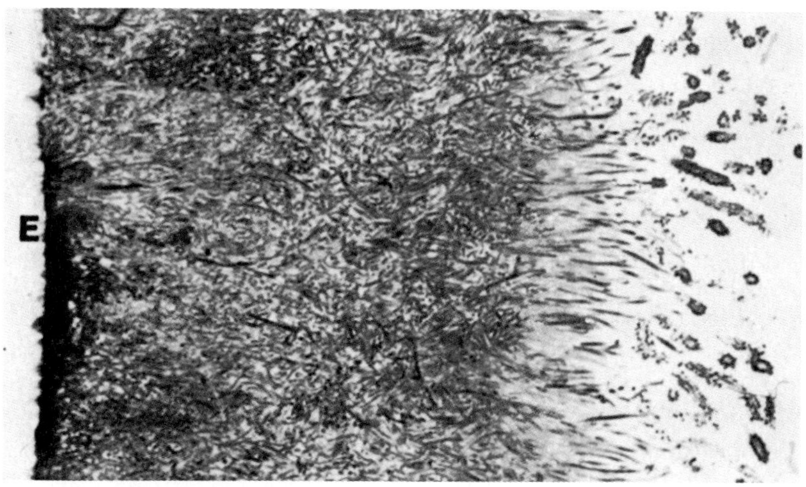

Figure 34–11. Dense, predominantly filamentous bacterial mass on the supragingival surface associated with periodontitis. E, enamel space. ×850. *(From Listgarten MA.* J Periodontol. *1976; 47:8.)*

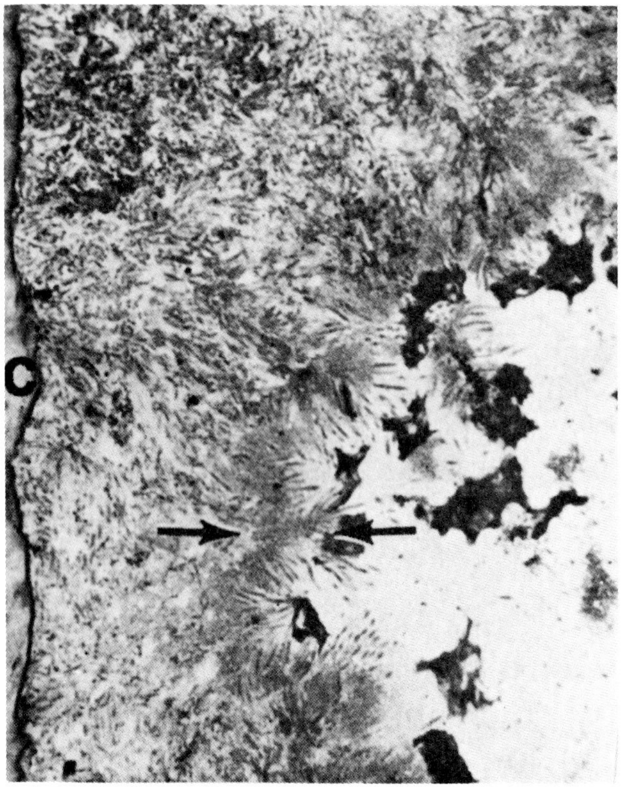

Figure 34–12. Periodontitis. Subgingival flora. The surface of the adherent flora is covered by a pallisading layer of test-tube brush formations and spirochetes (between arrows). The adherent flora is less filamentous than the supragingival flora and shows no particular orientation with respect to the cementum surface (C). The less dense area in the lower right segment is nonadherent plaque. ×600. *(From Listgarten MA.* J Periodontol. *1976; 47:11.)*

Even though microscopic observation of the periodontal microbiota has shown increased numbers of spirochetes and motile rods at diseased sites, it is still not clear if these organisms are active in causing periodontal breakdown or if they more appropriately serve as indicator organisms that increase in proportion as a result of the disease. Determination of the exact role played by spirochetes has been hampered by the difficulties associated with the cultivation of these strict anaerobes and the inability to establish these organisms in laboratory animals that may serve as models for periodontal diseases.

Cultivable Bacterial Types. As in gingivitis plaque, the material collected from pockets associated with adult periodontitis contains a higher percentage of cultivable gram-negative anaerobic rods than does healthy gingival sulcus material. In advanced adult periodontitis, this bacterial type may compose 75% of the cultivable organisms present, with gram-positive anaerobic rods comprising the second most predominant group (Table 34–5).

Specific Cultivable Bacteria

BACTEROIDES. Numerous bacteroides have been isolated from adult periodontitis pockets. *Bacteroides gingivalis* and *B. intermedius* are frequent isolates from these sites and usually are in higher concentrations than in healthy sites. A study on a small number of patients with evidence of progression of their moderate to advanced periodontal destruction has shown that sites associated with recent bone loss were characterized by higher proportions of *B. gingivalis* and *B. forsythus* than were inactive sites. There is serologic evidence for the involvement of *B. gingivalis* in adult periodontitis. Patients with chronic adult periodontitis or generalized juvenile periodontitis have higher mean antibody titers to *B. gingivalis* than do patients with juvenile periodontitis, ANUG, or nondiseased gingiva. *Bacteroides gingivalis, B. melaninogenicus,* and *B. intermedius* produce potentially harmful products (Table 34–3) and cause alveolar bone destruction as monocontaminants in gnotobiotic rats. Thus, it appears that the black-pigmented *Bacteroides* are among those oral bacteria that at least contribute to tissue destruction in adult periodontitis.

FUSOBACTERIUM NUCLEATUM. *Fusobacterium nucleatum* in many instances is the most frequently isolated gram-negative anaerobic rod in adult periodontitis sites. It possesses potentially pathogenic properties, produces harmful substances (Table 34–3), and induces periodontal disease as a monocontaminant in gnotobiotic rats.

EIKENELLA CORRODENS. *Eikenella corrodens* has been shown to occur more frequently and in higher concentrations at adult periodontitis sites than at healthy gingival sites. Rats monoinfected with *E. corrodens* develop severe alveolar bone resorption.

ACTINOBACILLUS ACTINOMYCETEMCOMITANS. *Actinobacillus actinomycetemcomitans* has been recovered from adult periodontitis lesions. The participation of this bacterium in tissue destruction is likely, since it is recovered more frequently from progressing lesions than from nonprogressing lesions.

5 WOLINELLA RECTA. *Wolinella recta* is present in many adult periodontitis sites at higher concentration than in healthy sites. This gram-negative rod also induces alveolar bone resorption as a rat monocontaminant.

TREPONEMA DENTICOLA. The association of spirochetes with periodontal diseases has been documented by microscopic observation of subgingival material. Quantitative culturing is very difficult. Recently, the first quantitative evidence of a positive relationship between a specific spirochete and severe periodontitis was obtained. An ELISA technique using monoclonal antibody to a serovariety of *T. denticola* demonstrated significantly elevated levels in plaque from deep pockets in patients with severe periodontitis, relative to healthy controls and a group with moderate disease.

GRAM-POSITIVE BACTERIA. *Peptostreptococcus micros* may be present in one half of the adult periodontitis sites and is, when present, in concentrations usually higher than in material from healthy sulci. This organism also is a common isolate from a variety of anaerobic infections at other body sites. Ten or more species of *Eubacterium*, including *Eubacterium nodatum*, *Eubacterium timidum*, *Eubacterium suburreum*, and *Eubacterium brachy*, may be present at adult periodontal disease sites. Collectively, they may constitute 20% of the organisms present. The potential role of *Eubacterium* in periodontal disease remains unknown, but it can constitute a significant portion of the periodontitis flora.

Juvenile Periodontitis

Juvenile periodontitis was first described under the name periodontosis in 1923. Since then, considerable controversy has existed about the possible etiologic factors involved, diagnosis, and its localized or generalized occurrence in the mouth. In general, localized juvenile periodontitis (LJP) occurs in the adolescent and is seen more frequently in females than in males. It has a familial association, and it may occur in 0.1 to 3% of teenagers and young adults. The disease is distinguished from other forms of periodontitis by a very rapid bone loss confined to the molar–incisor area and the fact that it usually is associated with minimal amounts of plaque or clinically visible gingival inflammation (Fig 34–13).

Evidence is accumulating that most patients with LJP have a defect in the functioning of the neutrophil granulocytes. Collective results from several studies involving a total of 111 patients show that about 70% of these patients have peripheral blood neutrophils with a reduced chemotaxis function. The chemotaxis is depressed to a variety of chemotactic factors and appears to be long lasting, since it has been demonstrated in postdisease states and is not reversed by therapy.

Microscopic Observations of Plaque. Material on the cementum of teeth extracted from patients with LJP exhibits a relatively sparse bacterial flora that microscopically appears to contain mainly coccoid and filamentous cells with a gram-negative cell wall (Fig 34–14).

Predominant Microorganisms

Darkfield Microscopy. Microscopic observations of pocket material from juvenile periodontitis patients reveal increased percentages of spirochetes and motile rods when compared to material from healthy sulci (Table 34–4).

Cultivable Bacterial Types. Diseased sites in juvenile periodontitis patients contain a different type of flora from healthy sites (Table 34–5). The predominant cultivable types are similar to those in adult periodontitis, since in both of these diseases the pocket flora consists predominantly of gram-negative anaero-

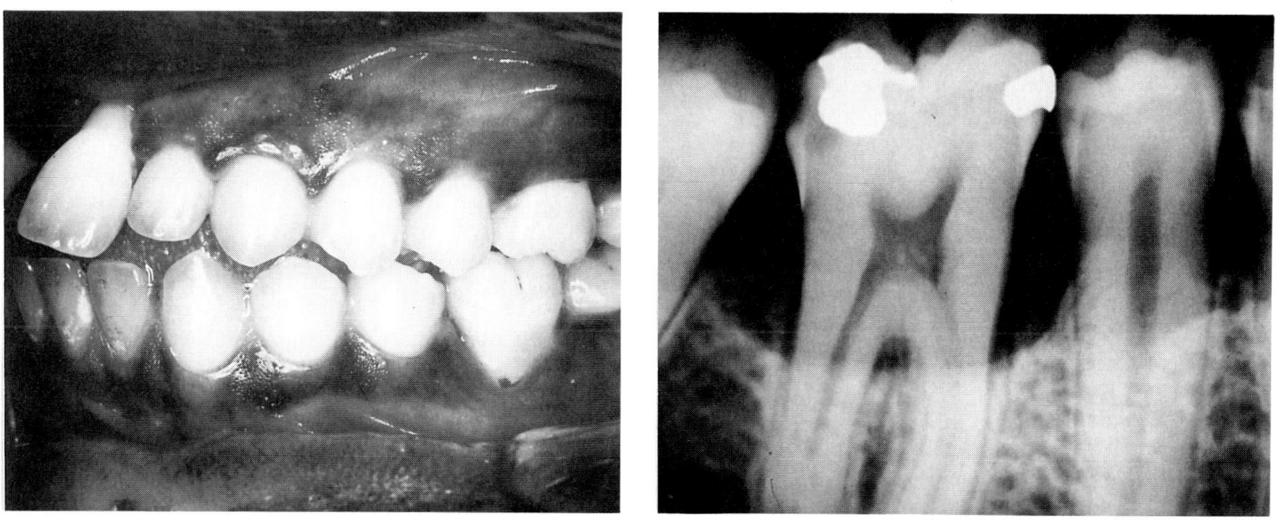

A B

Figure 34–13. A. Localized juvenile periodontitis showing a minimal amount of plaque and clinically visible inflammation around mandibular first molar. **B.** Radiograph showing lunar-shaped bone resorption around mandibular first molar. *(Courtesy of Dr. Timothy J. O'Leary, Indiana University, Indianapolis.)*

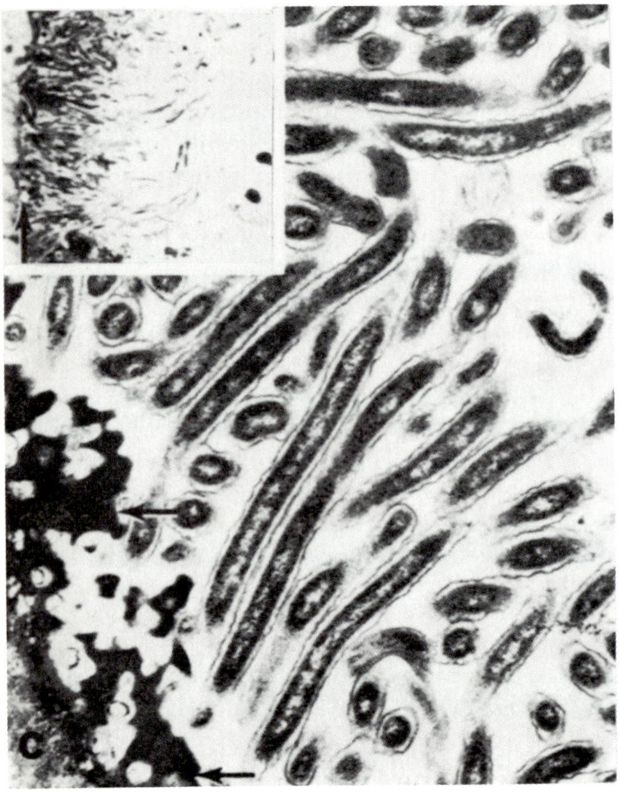

Figure 34–14. Juvenile periodontitis. Relatively sparse flora associated with cementum surface (arrow). ×1100. **Inset.** Electron micrograph of specimen shown. Thin filaments with gram-negative cell walls are oriented more or less perpendicularly to the dense cuticle (arrows) covering the cementum surface (C). ×13,000. *(From Listgarten MA.* J Periodontol. *1976; 47:17.)*

bic rods, followed by gram-positive anaerobic rods as the second most predominant group.

Specific Cultivable Bacteria (Table 34–6)

ACTINOBACILLUS ACTINOMYCETEMCOMITANS. Culturing studies and results of serum antibody response by patients with localized juvenile periodontitis have suggested a strong association of *A. actinomycetemcomitans* with this form of periodontitis. There is an increased prevalence of oral *A. actinomycetemcomitans* and elevated antibody levels to this species in LJP patients and their families. This bacterium is found in large numbers in the periodontal lesions of LJP patients but either is not present or is found in low numbers in healthy gingival sites. There is good correlation between elimination of *A. actinomycetemcomitans* from subgingival plaque and successful treatment of LJP. This bacterium appears to invade the gingival connective tissue adjacent to periodontal pockets, where it may produce numerous harmful substances (Table 34–3), such as collagenase, leukotoxin (LT), endotoxin, phosphatase, and a substance that interferes with proliferation of endothelial cells.

The LT produced by *A. actinomycetemcomitans* kills PMNs and monocytes, and this may alter the PMN defense against bacteria and allow disease production at subgingival sites. On the other hand, patients with juvenile periodontitis have LT-neutralizing antibody activity in their sera, some of which undoubtedly is present at the disease sites containing gingival crevice fluid. If, indeed, this LT is produced and is active during the disease process, timing and extent of the antibody response to the LT may be most important in determining the course of the disease.

FUSOBACTERIUM NUCLEATUM. *Fusobacterium nucleatum* may be one of the predominant isolates from LJP pockets and may be present at these disease sites more frequently and in higher concentrations than in healthy gingival sulci. This is not unique to LJP, since this organism also may be present in high numbers in other forms of periodontitis. The organism produces several potentially harmful substances (Table 34–3).

Rapidly Progressive Periodontitis

Rapidly progressive periodontitis is a rare form of periodontal disease that exhibits many of the same features as adult periodontitis, but the overall disease rate is much more rapid. The disease may progress with or without indefinite periods of remission to tooth loss within a few months. This disease is seen predominantly in the 20- to 35-year age group but may occur at any age past puberty. This rapidly progressing form of periodontitis may be related to defects in host cell defense mechanisms and possibly to differences in the periodontal flora when compared to that of the chronic form, adult periodontitis.

Bacteroides gingivalis, A. actinomycetemcomitans, and spirochetes have been associated with this form of periodontal disease, but other microorganisms may be important as well. Patients with rapidly progressive periodontitis have exhibited high serum antibody titers to *B. gingivalis* and *A. actinomycetemcomitans,* and fewer patients have high titers to other *Bacteroides* or *W. recta.*

Prepubertal Periodontitis

Recently, investigators have presented descriptive information on a rare form of periodontitis that affects deciduous teeth in young children. The disease entity is called prepubertal periodontitis, and it is associated with abnormalities in leukocyte chemotaxis. The localized form is characterized by minimal inflammation and plaque but rapid bone loss. The generalized form manifests acute gingival inflammation around all of the teeth, accompanied by gingival proliferation and recession and by rapid bone loss. Microbiologic analyses of diseased sites reveal high levels of *B. intermedius, A. actinomycetemcomitans, Capnocytophaga,* and *E. corrodens.*

Refractory Adult Periodontitis

Although most patients with adult periodontitis respond to surgical or nonsurgical therapy, some will not improve with this conventional treatment. This condition has been referred to as refractory adult periodontitis. Although some refractory adult periodontitis patients may have intrinsic defects in PMN chemotaxis, it is not yet clear if this is a separate form of periodontal disease with different contributing factors or if there is a different specific microbial etiology involved. These lesions harbor one or more combinations of *A. actinomycetemcomitans, B. gingivalis,* and *B. intermedius.*

Other Forms of Periodontitis

Some adolescents experience a generalized form of periodontitis, with rapid bone loss affecting more teeth than just the first molars and incisors. This has been referred to by some as generalized (in contrast to localized) juvenile periodontitis, but microbiologic and immunologic differences in the generalized versus the localized forms have been detected. Some teenagers with LJP have progressed to a more generalized disease. On the other hand, many young individuals with a generalized form did not have a detectable molar–incisor onset. Thus, there is still much to be discovered about differentiation and progression of the various forms of periodontal disease.

Unique forms of gingivitis and periodontitis have been described in persons infected with HIV. The HIV-associated gingivitis has been described as being an atypical gingivitis that is bright red and edematous and extends beyond the attached gingiva to the alveolar mucosa. Other unusual features include spontaneous bleeding, petechia-like lesions, and a distinct red border. HIV-associated periodontitis has been described as ANUG superimposed on a lesion with rapid destruction of the periodontal ligament and rapid bone loss. Patients complain of pain and exhibit spontaneous bleeding, interproximal necrosis and cratering, and extremely rapid bone loss. Although these clinical descriptions differ from those of typical gingivitis and periodontitis, it is not known if they represent different forms of these diseases. The microbiology of the HIV-associated disease appears to be similar to that of adult periodontitis. There is no known direct etiologic relationship between the virus and these diseases. It may be, as is the case with AIDS, that the immunocompromised status predisposes to a different progression of the disease than that seen in normal subjects or predisposes to periodontal infections by other opportunistic microorganisms.

PERIODONTAL DISEASE AND ROOT CARIES

Although the prevalence of human root surface caries has not been fully assessed, it is clear that at least an anatomic relationship exists between root caries and periodontal disease. Recession of gingival tissue as a result of periodontal disease or for other reasons exposes the cemental tooth surface to the oral environment and destructive products of plaque. Root caries starts in cementum, close to or at the cemental–enamel junction, and appears only after this site is exposed to the oral environment. Thus, conditions that influence gingival recession will likely influence the potential for development of root surface caries.

Although root caries (like the inflammatory periodontal diseases) is an infectious disease, its specific microbial etiology is not yet known. Several strains of *Actinomyces* cause both root caries and periodontal bone destruction as monocontaminants in gnotobiotic rats. *Streptococcus mutans* also may cause root caries in this animal model. Nevertheless, much more information is needed on the microbiology of the human disease before etiology or even specific mechanisms of dentin destruction can be described. Thus, if microbiologic relationships exist between root caries and periodontal disease, they are currently undescribed.

MICROBIOLOGY AND THE DIAGNOSIS OF PERIODONTAL DISEASES

The various clinical symptoms of the inflammatory periodontal diseases have been described earlier in this chapter and in numerous other texts. Although the traditional clinical criteria of visual observation, bleeding tendency, probing depth, and radiographic analysis will likely remain important to the diagnosis of these diseases, they may be inadequate for determining active disease sites in periodontitis, quantitatively monitoring the response to therapy, and measuring the degree of susceptibility to future tissue breakdown. Thus, a broad-based attempt is being made to develop objective measures to address these inadequacies that involves microbiologic, immunologic, and biochemical analyses of saliva, blood, plaque, or gingival crevice fluid.

The major and still unresolved problem in diagnosis has been the inability to identify an active, progressing periodontal lesion. Before one can determine the etiologic agent of a disease, one has to first understand and define the disease process. Until a definitive clinical diagnosis of an active lesion can be made, microbiologic methods can serve only as suggestive indicators of disease.

The microbiologic approaches to diagnosis and prognosis include darkfield microscopy and tests for specific bacteria and their products (*see* Fig 32-1). Darkfield microscopy was one of the first diagnostic tests used in periodontics, and the initial results suggested that there was a positive correlation between disease activity and increased numbers of spirochetes and motile bacteria (Table 34–4). Later studies, however, proved that rather than being an indicator of disease activity, these organisms might simply be an indication of conditions that favor their growth. Although the presence of spirochetes in a gingival pocket is not evidence of ongoing disease, an increase in numbers of these bacteria in sulci or pockets suggests the development of conditions conducive for active periodontal disease.

More recent diagnostic tests involve the three prime suspects in the etiology of periodontal diseases, *B. gingivalis, B. intermedius,* and *A. actinomycetemcomitans.* Since these bacteria may be found in low numbers in the absence of disease, the diagnostic tests are based on the presence above certain threshhold levels of any or all of these three species. Specific methods for culturing with rapid identification have been developed for these three species. Since, as noted before, the etiology of the diseases is still open to question, they cannot be used to definitively diagnose active lesions. Clinical studies indicate that they can be used as prognostic aids, in that their presence above certain threshhold concentrations is strong indication that the lesions are or are about to begin progressing. Culturing tests have an advantage over other diagnostic tests in that antibiotic sensitivity tests can be carried out on the isolated bacteria. A disadvantage is that special handling is needed to ensure the survival of the very fastidious, anaerobic bacteria.

Immunologic tests using monoclonal antibodies or highly specific polyclonal antisera have been developed for these bacteria. Subgingival plaque samples are placed on a glass slide and assayed using immunofluorescence. DNA probes also have been developed for diagnostic purposes. This method is based on the very specific hybridization of the DNA of plaque bacteria with the species-specific cloned DNA probes from known bacteria. DNA probes, as well as the immunologic tests, are highly specific and sensitive, and there is no need for concern for survival of fastidious bacteria in the plaque sample. Because live bacterial cultures are not maintained, the specimens cannot be used for antibiotic sensitivity testing.

Another approach to rapid identification of an active lesion has been development of tests that detect specific microbial products that may be unique to a given species or group of bacteria associated with progressive disease. One method being evaluated is the rapid detection of trypsinlike protease activity in subgingival plaque samples. This enzyme activity has been associated with *B. gingivalis* and *T. denticola.* Other bacterial and host-related inflammatory factors also are being studied.

TREATMENT OF PERIODONTAL DISEASE

Treatment of peridontal diseases is aimed at removing and preventing further accumulation of plaque near periodontal tissues. Treatment of simple gingivitis involves removal of accumulated material in and near the gingival sulcus area by scaling and tooth polishing. This, followed by good oral hygiene, allows the gingivitis tissue to return to its normal healthy state (Fig 34–5).

Successful treatment of ANUG also involves mechanical plaque removal procedures, elimination of predisposing factors, and, in some instances, tetracycline or metronidazole therapy.

Treatment of periodontitis also initially consists of mechanically removing calculus and the microbial mass lodged in periodontal pockets by scaling and root planing the diseased sites. After consideration of possible predisposing factors, such as diabetes and immune disorders, the patient is given oral hygiene instructions and is recalled periodically for additional cleaning. If pockets are deep or if furcations of multirooted teeth are involved, surgical access to the site may be necessary for adequate plaque removal. These procedures usually result in stopping the progression of the disease and eliminating inflammation at the disease site. Long-term success in preventing recurrences is dependent on the patient's maintaining good oral hygiene.

If periodontitis patients respond with clinical improvement to the mechanical plaque removal procedures, the use of antibiotics in conjunction with these procedures usually provides no additional benefit. However, use of tetracycline or metronidazole in adult periodontitis patients who did not respond to mechanical plaque removal therapy has resulted in clinical improvement in some instances. Some patients with juvenile periodontitis have been shown to respond to tetracycline therapy. A major problem in the antimicrobial treatment of patients with periodontitis is delivering the antimicrobial agent to the disease site so that it will remain in contact with the microorganisms in deep periodontal pockets. This may help explain the lack of success in treating periodontitis patients with systemically administered antibiotics in that sufficient antibiotic concentration may not be achieved in deep pockets. On the other hand, there may be other explanations, since tetracycline administered orally as 250 mg every 6 hours achieves a level of 4 to 8 μg per mL of gingival crevice fluid (about three times that achieved in blood). However, concentrations sufficient to inhibit causative organisms throughout the periodontal pocket may or may not be maintained in all cases.

Another combined mechanical–antimicrobial approach to treating periodontitis is known as monitored modulated therapy, or the Keyes technique. It is aimed at controlling the sulcus pocket microorganisms by mechanical–antimicrobial methods with little emphasis on surgical pocket elimination. Following in-office calculus removal, curettage, and irrigation, patients perform daily flossing and sulcular toothbrushing at home with a thick mixture of baking soda moistened with a few drops of water and 3% hydrogen peroxide. With frequent recalls, the patient's progress is monitored by microscopic observation of pocket microorganisms in attempts to detect desired reductions or elimination of spirochetes and motile forms. If these reductions do not occur, a repeat of the previous treatment with added antibiotic therapy may be instituted. Verification of the improved success of this treatment approach has thus far been weak, in that no beneficial effect on the patient has been clearly substantiated beyond that normally obtained by conventional scaling, root planing, and home care procedures provided by most general dentists.

PREVENTION OF PERIODONTAL DISEASES

Prevention of periodontal disease is based on eliminating the accumulation of microorganisms near the gingival tissue. Plaque removal has been shown to be consistently effective in preventing periodontal disease.

The degree of plaque removal required for prevention varies among individuals, but plaque removal must occur frequently to achieve prevention. The only methods for plaque removal currently available to the general public are mechanical in nature and include toothbrushing, flossing, and professional cleaning (scaling and root planing). Since the last can be provided to most people only on a periodic basis, prevention is truly in the hands of the individual. If the individual is not regularly attentive to oral hygiene practices or is not familiar with the proper procedures for good oral hygiene, prevention will not occur. Indeed, this is the current situation in hundreds of millions of people! Thus, a key ingredient in our only known effective and safe method of periodontal disease prevention is still education of the individual in relation to dental health, good oral hygiene practices, and regular visits to the dental office.

Because mechanical plaque removal has not been successful in preventing periodontal disease on a wide scale, several other approaches are being investigated.

Numerous types of topical antimicrobial agents and antibiotics (eg, penicillin, vancomycin, kanamycin, actinobolin, tetracycline, spiromycin, iodophors, quaternary ammonium compounds, chlorhexidine) have been investigated as means of preventing plaque accumulation. However, each has one or more properties or activities that either are undesirable or are as yet untested in relation to wide-scale and effective use in prevention. For example, individuals taking penicillin may experience decreased gingivitis. Nevertheless, advocating wide-scale use of penicillin for prevention of gingivitis would not be wise because this pratice would select out penicillin-resistant organisms throughout the population and reduce the effectiveness of this important antibiotic in treating life-threatening diseases.

Oral antiseptics have received a great deal of study either as oral rinses or irrigants to be used as adjuncts to mechanical cleansing. Although many different agents have been tested, the Council on Dental Therapeutics of the American Dental Association has accepted only two types of antimicrobial mouthrinses for the prevention of gingivitis. One type contains thymol, eucalyptol and other substances in an alcohol base, and the other contains chlorhexidine gluconate.

The effectiveness of the chlorhexidine gluconate is related to its unique ability to express antimicrobial activity while bound to oral surfaces. This property is known as substantivity and allows the agent to maintain reduced levels of microorganisms in the mouth for a longer period of time than that achieved by other oral antimicrobial agents. Chlorhexidine, which requires a prescription for use in the mouth, may stain the teeth. However, the stain can be removed with a dental prophylaxis.

Other microbiologic approaches being investigated for the prevention of periodontal diseases include immunization, substitution of oral pathogenic strains of bacteria with nonpathogenic strains, and altering and interfering with the mechanisms by which bacteria colonize the gingival sulcus.

SUGGESTED READINGS

Dzzink JL, Socransky SS, Haffajee AD. The predominant cultivable microbiota of active and inactive lesions of destructive periodontal diseases. *J Clin Periodontol.* 1988; 15:316–323.

Genco RJ, Mergenhagen SE, eds. *Host–Parasite Interactions in Periodontal Disease.* Washington, DC: American Society for Microbiology; 1982.

Genco, RJ, VanDyke TE, Levine MJ, Nelson RD, Wilson ME. Molecular factors influencing neutrophil defects in periodontal disease. *J Dent Res.* 1986; 65:1379–1391.

Johnson BD, Engel D. Acute necrotizing ulcerative gingivitis: A review of diagnosis, etiology and treatment. *J Periodontol.* 1986; 57:141–150.

Listgarten MA. Direct microscopy of periodontal pathogens. *Oral Microbiol Immunol.* 1986;1:31–36.

Listgarten MA. Nature of periodontal disease: Pathogenic mechanisms. *J Periodont Res.* 1987; 22:172–178.

Moore WEC, Holdeman LV, Smibert RM, Hash DE, Burneister JA, Ranney RR. Bacteriology of severe periodontitis in young adult humans. *Infect Immun.* 1982; 38:1137–1148.

Page RC, Schroeder HE. *Periodontitis in Man and Other Animals.* Basel, Switzerland: Karger; 1982.

Page RC. Gingivitis. *J Clin Periodontol.* 1986; 13:345–355.

Roitt IM, Lehner T. *Immunology of Oral Diseases.* Oxford: Blackwell Scientific Publications; 1983.

Slots J. Subgingival microflora and periodontal disease. *J Clin Periodontol.* 1979; 6:351–382.

Slots J, Genco RJ. Black-pigmented *Bacteroides* species, *Capnocytophaga* species, and *Actinobacillus actinomycetemcomitans* in human periodontal disease: Virulence factors in colonization, survival and tissue destruction. *J Dent Res.* 1984; 63:412–421.

Slots J, Listgarten MA. *Bacteroides gingivalis, Bacteroides intermedius* and *Actinobacillus actinomycetemcomitans* in human periodontal diseases. *J Clin Periodontol.* 1988; 15:85–93.

Tanner ACR, Haffer C, Bratthall GT, Visconti RA, Socransky SS. A study of the bacteria associated with advancing periodontitis in man. *J Clin Periodontol.* 1979; 5:278–307.

Van Winkelhoff AJ, Van Steenbergan TJM, De Graaff J. The role of black-pigmented *Bacteroides* in human oral infections. *J Clin Periodontol.* 1988; 15:145–155.

Zambon JJ, Christersson LA, Genco RJ. Diagnosis and treatment of localized juvenile periodontitis. *J Am Dent Assoc.* 1986; 113:295–300.

CHAPTER 35

Microbiology of Pulp and Periapical Infections

Robert R. White

INTRODUCTION
RESISTANCE FACTORS OF THE PULP CHAMBER
IMMUNOLOGY
ROUTES OF MICROBIAL INVASION
MICROBIAL VIRULENCE FACTORS
MICROBIAL FLORA OF PULP INFECTIONS
ENDODONTIC CULTURING
Endodontic Media
SUGGESTED READINGS

INTRODUCTION

Microorganisms are the cause of almost all pulp and periapical problems. Blood-borne bacterial infections may be the initiating factors leading to injury and death of the dental pulp or periapical tissues, but most often they occur as sequels to predisposing insults, such as dental caries or mechanical trauma, that comprise the integrity of these tissues. Successful management of endodontic diseases lies first in recognizing the role of microorganisms in the etiology of these diseases, followed by removal of the organisms and reestablishment of a sterile, intact pulp chamber sequestered from further microbial contamination.

The microbes found associated with pulpitis are of medical significance for several reasons. From the dental viewpoint, their most important role is that they are the agents that cause pulp injury and death. In addition, after instrumentation of an involved pulp chamber, microorganisms left in the chamber or oral contaminants may cause postoperative complications. Finally, the infected pulp can serve as a focus of infection that seeds bacteria to other tissues of the body. The microbes may spread through the periapical tissues and continue throughout the orofacial tissues, or they may enter the bloodstream and infect tissues distant from the oral cavity (hematogenous dissemination). Hematogenous dissemination also can occur if an endodontic instrument is forced beyond the apex of the tooth, and infectious material is extruded into the periapical tissues.

RESISTANCE FACTORS OF THE PULP CHAMBER

The protective elements of salivary, gingival, and mucosal secretions described in Chapters 8 and 9 serve as external resistance factors that prevent initial colonization and invasion of the hard tissues surrounding the pulp. The vascular system within the pulp chamber is a continuation of the systemic circulation, and, therefore, the resistance factors found in the rest of the body are available for defense of the pulp tissues. These systemic factors include both specific and nonspecific components, such as macrophages, neutrophils, lymphocytes, complement, and all classes of immunoglobulins. These immune factors may be protective, but they also may mediate harmful reactions.

The pulp chamber possesses several unique resistance factors. Enamel and dentin represent the first line of defense against external invasion of the pulp. These mineralized tissues are relatively impervious to most pathogens, but they can be compromised by cariogenic bacteria or mechanical trauma. Despite their susceptibility to caries and trauma, when one considers the many potential pathogens that reside in or pass through the oral cavity, it is obvious that enamel and dentin are very effective barriers to infection.

If a carious lesion progresses into these hard tissues, the cells within the pulp chamber can mount two additional unique defensive responses. As the microorganisms or their toxic products permeate the dentin, osteoblasts associated with the affected dentinal tubules form sclerotic dentin that occludes the tubule and impedes penetration of the microbes or their toxins. The sclerotic dentin, however, may serve only as a temporary barrier because it is subject to the same demineralizing activity that destroyed the overlying enamel and dentin.

The invasion of bacteria into the dentin also induces the production of reparative or irregular secondary dentin in the pulp chamber at the pulpal openings of the affected dentinal tubules (Fig 35–1). Because reparative dentin does not contain tubules, it hinders the entry of not only bacterial cells but also soluble bacterial factors. Despite its protective effects, dentin may be detrimental to the health of the pulp tissues. Even before there is microbial penetration of the pulp chamber, toxic bacterial products can diffuse through the dentinal tubules into the pulp chamber. Phagocytes, however, cannot migrate through the tubules to destroy the bacteria. Thus the toxins can enter the chamber and injure the pulp tissues before the invading bacteria can be neutralized by phagocytes or other internal resistance factors in the pulp.

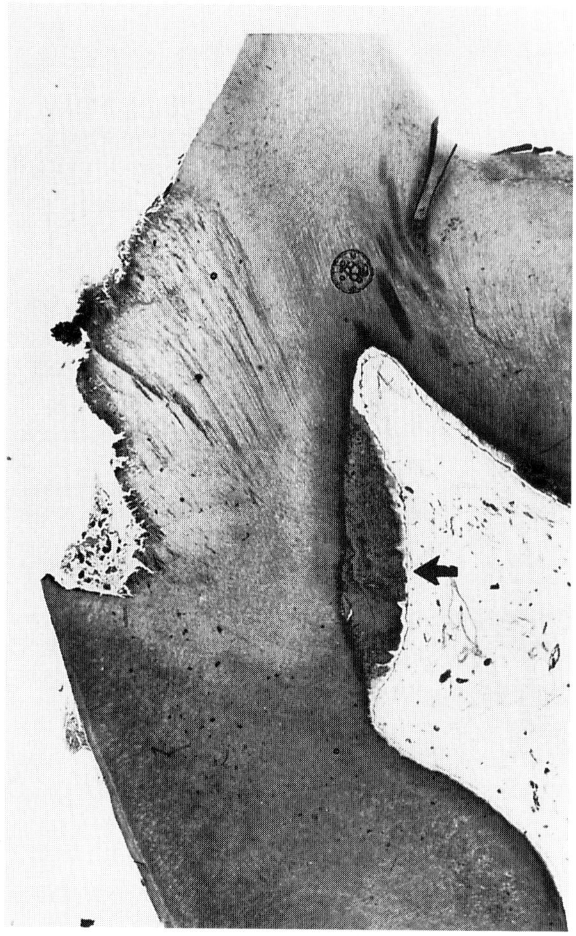

Fig 35–1. Reparative dentin formed in the pulp chamber beneath a carious lesion. *(From Trowbridge HO.* J Endodont *1981; 7:52.)*

IMMUNOLOGY

The immunologic status of the pulp and periapical tissues is similar to that of other tissues. Whereas immunocytes and antibodies are absent or present in only very low concentrations in the healthy state, increased levels of these and other immunologic factors are found in diseased pulp and periapical tissues. Involved pulp tissue and periapical granulomas and cysts contain the immunologic components associated with other antigenically stimulated tissues. The levels of immunoglobulins, complement components, immunoglobulin-producing plasma cells, and T and B lymphocytes increase significantly.

Animal studies have demonstrated that not only direct application of antigens to exposed pulps but also antigens percolating through the dentinal tubules can stimulate an immune response and, on subsequent challenges through the same routes, immunologic reactions. This indicates that not only direct carious exposure but also shallow dentinal lesions can allow access to the antigens of bacteria in the lesion. The pulp tissues can respond also to other immunologic stimuli, either antigenic or haptenic, that gain access through the enamel or dentin.

Little is known concerning the relative protective or injurious roles of the immune components in these diseased tissues, but there is no reason to believe that they are different from the rest of the body's tissues. A single report concerning an immunodeficient patient suggests that a competent immune system may retard bacterial invasion of the pulp chamber. The potential for hypersensitivity reactions against bacterial antigens is described subsequently.

ROUTES OF MICROBIAL INVASION

The pulp tissues are enclosed in a chamber that is relatively impermeable to microbial invasion, but it is not resistant to entry by all microorganisms. The obvious portals of entry and the ones that account for most pulp infections are carious lesions. Infection can occur following direct carious exposure of the pulp chamber to the oral cavity or by migration of bacteria through dentinal tubules that are exposed by the advancing carious lesion (Fig 35–2). Pulp infections also can occur from oral bacterial contamination following accidental pulp exposures during clinical instrumentation or fractures of the tooth.

The pulp may become infected as a sequel to periodontal disease. As the periodontal pocket extends apically, lateral and accessory canals may be exposed and permit bacteria to enter the chamber. When the pocket reaches the apex of the tooth, the apical foramen may serve as a portal of entry into the pulp chamber. In addition, loss of the cementum as a result of resorption during periodontal disease or periodontal scaling may expose the openings of dentinal tubules below the cementoenamel junction and allow microorganisms to enter the pulp chamber.

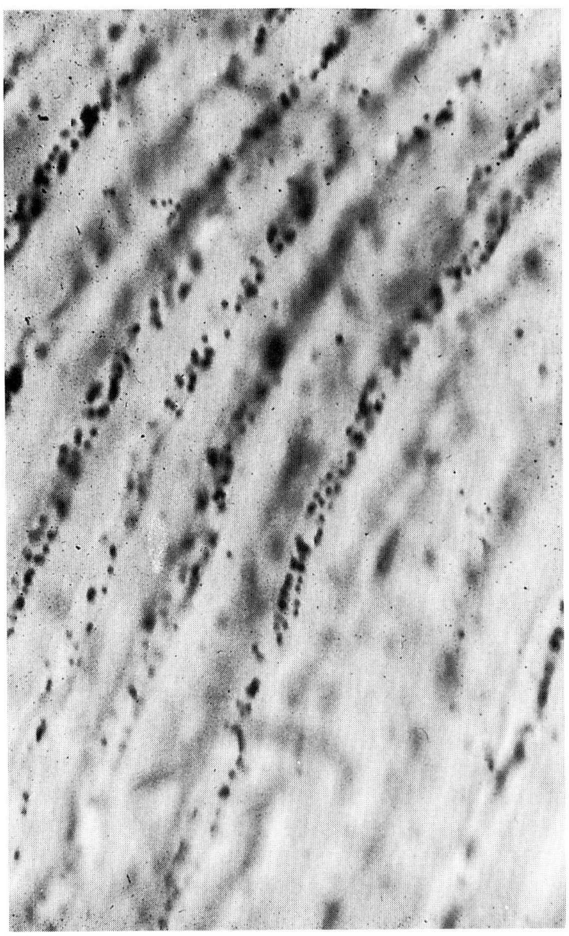

Fig 35–2. Bacteria in the dentinal tubules adjacent to a carious lesion. *(Courtesy of L.R. Brown, University of Texas Health Science Center at Houston, Dental Branch.)*

Periapical lesions on adjacent teeth may be sources of infection. The infectious process may extend into the tissues supporting an adjacent tooth, and the microorganisms then may invade the tooth through apical or lateral canals or dentinal tubules, as described previously.

Blood-borne microorganisms also may infect the pulp chamber. This process, called anachoresis, probably does not occur in healthy teeth, through which blood-borne bacteria pass unhindered. However, an inflamed pulp may predispose to bacterial localization and subsequent injury to the pulp tissues. Disruption of the normal blood flow and the structural integrity of the inflamed pulp's vascular tissues may enable blood-borne bacteria to escape from the vessel and colonize the extravascular areas of the pulp. Animal studies have shown that one can increase the degree of pulpal infection by blood-borne bacteria by artificially increasing inflammation of the pulp tissues. Inflammatory responses that may predispose to anachoresis in the pulp chamber can occur naturally. For example, mechanical trauma or toxic bacterial products percolating through the dentinal tubules in advance of a carious lesion may cause inflammation that could predispose to pulpal infection.

MICROBIAL VIRULENCE FACTORS

The microbes usually involved in pulp and periapical infections are of relatively low virulence, but several potential virulence factors have been associated with them. Gram-negative bacteria containing endotoxin are common in pulp and periapical infections, and there are several reports associating the severity of pulp or periapical inflammation with the concentrations of endotoxin present in the lesion. Table 35–1 illustrates the results of one study. Note the correlation between increasing severity of pathosis and levels of endotoxin extracted from the involved tissues, a corre-

TABLE 35–1. ENDOTOXIN CONTENT OF ENDODONTICALLY INVOLVED TEETH

Clinical Group	Mean Endotoxin Concentration (μg/mL)
Vital, asymptomatic	0.007
Vital, symptomatic	0.075
Pulpless, asymptomatic	0.192
Pulpless, symptomatic	1.070

From Schein B, Schilder H. J Endodontol. *1975; 1:19.*

lation that suggests that endotoxin may be a factor injuring the pulp tissues. In addition, teichoic acids and peptidoglycans, which possess endotoxin-like activity, also are products of the bacteria in pulp infections. Exotoxin-producing bacteria such as staphylococci are found in some endodontic infections, but there is no evidence of pathology resulting from their exotoxins.

Bacteria isolated from pulp and periapical infections have been shown to produce numerous enzymes that are suspected of being involved in pathologic processes. For example, *Bacteroides* produce collagenase, proteases that can hydrolyze immunoglobulins A, G, and M, and hyaluronidase, fibrinolysin, and alkaline and acid phosphatases, among other enzymes. Similar enzymes are produced by many of the other bacteria listed in Table 35–2. Although many of these enzymes are potentially harmful, none has been identified specifically as playing a definitive role in endodontic infections.

Metabolic end products that may be injurious to pulp and periapical tissues are produced by many of the bacteria associated with endodontic lesions. These include ammonia, hydrogen sulfide, toxic amines, and organic acids.

Bacterial antigens also can stimulate immune responses that lead to hypersensitivity reactions within the pulp chamber. The immunologic components that mediate immune hypersensitivity reactions are present in dental pulp, and these may be involved in the inflammatory reactions within the chamber. Several investigators have reported that there are disproportionately high levels of IgE-forming cells in periapical lesions, and others found high levels of circulating IgE in patients with periapical disease. This suggests that there is an association between type I, local anaphylactic reactions and endodontic disease. The presence of immune complexes containing immunoglobulins, complement, and specific bacterial antigens (ie, *Actinomyces viscosus, Bacteroides gingivalis,* and *Bacteroides intermedius*) in diseased pulp and periapical tissues indicates that type III or Arthus-like reactions occur. Several studies have demonstrated that T lymphocytes predominate in these chronic lesions, and their presence suggests that type IV or lymphokine-mediated delayed-type hypersensitivity reactions involving bacterial antigens may contribute to the disease processes.

TABLE 35–2. BACTERIA ISOLATED FROM INTACT TEETH WITH NECROTIC PULPS

Anaerobic gram-positive rods
Eubacterium alactolyticum
Arachnia proprionica
Propionibacterium acnes
Lactobacillus sp.
Anaerobic gram-negative rods
Bacteroides intermedius
Bacteroides oralis
Bacteroides ruminicola
Bacteroides sp.
Camplyobacter sputorum
Fusobacterium nucleatum
Fusobacterium sp.
Anaerobic gram-positive cocci
Peptostreptococcus anaerobius
Peptostreptococcus intermedius
Peptostreptococcus micros
Anaerobic gram-negative cocci
Veillonella parvula
Facultative bacteria
Actinomyces sp.
Lactobacillus sp.
Streptococcus sp.
Staphylococcus aureus

From Wittgow WC, Sabiston CB. J Endodontol. *1975; 1:168.*

MICROBIAL FLORA OF PULP INFECTIONS

Pulp infections share several characteristics with the other common dental infections, caries and periodontal diseases. The first is that they usually are caused by indigenous organisms; that is, they are caused by members of the normal microbial flora of the body. Second, as noted previously, the pathogens are of relatively low virulence. Finally, no single bacterium has been identified as the single cause of the disease or diseases. The same questions of microbial specificity associated with dental caries and periodontal diseases occur in pulp and periapical infections. The problem is accentuated in pulp infections. Because there is so little known about the specific etiologic agents of pulp infections in general, they are most correctly identified as nonspecific infections.

Most pulp infections are polymicrobic, averaging 5 to 6 taxa per infection and ranging as high as 13 taxa. If one considers the total numbers of bacteria isolated from dental pulps, one group of bacteria, streptococci, predominates. However, if the pulp lesions are differentiated according to specific clinical and laboratory criteria, a different microbial picture emerges. Different bacterial types can be associated with different clinical entities.

Some differentiating criteria are as follows. One is whether the pulp is open to the oral cavity or has an intact crown. The former would enhance the growth of aerobic oral bacteria, whereas the latter would enhance the growth of anaerobes. A second determinant would be whether the tooth is vital or nonvital. A vital tooth would still be receiving oxygenated blood, whereas a nonvital one would not. The latter would favor the growth of anaerobic bacteria. A third determinant would be the time of sampling. Cultures taken immediately on opening the chamber would most likely contain the microorganisms that actually caused the pulpitis. Cultures taken during or after instrumentation may contain oral contaminants, especially streptococci. Finally, the bacterial culturing techniques must be considered. Many of the pulp pathogens, especially the anaerobes, are fastidious and require special handling in order to be successfully cultivated in the clinical laboratory.

If one considers these criteria in analyzing the etiology of pulp and periapical infections, several generalities become apparent. The first is that because optimal aseptic and anaerobic techniques were not used, much of the older literature concerning the microflora of the pulp is biased in favor of facultative oral microorganisms. Thus, when reviewing the older literature, one finds that the organisms that were isolated most often from root canal cultures in general, without qualification as to the criteria noted here, were streptococci. These were predominantly alpha or viridans streptoccocci. Staphylococci also have been found in relatively high numbers, but since these organisms are common skin inhabitants, in most cases they probably represented contamination of the lesion or the clinical specimen.

Streptococci predominate in pulp lesions with direct exposure to the oral cavity. This would be expected, because these bacteria predominate in the oral environment that is the source of the infection or contamination of these lesions. Many different species of streptococci, including *Streptococcus salivarius, Streptococcus faecalis,* and *Streptococcus mitis,* have been isolated from endodontic cultures taken from these lesions. Other microbes that are found frequently in exposed pulpal lesions include staphylococci, bacilli, corynebacteria, coliform bacteria, anaerobes, and the yeast, *Candida albicans.*

The pulp chambers of vital teeth with intact crowns contain primarily aerobic bacteria. Apparently, the vital pulp is still receiving enough oxygen to retard the growth of anaerobes. Eventually, with increasing involvement, the pulp tissues will necrose and allow growth of obligate anaerobes. The microbes found in intact vital pulp chambers resemble those found in exposed pulps.

Necrotic, nonvital teeth with intact crowns most frequently are infected with strict or obligate anaerobes. In some studies, as many as 90% of all of the bacteria isolated were strict anaerobes, and in some teeth, all of the bacteria isolated were strict anaerobes. The bacteria identified in these lesions resemble the flora associated with subgingival plaque, suggesting that the gingival sulcus or pocket was the initial source of the infection. For example, in a typical study (Table 35–2), 31 of 36 intact teeth with necrotic pulps were found to be infected, and 31 of these teeth were infected with anaerobic bacteria. The anaerobes represented 75% of the total bacterial isolates. In addition to the microbes shown in Table 35–2, many other bacteria, including spirochetes and other anaerobes, fungi, and viruses, have been found in these lesions.

The few studies of the microbial flora of periapical infections indicate that the bacteria present in these lesions are very similar to those found in intact, necrotic teeth. Strict anaerobes predominate, and the species present resemble those found in subgingival plaque associated with periodontal diseases.

Although pulp and periapical infections are nonspecific, one genus does appear to be of special significance in terms of severity and pain. Several investigators have reported an association between the presence of *Bacteroides* species and pain and tissue destruction in endodontic lesions. Species most frequently found include the black-pigmented species, *Bacteroides intermedius, Bacteroides denticola* and *Bacteroides endodontalis,* and the nonpigmented species, *Bacteroides buccae* and *Bacteroides oris.* Preliminary evidence indicates that *B. endodontalis* is present only in endodontic infections or in abscesses of endodontic origin. Although *Bacteroides* species are highly suspect, further clinical studies are needed to determine the exact role of *Bacteroides* species in endodontic infections.

ENDODONTIC CULTURING

The purpose of endodontic therapy has been described as the restoration of the involved tooth to its proper form and function in a healthy state. If it is to be healthy, it must be free of microbes, and the most practical method of determining if the bacteria have been destroyed or removed by instrumentation and medication is by bacteriologic culturing. Some clinicians believe that culturing is the only way of determining if an instrumented root canal is free of viable bacteria (or at least determining that the bacterial count has been reduced to minimal and hopefully harmless numbers). Proponents of routine culturing admit that it is a less than perfect method but believe that it is much better than doing nothing. The validity of this argument has been questioned by others who believe that endodontic culturing is of little actual value, since (1) several investigators have reported that bacteria are frequently present in root canals that display negative cultures, and (2) the techniques used are subject to contamination from oral flora, resulting in misleading interpretations of the actual conditions within the chamber. The clinician, however, should not confuse the issues. There may be disagreement concerning the need for routine culturing, but there is no disagreement concerning the need to attempt to sterilize the canal (or at least reduce the bacterial flora to minimal numbers) and to constantly practice aseptic techniques when undertaking endodontic procedures.

There are cases in which endodontic culturing is desirable. It can be used as a means of evaluating aseptic technique and instilling operator confidence in his or her sterile instrumentation. Thus, it should be used in the initial student instruction in endodontic procedures. Culturing also is useful to assist in managing problems, such as septic pulp exposures, acute pulpitis, or cellulitis, and compromised patients. The clinician who incorporates culturing in these cases will be better prepared to manage postoperative complications that might occur. Culturing can be used as a guide for selective use of antibiotic therapy when required. This is often carried out routinely in the latter cases and should be used when one encounters a refractory lesion that does not repond to routine endodontic therapy.

Endodontic Culture Media

Culture and antibiotic sensitivity testing are best delegated to a clinical laboratory. The dentist simply collects the specimen, places it in an appropriate medium, and delivers it to a clinical laboratory for further processing. The media used to collect specimens may serve either as a transport medium or combine the functions of transport and growth of the bacteria. As the name implies, transport media are used to secure the microbial specimen and maintain its viability until it can be delivered to a clinical microbiology laboratory for further processing. Transport media are formulated so that bacteria will survive but will not readily grow in them. The latter property prevents rapidly growing bacteria such as streptococci from overgrowing other, possibly more medically significant, bacteria. Endodontic and most other oral specimens should be carried in anaerobic transport media.

The medium most commonly used for both transport and cultivation of specimens is enriched thioglycollate medium. Thioglycollate medium enhances survival of anaerobic bacteria because it contains a reducing agent (thioglycollate) that ties up any oxygen that may diffuse into the medium. It also may contain a dye, such as methylene blue, which indicates the relative oxygen content or oxidation-reduction potential (Eh) of the broth. Excessive levels of oxygen or a high Eh within the medium are detrimental to anaerobes. Finally, the medium contains additional nutrients, such as hemin and vitamin K, needed by fastidious bacteria. This medium will, under anaerobic conditions, support growth of most of the endodontically significant bacteria and can be used to initially assess the microbial status of the pulp chamber. If growth occurs, this medium can serve as a source for isolation and further characterization of the bacteria.

SUGGESTED READINGS

Chow AW, Roser SM, Brady FA. Orofacial odontogenic infections. *Ann Intern Med.* 1978; 88:392.

Farber PA. Endodontic microbiology. I. Etiology. *J Endodontol.* 1988; 14:363.

Haapsalo M. *Bacteroides* species in root canal infections. *Endodont Dent Traumatol.* 1989; 5:1.

Haapsalo M, Ranta H, Ranta KT. Facultative gram-negative enteric rods in persistant periapical infections. *Acta Odontol Scand.* 1983; 41:19.

Maurice JG. Microbiologic aspects of endodontics. In: Orland FJ, ed. *Microbiology in Clinical Dentistry.* Boston: JG Wright—PSG; 1982.

Pekovic DD, Fillery ED. Identification of bacteria in immunopathologic mechanisms of human dental pulp. *Oral Surg.* 1984; 57:652.

Sabiston CB, Grigsby WR. The microbiology of dental pyogenic infections. *CRC Crit Rev Clin Lab Sci.* 1977; 8:213.

Sundqvist G. Bacteriological Studies of Necrotic Dental Pulps. Thesis, Umea, Sweden, 1976.

Torabinejad M, Eby WC, Naidorf IJ. Inflammatory and immunological aspects of the pathogenesis of human periapical lesions. *J Endodontol.* 1985; 11:479.

Trowbridge, HO. Pathogenesis of pulpitis resulting from dental caries. *J Endodontol.* 1981; 7:52.

Index

Abscesses, 155, 176, 223, 332
Acid-fast staining, 4
Acidic proline-rich protein, 327
Acquired immunodeficiency syndrome (AIDS), 118, 313–316
  cytomegalovirus infection and, 272
  fungal infection and, 239
  Mycobacterium avium-intracellulare and, 185–186
  oral candidiasis and, 242, 248
  periodontal infections and, 381
  progressive multifocal leukoencephalopathy and, 279
  -related complex (ARC), 314
  tuberculosis and, 183
Actinobacillus actinomycetemcomitans, 332
  adult periodontitis and, 378
  bone resorption and, 364
  collagenases and, 362*t*, 363
  diagnosis of periodontal disease and, 382
  elevated antibody levels in periodontal disease and, 369
  immunosuppression by, 364
  juvenile periodontitis and, 150, 368, 380
  leukotoxin and, 361
  prepubertal periodontitis and, 381
  rapidly progressive periodontitis and, 380
  refractory adult periodontitis and, 381
  virulence of and periodontal disease, 365–366
Actinobolin, prevention of periodontal disease and, 383
Actinomyces, 209–212, 323
  adherence of, 324
  coaggregation and, 326, 361, 365
  experimental gingivitis and, 375
  healthy gingiva and, 371–372
  israelii, 332, 364–365, 375
  naeslundii, 364–365, 375
Actinomyces (*cont.*)
  odontolyticus, 364–365, 375
  periodontal disease and, 364–365
  root caries and, 348, 381
  selective media for, 320
  viscosus
    adherence and, 360
    bacteriocins and, 338
    gingivitis and, 375
    lactoperoxidase system and, 338
    low pH and, 346–347
    root caries and, 348
    virulence of and periodontal disease, 364–365
Actinomycetes, 209–213, 328
Actinomycetoma, 212
Active transport, 21–22
Acute
  necrotizing ulcerative gingivitis (ANUG), 373*t*, 375–376
    Bacteroides intermedius and, 369
    Entamoeba gingivalis and, 333
    spirochetes and, 208, 361, 369
  respiratory disease (ARD), 276
Acycloguanosine (Acyclovir, Zovirax), 260, 270, 271
ADCC. *See* Antibody-dependent cell mediated cytotoxicity
Adenine arabinoside (Vidarabine), 260, 270
Adenosatellite viruses (Dependovirus), 280
Adenosine
  diphosphate (ADP) ribosylating toxins, 141
  triphosphate (ATP), 26
Adenoviruses, 255, 257, 258, 275–276
Adherence, 137–138, 335
  colonization of subgingival sites and, 360–364
  electrostatic interaction and, 325
  Enterobacteriaceae and, 191
  group A streptococci and, 159
  oral microbes and, 323–327*f*
Adhesins, 137–138, 324, 325
Adjuvants, 115, 132, 171, 183
Adsorption, viruses and, 254
Aerobic bacteria, 19, 233, 389
Aerotolerant anaerobes, 19, 25
Agammaglobulinemias, 117
Agglutination, 121
  tests, 98
Agglutinins, 95
Aggregation, 323–327*f*, 326
AIDS. *See* Acquired immunodeficiency syndrome
Alcohol as antiseptic, 61
Alcoholism, pneumococcal infection and, 162
Aldehydes, 60
Allergens, 124
Allergic reactions, 119, 123–129. *See also* Anaphylactic reactions; Hypersensitivity
  immunoglobulin antigens and, 120
  lymphokines and, 114
  syphilis and, 205, 207
Alloantigens, 105
Allografts, 129, 130
Allosteric enzymes, 36
Alphaherpes, 266
Amantadine, 260, 285
Amikacin, 74
Amino acids, energy from, 31
Aminoglycosides, 74, 80, 149, 161, 200, 227
Amoxicillin, 70, 168, 192
Amphotericin B, 77–78
  aspergillosis and, 248
  blastomycosis and, 246
  candidal infections and, 244
  coccidioidomycosis and, 247
  cryptococcosis and, 247
  histoplasmosis and, 245
  phagocytosis and, 147
  zygomycosis and, 247
Ampicillin, 70, 148
  Brucella and, 230
  E. coli urinary tract infections and, 194

Page numbers followed by *t* refer to tables. Page numbers followed by *f* refer to figures.

Ampicillin (*cont.*)
gonorrhea and, 168
listeriosis and, 232
meningitis and, 233
oral infection and, 80
pseudomembranous colitis and, 177
Salmonella infections and, 192
shigellosis and, 193
staphylococcal infections and, 156
Anachoresis, 338, 387
Anaerobic bacteria
actinomycetes, 210
adult periodontitis and, 378
Bacteroides, 197–200
clostridia, 174
cultivation of, 226–227, 320
dental plaque and, 328, 331
energy production of, 25
Eubacterium, 332
Fusobacterium, 332
gingivitis and, 374
juvenile periodontitis and, 379–380
lincomycin and, 73
Peptostreptococcus, 162, 332
pulp infections and, 389
specimens of, 226
subgingival plaque and, 329
tricarboxylic acid cycle and, 32
Anaerobiosis, 223–227
Anaphylactic reactions, 123–125, 285, 370, 388. *See also* Allergic reactions; Hypersensitivity
Anaphylatoxins, complement and, 94
Anergy, fungal infection and, 239
Animal pathogens transmissible to humans, 229–232
Antiadherence antibodies, 95
Antibiosis, 333
Antibiotics, 67–82
cell wall inhibitors, 68–73
dangers of indiscriminate use of, 80
definition of, 68
effect of on the host-parasite relationship, 148–149
measurement of microbial susceptibility to, 80–81
periodontal diseases and, 337
plaque control and, 337
resistance to, 78–79
Actinomyces and, 212
aminoglycocides and, 74
conjugation and, 49–50
extrachromosomal genetic elements and, 14
mutation and, 46–47
pili and, 8
Antibiotics (*cont.*)
resistance to (*cont.*)
staphylococci and, 156
tetracyclines and, 75
transposons and, 47–48
secondary infections and, 248, 323
spirochetes and, 333
use of for oral infection, 79–80
Antibodies, 88–92
antiadherence, 122
capsid proteins and, 252
enzymes and, 122
fluorescent, test, 98
hepatitis B virus and, 306–307
human immunodeficiency virus and, 315
labeled, test, 98
monoclonal, 100–101
oral cavity and, 91–92
periodontal disease and, 368–369
protective immunity mediated by, 121–122
saliva and, 338
viruses and, 259
Weil-Felix reaction and, 216
Antibody-dependent cell-mediated cytotoxicity (ADCC), 108, 125, 132, 259
Anticodons, 41
Antifungal agents, 77–78
Antigenic
determinants, 86–87
shift, 284
Antigens, 86–88
-antibody complexes, 369, 371
binding site, 89
hepatitis B virus and, 306–307
human immunodeficiency virus and, 315
periodontal disease and, 364, 368
-presenting cells (APC), 109
sources of, 87–88
tumor-specific, 132
Antiglobulins, 89
Antihistamines, 124
Antimicrobials, disinfecting and sterilizing agents, 57–62
Antirabies globulin (RIG), 260
Antiseptic, definition of, 56
Antithymocyte sera, 118
Antitoxin, 95, 121
botulism and, 175
Clostridium perfringens and, 177
diphtheria and, 170
tetanus and, 176
Antiviral protein (AVP), 261
ANUG. *See* Acute necrotizing ulcerative gingivitis
APC. *See* Antigen-presenting cells
Aphthous ulcers, recurrent, 126, 131
Aplastic crisis, 280
Appendix, 105
ARA-A, varicella-zoster virus and, 271
Arboviruses, 297
ARC. *See* Acquired immunodeficiency syndrome-related complex
ARD. *See* Acute respiratory disease
Arenaviruses, 257
Arthralgia, 127
Arthritis
rheumatoid, 131, 280
rubella and, 298
septic, 233
serum sickness and, 127
Arthrobacter, root caries and, 348
Arthrospore, 238
Arthus reaction, 126–127, 367–368
Aschoff bodies, 160
Asepsis, 56, 63–64
Aspergillosis, 247–248
Aspermatogenesis, 131
Asthma, 123, 124
Astrocytes, 109
Athlete's foot, 248
Atopic reactions, 124
ATP. *See* Adenosine triphosphate
Atrophic candidiasis, 242–244
Autogenous infections, 62
Autografts, 129, 130
Autoimmunity, 130–131
AVP. *See* Antiviral protein
Axial filaments, 8
Azathioprine, 118
Azidothymidine (AZT), 260, 316

Babes-Ernst granules, 14, 169
Bacille Calmette-Guerin (BCG) tuberculosis vaccine, 121, 147, 185
Bacitracin, 72–73, 158, 178, 320, 355
Bacteria
caries development and, 345–348
cell membranes of, 12–14
cell surfaces of, 6–8
cytoplasm of, 14–16
size and shape of, 2–3
structure of, 1–16
ultrastructure of, 6–16
Bacteriocins, 338
Bacterionema, 212
Bacteroides, 197–200, 323
adherence and, 323–324
adult periodontitis and, 378
coaggregation and, 326
corrodens, 331

Bacteroides (*cont.*)
fragilis,198, 225, 363
gingivalis, 198–199
adult periodontitis and, 378
bone resorption and, 364, 365–366
collagenases and, 362*t*, 363
commensalism and, 322
diagnosis of periodontal disease and, 382
elevated antibody levels and, 369
rapidly progressive periodontitis and, 380
refractory adult periodontitis and, 381
virulence of and periodontal disease, 365–366
gingivitis and, 374–375
healthy gingiva and, 371–372
intermedius, 200
adult periodontitis and, 378
bone resorption and, 366
diagnosis of periodontal disease and, 382
elevated antibody levels and, 369
gingivitis and, 374–375
prepubertal periodontitis and, 381
pulp infections and, 389
refractory adult periodontitis and, 381
virulence of and periodontal disease, 356–366
pulp infections and, 389
virulence of and periodontal disease, 365–366
BALT. *See* Bronchus-associated lymphoid tissues
Barrier technique, 64, 316
Bauer-Kirby procedure, 81
BCG. *See* Bacille Calmette-Guerin tuberculosis vaccine
Behcet's syndrome, 126, 131
Beta-hemolytic streptococci, 158
Betaherpes, 266
Beta-lactamase, 225
BFP. *See* Biologic false positive
BI. *See* Biologic indicators
Biguanines, 61
Biologic
false positives (BFP), 206
indicators (BI), 63
Biosynthesis, 33–38, 36–37
Bites, anaerobic infections and, 226
BK virus, 279
Black-pigmented *Bacteroides* (BPBs), 365–366
Blastomycosis, 246–247
Blood
flow, anaerobiosis and, 223–224
group reactions, 125
B lymphocytes, 104–105, 108
antibiotics and, 148
endotoxins and, 142
Epstein-Barr virus and, 273
gingivitis and, 374
human immunodeficiency virus and, 313
humoral immunodeficiency and, 117
immunoglobulins and, 109
periodontal disease and, 369
Boiling water disinfection, 58
Boils, staphylococci and, 155
Bone
marrow, 104
resorption, 359, 363, 363–364, 379
Bordetella, 233–234
Bordet-Gengou medium, 233
Borrelia
burgdorferi, 208
recurrentis, 207
Botulism, 120, 121, 173, 174–175
BPBs. *See* Black-pigmented *Bacteroides*
Brightfield microscopy, 4
Brill-Zinsser disease, 217
Broad Street pneumonia, 235
Bronchiolitis, 286
Bronchitis, 220, 276, 286
Bronchus-associated lymphoid tissues (BALT), 105, 112–114
Brown's classification, 158
Brucella, 229–230
Brucellosis, 229
Brushing, 337, 351
Bruton's agammaglobulinemia, 117
Bubo, 231
Bubonic plague, 230–231
Bunyaviruses, 257
Burkitt's lymphoma, Epstein-Barr virus and, 259, 273, 274, 312
Bursa of Fabricus, 104

C′. *See* Complement
Calculus, 326, 335–337
chronic gingivitis and, 372
formation of, 212
lipids and, 335
subgingival plaque and, 329
Caliciviruses, 257
CAMP test, 161
Campylobacter
enteritis, 194–195
jejuni, 194
selective media for, 320
Cancer
cytomegalovirus and, 273
cytotoxic T lymphocytes and, 108
Epstein-Barr virus and, 273, 274
hepatitis B virus and, 306
immunology and, 131–132
papillomaviruses and, 277
Candida albicans, 238, 240–244
Candidiasis, 240–244, 248
acquired immunodeficiency syndrome (AIDS) and, 314, 316
antibiotic agents for, 77
atrophic, 242–244
secondary infection and, 80, 323
Capnocytophaga, 331
coaggregation and, 326
dental plaque and, 331
gingivalis, 331, 375
healthy gingiva and, 372
ochracea, 331, 364, 366
prepubertal periodontitis and, 381
sputigena, 331, 336, 368
virulence of and periodontal disease, 366
Capsid, 252
Capsomeres, 252
Capsule, 6–7
Carbenicillin, 71, 194, 200, 227
Carbohydrates, 27–31
caries and, 342
composition of dental plaque and, 334
dental caries and, 349, 352
spirochetes and, 202
Carbon dioxide (CO_2), bacterial growth and, 19
Carbuncles, staphylococci and, 155
Carcinogenesis, viral, 311–312
Carcinoma, primary hepatocellular (PHC), 306
Caries, 341–355
actinomycetes and, 209, 213
activity tests, 354–355
brushing and flossing and, 337
carious lesions, 342
cost of, 341
declining prevalence of, 354
Enterococcus faecalis and, 161
genetic influence on, 143
immunity to, 122
interrelationship among host, diet and bacteria and, 342–348
lactobacilli and, 332, 333
local immunodeficiency and, 121
low pH and, 323
lysogeny and, 262
oral microflora and, 322–323
plaque and, 337
prevention of, 351–354

Caries (*cont.*)
 pulp and periapical problems and, 385
 risk assessment, 355
 role of lactic and other acids in, 349–351, 352*f*
 root surface, 329, 331, 342, 348–349*f*, 381
 selective immunoglobin A deficiency and, 117
 selectivity of bacteria by tooth area and, 348, 349*t*
 Streptococcus mutans and, 150, 157, 163
 tetanus and, 176
 theories of development of, 342, 346
 vaccine against, 114, 120
 viridans streptococci and, 161
Carrier state, 136, 156, 192–193
CD. *See* Cluster differentiating antigens
Cefoxitin, *Bacteroides fragilis* and, 200
Cell
 envelope, 8–14
 -mediated immune response (CMI), 103, 114–115
  allergic reactions and, 123
  Brucella and, 230
  fungal infection and, 239
  graft rejection and, 129
  human immunodeficiency virus and, 314
  leprosy and, 186
  measles and, 288
  methods of assessing, 115–116
  mycobacteria and, 185
  periodontal disease and, 368–370, 371
  resorption of bone and, 363
  syphilis and, 207
  tuberculosis and, 183
  tumors and, 132
 membranes, 12–14
 wall, 9–12, 34, 220
Cellulitis, 227*f*
Centipeda periodontii, 364
Cephalosporins, 72
 allergic reactions to, 124
 anaerobic infections and, 227
 phagocytosis and, 149
 resistance to, 79
Cervical carcinoma, 312, 313
Cervicofacial lesions, *Actinomyces* and, 211
CFA. *See* Colonization factor antigens
CGD. *See* Chronic granulomatous disease
Chancre, 203
Chancroid, 233
Chediak-Higashi syndrome, 368
Chemiclave, 58, 60
Chemiosmotic hypothesis (Mitchell), 33
Chemoheterotrophs, 18–25
Chemoparasitic theory of caries development, 342
Chemotaxis, 94, 140, 146
Chickenpox, 270–271
Chlamydiae, 75, 217–220
Chlamydospore, 238, 240, 241*f*
Chloramphenicol, 75–76, 79
Chlorhexadine, 383
Chlorhexidine, 61, 337, 383
Chlorine, 60
Cholera, 191, 193
Chromosomal antibiotic resistance, 79
Chronic
 benign agranulocytopenia, 368
 granulomatous disease (CGD), 148
Ciprofloxacin, 77
CJD. *See* Creutzfeld-Jakob disease
Clindamycin, 73–74
 anaerobic infections and, 227
 Bacteroides and, 200
 oral infection and, 80
 phagocytosis and, 149
 pseudomembranous colitis and, 177, 178
 resistance to, 79
 secondary infections and, 80
 staphylococcal infections and, 156
Clofazimine, leprosy and, 186
Clonal
 anergy, 116
 deletion, 116
 selection, 109
Clostridium, 173–178
Clotrimazole, 244, 248
Cloxacillin, 70
Cluster differentiating (CD) antigens, 106
CMI. *See* Cell-mediated immune response
CMV. *See* Cytomegalovirus
Coagglutination, group A streptococci and, 160, 163
Coaggregation, 326, 360, 361
Coagulase, 154
Coccidioidomycosis, 247
Coccoid cells, periodontitis and, 377–378
Codons, 41
Cold sores, 269
Coliform diseases, 194
Collagenase, 363, 368, 380
Colonization, 135–136, 323–327*f*
 factor antigens (CFA), 191
Colorado tick fever, 295
Commensalism, 135, 333
Complement (C′), 92–94, 121, 144–145
 bacterial substances that activate, 364
 bone resorption and, 364, 371
 cascade, histocompatibility and, 105
 endotoxins and, 363
 fixation, 98, 259
 lysis and, 122
 lysozyme and, 144
 -mediated cell lysis, 132
 oral cavity and, 94
 periodontal disease and, 369, 371
 viruses and, 259
Conconavalin A (Con A), 111
Condylomas, 277, 313
Congenital
 rubella syndrome (CRS), 298
 thymic aplasia, 117
Conidia, 238
Conjugated antigen, 87
Conjugation, 49–51*f*
Conjunctivitis, 276, 284
Constitutive genes, 42
Contact dermatitis, 127, 128
Cord factor, 182–183
Corncob formation, 326, 327*f*
Coronaviruses, 295
Corticosteriods, 235
Corticosteroids, 118, 128, 242*f*, 248
Corynebacteria, 169–172
 prophage and, 262
Cowpox, 281
Coxsackievirus, 258, 293
CPE. *See* Cytopathic effect
C-reactive protein (CRP), 162
Creutzfeld-Jakob disease (CJD), 317
Cromolyn sodium, 124
Cross-infection, 62, 164
Croup, 276, 286
CRP. *See* C-reactive protein
CRS. *See* Congenital rubella syndrome
Cryptococcosis, 247, 314
CTL. *See* Cytotoxic T lymphocytes
Culturing of oral microflora, 320, 359–360, 382, 389–390
Cyclophosphamide, 118
Cyclosporine, 118
Cytokines, 106–107
Cytolytic toxins, 141
Cytomegalovirus (CMV), 140, 258, 265, 271–273, 273
Cytopathic effect (CPE), 258
Cytoplasm, bacterial, 14–16
Cytotoxic
 cells
  assays, 116
  cell-mediated immune response and, 114

Cytotoxic (*cont.*)
endotoxins, 362
hypersensitivity, 125–126
T lymphocytes (CTL, T-c), 106, 108, 114–115, 128–129, 132, 259
Cytotoxin
Campylobacter jejuni and, 194
enteropathogenic *E. coli* and, 193
Mycoplasma pneumoniae, 220

Dane particle, 304
Dapsone, 186
Darkfield microscopy, 4–5
adult periodontitis and, 377–378
diagnosis of periodontal diseases and, 382
gingivitis and, 374
juvenile periodontitis and, 379
leptospires and, 207
spirochetes and, 320
syphilis and, 205–206
Deafness, congenital rubella syndrome and, 298
Deamination, 31
Decayed, missing or filled teeth (DMFT), 341
Degranulation, 146
Delayed-type hypersensitivity (DTH), 108, 114, 127–128
Deletion mutation, 46
Delta agent, 308
Dendritic cells, 109
Dengue fever, 299
Dental fluorosis, 352
Dentin, 386
Dentinal tubules, 342, 386
Denture stomatitis, 243
Deoxyribonucleic acid (DNA), 14, 39–43*t*
synthesis of, 35–38, 37–38
tumor viruses and, 312–313
viral replication and, 254–255, 256*f*, 257
viruses and, 251–252
Dependovirus, 280
Dermatophytes, 248
Desensitization, 124–125
Desiccation, 59
Deuteromyces, 237
Dextrans, 334, 335, 364
Dextrins, 350
Diabetes mellitus, 247, 298, 366
Diagnosis of periodontal disease, 381–382
Dicloxacillin, 70
Dietary factors in caries development, 344–345, 346*f*
Diffusion, 21
method of testing for antimicrobial activity, 81
DiGeorge syndrome, 117
Dilution tests for antimicrobial activity, 81
Diphtheria, 120, 121, 169–172
cholera and, 191
exotoxins and, 141
prophage and, 262
Diphtheroids, 171–172
Diploid cell strains, 254
Disinfection, 56, 63–65, 253
DMFT. *See* Decayed, missing or filled teeth
Domains, immunoglobulin, 90
Double
diffusion in agar test, 96–97
-stranded circular DNA, 257
-stranded linear DNA, 257
Doxycycline, 75, 80, 200
Dry heat sterilization, 58–59
DTF. *See* Lawrence's dialyzable transfer factor
DTH. *See* Delayed-type hypersensitivity
Duplication mutation, 46
Dyes for disinfecting, 62
Dysentery, 193, 262

EAC. *See* Erythrocyte-antibody-complement rosetting
Eastern equine encephalitis virus (EEE), 299
EB. *See* Elementary body
EBV. *See* Epstein-Barr virus
ECF-A. *See* Eosinophil chemotactic factor of anaphylaxis
Echovirus, 293–294
Eclipse phase, 257, 262
EEE. *See* Eastern equine encephalitis virus
Eh. *See* Oxidation-reduction potential
Eikenella
corrodens, 331, 366, 378, 381
dental plaque and, 331
healthy gingiva and, 372
virulence of and periodontal disease, 366
Electron
microscopy, 5–6
transport system (ETS), 32–33
Electrostatic interaction, 325
Elek test, 170
Elementary body (EB), chlamydiae and, 218
ELISA. *See* Enzyme-linked immunosorbent assays
EMB. *See* Eosin-methylene blue agar
Embden-Meyerhof-Parnas pathway, 27–28, 36
Enamel, 386
carbohydrate metabolism and, 38
decalcification, 349
hypoplasia, 205
Encephalitis, 131, 281, 295, 299
Encephalomyelitis, measles and, 288
Endemic disease, 149
Endocarditis, 62
Actinobacillis actinomycetemcomitans and, 365
Actinomyces israelii and, 332
antibiotics to prevent, 80
bacterial, 139–140
Corynebacteria and, 172
infective, 161–162
Q fever and, 217
streptococci and, 157, 163, 164
Endodontic culture media, 390
Endospores, 14–16
Endotoxins, 34–35, 141–143
anaerobic infections and, 225
gingival tissue and, 150, 359
periodontal disease and, 361–363
phagocytosis and, 139
pulp infections and, 387–388
Energy production, 25–33
Entamoeba gingivalis, 332–333
Enteric fever, 192
Enteritis, 293
Enterobacteriaceae, 189–195
Enteropathogenic *Escherichia coli* (EPEC), 193
Enterotoxigenic *Escherichia coli* (ETEC), 193
Enterotoxin, 141
Campylobacter jejuni and, 194
cholera and, 193
Clostridium difficile and, 177
Clostridium perfringens and, 177
Escherichia coli and, 191
enteropathogenic *Escherichia coli* and, 193
Staphylococcus aureus and, 154
Enteroviruses, 291
Entner-Doudoroff pathway, 27, 28, 29*f*
Entry of microorganism, 137
Envelope, viruses and, 253
Enzyme-linked immunosorbent assays (ELISA), 99–100, 160, 259, 315
Enzymes
inhibition of, 57
periodontal disease and, 363
pulp infections and, 388
regulation of
activity of, 36
synthesis of, 36–37
Eosin-methylene blue agar (EMB), 190

Eosinophil chemotactic factor of anaphylaxis (ECF-A), 124
Eosinophils, 146
EPEC. *See* Enteropathogenic *Escherichia coli*
Epidemic, 149
Epidemiology, 149–150
Epidermodysplasis verruciformis (EV), 313
Epiglottitis, 233
Epinephrine, 124
Episomes, 14
Epitactic mechanism of calculus formation, 337
Epstein-Barr virus (EBV), 265–266, 273–274
  antigen in, 88
  Burkitt's lymphoma and, 259, 273, 274, 312
  cancer and, 274
  human immunodeficiency virus and, 314
  pathogenesis of, 258
Equine encephalitis viruses, 299
E-rosetting, 107
Erysipleas, 160
Erythema
  infectiosum, 280
  multiforme, 270
Erythrocyte-antibody-complement (EAC) rosetting, 108
Erythromycin, 73
  oral infection and, 80
  phagocytosis and, 149
  resistance to, 79
Escherichia coli
  dental unit water supplies and, 195
  diarrheal diseases caused by, 193–194
ETEC. *See* Enterotoxigenic *Escherichia coli*
Ethambutal, tuberculosis and, 185
Ethionamide, leprosy and, 186
Ethylene oxide, 59–60
ETS. *See* Electron transport system
Eubacterium, 7–8, 332, 365, 379
Eucalyptol, 383
EV. *See* Epidermidodysplasis verruciformis
Exfoliatin, 154
Exoenzymes, 21
Exotoxins, 141
  Bordetella pertussis and, 233
  Clostridium and, 225
  corynebacterium and, 169–170
  Enterobacteriaceae and, 190
  gangrene and, 177
  periodontal disease and, 361
Extrachromosomal antibiotic resistance, 79
Eyewear, 64

Fab fragments, 90
Facilitated diffusion, 21, 22*f*
Factor
  B, 93
  D, 93
  V, 232
  X, 232
Facultative anaerobes, 19
  actinomycetes, 210
  dental plaque and, 331
  energy production of, 25
  Listeria monocytogenes, 232
  mycoplasmas, 220
  pneumococci, 162
  staphylococci, 154
Fatty acids, energy from, 31
FC fragment, 90
Feline leukemia virus, 312
Fermentation, 25–26
  Capnocytophaga and, 331
  group translocation and, 22–23
  pyruvate and, 30
  staphylococci and, 154
  Streptococcus mutans and, 320, 347
  yeasts and, 239
Fetal
  liver, 104
  tolerance, 116
Fever blisters, 269
Fibroblasts, interferon and, 261
Fibrolysin, 154
Fifth disease, 280
Filtraton sterilization, 59
Fimbriae, 8, 137–138
  adhesins and, 325
  Enterobacteriaceae and, 191
  group A streptococci and, 159
  Streptococcus pyogenes and, 158
5-fluorocytosine (5-FC), 78, 244
Flagella, 7–8, 201, 333
Flagellin, 7
Flavoproteins, 32
Fleas, *Yersinia pestis* and, 231
Flies, tularemia and, 231
Floppy baby syndrome, 175
Flossing, 337, 351
Fluorescent antibody staining, 320
  test, 98–99, 100*f*
Fluoride
  caries rates and, 354
  caries resistance and, 343
  control of plaque and, 337
  cost of caries and, 341
  prevention of caries and, 352–353, 355
  root caries and, 348
  stannous, 334
Folic acid, sulfonamides and, 77
Formaldehyde, 60
Formic acid, caries and, 349
F protein, 285, 286

Frame-shift mutation, 46
Francisella, 231
Freund's adjuvant, 115
Fructan, 349–350
Fructose, dental plaque and, 351
FTA-ABS test, 206
Fungal infections, 128, 237–249
Fungi Imperfecti, 237
Furuncles, 155
Fusiform bacteria, 374
Fusobacterium, 323, 332
  coaggregation and, 326
  gingivitis and, 374
  healthy gingiva and, 372
  nucleatum, 332
    adult periodontitis and, 378
    bone resorption and, 366
    gingivitis and, 374
    immunosuppression by, 364
    juvenile periodontitis and, 380
    mitogenicity of, 369
  virulence of and periodontal disease, 366
Fusospirochetal infection, 375–376

GALT. *See* Gastrointestinal-associated lymphoid tissues
Gammaglobulins, 117, 120
Gammaherpes, 266
Gangrene, 176–177
Gaseous sterilization, 59–60
Gastroenteritis, coronavirus and, 295
Gastrointestinal-associated lymphoid tissues (GALT), 104, 105, 112–114
Generalized transduction, 51
Genetic
  antibiotic resistance, 79
  engineering, 50
  exchange, 48–53
Genetics, 39–54, 45–53, 143, 343
Genital warts, 277
Genotype, 45
Gentamicin, 74, 80, 194, 231, 232
Ghon complex, 184
Gingiva, healthy, 371–372
Gingival
  connective tissue, 358
  crevice microflora, 322*t*, 331, 360–361
  hyperplasia, cyclosporine and, 118
  sulci, 320, 323, 358
Gingivitis, 357
  actinomycetes and, 213
  acute necrotizing ulcerative (ANUG), 332–333, 361, 373*t*, 375–376
  antibody and, 91

Gingivitis (*cont.*)
Bacteroides and, 365–366
Bacteroides intermedius and, 199, 200
chlorhexadine mouthwashes and, 61
chronic, 372–375
Entamoeba gingivalis and, 333
histologic characteristics, 373–374
human immunodeficiency virus (HIV) and, 381
lymphocytes and, 368
microbial etiology of, 359–360
oxidation-reduction potential and, 20
plaque and, 337, 373
pregnancy and, 143–144
spirochetes and, 208
streptococci and, 164
Trichomonas tenax and, 333
Gingivostomatitis, herpetic, 267, 268*f*
Glaucoma, 298
Global regulatory networks, 44–45
Glomerular capillary thrombosis, 143
Glomerulonephritis, 127, 131, 159, 160
Gloving, 64
Glucans, 334, 335, 349–350, 353, 360
Glucose, dental plaque and, 351
Glucosyltransferase (GTF), 353
Glutaraldehyde, 60
Glycocalyx, 6–7, 138
Glycolytic pathway, 27
Glyoxalate shunt, 32
Gonorrhea, 167–168
Goodpasture's syndrome, 131
Graft rejection, 106
Graft-versus-host (GVH) disease, 130
Gram-negative bacteria, 189–195
adult periodontitis and, 378
calculus and, 336
cause of periodontal diseases and, 361
cell envelope of, 11*f*–12
complement cascade and, 145
conjugation and, 49
dental plaque and, 331
endotoxins and, 141–143
gingival crevice microflora and, 331
gingivitis and, 374
healthy gingiva and, 371–372
juvenile periodontitis and, 379
lipopolysaccharide synthesis and, 34–35
periodontal disease and, 363
Gram-negative bacteria (*cont.*)
periodontal pocket debris and, 359
virulence of and periodontal disease, 365–366
Gram-positive bacteria
calculus and, 336
cause of periodontal diseases and, 361
cell walls of, 9–12
coronal plaque and, 332*t*, 331
healthy gingiva and, 371–372
lysozyme and, 144
periodontal pocket debris and, 359
virulence of and periodontal disease, 364–365
Gram staining, 3–4
actinomycetes and, 211
cell envelope and, 8–9
Griseofulvin, 78, 248
Group translocation, 22–23
Growth, bacterial, 18–25
Gummas, 205, 207
GVH. *See* Graft-versus-host disease

Haemophilus, 232–233
dental plaque and, 331
gingivitis and, 375
Hageman factor, 124, 225
Hairy leukoplakia, 314, 316
Haloprogin, 248
Handcleaning, 64
Hansen's disease, 186
H antigen, 7
Haptens, 86, 87, 128, 131
Hashimoto's thyroiditis, 131
HAV. *See* Hepatitis A virus
Hay fever, 123, 124
HBIG. *See* Hepatitis B immune globulin
HBV. *See* Hepatitis B virus
Heat-shock response, 45
Heavy metals for disinfection, 61
Helper T lymphocytes (T-h), 106, 107, 109–110, 313, 314
Hemagglutination inhibition, 259
Hemagglutinin, 253, 283, 284–285
Hemolysins, 158, 159
Hemolytic
anemias, 131
disease of the newborn, 125
Hemorrhagic dengue, 299
Hepadnavirus, DNA in, 257
Heparinase, 225
Hepatitis, 303–309
A virus (HAV), 259, 304
B virus (HBV), 62, 120, 304–308
heat and, 253
immune globulin (HBIG), 260
Hepatitis (*cont.*)
B virus (HBV) (*cont.*)
liver cancer and, 259
pathogenesis of, 258
primary hepatocellular carcinoma and, 313
vaccine for, 260
C, 308–309
chronic, 305
non A, non B (NANB), 308–309
Herd immunity, 149
Hereditary fructose intolerance (HFI), 344–345
Herpangina, coxsackievirus and, 293, 294*f*
Herpesvirus, 265–274
acquired immunodeficiency syndrome (AIDS) and, 316
chemotherapy for, 260
DNA replication in, 255, 257
immunosuppressive properties of, 259
inclusion bodies and, 258
labialis, 267, 269, 270
simplex, 258, 266–270, 314
1 (HSV-1), 265–266, 267
2 (HSV-2), 259, 265–266, 269, 312
Herpetic
keratitis, 268–269
whitlow, 268
Hetacillin, 70
Hexose monophosphate shunt, 27
Hexoses, as energy source, 27
HFI. *See* Heriditary fructose intolerance
High dose tolerance, 116
Histamine, 123, 124, 143, 146
-sensitizing factor, 233
Histocompatibility, 105–106, 129–130
Histoplasma capsulatum, 244–246
Histoplasmosis, 244–246
Histotoxic clostridia, 176–177
HIV. *See* Human immunodeficiency virus
HLA. *See* Human leukocyte antigens
Hodgkin's disease, 271
Host resistance, 143–149, 343–344
HPV. *See* Human papillomaviruses
HSV-1. *See* Herpesvirus, simplex 1
HSV-2, *See* Herpesvirus simplex 2
HTLV. *See* Human T lymphocytotrophic viruses
Human
immunodeficiency virus (HIV), 118, 313–316
azidothymidine (AZT) and, 260
fungal infection and, 239

Human (*cont.*)
immunodeficiency virus (*cont.*)
gingivitis and, 381
immunosuppressive properties of, 140, 259
infection control and, 62
pathogenesis of, 258
tuberculosis and, 183
leukocyte antigens (HLA), 105, 129–130
papillomavirus (HPV), 312–313, 314
T lymphocytotrophic viruses (HTLV), 259
T lymphocytotropic viruses (HTLV), 312
Humoral immunity, 103–104, 104–105, 111–114
allergic reactions and, 123
immunodeficiencies, 117
resportion of bone and, 363
tumors and, 132
viral infections and, 259
Hutchinsonian triad, 205
Hyaluronidase, 159, 363
Hydrocarbons, energy from, 31
Hydrocephalus, 295
Hydrophobia, 300
Hyperacute rejection, 129
Hyperplastic candidiasis, 243–244
Hypersensitivity, 123–129. *See also* Allergic reactions; Anaphylactic reactions
cephalosporins and, 72
complement and, 94
delayed-type (DTH), 108
fungal antigens and, 239
immunopathogenesis of periodontal disease and, 370
measles and, 288
penicillins and, 69, 71
pulp infections and, 388
scarlet fever and, 159
Streptococcus mutans vaccines and, 353
tuberculin skin test and, 184
vaccines and, 120
Hyphae, 237
Hypogammaglobulinemias, 117, 118

Iatrogenic infections, 226, 248
Icteric leptospirosis, 207
Identification of oral microflora, 320, 359–360
Idiotypic determinants, 111
Idoxuridine (IDU), 260, 270
IgA. *See* Immunoglobulin A
IgD. *See* Immunoglobulin D
IgE. *See* Immunoglobulin E
IgG. *See* Immunoglobulin G
IgM. *See* Immunoglobulin M
IL-1. *See* Interleukin 1
IL-2. *See* Interleukin 2
IM. *See* Mononucleosis, infectious
Imidazoles, 78, 239–240, 244
Immune
complex, 95, 126–127
globulin
hepatitis A (HAV) and, 304
hepatitis B (HBIG) and, 307–308
rabies (RIG) and, 301
rubella and, 298
vaccinia virus infection and, 281
response, 85–86, 109–111
adverse reactions and periodontal disease, 364
cell-mediated, 114–115
cellular interactions in, 109–110
control of, 110–111
fungal infection and, 239
humoral, 111–114
immunologic injury in periodontal disease and, 370–371
interferons and, 261
molecules and cells in, 105–109
organs and tissues in, 104–105
periodontal disease and, 368–371
specificity of, 87
tolerance, 108, 115, 116–117
unresponsiveness, 116–118
sera, allergic reactions to, 124
Immunity
acquisition of, 119–121
Haemophilus influenzae and, 233
herd, 149
lymphogranuloma venereum and, 219
meningococci and, 167
protective, 121
relapsing fever and, 207
Rocky Mountain spotted fever and, 216
shigellosis and, 193
syphillis and, 205, 207
trachoma and, 219
typhoid fever and, 192
in vitro correlates of, 115–116
whooping cough and, 234
Immunization, 109, 111, 115
diphtheria and, 169
oral vs. parenteral, 113
Rocky Mountain spotted fever and, 216
Immunoblot assays, 100
Immunodeficiency diseases, 117–118
Immunodepression, 118
adenovirus and, 275
candidiasis and, 241
caused by microorganisms, 140–141, 271, 364
cryptococcosis and, 247
cytomegalovirus and, 272
Epstein-Barr virus and, 274
tumors and, 131–132
Immunoelectrophoresis, 98
Immunogenicity, 86
Immunoglobulin, 88–92
clonal selection and, 109
D (IgD), 90
E (IgE), 91, 123, 124–125
G (IgG), 90–91, 121
Brucella and, 230
desensitization and, 124–125
hemolytic disease of the newborn and, 125
hepatitis A virus and, 304
humoral immune response and, 112
killer cells and, 108
lysis and, 122
natural passive immunity and, 120
oral microbial ecology and, 338
protein A and, 154
tumors and, 132
type III hypersensitivity and, 126
A (IgA), 91, 121. *See also* Secretory immunoglobin A (SIgA)
humoral immune response and, 112
lysozyme and, 144
memory response, 112–114
natural passive immunity and, 120
Neisseria and, 167
phagocytosis and, 146
syphilis and, 206
tumors and, 132
M (IgM), 90, 121
Brucella and, 230
hepatitis A virus and, 304
lysis and, 122
syphilis and, 206
T-dependent antigen and, 111
type III hypersensitivity and, 126
periodontal disease and, 368–369
Immunologic tests, 382
Immunology
pulp and periapical tissues and, 386
transplantation and, 129–130
tumor, 131–132

Impetigo, 154, 155, 160
Incineration, 59
Incisors, hypoplasia of, 205
Inclusion
  bodies, 258, 300
  conjunctivitis, 219
  granules, 14
Inducer T cell, 108
Inducible genes, 42
Induction, enzyme synthesis and, 36–37
INF. *See* Interferons
Infant
  botulism, 175
  pneumonia, 219
Infection control, 62–65
Inflammation, 145, 203
Influenza virus, 121, 283–285
  amantadine and, 260
  human immunodeficiency virus and, 313
  pathogenesis of, 258
  rimantadine and, 260
INH. *See* Isoniazid
Interferons (INF), 261–262*f*
  cancer and, 132
  immune response and, 108, 114, 122
  respiratory papillomas and, 279
  rhinovirus and, 294
  vaccinia virus infections and, 281
Interleukin
  1 (IL-1), 109
  2 (IL-2), 108, 110, 132
Intracellular
  polysaccharide (IPS), 334
  resistance, 147
Invasiveness, 138–141
Inversion mutation, 46
Iodine, 60
Iodophors, 383
IPS. *See* Intracellular polysaccharide
ISG. *See* Standard immune serum globulin
Isoagglutinins, 125
Isografts, 129, 130
Isoniazid (INH), 77, 185

Japanese B encephalitis virus, 299
J-chain, 91, 113
JC virus, 279, 317

Kanamycin, 74, 198, 383
  vancomycin agar (KVA), 198
Kaposi's sarcoma, 313, 314, 315*f*, 316
Keratoconjunctivitis, epidemic, 276
Ketoconazole, 78
  blastomycosis and, 246
  candidiasis and, 244
  coccidioidomycosis and, 247
  dermatophytic infections and, 248
  histoplasmosis and, 245
Keyes technique, 383
Killer cells, 108, 114–115. *See also* Natural killer cells
Klebsiella, 191, 194, 195
Koch, Robert, 136
Koch's postulates, 136, 345
Koplik's spots, 288
Kupffer cells, 109
Kuru, 317
KVA. *See* Kanamycin vanocomycin agar

Labeled antibodies tests, 98
Lactic acid, dental caries and, 349–351, 352*f*
Lactobacilli, 322
  activity tests for, 354–355
  adherence and, 323, 348
  caries and, 347–348
  caries etiology and, 355
  coronal caries and, 346
  fluoride and, 353
  lactic acid and, 349
  lactoperoxidase system and, 338
  low pH and, 323, 347
  plaque development and, 328
  selective media for, 320
Lactobacillus, 323, 332
Lactoferrin, 143, 144, 147, 338
Lactoperoxidase system, 338
Lactose catabolism, 42–44*f*
Lag period, 111
Lancefield classification, 157, 347
Langerhans cells, 109, 128
Large granular lymphocytes, 108
Latex agglutination
  passive agglutination assays, 98
  streptococci and, 160, 163
Lattice theory, precipitation reaction and, 96
Lawrence's dialyzable transfer factor (DTF), 115
Lazy leukocyte syndrome, 368
L cells, 108
Legionella, 234–236
Legionnaires' disease, 149, 234–236
Leprosy, 128, 181, 186, 206
Leptospirosis, 207
Leukemia, 117–118, 311
  adult T cell, 312
  aspergillosis and, 248
  candidiasis and, 241
  chickenpox and, 270
Leukemia (*cont.*)
  cryptococcosis and, 247
  hairy-cell, 312
  interferons and, 132
  progressive multifocal leukoencephalopathy and, 279
  serum sickness and, 127
vaccine, 132
Leukocytes
  gingivitis and, 373–374
  interferon and, 261
Leukoplakia, hairy, 314, 316
Leukotoxin (LT), 361, 365, 380
Levan, 334, 335, 364
L forms, streptococci and, 158
LGV. *See* Lymphogranuloma venereum
Lice, 207, 217, 231
Lincomycin, 73–74
Lipid, composition of dental plaque and, 334–335
Lipopolysaccharide (LPS), 12, 366
  bone resorption and, 364
  complement activation and, 364
  periodontal disease and, 361–363, 365
  synthesis of, 34–35
Lipoteichoic acid, 159
Listeria, 232
Listeriosis, 232
Liver, 104
LJP. *See* Periodontitis, juvenile, localized
Lockjaw, 176
Low
  dose tolerance, 116
  pH, dental caries and, 349–351, 352*f*
  temperature disinfection, 59
LPS. *See* Lipopolysaccharide
LT. *See* Leukotoxin
Lupus erythematosus, systemic, 127, 131
Lyme disease, 208
Lymphadenopathy, 204, 314
Lymph nodes, 139
Lymphocytes, 103, 145
  gingivitis and, 368
  interferon and, 261
  protective immunity mediated by, 122–123
  transformation tests, 116
Lymphocytosis-promoting factor, 233
Lymphogranuloma venereum (LGV), 219
Lymphokines
  assays, 116
  cell-mediated immune response and, 114

Lymphokines (*cont.*)
osteoclast-activating factor (OAF), 116, 364
periodontal disease and, 369–370, 371
produced by T cells, 110
release of, complement and, 93
Lymphoma, 311
aspergillosis and, 248
candidiasis and, 241
cryptococcosis and, 247
progressive multifocal leukoencephalopathy and, 279
reoviruses and, 295
Lysins, 95, 122
Lysogeny, 170, 262
Lysosomal enzyme release, 94
Lysosomes, 146
Lysozyme, 143, 144, 147, 338

MacConkey agar, 190
Macrolide antibiotics, 73
Macrophages, 108–109, 146
cell-mediated immune response and, 122, 145
endotoxins and, 142
fungal infection and, 239
histocompatibility and, 105
leukocidin and, 154
primary immune response and, 109
prostaglandins and, 364
tumors and, 132
Major histocompatibility complex (MHC), 105–106
Malaria, 140, 143, 206
Malta fever, 229
Mammary tumors, 311
Mannitol, 154, 320, 347
Mantoux test, 184
Masks, 64
Mastitis, 155
Material alba, 326
MBC. *See* Minimal bacterial concentration
Measles, 259, 285, 287–288
immunosuppressive properties of, 259
pooled gamma-globulin and, 259
subacute sclerosing panencephalitis and, 317
vaccine for, 260
Membranolysis, complement and, 94
Memory cells, 108, 112, 114
Meningitis, 155
coxsackievirus and, 293
echovirus and, 293, 294
Haemophilus influenzae and, 233
Meningitis (*cont.*)
Neisseria meningitidis and, 165, 166–167
pneumococci and, 163
poliomyelitis and, 292
Meningoencephalitis, 232, 287
Mesosomes, 13–14
Messenger ribonucleic acid (mRNA), 41, 257
Metabolic regulation, 36–38
Metabolites
periodontal disease and, 363
pulp infections and, 388
Metachromatic granules, 14
Methicillin, 69, 156
Methylxanthines, 124
Metronidazole, 178, 200, 337, 382
Mezlocillin, 71
MHC. *See* Major histocompatibility complex
MIC. *See* Minimal inhibitory concentration
Miconazole, 78, 248
Microscopy, 4–6
Milker's nodes, 281
Miller, W.D., 342
Minimal
bacterial concentration (MBC), 81
inhibitory concentration (MIC), 81
Minocycline, 75, 80, 200
Mitis-salivarius agar (MSA), 320, 355
Mitogens, 111
Molars, hypoplasia of, 205
Molecular weight, immunogenicity and, 86
Molluscum contagiosum, 280, 281
Monitored modulated therapy, 383
Monoclonal antibodies, 100–101, 270
Monocyte-macrophages, 146
Monokines, 107
Mononucleosis
biologic false positives and, 206
Burkitt's lymphoma and, 312
chronic syndromes, 274
human immunodeficiency virus and, 313
infectious (IM), 272, 273–274
Mosquitoes, 298–299
Motility of bacteria, 7–8
Moxalactam, 200
M protein, 159, 283
mRNA. *See* Messenger RNA
MSA. *See* Mitis-salivarius agar
Mucormycosis, 247
Mucosal immune response, 112–114. *See also* Secretory immunoglobin A (SIgA), 193
Mulberry molars, 205
Mumps, 259, 285, 286–287
Mutans, 334, 335, 346
Mutation, 45–49, 284
Mycelium, 237–238
Mycobacteria, 181–187
Mycobacterium tuberculosis, 62, 182, 183–185
Mycology, 237–249
Mycoplasma, 75, 220–221, 320
Myelomas, 117–118
Myocarditis, coxsackievirus and, 293
Myxoviruses, 258, 283–289

NAD. *See* Nicotinamide adenine dinucleotide
NADP. *See* Nicotinamide adenine dinucleotide phosphate
Nalidixic acid, 77
NANB. *See* Hepatitis non A, non B
Nasopharyngeal carcinoma, Epstein-Barr virus and, 273, 274, 312
Natural killer (NK) cells, 108
interferons and, 261
tumors and, 132
viral infections and, 259
Negri bodies, rabies and, 300
Neisseria, 165–172, 323, 327
Neomycin, 74
Neuraminidase, 253, 283, 284–285
Neurotoxins, 141
Neutralization assays, 259
Neutrophils, 146
NGU. *See* Nongonococcal urethritis
Nicotinamide adenine dinucleotide (NAD), 27
Nicotinamide adenine dinucleotide phosphate (NADP), 27
Nitrofurans, 77
Nitrofurantoin, 194
NK. *See* Natural killer cells
Nocardia, 212, 323
Nocardiosis, 212
Nomarski microscopy, 5
Nongonococcal urethritis (NGU), 219, 221
Norfloxacin, 77
Nosocomial infections, 74
antibiotid resistance and, 50, 74
Clostridium difficile and, 178
Legionella and, 234
mutation and, 47
penicillins and, 70
Pseudomonas aeruginosa and, 194
respiratory syncytial virus and, 286
staphylococci and, 153
Staphylococcus aureus and, 155

N protein, 300
Nucleic acid hybridization, 270
Nucleoside analogs, 260
Nucleus, 14
Null cells, 108
Nutritional specificity of pathogens, 138–139
Nystatin, 77, 243, 244

OAF. *See* Osteoclast-activating factor
O antigens, 12
Obligate
  aerobes, 19, 25
  anaerobes, 19, 31
Odor, anaerobic infections and, 225
Oncogenes, 312
Operons, 43–44
Opisthotonos, 176
Opsonins, 95, 121–122, 146
Opsonization
  complement and, 94, 139, 145
  Immunoglobin G (IgG) and, 90
  recognition and, 146
  type II allergic reactions and, 125
Oral
  cancers, 313
  cavity, 224
  disease, 111
  ecology, 338
  lesions, 204–206, 207
  microflora, 319–339
    changes in from birth to death, 323
    factors that effect, 320–323
    pathogenic potential of, 338
    sampling for, 320
  tolerance, 113
Orbiviruses, 257, 295
Orchitis, 286
Orf virus, 281
Ornithosis, 219
Orofacial infections, 226, 227
Orthomyxoviruses, 255, 257, 283–285
Osteoclast-activating factor (OAF), 116, 364
Osteomyelitis, 155
Otitis media, 160, 163, 232, 288
Ouchterlony test, 97
Oxacillin, 70, 156
Oxidation
  -reduction potential (Eh), 20, 26, 223, 323, 338
  terminal, 31–33
Oxidative phosphorylation, 33
Oxidizing agents for disinfecting, 61
Oxygen
  bacterial response to, 19–21*f*
  -dependent reactions in phagocytosis, 147, 225

PAF. *See* Platelet-activating factor
Papillomatosis, 243
Papillomaviruses, 277–278
Papovaviruses, 255, 257, 276–279
Para-aminosalicylic acid, 185
Parainfluenza virus, 285–286
Paramyxoviruses, 255, 257, 285–288
Parotids, mumps and, 286–287*f*
Parvovirus, 257, 280
Passive
  diffusion, 21
  immunity, 271, 286, 298, 307–308
Pasteurization, 58
Pathogenicity, 136–143
PBHB granules. *See* Polybetahyroxybutyrate granules
PBLs. *See* Peripheral blood lymphocytes
PCR. *See* Polymerase chain reaction
Pellicle, 326
Pelvic inflammatory disease (PID), 167, 221
Pemphigus vulgaris, 131
Penicillin, 68–72
  allergic reactions to, 124, 125
  binding proteins, 71
  calculus and, 336
  hypersensitivity to, 71
  mode of action of, 72
  prevention of periodontal disease and, 383
  resistance to staphylococci and, 153, 156
Penicillinase-producing *Neisseria gonorrhoeae* (PPNG), 168
Penile intraepithelial neoplasia, 313
Pentose phosphate pathway, 27, 28, 29*f*
Peplomer, 253
Peptidoglycan, 9–10, 34
Peptostreptococcus, 162, 332, 365, 375, 379
Periapical infections, 225–226, 385–390
Pericarditis, coxsackievirus and, 293
Periodic acid-Schiff reaction, 244
Periodontal
  disease
    allergic reactions and, 123, 125, 127, 128
    anaerobic bacteria and, 225–226, 227, 323
    bacteria associated with, 320, 321*f*
    B lymphocytes and, 369
    B lympocytes and, 111
    brushing and flossing and, 337
    calculus and, 337

Periodontal (*cont.*)
  disease (*cont.*)
    caries and, 342
    diagnosis of, 381–382
    Eikenella corrodens and, 331
    endotoxin and, 143
    enzymes and, 38
    fusobacteria and, 332
    growth of bacteria and, 361
    human leukocyte antigen (HLA) association and, 106
    hyaluronidase and, 150
    immune response and, 145, 366–371, 369, 370
    immunization and, 370
    immunologic injury in, 370–371
    local immunodeficiency and, 121
    lysogeny and, 262
    nonspecific plaque hypothesis, 359
    prevention of, 383
    pulp infections and, 389
    root surface caries and, 348
    specific plaque hypothesis, 359
    spirochetes and, 208, 332
    treatment of, 80, 382–383
    types of, inflammatory, 371–381
  ligament, 358
  microbiology, 357–383
  pocket, 197, 358, 376, 387
  syndrome, acute, 316
Periodontitis, 150, 357
  adult, 376–379
  anaphylactic reactions and, 370
  Bacteroides gingivalis and, 199, 200, 369
  bone resorption and, 363, 379
  Clostridium and, 178
  Entamoeba gingivalis and, 333
  juvenile, 379–380
    Actinobacillis actinomycetemcomitans and, 150, 236, 361, 365, 369
    Actinomyces actinomycetemcomitans and, 332
    Capnocytophaga and, 331
    depressed neutrophil chemotaxis and, 368
    localized (LJP), 379
    neutrophils and, 370
    Trichomonas tenax and, 333
  microbial etiology of, 359–360
  Mycoplasma and, 221
  posttreatment healing of, 363
  prepubertal, 366, 380–381
  rapidly progressive, 380
  refractory adult, 381

Periodontitis (*cont.*)
T lymphocytes and, 368
Trichomonas tenax and, 333
Peripheral blood lymphocytes (PBLs), 370
Peritonitis, 199
Peroxidase, 144
-thiocyanate-H_2O_2 systems, 143
Peyer's patches, 105
PGE. *See* Type E prostaglandins
pH, 19, 338
PHA. *See* Phytohemagglutinin
Phage lambda, 47, 48*f*, 52
Phages, 52–53, 169–170, 262
Phagocytosis, 145–148
agglutination and, 121
complement action and, 145
dentinal tubules and, 386
encapsulated bacteria and, 7, 198, 232
entry of parasites and, 137, 218
Immunoglobin G (IgG) and, 90
type II allergic reactions and, 125
Phagosome, 146
Pharyngoconjunctival fever, 276
Phase contrast microscopy, 5, 320
PHC. *See* Carcinoma, primary hepatocellular
Phenols, 61
Phenotype, 45
Phosphofructokinase (PKF), 36
Phospholipids, energy from, 31
Phosphoroclastic cleavage, 30
Phosphorylation, 26
Phycomycosis, 247
Physiology, bacterial, 17–38
Phytohemagglutinin (PHA), 111
Picornaviruses, 257, 291–294
PID. *See* Pelvic inflammatory disease
Pili, 8, 137–138, 158, 167, 198
Piperacillin, 71
Pittsburgh pneumonia agent (PPA), 235
PK. *See* Pyruvate kinase
PFK. *See* Phosphofructokinase
Plaque, dental, 326–338
Actinomyces and, 324
acute necrotizing ulcerative gingivitis and, 375–376
adherence and, 335
bacterial metabolites and, 363
Bacteroides and, 324
bone resorption and, 359
Bordetella and, 236
calculus and, 326
caries and, 342
chemical composition of, 334–335
composition of coronal, 332*t*, 331
control of, 337–338
Plaque, dental (*cont.*)
development of, 326–329
Eubacterium and, 332
gingival sulcus and, 358
gingivitis and, 372, 373, 374–375
Haemophilus and, 236
juvenile periodontitis and, 379–380
Legionella and, 236
lung abscesses and, 226
microbial composition of, 329–333, 333, 334*f*
oxidation-reduction potential and, 323
periodontitis and, 377
pH of, 351
removal of, 351–352
Streptococcus mutans and, 346
subgingival, 328–329
supragingival, 326–328
Plasma cells, 108
Plasmids, 14, 49, 191, 262
Platelet-activating factor (PAF), 123
Pleuropneumonia organisms (PPO), 220–221
PMC. *See* Pseudomembranous colitis
PML. *See* Progressive multifocal leukoencephalopathy
PMNs. *See* Polymorphonuclear neutrophils
Pneumonia, 120, 155
congenital rubella syndrome and, 298
infant, 219
influenzal, 283
Legionella pneumophila and, 235
measles and, 288
Mycoplasma pneumoniae and, 220–221
parainfluenza virus and, 286
reoviruses and, 295
respiratory syncytial virus and, 286
tularemia and, 231
TWAR strains and, 220
Pneumonitis, 281, 298
Poison ivy, 128
Pokeweed mitogen (PWM), 111
Poliovirus, 291–293
antibody and, 259
hepatitis A virus and, 304
synthesis of RNA in, 255, 256*f*
vaccine for, 260
Poly-betahydroxybutyrate (PBHB) granules, 14
Polycistronic messenger ribonucleic acid (mRNA), 43
Polyclonal activators, 111
Polymerase chain reaction (PCR), 270
Polymicrobic anaerobic infections, 224
Polymorphonuclear
leukocytes, 145, 154
neutrophilic granulocytes, 367–368, 373–374
neutrophils (PMN), 147
neutrophils (PMNs), 126, 146, 225
lactoferrin and, 144
leukotoxin and, 361
Polysaccharides, 14, 35, 334
Pontiac fever syndrome, 235–236
Poxviruses, 255, 257, 280–281
PPA. *See* Pittsburgh pneumonia agent
PPD. *See* Purified protein derivative
PPNG. *See* Penicillinase-producing *Neisseria gonorrhoeae*
PPO. *See* Pleuropneumonia organisms
Precipitation
reaction, 95–96
tests, 96–98
Precipitins, 95
Prevention of
dental caries, 351–354
periodontal disease, 383
Primary cell cultures, 254
Prions, 252, 317
Progressive
degenerative panencephalitis, 298
multifocal leukoencephalopathy (PML), 279, 317
rubella panencephalitis, 317
Properdin system, 93
Prophage, 262
Propionibacterium, 365
Prostaglandins, 124, 364, 368
Proteases, 145
Protective immunity, 121–123
Protein
A, 154
composition of dental plaque and, 334
denaturation, 57
energy from, 31
NP, 285
spike, 253
synthesis, 35–36, 38, 41, 73–76
Proteolytic chelation theory of caries development, 342
Proteus, dental unit water supplies and, 195
Prothiaramide, 186
Protoplasts, 12
Protozoa, 332–333
Proviruses, 258

Pseudomembranous
candidiasis, 242
colitis (PMC), 177
Pseudomonas, 7–8, 194, 195
Psittacosis, 138, 219
Pulp
chamber, resistance factors of, 385–386
infections, 385–390
anaerobic bacteria and, 225–226
microbial flora of, 388–389
routes of microbial invasion, 387
Purified protein derivative (PPD), 184
Purines, energy from, 31
PWM. *See* Pokeweed mitogen
Pyridine nucleotides, 26–27
Pyrimidines, 31
Pyrophosphate, 338
Pyruvate, 28–32
kinase (PK), 36
Pyruvic acid, 349

Q fever, 217
Quaternary ammonium compounds, 61, 337, 383
Quinolones, 77

Rabies, 121, 258, 260, 300–301
Radial immunodiffusion, 97
Radiation sterilization, 59
Radioimmunoassays (RIA), 99
Rapid plasma reagin (RPR) test for syphilis, 206
RB. *See* Reticulate body
Receptor-mediated endocytosis, 137
Recognition of self antigens, 130
Recombination, 47–48
Redox potential. *See* Oxidation-reduction potential (Eh)
Relapsing fever, 207–208
Reoviruses, 257, 295
Replica plating, 46–47
Repressible genes, 42
Repression, 36–37, 44–45
Repressors, 43
Reservoirs of infection, 149
Respiration, 25–26
Respiratory
burst, 147
papillomatosis, 279
syncytial virus (RSV), 258, 285, 286
Reticulate body (RB), 218
Retroviruses, 255, 257, 259, 312, 313
Rhabdoviruses, 255, 257, 299–301
Rheumatic fever, 131, 139, 159, 160, 161
Rheumatoid arthritis, 280
Rhinoviruses, 291, 294
RIA. *See* Radioimmunoassays
Ribavirin (Virazole), 260, 286
Ribonucleic acid (RNA), 41
ribosomal (rRNA), 41
synthesis of, 37–38
viruses and, 251–252, 254–257, 312
Ribosomes, 14, 41
Rickettsiae, 75, 75–76, 147, 215–217
Rickettsialpox, 216
Rifampin, 76, 167, 185, 186, 233, 235
RIG. *See* Antirabies globulin; Immune globulin, rabies
Rimantidine, 260
Ring test, 96
Ringworm, 248
Riscus sardonicus, 176
RNA. *See* Ribonucleic acid
Rocket immunoelectrophoresis, 98
Rocky Mountain spotted fever, 216
Rogosa's SL agar, 354–355
Root canals, 332
Rotaviruses, 257, 295
Roth, Genevieve, 331
Rothia dentocariosa, 328. See also *Viellonella Rothia dentocariosa,* 331
RPR. *See* Rapid plasma reagin test
rRNA. *See* Ribonucleic acid, ribosomal
RSV. *See* Respiratory syncytial virus
Rubella, 258, 297–298, 317
Rubeola, 285, 287–288
Runyon classification, 182

Sabin attenuated virus vaccine, 293
Sabouraud's medium, 239
St. Louis encephalitis virus (SLE), 299
Saliva
antibody in, 91–92
antimicrobial factors in, 144
buffering activity of, 351
caries etiology and, 343
Salivary peroxidase system, 144
Salk polio vaccine, 121, 293
Salmonella, 191–193, 262
Sanguinarine, 337–338
Sarcoidosis, 247
Sarcomas, 311
Satellite bubo, 204
Scalded skin syndrome, 154, 155
Scanning electron microscopy (SEM), 5–6
Scarlet fever, 159, 160, 161, 262
Schick test, 171
SCID. *See* Severe combined immunodeficiency disease
Secondary infections
candidiasis as, 80, 248, 323
pseudomembranous colitis as, 178
Staphylococcus aureus and, 155
Secretory immunoglobin A (SIgA), 92. *See also* Immunoglobin A; Mucosal immune response
caries and, 353
meningococci and, 166
oral microbial ecology and, 338
respiratory syncytial virus and, 286
response, 112–114
shigellae and, 193
Selenomonas, 372
Self
-infection, 164
-recognition, 108, 116
SEM. *See* Scanning electron microscopy
Sepsis, 56
Serology, 94–101
Serotonin, 123, 143
Serpentine cords, 182–183
Serum sickness, 127
Severe combined immunodeficiency disease (SCID), 117
Sex pili, 50, 191
Shellfish, hepatitis A virus and, 304
Shigella, 193, 262
Shingles, 270–271
Shwartzman reaction, 94, 143
Sickle cell anemia, 143, 280
Siderophores, 138, 140
SIDS. *See* Sudden infant death syndrome
SIgA. *See* Secretory immunoglobin A
Single-stranded linear DNA, 257
Sinusitis, 160, 288
Sjogren's syndrome, 126, 131
Skin reactive factor, 122
SLE. *See* St. Louis encephalitis virus
Slime layer, 6–7
Slow
reacting substance of anaphylaxis (SRS-A), 123–124
virus diseases, 317
Smallpox, 260, 280–281
vaccine (Jenner), 121, 260
Snacking, caries and, 345, 355
SOD. *See* Superoxide dismutase

Sorbitol, 320, 347, 351, 352
SOS system, 45
Specificity, 95, 96*f*
Specific soluble substance (SSS), 162
Spectinomycin, 168
Spheroplasts, 12
Spirochetes, 201–208, 322, 323
  acute nectotizing ulcerative gingivitis and, 375–376
  adherence and, 323–324
  axial filaments of, 8
  gingivitis and, 374
  healthy gingiva and, 371–372
  juvenile periodontitis and, 379
  lysis of, 122
  methods of sampling, 320
  periodontitis and, 377–378, 380
Spiromycin, 383
Spleen, 105
Sporangiospores, 238
Sporulation, 14–16
Spotted fever, 166
Squamous cell carcinoma, 313
SRS-A. *See* Slow reacting substance of anaphylaxis
SSPE. *See* Subacute sclerosing panencephalitis
SSS. *See* Specific soluble substance
Staining techniques, 3–4
Standard immune serum globulin (ISG), 259
Staphylococci, 153–156, 157, 323
Staphylokinase, 154
Starch granules, 14
Steam sterilization, 58
Steptomycin, 231
Sterilization, 56, 58, 63
Stickland reaction, 31
Strep throat, adenovirus and, 275–276
Streptococci, 157–164
  adherence of, 324–325
  calculus and, 336
  coaggregation and, 326, 361
  coronal caries and, 346
  diptheria and, 170
  experimental gingivitis and, 375
  fluoride and, 353
  healthy gingiva and, 371–372
  lactic acid and, 349
  low pH and, 323
  periodontal disease and, 365
  pulp infections and, 388
  selective media for, 320
Streptococcus
  anginosus, 375
  faecalis, 353–354, 389
  mitior, 322, 323, 338, 346–347
  mitis, 363, 375, 389
Streptococcus (*cont.*)
  mutans
    adherence of, 324, 335, 346
    age of host and, 323
    aggregation and, 326
    antibiotics and, 354
    bacitracin and, 320
    bacteriocins and, 338
    caries and, 157, 346–347, 355
    characterization of, 347
    development of plaque and, 327–328
    extracellular polysaccharide biosynthesis and, 35
    genetic engineering and, 50
    intraoral distribution of bacteria and, 322
    lactoferrin and, 338
    lactoperoxidase system and, 338
    low pH and, 346
    polysaccharide synthesis and, 335
    root caries and, 348, 381
    selective media for, 355
    vaccines against, 353–354
  pneumoniae, 48–49, 162
  pyogenes, 262
  salivarius, 322, 323, 346–347, 389
  sanguis, 322, 323
    adherence and, 324, 360
    development of plaque and, 327
    gingivitis and, 375
    lactoperoxidase system and, 338
    low pH and, 346–347
    root caries and, 348
Streptodornase, 159
Streptokinase, 159
Streptomycin, 74, 148, 185, 231
Stringent response, 45
Subacute sclerosing panencephalitis (SSPE), 259, 288, 317
Subgingival plaque, 328–329, 359, 389
Sucrose, 344–345, 346*f*, 349, 351
Sudden infant death syndrome (SIDS), 175
Sugar, caries and, 344–345, 346*f*
Sulfadiazine, 167, 219
Sulfa drugs, 149
Sulfanilamides, 194
Sulfonamides, 76–77, 79, 212, 219
Superoxide dismutase (SOD), 19–20
Suppressor T lymphocytes (T-s), 107, 108, 110–111
  autoimmunity and, 131
  Epstein-Barr virus and, 273–274
Suppressor T lymphocytes (*cont.*)
  low dose tolerance and, 116
  tumors and, 132
Supragingival plaque, 326–328, 359
Syphilis, 128, 202–207

Taxonomy, 1–2
T-c. *See* Cytotoxic T lymphocytes
TCA cycle. *See* Tricarboxylic acid cycle
T-dependent antigens, 110, 111
Teichoic acid, 364
TEM. *See* Transmission electron microscopy
Temperature, chemoheterotrophs and, 19
Terminal oxidation, 31–33
Tetanus, 120, 121, 173, 175–176, 178
Tetracyclines, 74–75, 79, 80, 149
T-h. *See* Helper T lymphocytes
Thalassemia, 280
Thioglycollate medium, 390
Thiol compounds, 141
Thrombocytopenias, 131, 298
Thrombophlebitis, 225
Thrush, 242, 314. *See also* Candidiasis
Thymol, 383
Thymosin, 107, 117, 132
Thymus, 104
Ticarcillin, 71
Ticks
  orbivirus, 295
  Q fever and, 217
  relapsing fever and, 207
  Rickettsiae and, 215
  togaviruses and, 298–299
  tularemia and, 231
Tineas, 248
Tissue cultures of viruses, 254
T lymphocytes, 104, 105, 107–108
  antibiotics and, 148
  Epstein-Barr virus and, 273–274
  fungal infection and, 239
  gingivitis and, 374
  receptor, 109
Tobramycin, 74, 80, 194
Togaviruses, 257, 297–299, 298–299
Tolnaftate, 248
Tonsils, 105
Tooth
  autografts, 130
  extraction, 176
  transplantation of, 130
Toxic shock syndrome, 154, 155
Toxigenicity, 138, 141–143
Toxins, 231, 361–363
Toxoids, 141
Toxoplasmosis, 314

Trachoma, 219
Transcription, 41, 42–44*f*, 43
Transduction, 51–53
Transfer
 factor, 132
 ribonucleic acid (tRNA), 41
Transformation, 48–49
Transition mutation, 46
Translation, 41–42*f*
Transmission
 electron microscopy (TEM), 5–6
 reservoirs of, 149
Transplantation immunology, 129–130
Transport mechanisms, 12, 13, 21–23, 27
Transposition, 47
Transposons, 47–48
Transversion mutation, 46
Trench mouth, 375–376
Treponemes, 202–207, 320, 364, 378–379
 Tricarboxylic acid (TCA) cycle, 31–32
 Trichomonas tenax, 332–333
 Trifluorothymidine, 270
 Trimethoprim, 76–77
 -sulfamethoxazole, 192, 193, 194, 233
Trismus, 176
tRNA. *See* Transfer RNA
T-s. *See* Suppressor T lymphocytes
Tuberculosis, 181, 183–185
 delayed-type hypersensitivity reactions and, 128
 histoplasmosis and, 244
 immune response to infection and, 145
 isoniazid and, 77
 rifampin and, 76
 streptomycin and, 74
 vaccine, 132
Tularemia, 231
Tumor
 immunology, 131–132
 viruses, 311–313
Type E prostaglandins (PGE), 364
Typhoid fever, 121, 191–193
Typhus, 217
Tzanck smear, 266*f*, 270

Ultrasonic vibrations, 59
Uncoating of viruses, 254–255
Undulant fever, 229
Universal precautions, 62–63
Uronic acids, 10
Uveitis, 131

Vaccines, 119–121
 adenovirus infections and, 276
Vaccines (*cont.*)
 antistreptococcal, 161
 caries and, 114, 346, 351, 353
 coronavirus and, 295
 coxsackievirus and, 293
 cytomegalovirus and, 273
 diphtheria and, 169, 171
 diploid cell strains and, 254
 echovirus and, 294
 gonorrhea and, 168
 Haemophilus influenzae and, 233
 hepatitis and, 304, 308, 309
 herpes simplex virus and, 270
 influenza, 285
 leptospires and, 207
 measles and, 288
 meningococci and, 167
 mumps and, 287
 parainfluenza virus and, 286
 periodontal disease and, 370
 plaque control and, 337
 pneumococcal, 163
 poliovirus infections and, 292, 293
 rabies, 301
 reoviruses and, 295
 rhinovirus and, 294
 rubella and, 298
 shigellae and, 193
 smallpox and, 280
 tetanus, 176
 tularemia and, 231
 tumors and, 132
 typhoid fever and, 195
 varicella-zoster virus and, 271
 viruses and, 260
 Wax-D and, 183
 whooping cough and, 234
 yellow fever and, 299
Vaccinia virus, 280–281
Vancomycin, 73, 156, 178, 383
 kanamycin vancomycin agar (KVA), 198
Varicella-zoster virus (VZV), 258, 260, 265–266, 270–271
VDRL. *See* Venereal Disease Research Laboratory test
VEE. *See* Venezuelan equine encephalitis virus
Veillonella, 323
 acid production by, 349
 coaggregation and, 326
 healthy gingiva and, 371–372
 plaque development and, 328
 Rothia dentocariosa root caries and, 328, 331348
Venereal Disease Research Laboratory (VDRL) test, 206
Venezuelan equine encephalitis virus (VEE), 299
Vidarabine (adenine arabinoside), 260–262
Vincent's infection, 375–376
Virazole, 260
Viridans streptococci, 161–162
Virions, 251, 253–254
Viroids, 252
Virulence, 136–143
 anaerobic infections and, 225
 exoenzymes and, 21
 extracellular polymers and, 7
 lysogeny and, 170
 periodontal bacteria and, 360–364
 phage conversion and, 52–53
 pulp infections and, 387–388
 serpentine cords, 182–183
 somatic pili and, 8
Viruses, 251–262
 alteration of the biochemical behavior of the cell by, 141
 animal virus growth, 253–254
 antiadherence immunity and, 122
 antigens in, 88
 antiviral chemotherapy, 260–262*f*
 bacterial, 262
 cell-mediated immune response and, 122
 complement and, 94, 145
 control and prevention of infections by, 259–260
 cytotoxic T lymphocytes and, 108, 114
 delayed-type hypersensitivity and, 128
 genomes of, 251, 252–253
 growth of, 257–258
 immunosuppression of host by, 140
 intracellular resistance and, 147
 invasion and replication of, 254–255
 lysis of, 122
 nature of, 251–252
 passive protection and, 259–260
 pathogenesis of, 258–259
 pneumococci and, 162
 reactions to physical and chemical agents, 253
 recombination and, 47, 48*f*
 structure and composition of, 252–253
 transduction and, 51–53
 variations in structure of, 253
 viral immunology, 259
VZV. *See* Varicella-zoster virus

Warts, 277
Waterhouse-Friderichsen syndrome, 166
Water supplies to dental units, bacterial contamination of, 195

Wax-D, 183
WEE. *See* Western equine encephalitis virus
Weil-Felix reaction, 216
Weil's disease, 207
Western blot analysis, 316
Western equine encephalitis virus (WEE), 299
Whooping cough, 121, 233–234
Wolinella, 331–332, 366, 378

Xenografts, 129, 130
X-linked infantile hypogammaglobulinemia, 117
Xylitol, 352

Yeasts, 238, 320
Yellow fever, 299
Yersinia, 195, 230–231

Ziehl-Neelsen staining method, 182
Zones of optimal proportions, 96–97
Zovirax (Acycloguanosine, Acyclovir), 260, 270, 271
Zygomycosis, 247